encyclopedia of
EXERCISE
ANATOMY

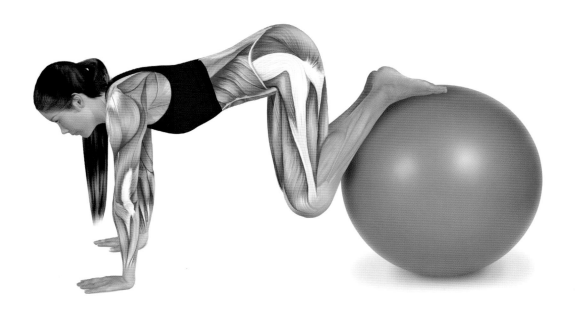

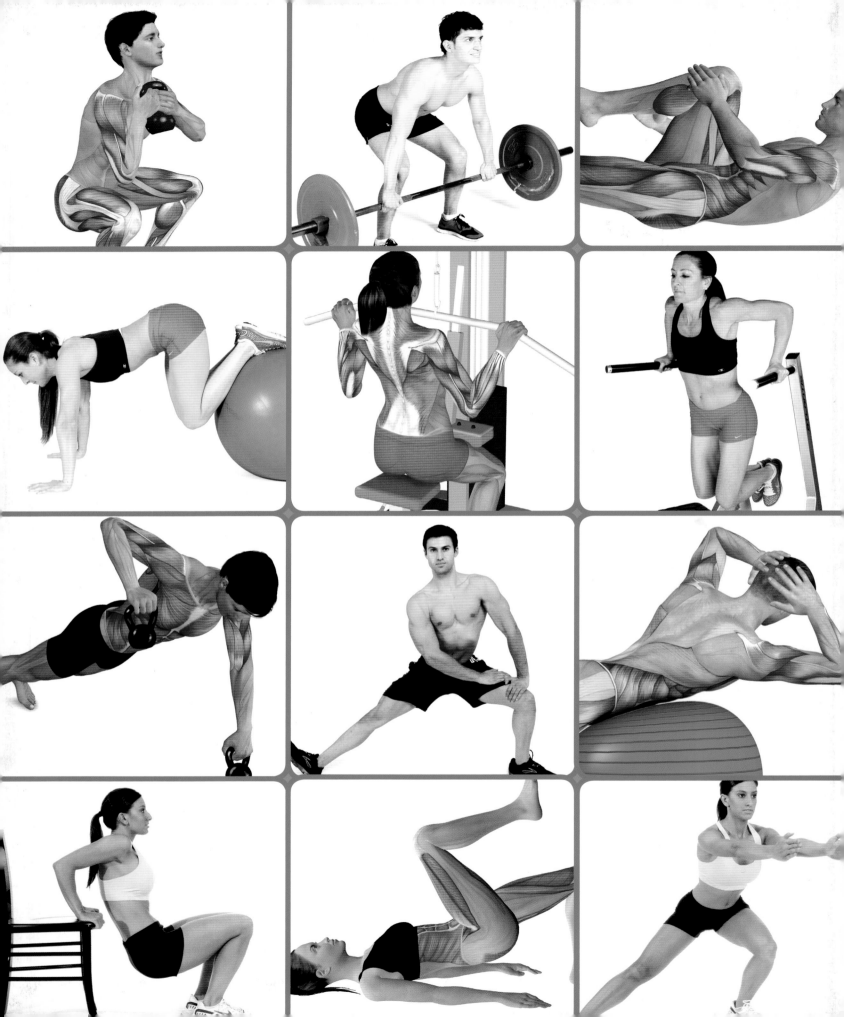

encyclopedia of
EXERCISE
ANATOMY

Hollis Lance Liebman

FIREFLY BOOKS

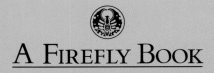

A FIREFLY BOOK

Published by Firefly Books Ltd. 2014

First printing

Publisher Cataloging-in-Publication Data (U.S.)

Liebman, Hollis Lance.
Encyclopedia of exercise anatomy / Hollis Lance Liebman.
[392] pages : col. ill., col. photos. ; cm.
Includes index.
ISBN-13: 978-1-77085-443-7
1. Exercise – Encyclopedias. 2. Muscles – Anatomy – Encyclopedias. I. Title.
613.7103 dc 23 RA781.L543 2014

Library and Archives Canada Cataloguing in Publication

Liebman, Hollis Lance, author
        Encyclopedia of exercise anatomy / Hollis Lance Liebman.
Includes index.
ISBN 978-1-77085-443-7 (bound)
        1. Exercise--Encyclopedias. 2. Muscles--Anatomy--Encyclopedias. I. Title. II. Title: Exercise anatomy.
RA781.L538 2014   613.7'103   C2014-902793-1

Published in the United States by
Firefly Books (U.S.) Inc.
P.O. Box 1338, Ellicott Station
Buffalo, New York 14205

Published in Canada by
Firefly Books Ltd.
50 Staples Avenue, Unit 1
Richmond Hill, Ontario L4B 0A7

Printed in China

This title was developed by
Moseley Road Inc.
123 Main St.
Irvington, NY 10533

President: Sean Moore
General Manager: Karen Prince
Art Director: Tina Vaughan
Ediorial Director: Damien Moore
Production Director: Adam Moore
Editorial assistance: Jill Hamilton, Jo Weeks
Design assistance: Mark Johnson Davies
Picture researcher: Jo Walton

Photographer: Fine Arts Photography, Jonathan Conklin/Jonathan Conklin Photography, Inc. TBC
Models: Melissa Grant, Michael Radon, Elaine Altholz, Peter Vaillancourt, Michael Galizia, Miguel Carrera, Tara DiLuca, Craig Ramsay, Monica Ordonez, TJ Fink (tjfink@gmail.com), Jenna Franciosa, David Anderson, Maria Grippi, Sara Blowers and Nicolay Alexandrov

SPORTS ICONS

- Archery
- Australian Rules Football
- Badminton
- Baseball
- Basketball
- Boxing
- Canoeing
- Climbing
- Cricket
- Cross Country Skiing
- Cycling
- Diving
- Equestrian
- Fencing
- Field Hockey
- Figure Skating
- Fly Fishing

- Football US
- Gaelic Football
- Golf
- Gymnastics
- Handball
- Hurling
- Ice Hockey
- Judo
- Karate
- Kayaking
- Lacrosse
- Mountain Biking
- Paddle Board
- Raquet Ball
- Rowing
- Rugby
- Running

- Sailing
- Shooting
- Skateboarding
- Skiing
- Snowboarding
- Soccer
- Squash
- Surfing
- Swimming
- Table Tennis
- Tennis
- Volley Ball
- Water Polo
- Water Skiing
- Wrestling
- **All Sports**

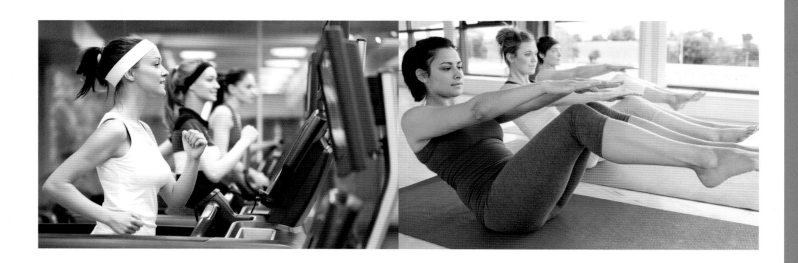

CONTENTS

Part 1 INTRODUCTION 10

Introduction 12

Upper-Body Anatomy 26

Lower-Body Anatomy 28

Part 2 EXERCISES & STRETCHES 30

Upper-Body Exercises 32

Barbell Deadlift 34

Barbell Row 36

Dumbbell Row 38

Dumbbell Pullover 40

Lat Pulldown 42

Scapular Range of Motion 44

Alternating Kettlebell Row 46

Alternating Renegade Row 48

Incline Bench Row 50

Rope Pulldown 52

Reverse Close-Grip Front Chin 54

Flat Bench Hyperextension 56

Rotated Back Extension 58

Barbell Bench Press 60

Roller Push-Up 62

Dumbbell Fly 64

Cable Fly 66

Dips 68

Push-Up 70

Push-Up Hand Walk-Over 72

Dumbbell Shoulder Press 74

Overhead Press 76

Rotation Exercises 78

External Rotation with Band 80

Lateral Raise 82

Shoulder Raise and Pull 84

Barbell Upright Row 86

Reverse Fly 88

Swiss Ball Reverse Fly 90

Front-Plate Raise 92

Barbell Shoulder Shrug 94

Biceps Curl 96

Alternating Hammer Curl 98

Barbell Curl 100

Single-Arm Concentration Curl 102

Rope Hammer Curl 104

Rope Pushdown 106

Lying Triceps Extension 108

Triceps Roll-Out 110

Chair Dip 112

Rope Overhead Extension 114

Wrist Flexion 116

Wrist Extension 117

Crunch 118

Plank 120

Side Plank 122

T-Stabilization 124

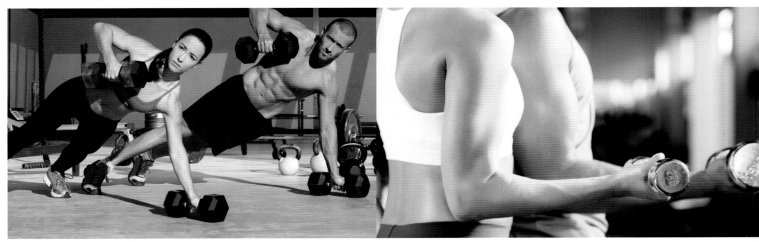

Swiss Ball Walk-Around	126	Single-Leg Calf Press	176
Swiss Ball Jackknife	128	Dumbbell Calf Raise	178
Medicine Ball Wood Chop	130	Dumbbell Shin Raise	180

Lower-Body Exercises   132   Core Exercises   182

Swiss Ball Wall Sit	134	Abdominal Kick	184
Barbell Squat	136	Abdominal Hip Lift	186
Dumbbell Lunge	138	Turkish Get-Up	188
Reverse Lunge	140	Bicycle Crunch	190
Lateral Low Lunge	142	Reverse Crunch	192
Dumbbell Walking Lunge	144	Cobra Stretch	194
High Lunge	146	Swiss Ball Pelvic Tilt	196
Crossover Step	148	Plank Press-Up	198
Goblet Squat	150	Seated Russian Twist	200
One-Legged Step-Down	152	Wood Chop with Resistance Band	202
Knee Extension with Rotation	154	Hip Abduction and Adduction	204
Star Jump	156	Swiss Ball Roll-Out	206
Mountain Climber	158	Thigh Rock-Back	208
Burpee	160	Swiss Ball Hip Crossover	210
Adductor Extension	162	V-Up	212
Hamstring Abductor	163	Medicine Ball Slam	214
Swiss Ball Hamstrings Curl	164	The Windmill	216
Inverted Hamstring	166		
Stiff-Legged Barbell Deadlift	168		
Hamstring Pull-In	170	**Stretches**	**218**
Sumo Squat	172	Chest Stretch	220
Stiff-Legged Deadlift	174	Shoulder Stretch	220
		Triceps Stretch	221

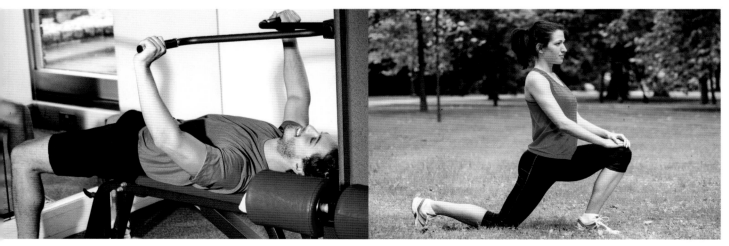

CONTENTS CONTINUED

Standing Biceps Stretch	221
Latissimus Dorsi Stretch	222
Spine Stretch	223
Supine Lower Back Stretch	224
Kneeling Swiss Ball Lat Stretch	225
Iliotibial Band Stretch	226
Hip-to-Thigh Stretch	227
Standing Hamstring Stretch	228
Lying Hamstring Stretch	229
Piriformis Stretch	230
Calf Stretch	232
Shin Release	233
Standing Quadriceps Stretch	234
Butterfly	235
Toe Touch	236
Child's Stretch	237
Unilateral Seated Forward Bend	238
Bilateral Seated Forward Bend	239
Seated Hip and Spine Stretch	240
Pretzel (Spinal Rotation) Stretch	242
Knee-to-Chest Flex	244
Wide-Legged Forward Bend	245

Pregnancy Stretches — 246
Torso Rotation	248
Hand-on-Knee Stretch	249

Lying Pelvic Tilt	250
Unilateral Good Morning Stretch	251
Cat Stretch	252
Downward-Facing Dog	253

Part 3 WORKOUTS — 254

Sport-Specific Workouts — 256
American Football	258
Archery	260
Australian Rules Football	262
Badminton	264
Baseball	266
Basketball	268
Boxing	270
Canoeing	272
Climbing	274
Cricket	276
Cross-Country Skiing	278
Cycling	280
Diving	282
Equestrianism	284
Fencing	286
Field Hockey	288
Figure Skating	290
Fly Fishing	292

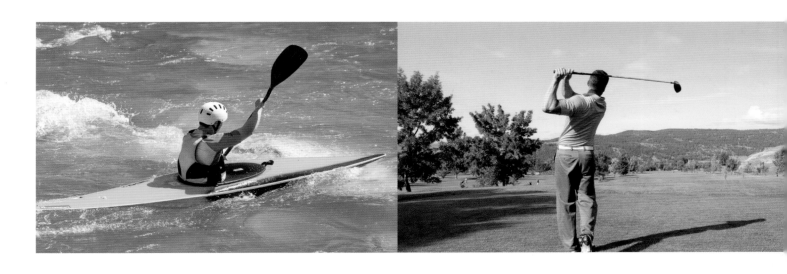

Gaelic Football 294
Golf 296
Gymnastics 298
Handball 300
Hurling 302
Ice Hockey 304
Judo 306
Karate 308
Kayaking 310
Lacrosse 312
Mountain Biking 314
Paddle Board 316
Racquetball 318
Rowing 320
Rugby 322
Running 324
Sailing 326
Shooting 328
Skateboarding 330
Skiing 332
Snowboarding 334
Soccer 336
Squash 338
Surfing 340
Swimming 342
Table Tennis 344

Tennis 346
Volleyball 348
Water Polo 350
Water Skiing 352
Wrestling 354

Functional Workouts 356

Healthy Back 358
Knee Problems 360
Office Fit 362
Belly Buster 364
Cardio Plan 366
Stronger Legs 368
Core Stability 370
Overall Strength 372
60+ 374
Weight Free 376
Full-Body Resistance 378
Bigger Arms 380
Stronger Chest 382
Strong Glutes 384

Part 4 APPENDIX 386

Glossary: General terms 388
Glossary: Latin terms 391
Credits & Acknowledgments 392

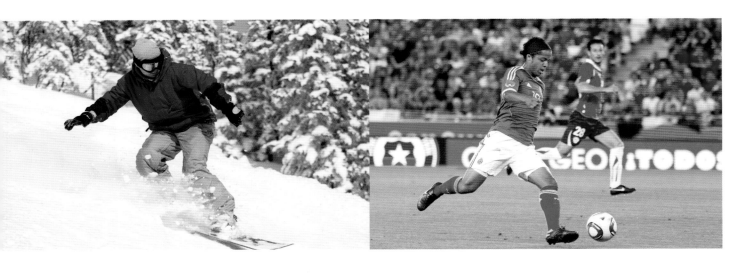

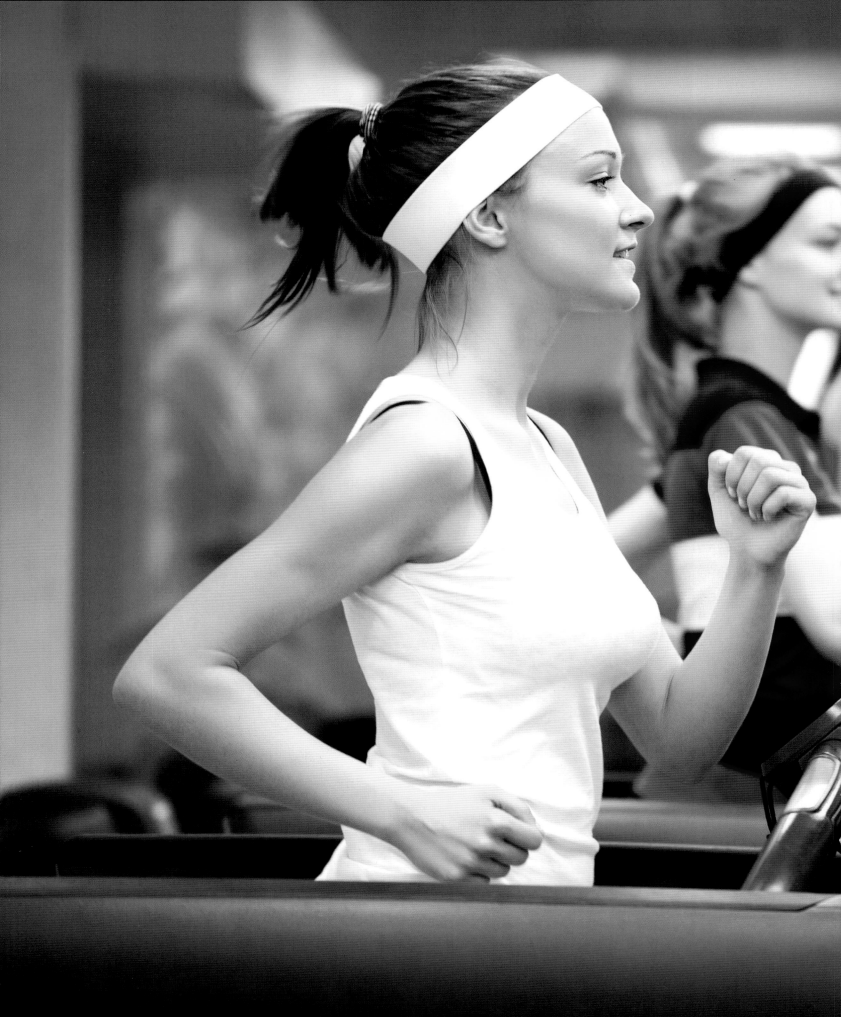

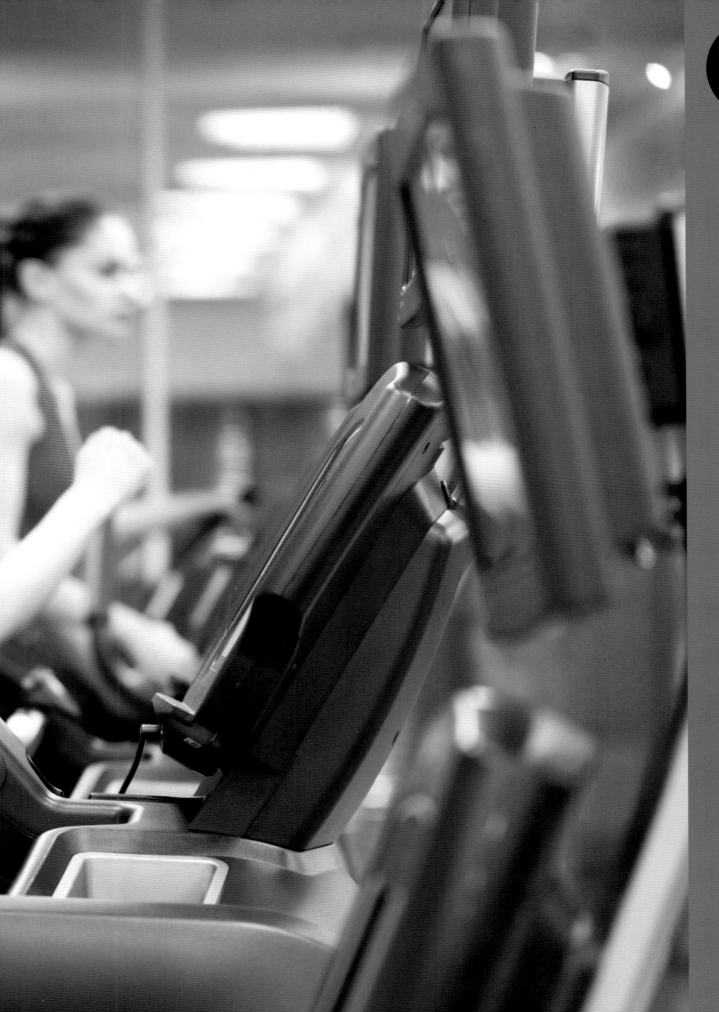

Part
1

Introduction

INTRODUCTION

The *Encyclopedia of Exercise Anatomy* features a comprehensive range of exercises for the whole body, along with detailed anatomical drawings to show exactly which muscles are being worked during each exercise. Whether you are interested in improving your sporting performance or toning specific parts of your body, this format allows you to target your exercise routines to achieve the desired results. To help you formulate an all-round routine, the book also includes workout routines that focus on improving performance in a number of popular sports as well as some to follow to help your body cope with particular stresses or build strength where it is lacking.

BUILDING STRENGTH WHERE IT'S NEEDED

Today nearly every sport across the globe uses resistance training to improve performance — long gone is the idea that weight training is only for those looking to increase muscle bulk. A quick peek into any gym will bear witness to how well stocked and versatile training facilities have become in recognition of the importance of strength and stamina in any fitness program. Sporting performance is improved, like most things in life, with repetition and practice. But the human body's musculature is complex, so the question is: what exercises should you be doing and what is best practice for your particular sport? The *Encyclopedia of Exercise Anatomy* is designed to answer that question. Whether you're a novice at tennis picking up the racquet for the first time, or a seasoned rugby player wishing to brush up on strengthening the particular muscles that provide much needed power in the scrum, this is the book for you.

Part 1 of the book includes detailed anatomical illustrations highlighting all the major muscles in the upper body (see pages 26–27) and all the major muscles of the lower body (see pages 28–29). Don't worry, you don't need to learn all the anatomical terminology, but the information is there for you to refer back to at any time. The more you work out, the more you will begin to understand about the way the human body works — and that can only be a good thing when your ambition is to achieve peak fitness.

Part 2 introduces over 100 exercises divided into four sections: upper body exercises, lower body exercises, core exercises and stretches. There is an in-depth guide for each exercise, including the muscle groups used, step-by-step instructions and pertinent performance tips. Once again, anatomical illustrations highlight the

Make sure that the gym you choose is well stocked with free weights as well as machines. Mirrors aren't there so that you can admire your increasingly sculpted body (well, not only for that!), they allow you to keep a close eye on your form as you perform each exercise.

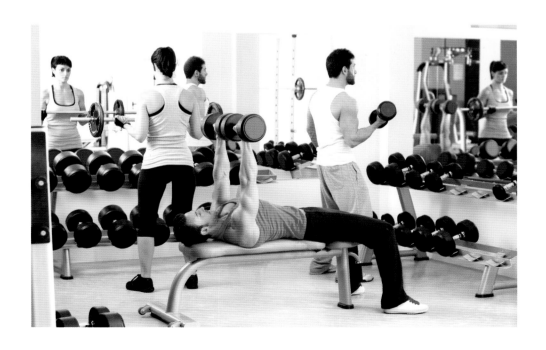

INTRODUCTION

key muscle groups involved in the exercise and annotation identifies the individual muscles being worked.

Part 3 of the book combines the individual exercises into highly effective programs. This section is divided into two subsections: the first dealing with 50 popular sports; the second dealing with functional workouts for specific nonsporting activities.

Following a brief overview of each sport and the muscles called into play, the sports programs are organized into three levels of intensity to meet the demands of every athlete, from beginner to advanced, and to provide those all-important goals to work toward — whatever your level of fitness. An alternative set of programs is provided to add interest and variety to your workout.

The remaining programs in the book focus on real-world scenarios such as workouts to help back or knee problems. This final exercise section also helps you target specific body areas that you want to enhance for purely aesthetic reasons, whether you're looking to build bigger, more powerful arms or sculpting a glorious derrière. As with the sport-specific section, there is an introductory paragraph that gives a brief overview of the muscles used; the exercise

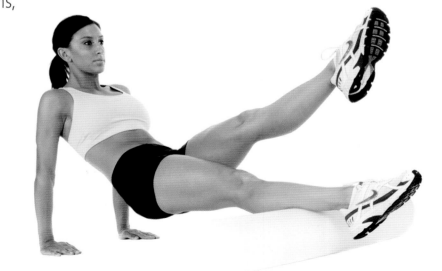

programs themselves are set at three different levels of intensity — in most cases an alternative program is provided for variety.

A WORD ON FORM

In order for you to get the most from this book, a few pointers should be taken into consideration. Remember that good form is paramount. Unless the exercise specifically calls for it, momentum should rarely, if ever, be used in order to get through a given set of movements. For maximum benefit, we are taxing a very specific set of muscles to enhance performance, and as such, proper range of motion and correct execution should always be our aim.

There can be a tendency to shorten a range of motion when the "burn" (lactic acid) builds during an intense portion of a set. If this is the case, simply rest for a few seconds to ward off the temporary fatigue rather than haphazardly advancing through the set. During a set of barbell curls, for example, don't be tempted to swing excessively using too much lower back in an effort to complete the repetitions — the next day, rather than having the slight ache in the arms that indicates a good workout, you may need ice on a strained lower back that keeps you out of the gym for a week!

Time is another important factor. You should only begin a new set when properly rested. Avoid rushing since it will not help you to achieve the optimum benefits; proceeding at a steady pace will ensure that you increase your strength and remain injury free. Training with

INTRODUCTION

a partner can be a great help in this department — you get to rest while your partner performs his or her set and you have someone to encourage you to complete each set and to keep a eye on your form.

MEASURING PROGRESS

In sport and exercise, progress can be made in myriad ways: shaving a few seconds off a previous best completion time; achieving an extra repetition or two with a particular weight; increasing the size of that weight; increasing the distance you run or the distance you throw a ball. The sport or activity you are training for defines the goals to be set. Improvement can be measured simply by how many times you hit your target each time you practice. Alternatively, if your goal is to develop a more toned body, then you can measure your success by how good you feel when you look in the mirror or your ability to slip into clothes you used to struggle to fasten.

Whatever your target, proceed with patience and don't be distracted or dismayed by how well other people are doing or how they look — the only true way to measure your progress is against your own performance. And keep your targets realistic; you can travel just as far with short steps. Find the program in this book that's the right one for you. Follow it at your own pace. If you are persistent and exercise regularly, in time, you'll find that you are one of the people that others start to look at wistfully and strive to emulate.

In sport, decreasing body fat and increasing quality muscle tissue have a direct effect on performance. From the lean long-distance cyclist to

Resistance machines are often recommended to novices in the gym. Their rigid design helps you to maintain good form at all times. Even so, get an expert to introduce you to each machine — to show you how it works, recommend the best weight and adjust the seat to the appropriate height.

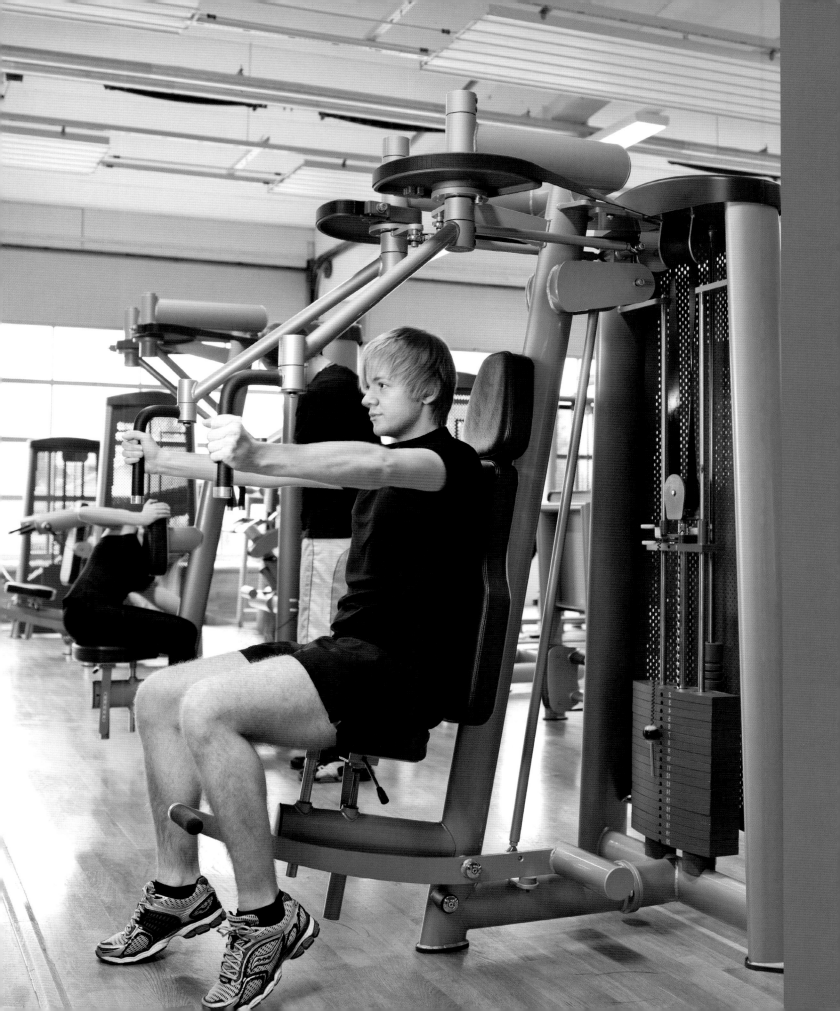

INTRODUCTION

the densely muscled rugby player, composition of the body plays an important role. Strength is generally associated with larger muscles, speed with lean muscles, and athletic performance with a combination of strength and speed as well as proficiency and control over those muscles. The truth is, whatever sport we enjoy — and to get the most out of life generally and remain injury free — we need to be strong and toned, but also flexible. Warming up and stretching are a vital part of your program. There is more about that later. Let's talk first about what you put into your body.

FUELLING ACTIVITY

There is a definite correlation between output and intake. Just as a performance car cannot expect to race successfully on anything less than premium fuel, so too must the human body be fed well for excellence in exercise. Eating good quality food that is largely unprocessed and still close to its natural state when consumed will pay dividends.

Carbohydrates

Carbohydrates enable muscles to work and can be broken into three subcategories:

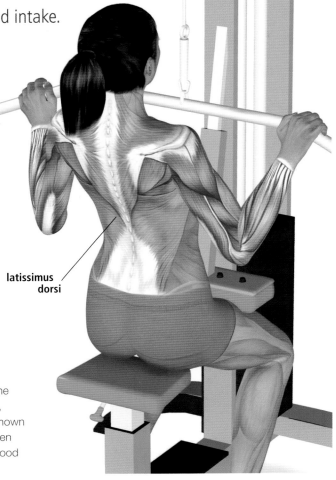

latissimus
dorsi

Progress is also made by gaining more control over the actual working muscles during exercise. For example, firing a muscle from the latissimus dorsi (commonly known as your "lats"), and not your biceps and forearms, when performing Lat Pulldowns (see page 42) is a sign of good form and a sure sign of good progress.

simple, complex and fibrous. Simple carbs, such as fruits and sugar, are broken down quickly by the body and provide short bursts of energy. Complex carbs take longer to break down, so they provide sustained energy for longer periods. Oats, quinoa, beans and brown rice are excellent examples of "clean" (unprocessed) complex carbohydrates. Fibrous carbs, such as broccoli and asparagus, aid digestion. Breads, pastas, cereals and flour are examples of processed carbs that convert quickly to sugar in the body, giving you an energy spike one minute but leading to a dramatic sugar-low the next.

If you are serious about your performance, you need to get your carbs in early in the day. Beginning your day without carbs will put an immediate limit on the amount of energy you can expend through the rest of the day. Trying to compensate by having a salad for lunch with its abundance of fibrous carbs but lack of complex carbs, will do little to help you through the afternoon. Arriving home ravenous in the evening, you will be tempted to devour excessive complex and simple carbs, which may lead your body to store them as fat. To avoid this vicious cycle make sure you eat a sensible breakfast of toast or unsweetened cereal and have some fruit too. If you can't face it first thing, take a sandwich with you to work and eat it as soon as you feel hungry. Have a lunch that includes fruit and/or vegetables, along with some carbohydrate, such as pasta or potatoes. Eat a balanced evening meal with some protein, such as lean meat or oily fish, as well as vegetables; don't eat too many carbohydrates, such as potatoes or pasta in the evening. If you are inclined to crave high fat or high sugar foods in the evening, have a glass of water or fruit juice to take the edge off your appetite before you eat your meal.

Fats

Forget the out-moded idea that all fats are evil, some are very important for healthy bodily function and regulation. Omega fats such as those found in fish are particularly good for you. It is the artery-clogging saturated fats, such as those found in fatty meats, that have little or no place in a healthy diet. Good fats are important for the health of your hair, skin and nails. These fats, including those found in nuts as well as olive oil, also provide a feeling of satiety, help to lubricate the joints and protect the heart.

Proteins

Protein enables muscles to grow bigger and stronger and, along with the proper training stimulus, allows an athlete to make the most of his or her body both on the field and in training. Complete sources of proteins — that is, sources that contain all of the amino acids — are eggs, poultry, beef, fish and protein supplements.

Try to consume protein from lean sources (egg whites, chicken and turkey breast and fish) since these are thought to preserve lean muscle mass.

MODERATION AND BALANCE

The most common mistake any aspiring athlete can make is to overtrain — breaking the body down to the point of exhaustion — and not consume enough fuel to power their body. As discussed earlier, it is never a good idea to skip breakfast or, at best, rely on a last-minute stimulant and source of sugar (coffee and fruit) — this is akin to travelling on an empty tank and will not allow your body to perform daily tasks let alone train for fitness and sport. Please take note that the only best time to have an intake of simple carbs such as sugar is following exercise, when glycogen (stored carbohydrates) needs to be quickly replenished. Following your sport or activity, a complex carb such as beans will take longer to refuel you than something that converts to sugar much quicker such as juice or fruit. For optimal results, the rest of the time it is best to consume small, frequent and healthy meals throughout the day. This will keep the body energized and help it to use stored adipose (fat) as fuel.

Generally speaking, a ratio of 40 percent protein, 40 percent carbohydrates and 20 percent fats should be the cornerstone of your nutritional intake. Additionally, tapering your carb intake, commencing with the largest portion early in the day, then switching to more fibrous or low calorie types as the day progresses will help to keep the fat furnace burning. For example, cereal, porridge or toast for breakfast, a sandwich or pasta salad for lunch and chicken salad or fish and vegetables for supper.

INTRODUCTION

If you are exercising to lose weight, it is important not to cut down drastically on food. The healthy aim for fat loss, if that is your aim, is 1 to 2 pounds (0.5 to 1 kg) per week and is best achieved through a consistent and complimentary combination of good nutrition (to fuel the body), proper weight training (to harden the body), and ample cardiovascular activity (to burn stored adipose).

GI rules

The Glycemic Index (GI) measures the rate at which carbohydrates affect the blood-sugar levels and is the key, nutritionally, to long-term fat loss. A lower GI number indicates a slower rate of digestion as well as a lower insulin demand by the body and, ultimately, less fat storage.

Fuel your exercise regime with a healthy, balanced diet, including fresh fish and vegetables, nuts and beans.

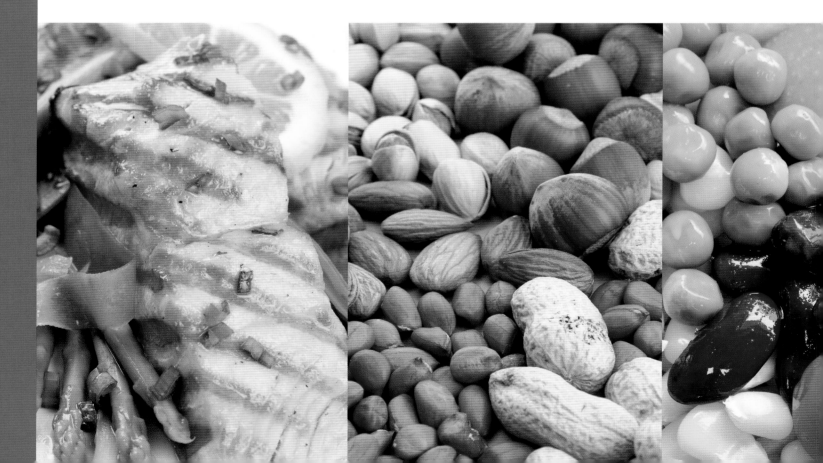

The GI classifies foods with a high GI at 70 or above. These include white bread, white rice, breakfast cereals and glucose. Those foods with a medium range of 56 to 69 include whole-wheat products, potatoes and sucrose. Foods scoring a low GI at 55 or less are most vegetables, including legumes and beans, whole grains, nuts and fructose. For a lean physique and balanced blood-sugar levels, low GI foods should make up the majority of carbohydrates you consume.

FLUID INTAKE

Last, but definitely not least, you must stay hydrated. Take water on board before, during and after exercise. Water is your body's principal chemical component and makes up about 60 percent of your body weight. Every system in your body depends on it. Lack of water can lead to dehydration, which means you don't have enough water in your body to carry out normal functions. Even mild dehydration can drain your energy and make you tired and lethargic.

Every day you lose water through your breath, perspiration, urine and bowel movements. For your body to function properly, you must replenish this water. You need 2 to 3 liters of water each day — much of this is obtained through normal eating and drinking — but

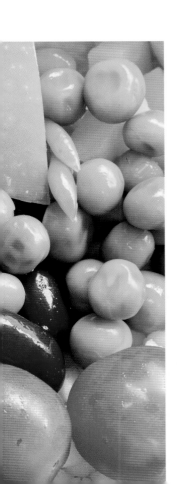

Drinking water is vital to keep yourself fit and energized whatever sport you perform. Get into the habit of drinking several glasses of water each day.

INTRODUCTION

this figure will increase or decrease depending on such variables as the weather and the amount of exercise you perform.

STRETCHING YOURSELF

The *Encyclopedia of Exercise Anatomy* is designed to be both user-friendly and progressive. Use it to help unlock the unlimited potential of your body and restore proper body balance, functionality and strength. Begin with a specific sport or functional workout and advance at your own pace through the programs.

Be sure to spend some time on the stretching portion of the book. Stretching is important for proper elongation of muscle tissue both during and after exercise as well as for releasing lactic acid — the by-product of muscles hard at work. In addition, the more flexible and pliable the tissue, the fuller the range of motion that can be achieved, and the higher the additional lean muscle tissue that can be developed, which directly assists sporting activity.

There exists a school of thought that states that stretching must precede exercise. It is, in reality, best to have warmed up prior to stretching. Often 5 to 10 minutes on a stationary bike is good preparation prior to stretching. During and after exercise are the ideal times to stretch as muscles are both warm and pliable at the time.

GOAL SETTING

It is interesting to note that the sporting section of the book is predominately geared toward athletic performance, whereas the functional workout section is geared toward both human everyday functionality and, where applicable, improving body tone. All pursuits start with goal planning and knowing where the road will ultimately take you. Armed with the mental "what?" this book is the "how." Together, you can achieve great things. Be safe and have fun.

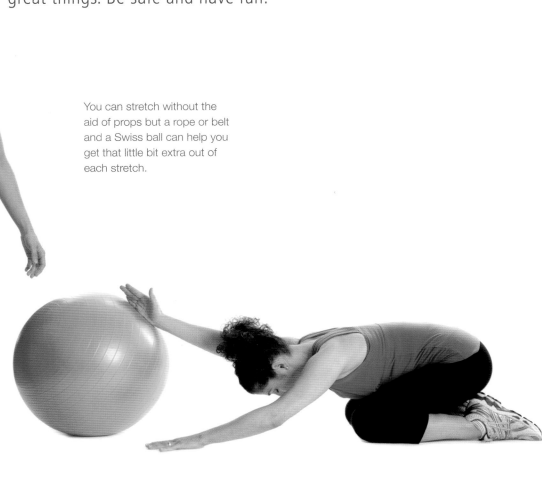

You can stretch without the aid of props but a rope or belt and a Swiss ball can help you get that little bit extra out of each stretch.

upper-body anatomy

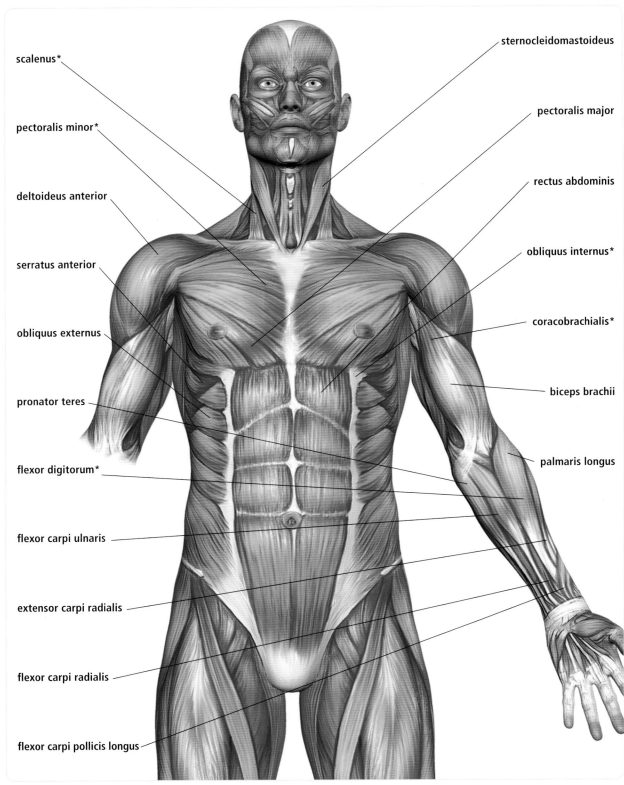

scalenus*

pectoralis minor*

deltoideus anterior

serratus anterior

obliquus externus

pronator teres

flexor digitorum*

flexor carpi ulnaris

extensor carpi radialis

flexor carpi radialis

flexor carpi pollicis longus

sternocleidomastoideus

pectoralis major

rectus abdominis

obliquus internus*

coracobrachialis*

biceps brachii

palmaris longus

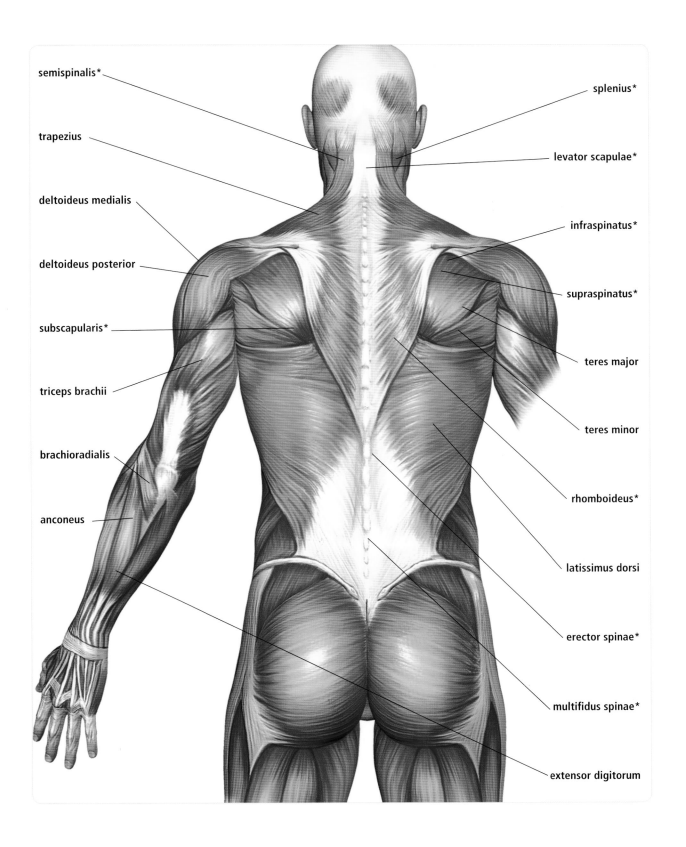

semispinalis*

trapezius

deltoideus medialis

deltoideus posterior

subscapularis*

triceps brachii

brachioradialis

anconeus

splenius*

levator scapulae*

infraspinatus*

supraspinatus*

teres major

teres minor

rhomboideus*

latissimus dorsi

erector spinae*

multifidus spinae*

extensor digitorum

lower-body anatomy

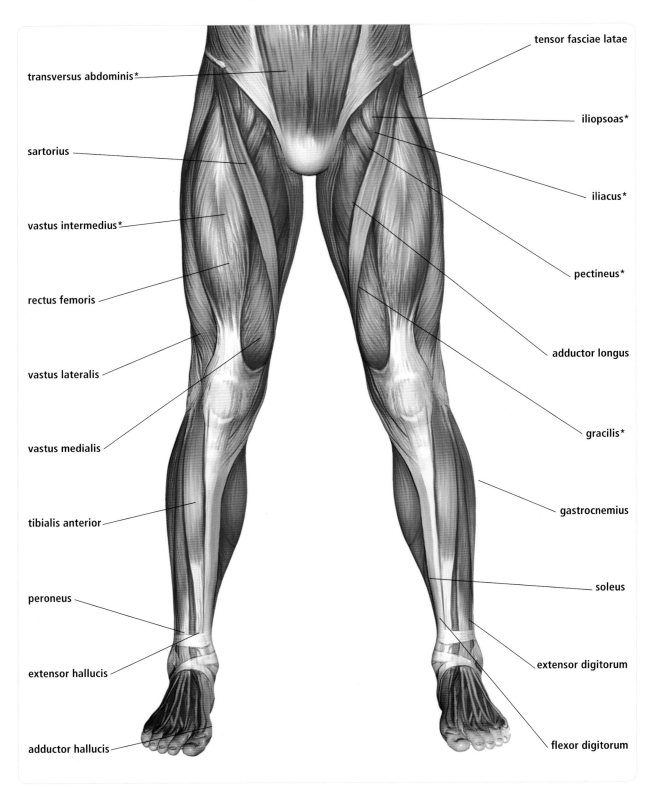

transversus abdominis*

sartorius

vastus intermedius*

rectus femoris

vastus lateralis

vastus medialis

tibialis anterior

peroneus

extensor hallucis

adductor hallucis

tensor fasciae latae

iliopsoas*

iliacus*

pectineus*

adductor longus

gracilis*

gastrocnemius

soleus

extensor digitorum

flexor digitorum

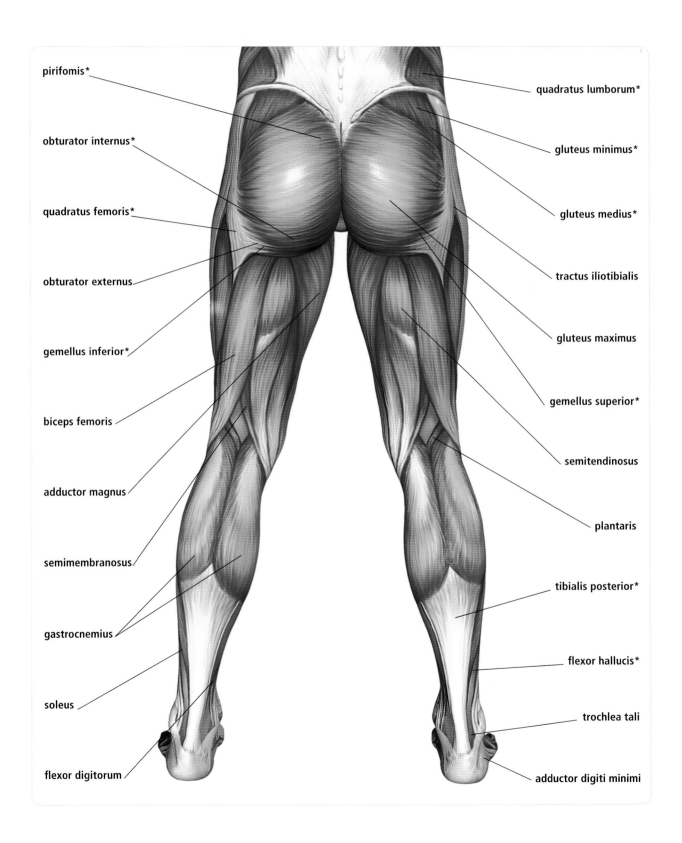

pirifomis*

obturator internus*

quadratus femoris*

obturator externus

gemellus inferior*

biceps femoris

adductor magnus

semimembranosus

gastrocnemius

soleus

flexor digitorum

quadratus lumborum*

gluteus minimus*

gluteus medius*

tractus iliotibialis

gluteus maximus

gemellus superior*

semitendinosus

plantaris

tibialis posterior*

flexor hallucis*

trochlea tali

adductor digiti minimi

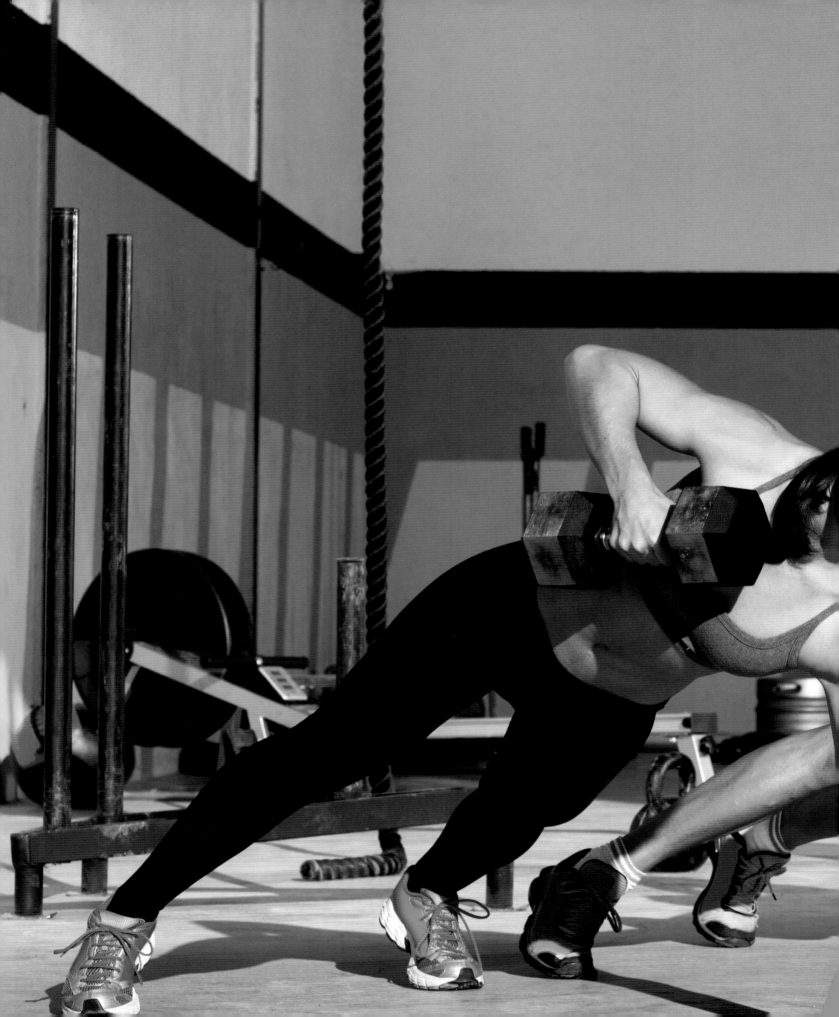

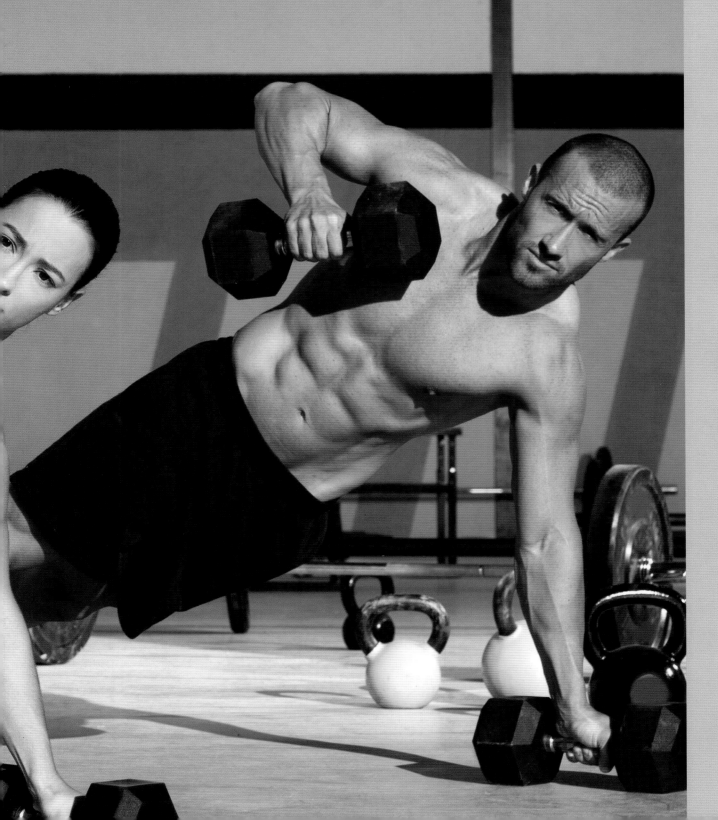

Part 2

Exercises & Stretches

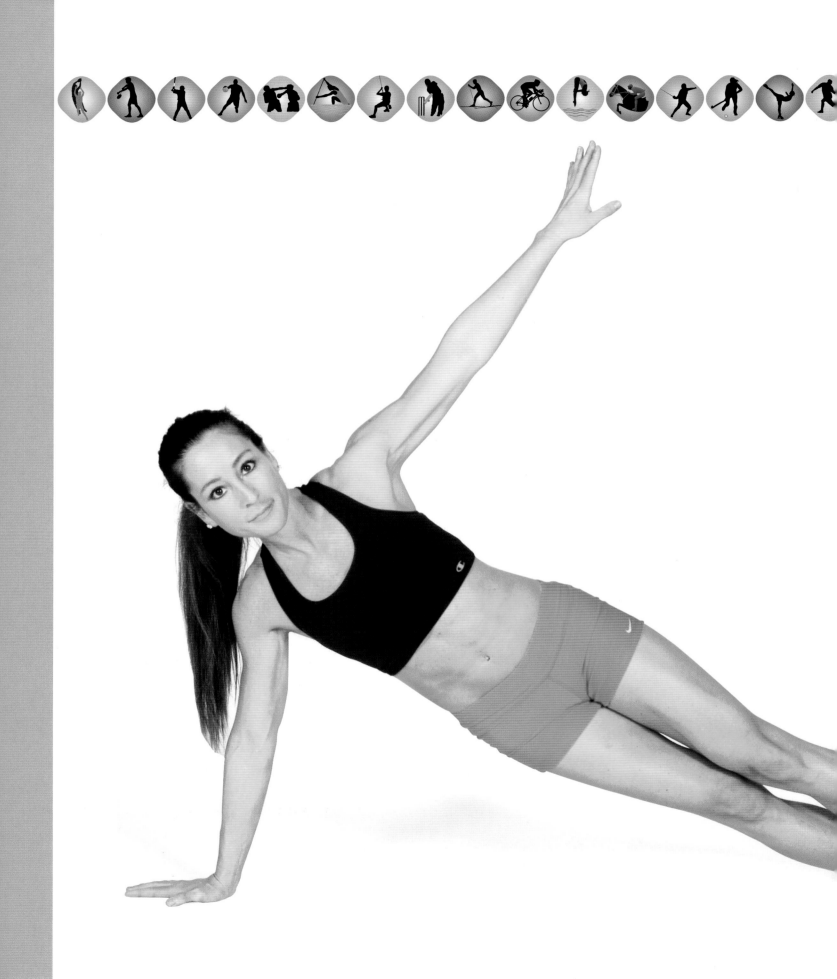

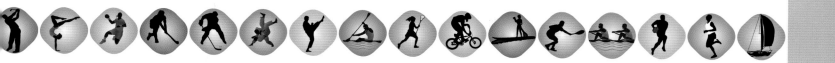

UPPER-BODY EXERCISES

The upper-body exercises provided here represent some of the most effective movements that have been proven to enhance your performance in a given sport or activity. All exercises are clearly defined and come with complete step-by-step instructions. This section includes exercises aimed at strengthening and toning all the muscles of the chest, back, shoulders and arms — enhancing these important muscle groups both in terms of aesthetics and performance. The routines provided later in the book use these exercises in the most effective combinations for specific sports or activities. However, feel free to dip into these pages and enjoy the individual exercises at any time to introduce variety into your workout. As always, it is important to pay strict attention to form to be sure to fire from the intended muscle rather than rely on ancillary help. All levels of experience are represented with plenty of variety. Enjoy!

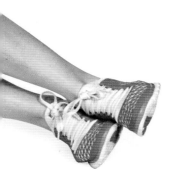

BARBELL DEADLIFT

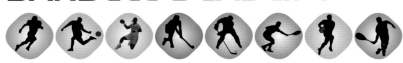

1 Begin standing with your feet shoulder-width apart in front of a barbell. Looking straight ahead, squat down and grab the barbell with a wide overhand grip; make sure your knees are close to the bar.

DO IT RIGHT
• Use your glutes to help with the movement.

AVOID
• Overarching your back.

TARGETS
• Back
• Quads
• Glutes
• Hamstrings
• Core
• Forearms
• Biceps

LEVEL
• Intermediate

BENEFITS
• Increases power and mass in the torso

NOT ADVISABLE IF YOU HAVE . . .
• Knee pain

MODIFICATIONS
• Easier: Use a very light bar or just your own body weight.
• More difficult: Bring your feet closer together to increase the range of motion required.

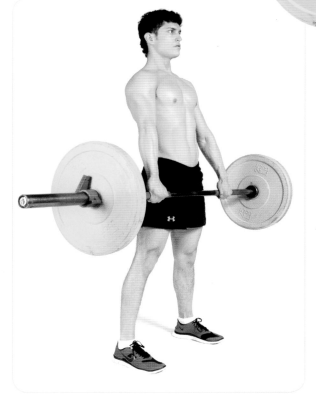

2 Push through your heels as you stand erect while holding the barbell below you at arms' length. Be sure to keep a straight back throughout this movement.

3 Stand fully erect while holding the completed movement, then reverse the process to carefully lower the barbell to the ground. Perform six to eight repetitions.

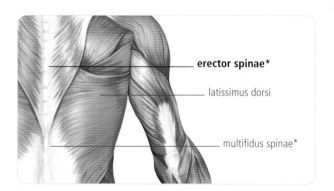

erector spinae*

latissimus dorsi

multifidus spinae*

BEST FOR

• erector spinae

ANNOTATION KEY

Bold text indicates target muscles
Grey text indicates other working muscles

* indicates deep muscles

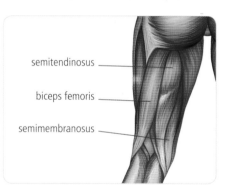

semitendinosus

biceps femoris

semimembranosus

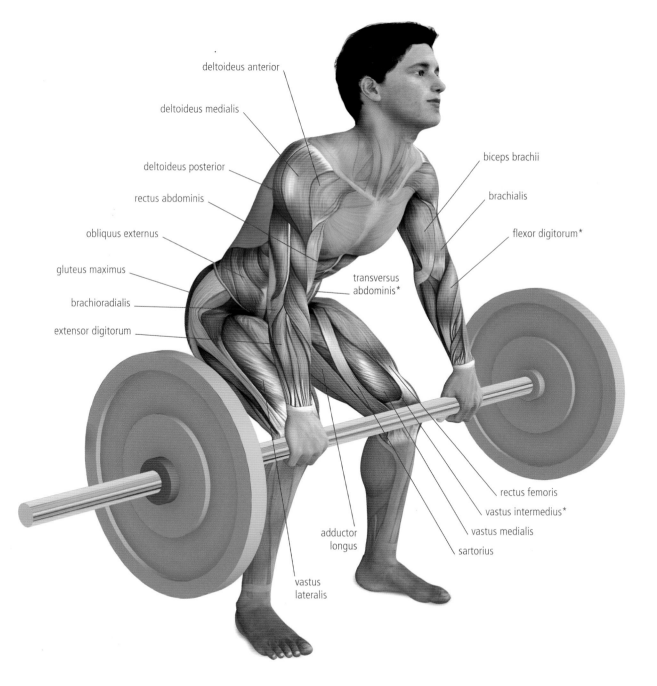

deltoideus anterior

deltoideus medialis

deltoideus posterior

rectus abdominis

obliquus externus

gluteus maximus

brachioradialis

extensor digitorum

biceps brachii

brachialis

flexor digitorum*

transversus abdominis*

rectus femoris

vastus intermedius*

vastus medialis

sartorius

adductor longus

vastus lateralis

BARBELL ROW

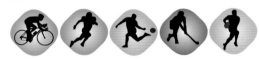

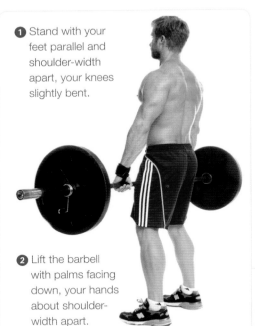

1 Stand with your feet parallel and shoulder-width apart, your knees slightly bent.

2 Lift the barbell with palms facing down, your hands about shoulder-width apart.

3 Bend at the waist to bring your torso forward, keeping a straight back until it is nearly parallel to the floor. The barbell should be directly in front of you, allowing your arms to hang perpendicular to the floor and your torso. This is the starting position.

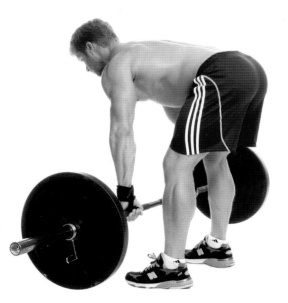

TARGETS
• Deltoids
• Back

LEVEL
• Intermediate

BENEFITS
• Increases power to shoulders, back and arms

NOT ADVISABLE IF YOU HAVE . . .
• Back problems

TRAINER'S TIPS
• Exhale as you lift the barbell, and inhale as you lower it to the starting position.
• Keep a slight bend of the knees, engaging your glutes and hamstrings.
• Use manageable weights for this exercise — heavy lifting can lead to bad form and possible back injury.

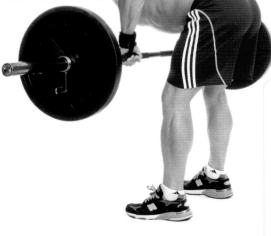

4 Lift the barbell toward your torso, keeping your elbows pointing in toward the sides of the body.

DO IT RIGHT
• Keep your torso horizontal throughout the exercise.

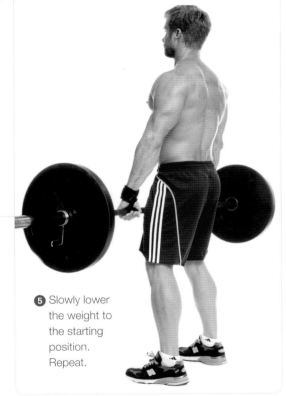

5 Slowly lower the weight to the starting position. Repeat.

AVOID
• Dropping your head during this exercise.

UPPER BODY: BARBELL ROW

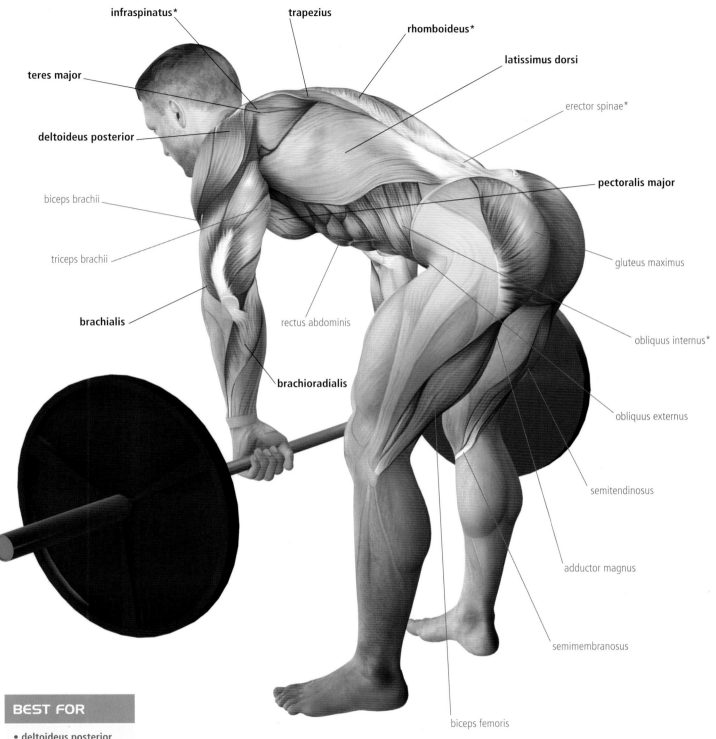

infraspinatus*

trapezius

rhomboideus*

latissimus dorsi

teres major

erector spinae*

deltoideus posterior

pectoralis major

biceps brachii

gluteus maximus

triceps brachii

rectus abdominis

obliquus internus*

brachialis

obliquus externus

brachioradialis

semitendinosus

adductor magnus

semimembranosus

biceps femoris

BEST FOR

- deltoideus posterior
- trapezius
- rhomboideus
- latissimus dorsi
- teres major
- infraspinatus
- brachialis
- brachioradialis
- pectoralis major

ANNOTATION KEY

Bold text indicates target muscles

Grey text indicates other working muscles

* indicates deep muscles

DUMBBELL ROW

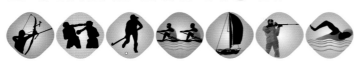

1 Holding a dumbbell in your left hand, stand next to an incline bench with your feet placed generously shoulder-width apart.

2 Lean forward, and place your right hand on the bench. Your back should be flat and your knees slightly bent. Your left hand should be holding the dumbbell in a hammer-grip position, with your elbow close to your ribs.

DO IT RIGHT
• Don't drop your chest.
• Keep your pelvis tucked in slightly and keep your back flat.

AVOID
• Drawing your elbow away from your rib cage.
• Using momentum to lift the dumbbell.

3 Draw your elbow toward the ceiling.

4 Lower the dumbbell to starting position, and repeat. Switch sides, and repeat all steps with your right hand holding the dumbbell.

TARGETS
• Middle back

LEVEL
• Intermediate

BENEFITS
• Increases power to shoulders and back

NOT ADVISABLE IF YOU HAVE . . .
• Back problems

TRAINER'S TIPS
• Wear wrist straps for greater stability.
• Keep a slight bend in your supporting arm.
• Relax your jaw.

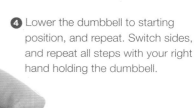

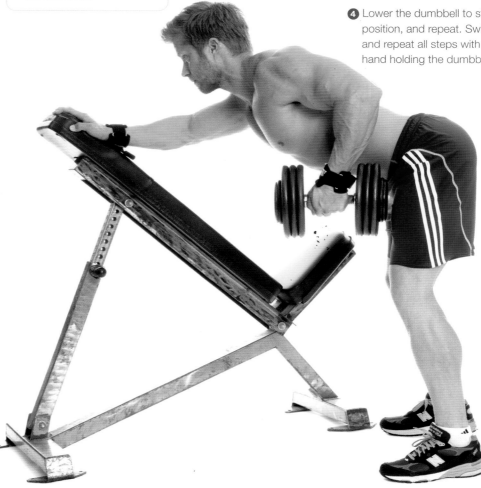

UPPER BODY: DUMBBELL ROW

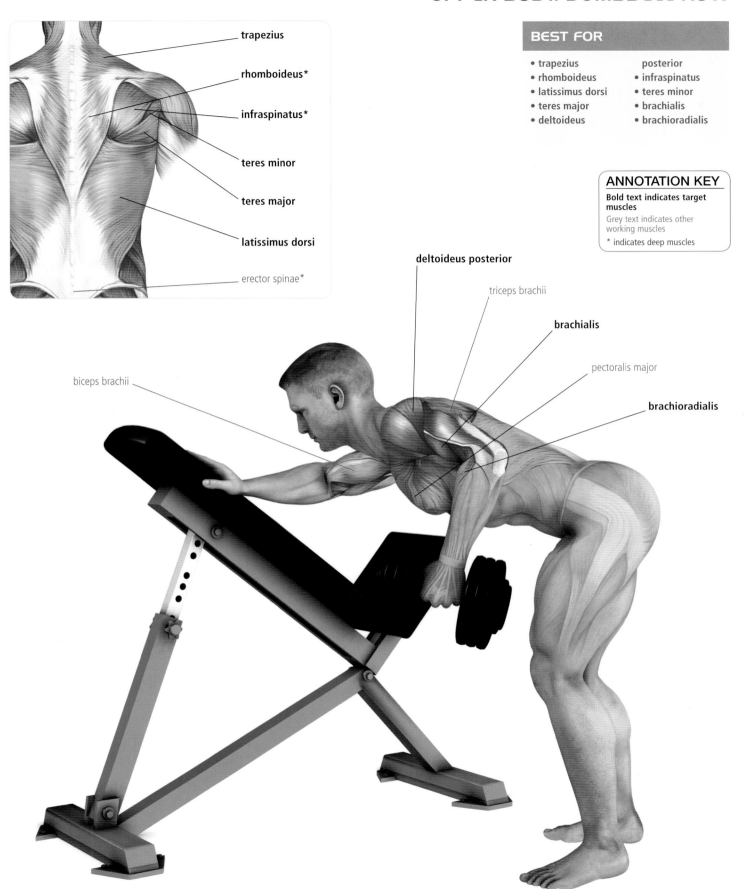

trapezius

rhomboideus*

infraspinatus*

teres minor

teres major

latissimus dorsi

erector spinae*

BEST FOR

- trapezius
- rhomboideus
- latissimus dorsi
- teres major
- deltoideus
- posterior
- infraspinatus
- teres minor
- brachialis
- brachioradialis

ANNOTATION KEY

Bold text indicates target muscles

Grey text indicates other working muscles

* indicates deep muscles

deltoideus posterior

triceps brachii

brachialis

pectoralis major

brachioradialis

biceps brachii

DUMBBELL PULLOVER

1. Lie on a flat bench with your head supported. Bend your legs and place your feet, shoulder-width apart, flat on the bench for extra lower-back support.

2. Hold a light dumbbell above your chest with your arms extended.

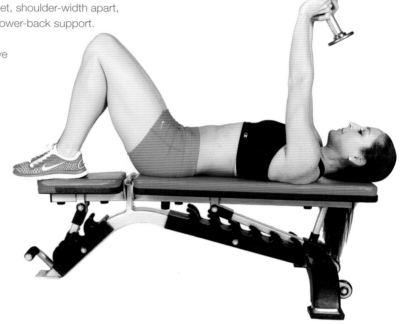

DO IT RIGHT
- Always bend your arms when performing this exercise.

AVOID
- Hitting your head with the dumbbell.

TARGETS
- Back
- Quads
- Glutes
- Hamstrings
- Core
- Forearms
- Biceps

LEVEL
- Beginner

BENEFITS
- Increases strength to shoulders, chest and arms.

NOT ADVISABLE IF YOU HAVE . . .
- Back problems
- Shoulder issues

TRAINER'S TIPS
- Do not let the dumbbell go too far forward. The starting position is directly above your chest and the dumbbell should not go any farther than that.

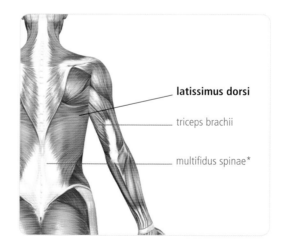

latissimus dorsi

triceps brachii

multifidus spinae*

pectoralis minor*

pectoralis major

serratus anterior

obliquus externus

rectus abdominis

transversus abdominis*

MODIFICATIONS

Easier: Use a very light dumbbell.

More difficult: Lay across a bench with only your head and shoulders supported (right).

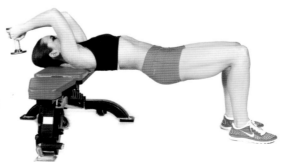

BEST FOR
- latissimus dorsi
- serratus anterior

ANNOTATION KEY

Bold text indicates target muscles

Grey text indicates other working muscles

* indicates deep muscles

❸ Moving your shoulders only and keeping a slight bend in your arms, slowly lower the weight down behind your head. Bring the dumbbell back to the starting position and repeat six to eight times.

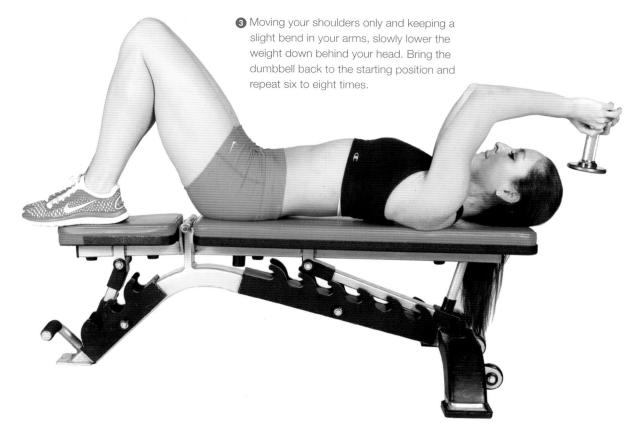

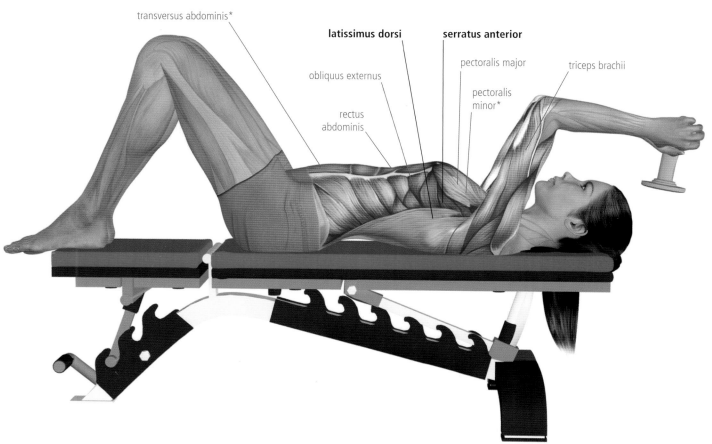

transversus abdominis*

latissimus dorsi

serratus anterior

obliquus externus

pectoralis major

triceps brachii

rectus abdominis

pectoralis minor*

LAT PULLDOWN

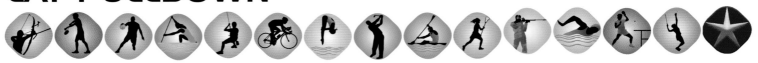

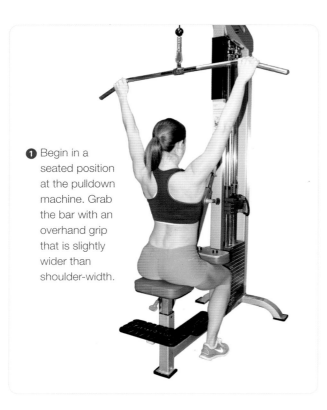

1 Begin in a seated position at the pulldown machine. Grab the bar with an overhand grip that is slightly wider than shoulder-width.

2 Pull the bar down to the very top of your chest.

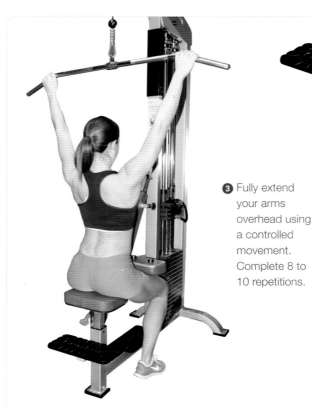

3 Fully extend your arms overhead using a controlled movement. Complete 8 to 10 repetitions.

TARGETS
- Back
- Forearms
- Biceps

LEVEL
- Beginner

BENEFITS
- Increases both strength and width in the back muscles

NOT ADVISABLE IF YOU HAVE . . .
- Back problems

MODIFICATIONS
- **Easier:** Try using a wider grip to reduce your range of motion.
- **More difficult:** A closer grip will increase your range of motion.

DO IT RIGHT
- Always sit up straight, maintaining a flat back.

AVOID
- Pulling the bar behind your neck.

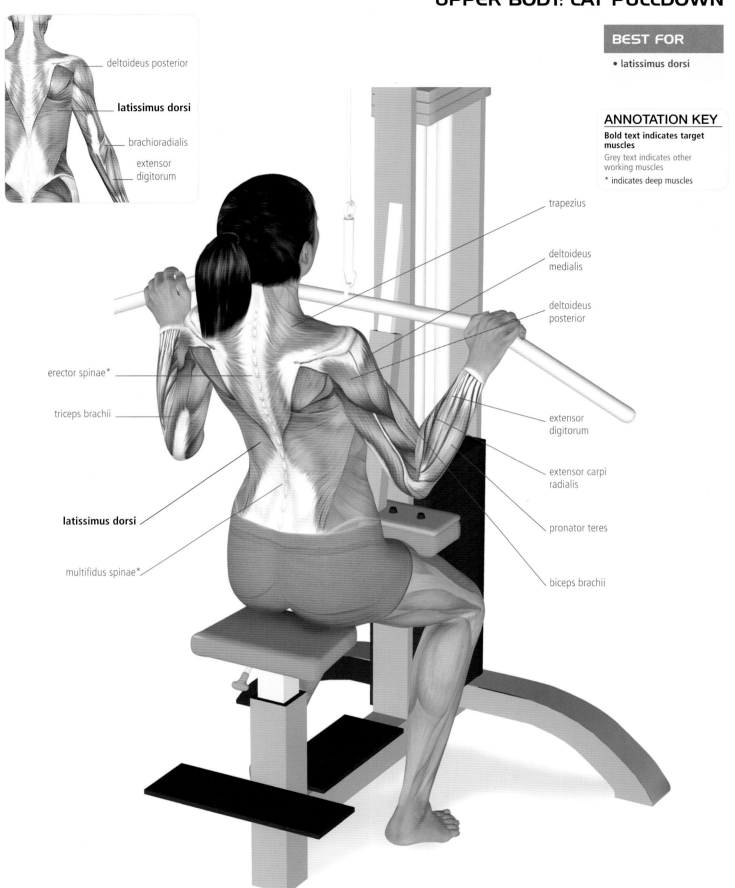

deltoideus posterior

latissimus dorsi

brachioradialis

extensor
digitorum

ANNOTATION KEY

Bold text indicates target muscles

Grey text indicates other working muscles

* indicates deep muscles

trapezius

deltoideus medialis

deltoideus posterior

erector spinae*

triceps brachii

extensor digitorum

extensor carpi radialis

pronator teres

latissimus dorsi

biceps brachii

multifidus spinae*

SCAPULAR RANGE OF MOTION

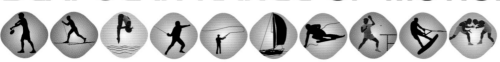

1 Sit or stand, keeping your neck, shoulders, and torso in a relaxed, neutral position. Keeping your chin level, look straight ahead.

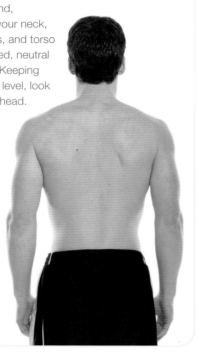

DO IT RIGHT
• Move your shoulders in a smooth, controlled manner.

AVOID
• Moving your torso.

2 With your arms at your side, bend your elbows slightly. Hold your hands with the palms facing inward.

3 Roll your shoulders forward, concentrating on separating your scapulae from your spine.

TARGETS
• Shoulders
• Scapula
• Neck

LEVEL
• Beginner

BENEFITS
• Improves range of motion
• Relaxes tight neck, shoulder, chest and upper-back muscles
• Stabilizes your shoulder blades

NOT ADVISABLE IF YOU HAVE . . .
• Shoulder issues

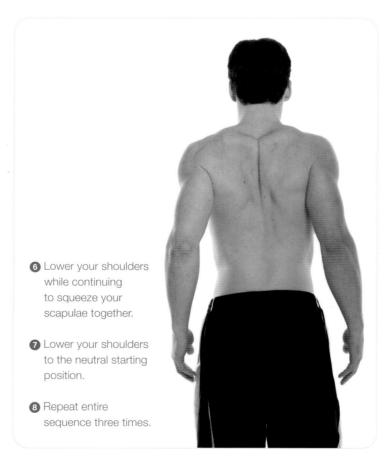

6 Lower your shoulders while continuing to squeeze your scapulae together.

7 Lower your shoulders to the neutral starting position.

8 Repeat entire sequence three times.

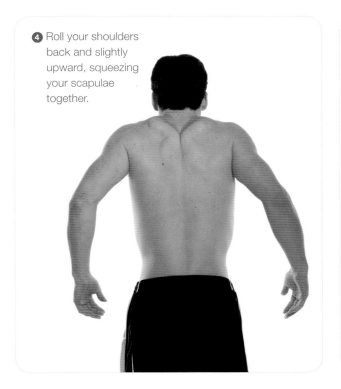

4 Roll your shoulders back and slightly upward, squeezing your scapulae together.

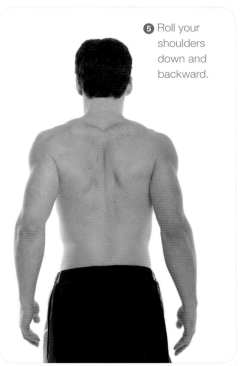

5 Roll your shoulders down and backward.

ANNOTATION KEY

Bold text indicates target muscles

Grey text indicates other working muscles

* indicates deep muscles

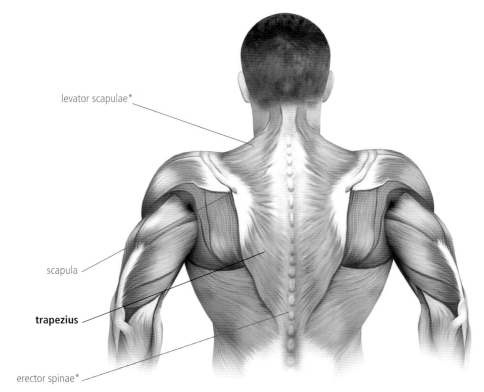

levator scapulae*

scapula

trapezius

erector spinae*

ALTERNATING KETTLEBELL ROW

1 Stand upright with your feet shoulder-width apart. Hold a pair of kettlebells in front of you with an overhand grip. Bend forward slightly at the waist, maintaining a flat back.

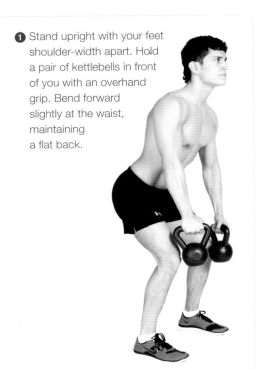

2 Bend your arm at the elbow, and pull your left hand up toward your abdomen, then lower it again.

DO IT RIGHT
• Maintain a flat back during the exercise.

AVOID
• Rotating your core.

TARGETS
• Middle back
• Biceps

LEVEL
• Beginner

BENEFITS
• Builds strength in the middle back

NOT ADVISABLE IF YOU HAVE . . .
• Back pain

MODIFICATIONS

Easier: Lift with both arms at the same time (below).

More difficult: Raise one leg off the floor for a tougher challenge.

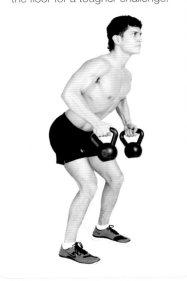

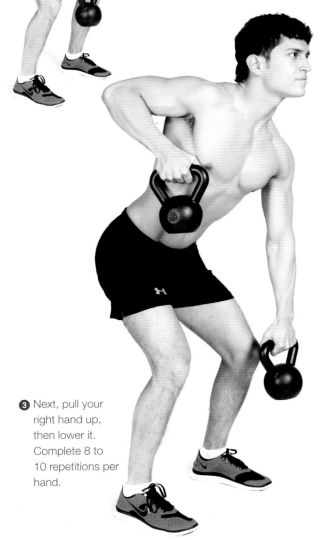

3 Next, pull your right hand up, then lower it. Complete 8 to 10 repetitions per hand.

UPPER BODY: ALTERNATING KETTLEBELL ROW

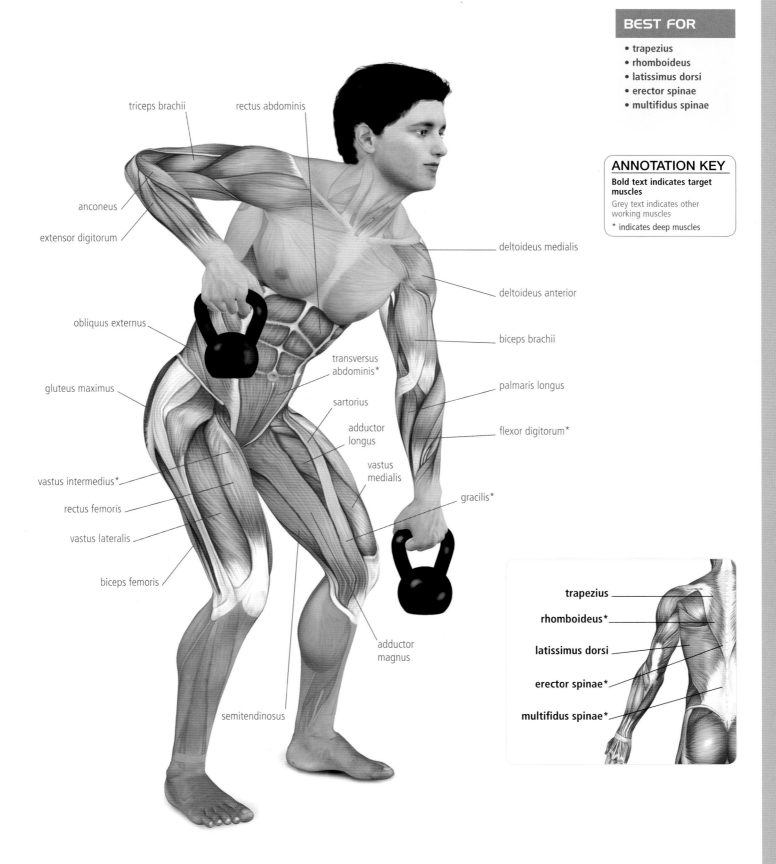

triceps brachii

rectus abdominis

anconeus

extensor digitorum

deltoideus medialis

deltoideus anterior

biceps brachii

obliquus externus

transversus abdominis*

palmaris longus

gluteus maximus

sartorius

adductor longus

flexor digitorum*

vastus medialis

gracilis*

vastus intermedius*

rectus femoris

vastus lateralis

biceps femoris

adductor magnus

semitendinosus

trapezius

rhomboideus*

latissimus dorsi

erector spinae*

multifidus spinae*

ALTERNATING RENEGADE ROW

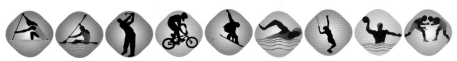

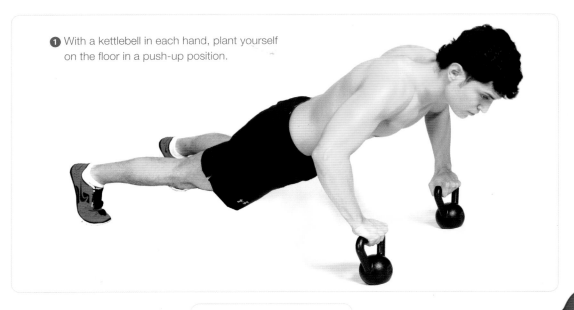

1 With a kettlebell in each hand, plant yourself on the floor in a push-up position.

DO IT RIGHT
- Keep your core stable and straight on.

AVOID
- Dropping or slamming the weight into the floor.

TARGETS
- Middle back
- Abdominals
- Biceps
- Chest
- Triceps

LEVEL
- Advanced

BENEFITS
- Builds strength in the middle back

NOT ADVISABLE IF YOU HAVE . . .
- Back problems or shoulder issues

TRAINER'S TIPS
- Forcefully push down on one kettlebell as if trying to force it into the ground. Make sure that you minimize rotation through your body as you pull the other kettlebell into your ribs.

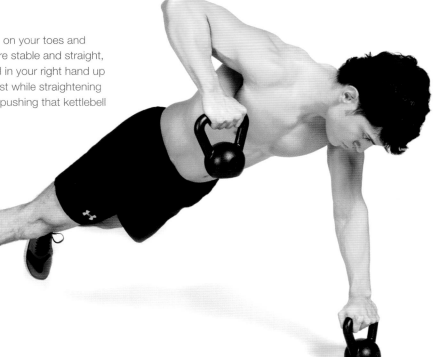

2 While staying up on your toes and keeping your core stable and straight, pull the kettlebell in your right hand up toward your chest while straightening the left arm and pushing that kettlebell into the floor.

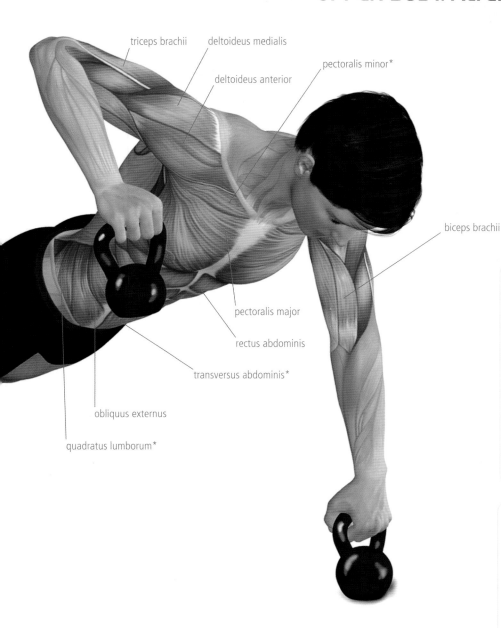

triceps brachii

deltoideus medialis

pectoralis minor*

deltoideus anterior

biceps brachii

pectoralis major

rectus abdominis

transversus abdominis*

obliquus externus

quadratus lumborum*

BEST FOR

- trapezius
- rhomboideus
- latissimus dorsi
- erector spinae
- multifidus spinae

ANNOTATION KEY

Bold text indicates target muscles

Grey text indicates other working muscles

* indicates deep muscles

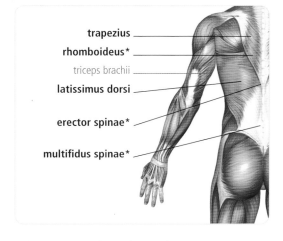

trapezius

rhomboideus*

triceps brachii

latissimus dorsi

erector spinae*

multifidus spinae*

MODIFICATIONS

Easier: Row with just one kettlebell while keeping the empty hand planted flat on the floor. Switch hands after 10 repetitions.

More difficult: Raise one leg off the floor (below) for a tougher challenge.

❸ Lower your right arm, then repeat the movement with the left. Complete 8 to 10 repetitions per arm.

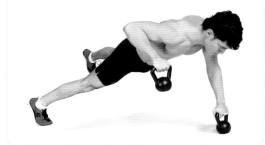

INCLINE BENCH ROW

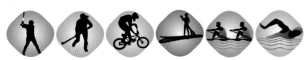

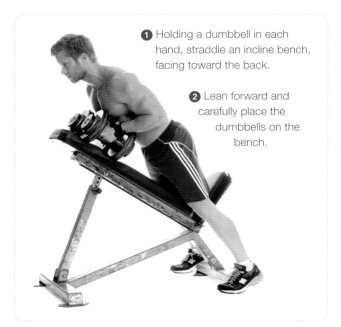

❶ Holding a dumbbell in each hand, straddle an incline bench, facing toward the back.

❷ Lean forward and carefully place the dumbbells on the bench.

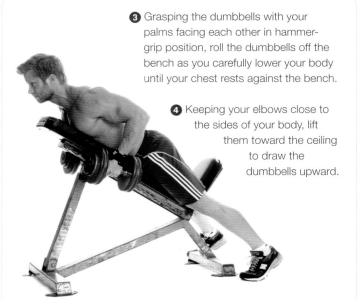

❸ Grasping the dumbbells with your palms facing each other in hammer-grip position, roll the dumbbells off the bench as you carefully lower your body until your chest rests against the bench.

❹ Keeping your elbows close to the sides of your body, lift them toward the ceiling to draw the dumbbells upward.

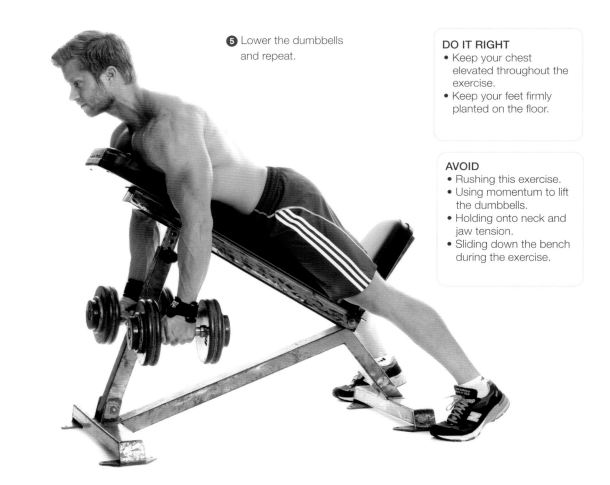

❺ Lower the dumbbells and repeat.

TARGETS
• Back
• Shoulders

LEVEL
• Advanced

BENEFITS
• Increases power and mass in the torso

NOT ADVISABLE IF YOU HAVE . . .
• Shoulder pain

TRAINER'S TIPS
• When getting into the starting position, place your pelvis on the bench first, then your stomach, and then your chest upon the dumbbells.
• To protect your back and shoulders, carefully drop the dumbbells when you have finished the exercise.

DO IT RIGHT
• Keep your chest elevated throughout the exercise.
• Keep your feet firmly planted on the floor.

AVOID
• Rushing this exercise.
• Using momentum to lift the dumbbells.
• Holding onto neck and jaw tension.
• Sliding down the bench during the exercise.

BEST FOR

- trapezius
- rhomboideus
- latissimus dorsi
- teres major
- deltoideus posterior
- infraspinatus
- teres minor
- brachialis
- brachioradialis
- pectoralis major

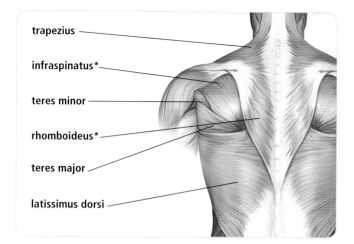

trapezius

infraspinatus*

teres minor

rhomboideus*

teres major

latissimus dorsi

MODIFICATION

Similar difficulty: Follow instructions for the Incline Bench Row, but hold the dumbbells with your hands facing behind you in.

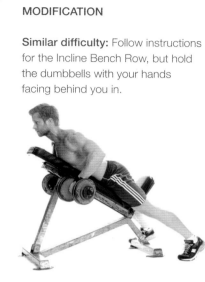

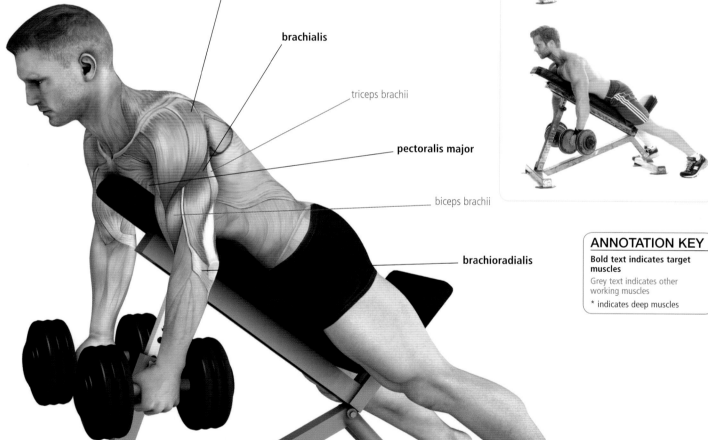

deltoideus posterior

brachialis

triceps brachii

pectoralis major

biceps brachii

brachioradialis

ANNOTATION KEY

Bold text indicates target muscles

Grey text indicates other working muscles

* indicates deep muscles

ROPE PULLDOWN

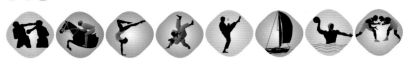

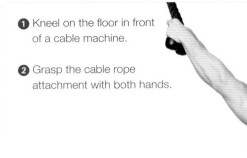

1 Kneel on the floor in front of a cable machine.

2 Grasp the cable rope attachment with both hands.

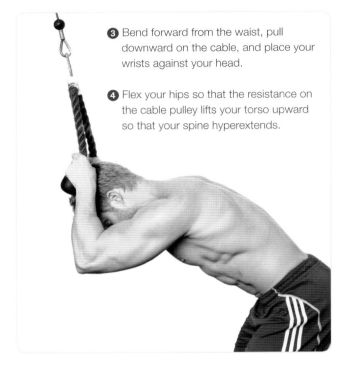

3 Bend forward from the waist, pull downward on the cable, and place your wrists against your head.

4 Flex your hips so that the resistance on the cable pulley lifts your torso upward so that your spine hyperextends.

TARGETS
- Upper abdominals
- Obliques

LEVEL
- Intermediate

BENEFITS
- Increases power and flexibility in the back

NOT ADVISABLE IF YOU HAVE . . .
- Back pain

TRAINER'S TIPS
- Do not hold your breath. Let air out of your lungs, and take short breaths when necessary.
- Do not use arm strength to execute movement.

DO IT RIGHT
- Focus on using your abdominal muscles.

AVOID
- Shifting your hips once the movement begins.

5 Keeping your hips stationary, flex your waist so that your elbows move toward the middle of your thighs. Return to starting position, and repeat.

MODIFICATION

Similar difficulty:
Follow steps 1 through 4, and then as you bend forward from the waist, twist to one side, moving your elbow toward the middle of the opposite thigh.

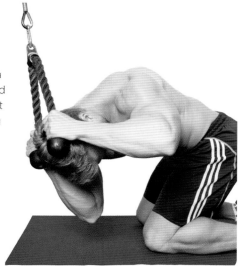

MODIFICATION

More difficult:
Follow previous instructions, but deepen the twist, aiming your elbow for the opposite knee.

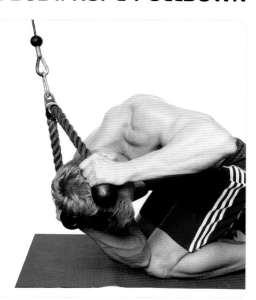

BEST FOR

- rectus abdominis
- obliquus internus
- obliquus externus

ANNOTATION KEY

Bold text indicates target muscles

Grey text indicates other working muscles

* indicates deep muscles

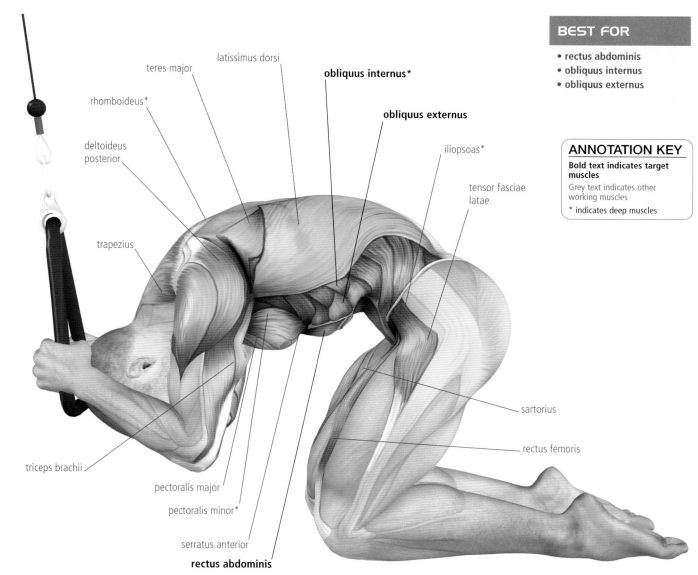

latissimus dorsi

teres major

obliquus internus*

rhomboideus*

obliquus externus

deltoideus posterior

iliopsoas*

tensor fasciae latae

trapezius

sartorius

rectus femoris

triceps brachii

pectoralis major

pectoralis minor*

serratus anterior

rectus abdominis

REVERSE CLOSE-GRIP FRONT CHIN

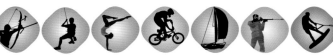

DO IT RIGHT
- Always perform a full range of motion.

AVOID
- Dropping your body weight suddenly.

TARGETS
- Lower back
- Forearms
- Biceps

LEVEL
- Intermediate

BENEFITS
- Increases both strength and width in the back muscles

MODIFICATIONS
- **Easier:** Have a partner assist you by supporting the weight of your legs.
- **More difficult:** Place a dumbbell between your lower legs for increased resistance.

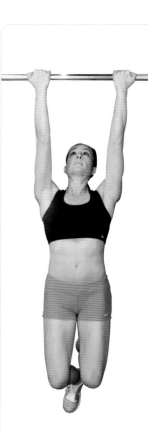

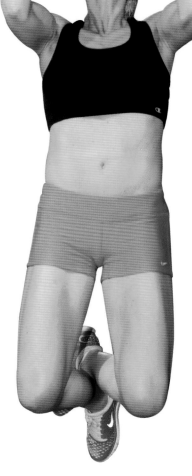

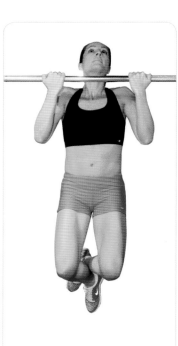

1 Standing in front of a pull-up bar, either reach up or step on a stool. Take an underhand close grip and hang below at arms' length.

2 Cross your legs at the ankles, and pull yourself up.

3 When your chin is as close to the bar as possible, lower yourself back to arms' length. Repeat 8 to 10 times.

BEST FOR

- **latissimus dorsi**
- **biceps brachii**

ANNOTATION KEY

Bold text indicates target muscles

Grey text indicates other working muscles

* indicates deep muscles

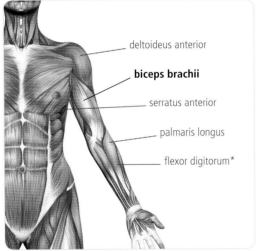

deltoideus anterior

biceps brachii

serratus anterior

palmaris longus

flexor digitorum*

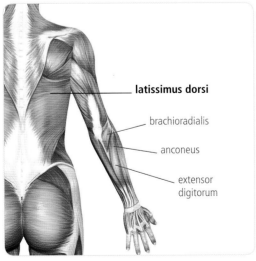

latissimus dorsi

brachioradialis

anconeus

extensor digitorum

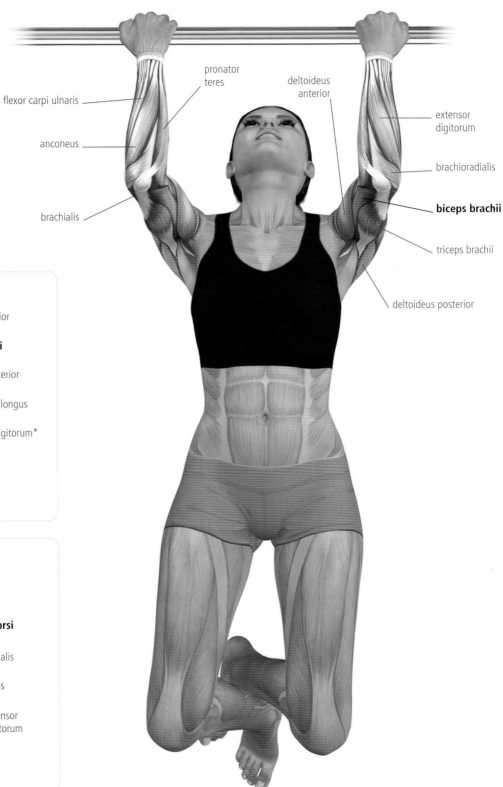

flexor carpi ulnaris

pronator teres

deltoideus anterior

extensor digitorum

anconeus

brachioradialis

brachialis

biceps brachii

triceps brachii

deltoideus posterior

FLAT BENCH HYPEREXTENSION

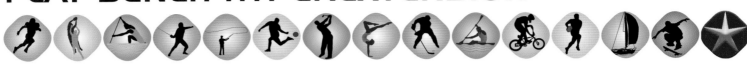

1. Lie supine on a flat bench with your sternum even with the bench's upper edge. Your upper chest and head should hang off the top of the bench.

2. Hook your feet under the bench, securing yourself in a stable starting position. Place your hands at the sides of your head, fingertips touching your ears.

DO IT RIGHT
- Maintain a constant engagement of the glutes and thighs while executing this exercise.
- Your lower body should remain taut throughout the movement.
- Keep your head in a neutral position.

AVOID
- Elevating your shoulders.
- Lifting your hip bones off the bench.

TARGETS
- Lower back

LEVEL
- Intermediate

BENEFITS
- Increases core strength and flexibility

NOT ADVISABLE IF YOU HAVE . . .
- Back pain

TRAINER'S TIPS
- Wear shoes that support a strong grip on the underside of the flat bench.

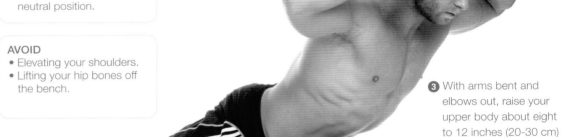

3. With arms bent and elbows out, raise your upper body about eight to 12 inches (20-30 cm) off the bench.

4. Slowly and carefully lower your body back to the starting position. Repeat 8 to 10 times.

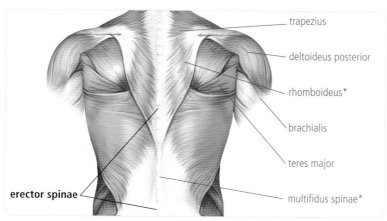

trapezius

deltoideus posterior

rhomboideus*

brachialis

teres major

erector spinae

multifidus spinae*

BEST FOR

- erector spinae
- gluteus maximus
- adductor magnus

ANNOTATION KEY

Bold text indicates target muscles

Grey text indicates other working muscles

* indicates deep muscles

semitendinosus

adductor magnus

biceps femoris

semimembranosus

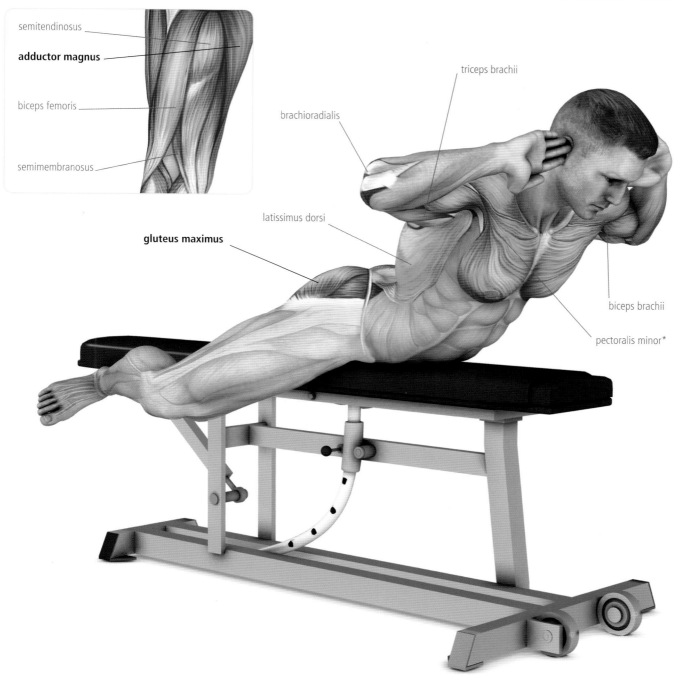

triceps brachii

brachioradialis

latissimus dorsi

gluteus maximus

biceps brachii

pectoralis minor*

ROTATED BACK EXTENSION

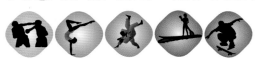

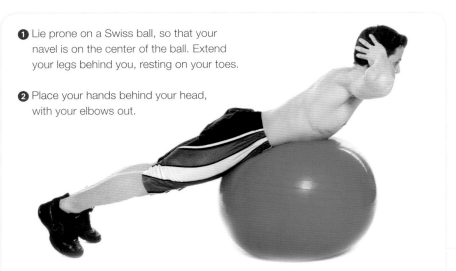

① Lie prone on a Swiss ball, so that your navel is on the center of the ball. Extend your legs behind you, resting on your toes.

② Place your hands behind your head, with your elbows out.

DO IT RIGHT
• Keep your toes firmly planted on the floor.
• Keep your arms out at a 90-degree angle to your body with your elbows bent.
• Widen your feet for increased stability.

AVOID
• Shifting your hips as you rotate — hold them square to the ball throughout the movement.

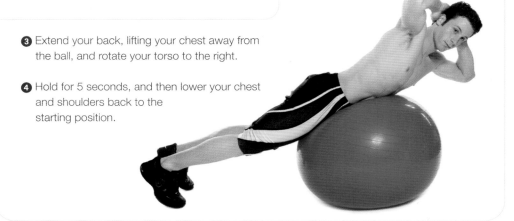

③ Extend your back, lifting your chest away from the ball, and rotate your torso to the right.

④ Hold for 5 seconds, and then lower your chest and shoulders back to the starting position.

TARGETS
• Obliques
• Back

LEVEL
• Advanced

BENEFITS
• Strengthens back muscles
• Strengthens obliques

NOT ADVISABLE IF YOU HAVE . . .
• Neck issues
• Lower-back pain

⑤ Repeat, extending your back and rotating your torso to the left. Repeat entire sequence three times in both directions.

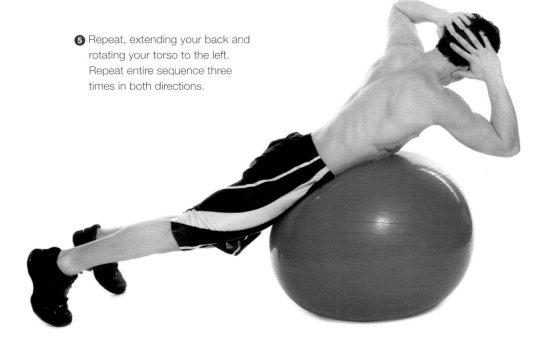

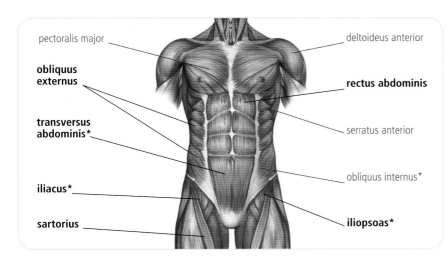

pectoralis major

deltoideus anterior

obliquus externus

rectus abdominis

transversus abdominis*

serratus anterior

iliacus*

obliquus internus*

sartorius

iliopsoas*

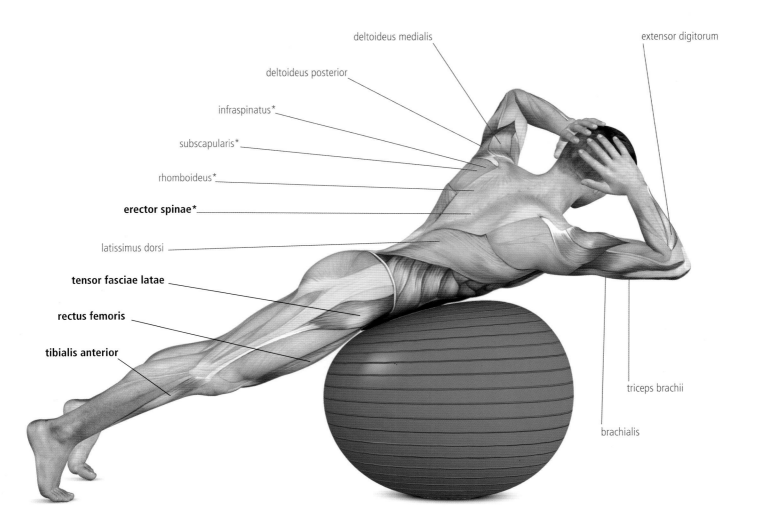

deltoideus medialis

extensor digitorum

deltoideus posterior

infraspinatus*

subscapularis*

rhomboideus*

erector spinae*

latissimus dorsi

tensor fasciae latae

rectus femoris

tibialis anterior

triceps brachii

brachialis

BARBELL BENCH PRESS

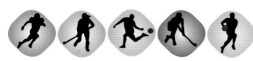

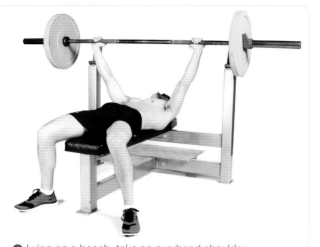

1 Lying on a bench, take an overhand shoulder-width grip on a barbell, and unrack it.

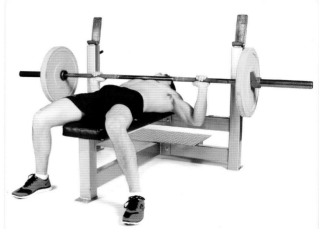

2 Lower the bar through a slow, controlled movement to your nipple line, inhaling as you do so.

TARGETS
- Pectorals
- Anterior deltoids
- Triceps
- Abdominals
- Upper back

LEVEL
- Intermediate

BENEFITS
- Increases power and mass in the chest

NOT ADVISABLE IF YOU HAVE . . .
- Wrist pain
- Shoulder pain
- Lower-back pain

TRAINER'S TIPS
- Be careful not to hyperextend your arms at the top range of movement — this will take the weight of the contracting muscles.

DO IT RIGHT
- Be sure to thrust your chest outward to complete the movement.

AVOID
- Bouncing the weight off your chest.

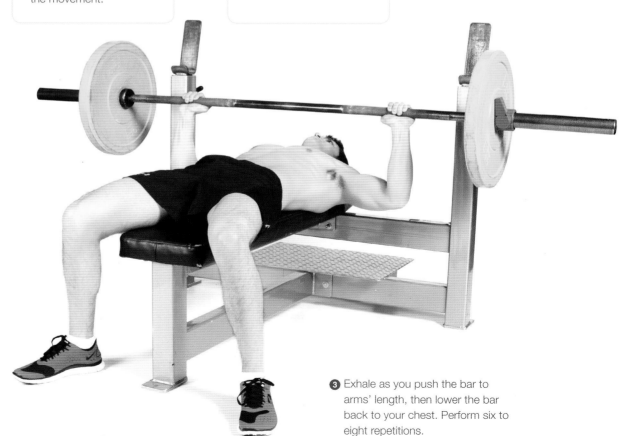

3 Exhale as you push the bar to arms' length, then lower the bar back to your chest. Perform six to eight repetitions.

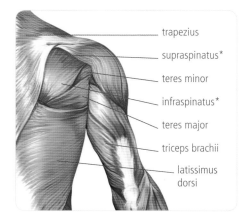

- trapezius
- supraspinatus*
- teres minor
- infraspinatus*
- teres major
- triceps brachii
- latissimus dorsi

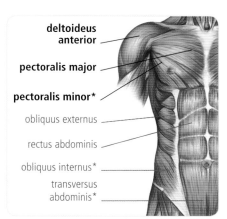

- **deltoideus anterior**
- **pectoralis major**
- **pectoralis minor***
- obliquus externus
- rectus abdominis
- obliquus internus*
- transversus abdominis*

MODIFICATIONS

Easier: Use a very light bar or your own body weight.

More difficult: Vary your grip width. A closer grip (below) makes the exercise more difficult, requiring greater effort.

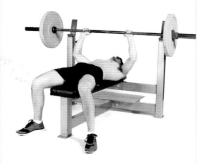

BEST FOR

- pectoralis major
- pectoralis minor
- deltoideus anterior

ANNOTATION KEY

Bold text indicates target muscles

Grey text indicates other working muscles

* indicates deep muscles

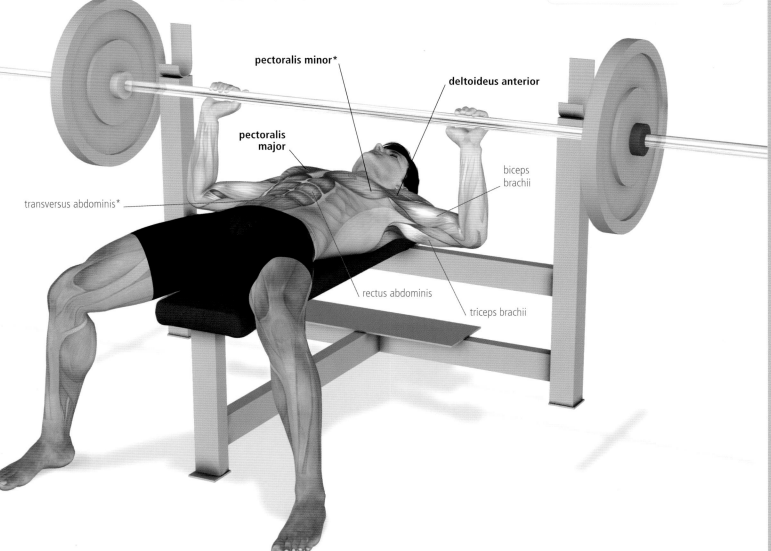

- **pectoralis minor***
- **deltoideus anterior**
- **pectoralis major**
- biceps brachii
- transversus abdominis*
- rectus abdominis
- triceps brachii

ROLLER PUSH-UP

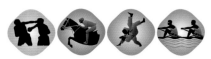

1 Kneel on the floor with the roller placed crosswise in front of you. Place your hands on the roller with your fingers pointed away from you. Press into a plank position, lifting your knees and straightening your legs.

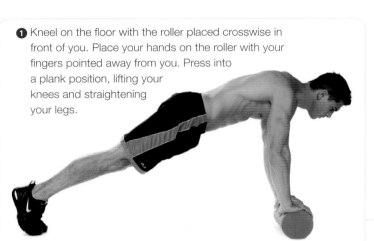

DO IT RIGHT
- Maintain a single plane of movement, with your body forming a straight line from shoulders to ankle.
- Keep your neck and shoulders relaxed throughout the exercise.

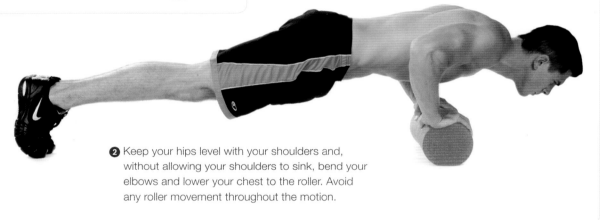

2 Keep your hips level with your shoulders and, without allowing your shoulders to sink, bend your elbows and lower your chest to the roller. Avoid any roller movement throughout the motion.

TARGETS
- Triceps
- Shoulder stabilizers
- Abdominals

LEVEL
- Advanced

BENEFITS
- Improves core, pelvic and shoulder stability

NOT ADVISABLE IF YOU HAVE . . .
- Wrist pain
- Shoulder pain
- Lower-back pain

AVOID
- Allowing your shoulders to lift toward your ears.
- Bending your knees.
- Raising or lowering your body in segments.

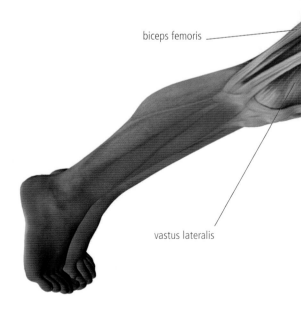

biceps femoris

vastus lateralis

3 Return to the starting position by pressing upward, straightening your elbows, and maintaining a straight spine. Repeat 15 times for two sets.

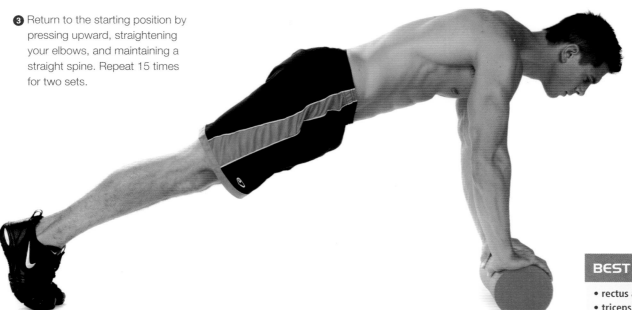

BEST FOR

- rectus abdominis
- triceps brachii
- deltoideus
- pectoralis major
- pectoralis minor
- biceps brachii
- teres minor
- teres major
- serratus anterior

ANNOTATION KEY

Bold text indicates target muscles
Grey text indicates other working muscles

* indicates deep muscles

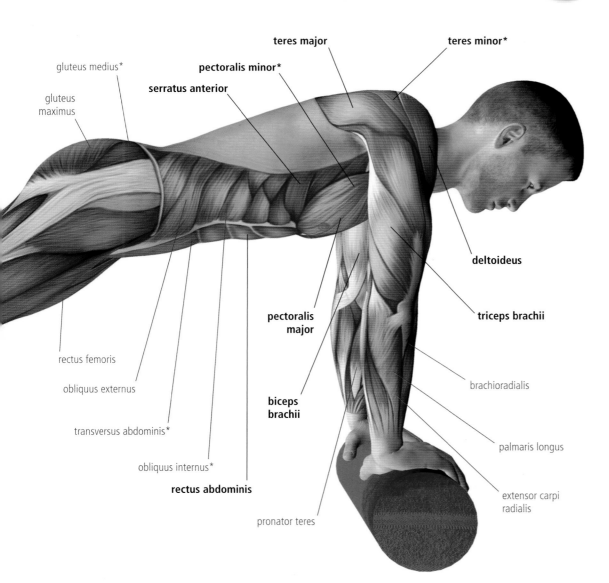

gluteus medius*

gluteus maximus

serratus anterior

pectoralis minor*

teres major

teres minor*

deltoideus

triceps brachii

rectus femoris

obliquus externus

pectoralis major

brachioradialis

transversus abdominis*

biceps brachii

palmaris longus

obliquus internus*

rectus abdominis

extensor carpi radialis

pronator teres

DUMBBELL FLY

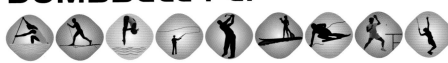

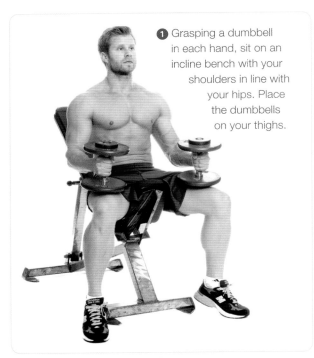

1 Grasping a dumbbell in each hand, sit on an incline bench with your shoulders in line with your hips. Place the dumbbells on your thighs.

2 Lie back on an incline bench, kicking up the dumbbells with your elbows in as you lift them to shoulder height.

3 Lift the dumbbells above your chest with your palms facing each other in hammer-grip position.

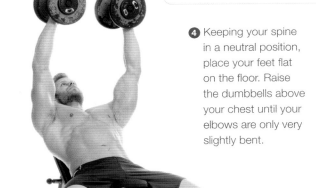

4 Keeping your spine in a neutral position, place your feet flat on the floor. Raise the dumbbells above your chest until your elbows are only very slightly bent.

TARGETS
• Middle chest

LEVEL
• Intermediate

BENEFITS
• Increases power and mass in the torso

NOT ADVISABLE IF YOU HAVE . . .
• Shoulder issues

TRAINER'S TIPS
• Kick into starting position.
• Keep your grip strong and your upper arms, both biceps and triceps, contracted.

DO IT RIGHT
• Ensure that your chest and rib cage rise as the dumbbells descend.
• Keep your spine and shoulders in the same position as you return to the starting position.
• Maintain your elbows on a horizontal plane, even with the bench, when you reach the lowest position.

AVOID
• Moving your head or chin forward or off the bench.
• Elevating your shoulders.
• Bending your elbows excessively as the dumbbells descend, or flattening them as the dumbbells ascend.

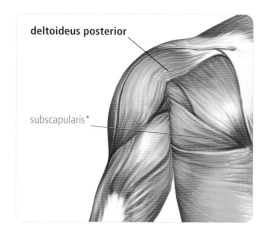

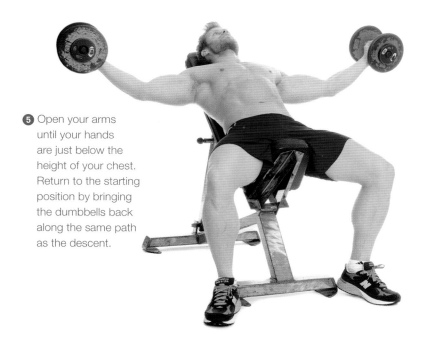

5 Open your arms until your hands are just below the height of your chest. Return to the starting position by bringing the dumbbells back along the same path as the descent.

deltoideus posterior

subscapularis*

ANNOTATION KEY
Bold text indicates target muscles
Grey text indicates other working muscles
* indicates deep muscles

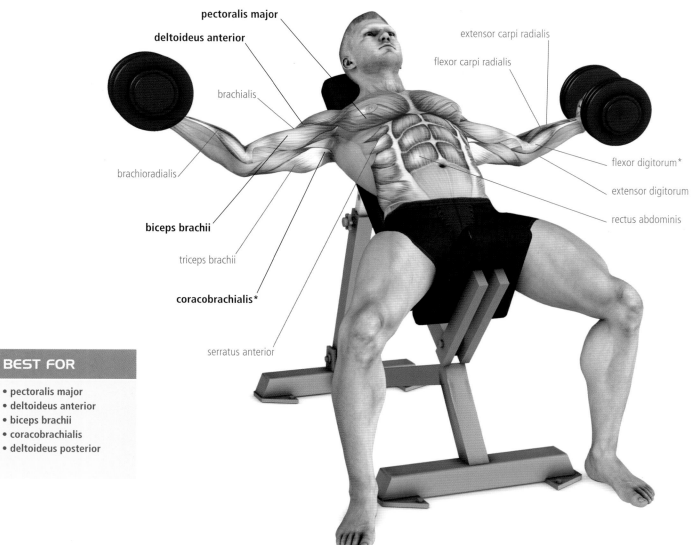

pectoralis major

deltoideus anterior

brachialis

extensor carpi radialis

flexor carpi radialis

brachioradialis

flexor digitorum*

extensor digitorum

rectus abdominis

biceps brachii

triceps brachii

coracobrachialis*

serratus anterior

BEST FOR

• pectoralis major
• deltoideus anterior
• biceps brachii
• coracobrachialis
• deltoideus posterior

CABLE FLY

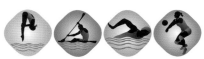

1 Stand between two high cable-machine uprights. Grasp an overhead handle grip in each hand, one at a time.

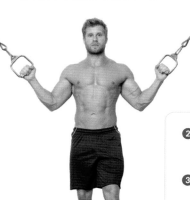

DO IT RIGHT
- Ensure your hands continue to face each other in the hammer-grip position.
- Extend your arms fully throughout the movement.

2 Center yourself between the cable uprights.

3 Take a full step back, bringing your hands toward your thighs.

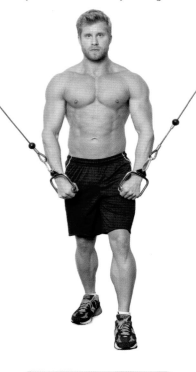

TARGETS
- Upper chest
- Deltoids

LEVEL
- Intermediate

BENEFITS
- Increases power to the shoulders and chest

NOT ADVISABLE IF YOU HAVE . . .
- Shoulder issues

TRAINER'S TIPS
- Start off with a light weight until you have mastered the movement and feel confident that you have the strength to execute it.
- Keep a slight bend in your elbow. This will ease the stress on your shoulder joint.

AVOID
- Extending your arms too far back — this will compromise your technique and could lead to a rotator-cuff injury.

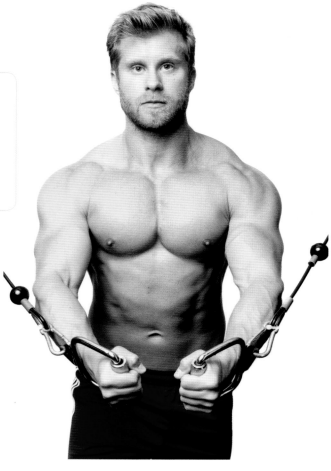

4 Step forward and start the exercise with your hands facing each other, just below the chest. Place one leg in front of the other and slightly lunge forward, putting your weight on your front foot.

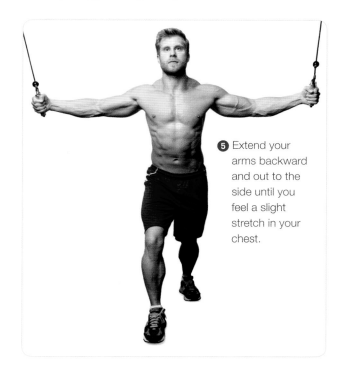

5 Extend your arms backward and out to the side until you feel a slight stretch in your chest.

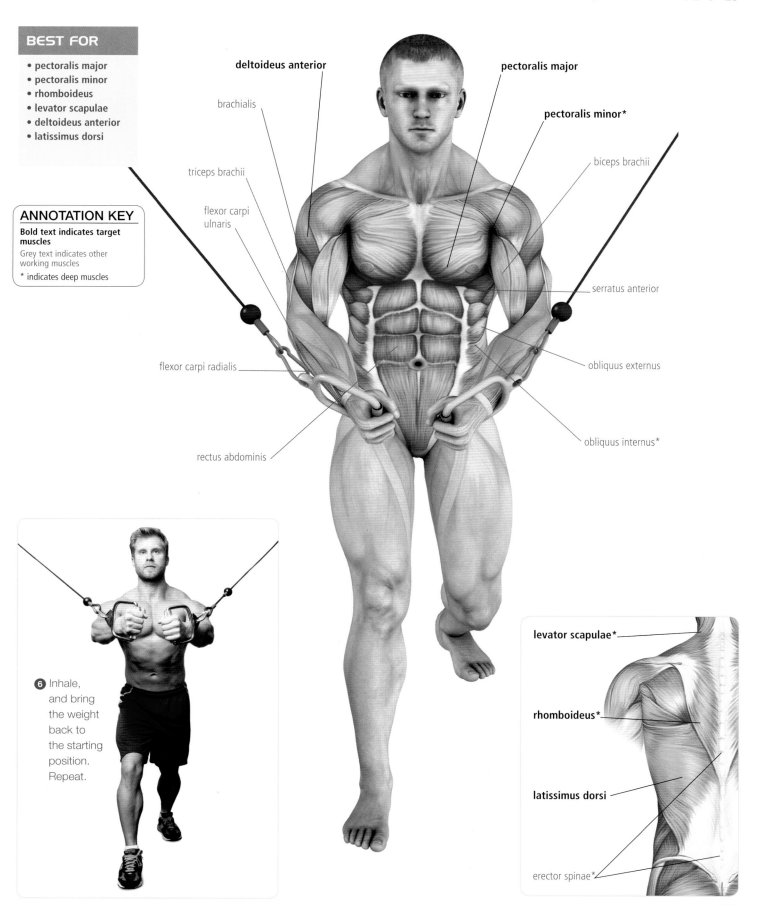

BEST FOR

- pectoralis major
- pectoralis minor
- rhomboideus
- levator scapulae
- deltoideus anterior
- latissimus dorsi

ANNOTATION KEY

Bold text indicates target muscles

Grey text indicates other working muscles

* indicates deep muscles

deltoideus anterior

brachialis

triceps brachii

flexor carpi ulnaris

flexor carpi radialis

rectus abdominis

pectoralis major

pectoralis minor*

biceps brachii

serratus anterior

obliquus externus

obliquus internus*

6 Inhale, and bring the weight back to the starting position. Repeat.

levator scapulae*

rhomboideus*

latissimus dorsi

erector spinae*

DIPS

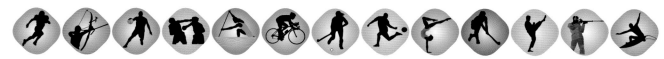

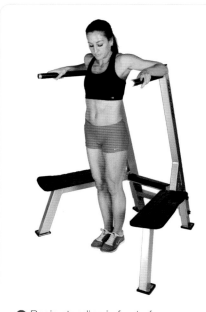

1 Begin standing in front of a dip station or parallel bars.

DO IT RIGHT
- Always complete a full range of motion.

AVOID
- Performing the exercise at excessive speed.

2 Place one hand on each bar, and grip as you push and extend your arms to full lockout.

TARGETS
- Pectorals
- Triceps
- Upper back
- Forearms
- Core

LEVEL
- Intermediate

BENEFITS
- Increases strength and mass in the upper body

MODIFICATIONS
- **Easier:** Have a partner support the weight of your legs.
- **More difficult:** Place a dumbbell between your lower legs for increased resistance.

3 Lower yourself until your upper arms are parallel to the ground, then push back up to the starting position. Complete 8 to 10 repetitions.

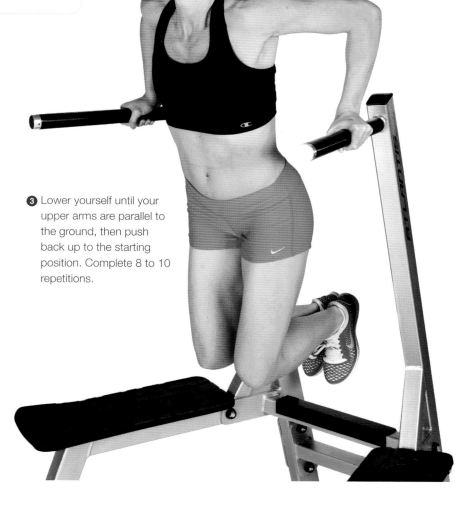

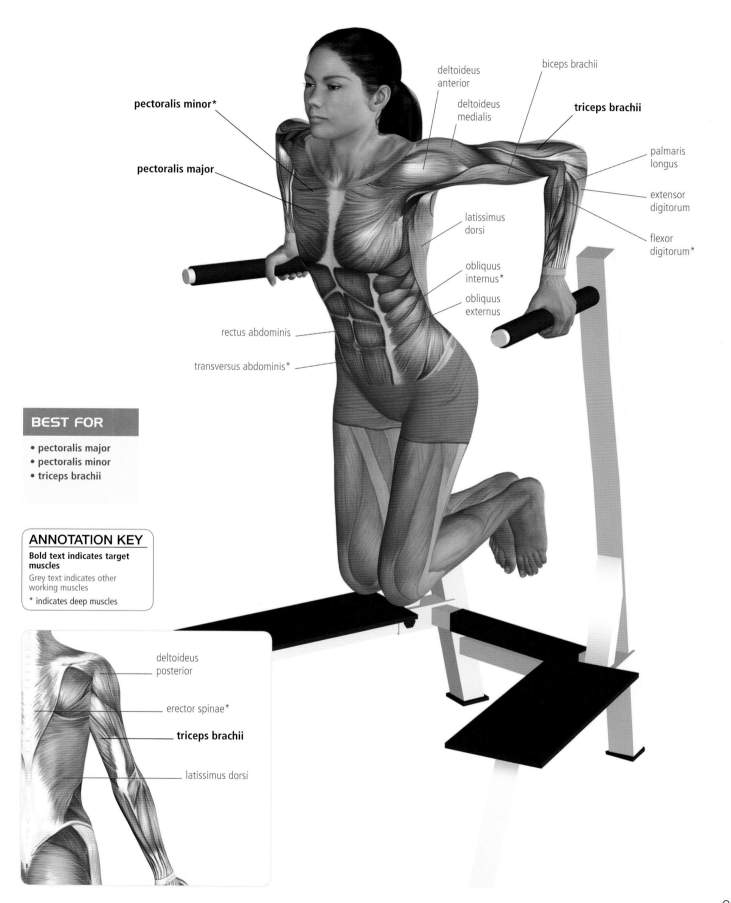

pectoralis minor*

pectoralis major

deltoideus anterior

deltoideus medialis

biceps brachii

triceps brachii

palmaris longus

extensor digitorum

flexor digitorum*

latissimus dorsi

obliquus internus*

obliquus externus

rectus abdominis

transversus abdominis*

BEST FOR

- **pectoralis major**
- **pectoralis minor**
- **triceps brachii**

ANNOTATION KEY

Bold text indicates target muscles

Grey text indicates other working muscles

* indicates deep muscles

deltoideus posterior

erector spinae*

triceps brachii

latissimus dorsi

PUSH-UP

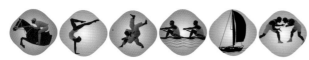

① Stand straight, inhale, and pull your navel to your spine.

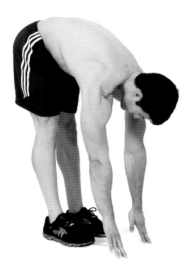

② Exhale as you roll down one vertebra at a time until your hands touch the floor in front of you.

③ Walk your hands out until they are directly beneath your shoulders in the plank position.

④ Inhale, and "set" your body by drawing your abdominals toward your spine. Squeeze your buttocks and legs together and stretch out of your heels, bringing your body into a straight line.

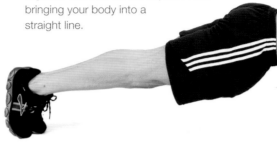

DO IT RIGHT
- Keep your neck long and relaxed as you perform the push-up.
- Ensure your buttocks stay tightly squeezed as you scoop in your abdominals for stability.

AVOID
- Allowing your shoulders to lift toward your ears.

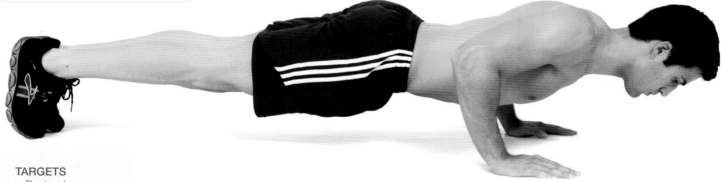

TARGETS
- Pectoral
- Triceps

LEVEL
- Intermediate

BENEFITS
- Strengthens core stabilizers, shoulders, back, buttocks, and pectoral muscles

NOT ADVISABLE IF YOU HAVE . . .
- Shoulder issues

⑤ Exhale and inhale as you bend your elbows and lower your body toward the floor. Then push upward to return to plank position. Keep your elbows close to your body. Repeat eight times.

⑥ Inhale as you lift your hips into the air, and walk your hands back toward your feet. Exhale slowly, rolling up one vertebra at a time into your starting position. Repeat the entire exercise three times.

MODIFICATIONS

Easier: Kneel with your hands on the floor in front of you, supporting your torso. Keeping your hips open, bend and straighten your elbows as if you were going to perform a push-up.

More difficult: Place your hands shoulder-width apart on an exercise ball. With the balls of your feet on the floor behind you, complete the push-up movement while maintaining stability on the ball.

More difficult: Place the balls of your feet on top of an exercise ball, while supporting your body with your hands on the floor in front of you. Use your abdominals to keep your body in a straight line and balance as you complete the push-up.

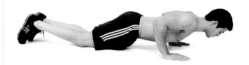
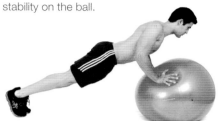
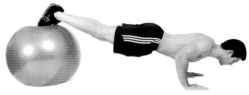

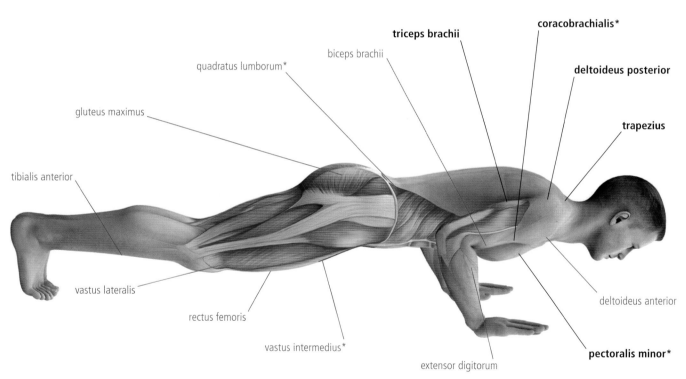

coracobrachialis*

triceps brachii

biceps brachii

quadratus lumborum*

gluteus maximus

deltoideus posterior

trapezius

tibialis anterior

vastus lateralis

rectus femoris

vastus intermedius*

extensor digitorum

deltoideus anterior

pectoralis minor*

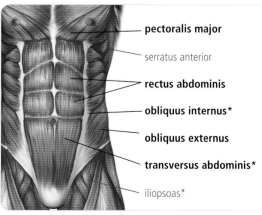

pectoralis major

serratus anterior

rectus abdominis

obliquus internus*

obliquus externus

transversus abdominis*

iliopsoas*

BEST FOR

- triceps brachii
- pectoralis major
- pectoralis minor
- coracobrachialis
- deltoideus posterior
- rectus abdominis
- transversus abdominis
- obliquus externus
- obliquus internus
- trapezius

ANNOTATION KEY

Bold text indicates target muscles

Grey text indicates other working muscles

* indicates deep muscles

71

PUSH-UP HAND WALK-OVER

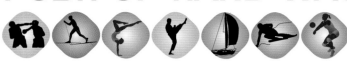

① Start in a plank position with your left hand on the floor and your right on an elevated box or step between 4 and 6 inches (10 and 15 cm) high.

② Keeping your torso rigid and your legs straight, bend your elbows into a push-up position.

③ Push back up, straightening your elbows to return to the starting position.

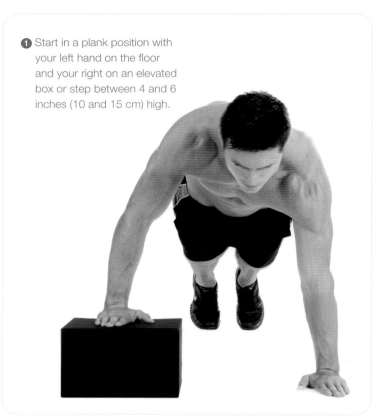

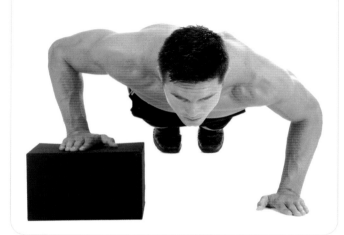

TARGETS
• Whole body

LEVEL
• Intermediate

BENEFITS
• Strengthens the pelvic, trunk and shoulder stabilizers

NOT ADVISABLE IF YOU HAVE . . .
• Shoulder pain
• Back pain
• Neck pain

DO IT RIGHT
• Ensure your hands align under your shoulders.

AVOID
• Dipping your shoulders to one side.
• Shifting your hips as your hands "walk."
• Craning your neck.

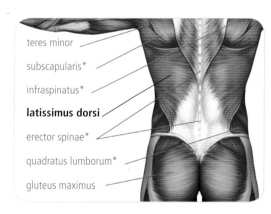

teres minor
subscapularis*
infraspinatus*
latissimus dorsi
erector spinae*
quadratus lumborum*
gluteus maximus

BEST FOR

• vastus medialis
• vastus lateralis
• vastus intermedius
• rectus femoris
• sartorius
• triceps brachii
• transversus abdominis
• gracilis
• trapezius
• latissimus dorsi
• iliopsoas
• iliacus
• tensor fasciae latae
• adductor longus

④ Lift your left hand off the floor, and place it beside your right on the top of the box.

⑤ Lift your right hand off the box, placing it on the floor about one shoulder width to the right.

⑥ Bend your elbows to perform another push-up, this time on the other side of the box.

⑦ Return to the top of the box and repeat. Perform five push-ups on each side.

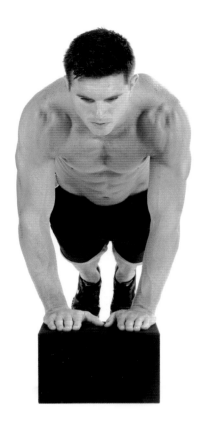

ANNOTATION KEY
Bold text indicates target muscles
Grey text indicates other working muscles
* indicates deep muscles

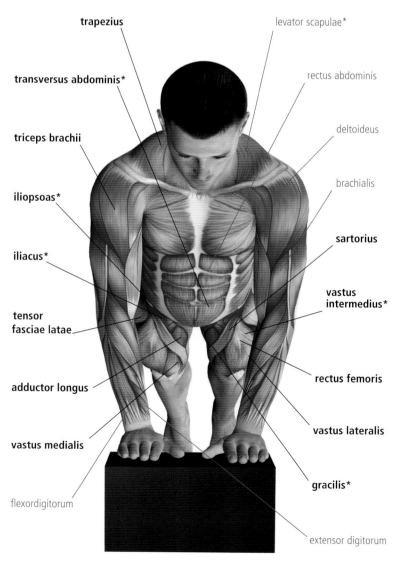

trapezius

levator scapulae*

transversus abdominis*

rectus abdominis

triceps brachii

deltoideus

iliopsoas*

brachialis

iliacus*

sartorius

tensor fasciae latae

vastus intermedius*

adductor longus

rectus femoris

vastus lateralis

vastus medialis

gracilis*

flexordigitorum

extensor digitorum

DUMBBELL SHOULDER PRESS

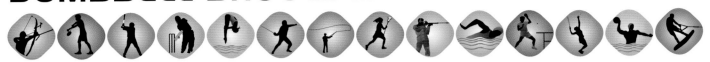

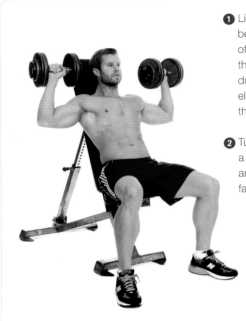

1 Lie back on an incline bench, and place a pair of dumbbells on your thighs to start. Kick up dumbbells with your elbows in, and then lift them to shoulder height.

2 Turn your elbows out in a 90-degree angle of the arms, with your palms facing forward.

DO IT RIGHT
• Ensure your chin remains over your shoulders during this exercise.

AVOID
• Hyperextending your back when pressing the dumbbells upward during the press motion of this exercise.

TARGETS
• Side deltoids

LEVEL
• Intermediate

NOT ADVISABLE IF YOU HAVE . . .
• Shoulder issues

TRAINER'S TIPS
• When you are finished with the set, bring your elbows back in, palms facing each other, and slowly lower the dumbbells back to your thighs.
• Relax your neck and jaw during the exercise.

3 Press the dumbbells upward into a pyramid position.

4 Slowly lower the dumbbells back to the starting position. Repeat 8 to 10 times.

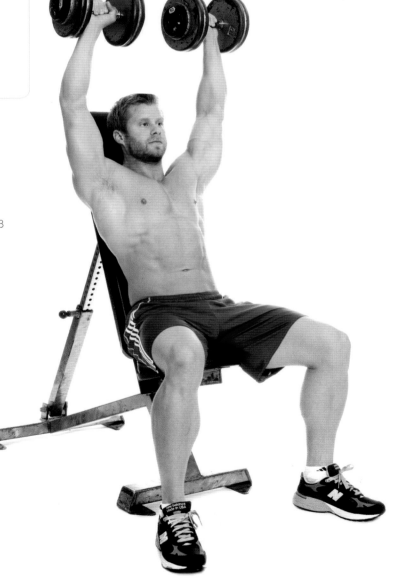

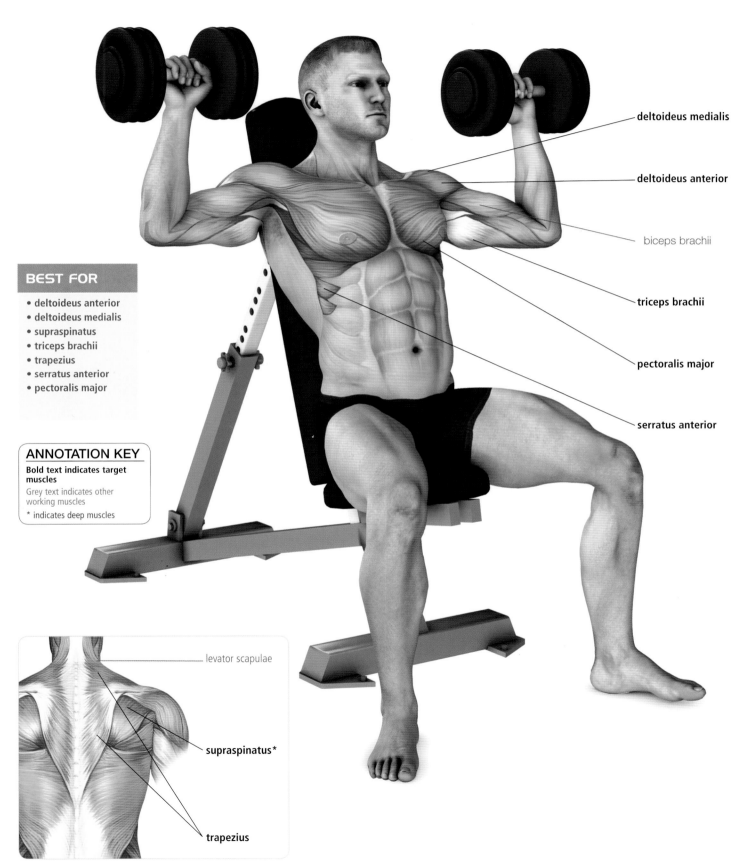

deltoideus medialis

deltoideus anterior

biceps brachii

triceps brachii

pectoralis major

serratus anterior

BEST FOR

- **deltoideus anterior**
- **deltoideus medialis**
- **supraspinatus**
- **triceps brachii**
- **trapezius**
- **serratus anterior**
- **pectoralis major**

ANNOTATION KEY

Bold text indicates target muscles

Grey text indicates other working muscles

* indicates deep muscles

levator scapulae

supraspinatus*

trapezius

OVERHEAD PRESS

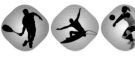

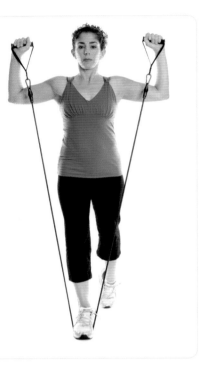

1 Stand upright with one leg extended about 1 foot (30 cm) behind you, heel off the ground. Position the resistance band beneath the foot of your front leg. Hold the handles in both hands, with arms bent, so that the resistance band is taut.

2 Straighten both arms so that they are extended to full lockout above your head a few inches in front of your shoulders.

TARGETS
• Shoulders
• Triceps

LEVEL
• Beginner

BENEFITS
• Strengthens and tones shoulders and upper arms

NOT ADVISABLE IF YOU HAVE . . .
• Shoulder issues

DO IT RIGHT
• Keep the rest of your body stable as you extend your arms.
• Keep looking forward throughout the exercise.
• Keep your abdominals engaged and pulled in.
• Extend both arms at the same time.

AVOID
• Twisting your torso.

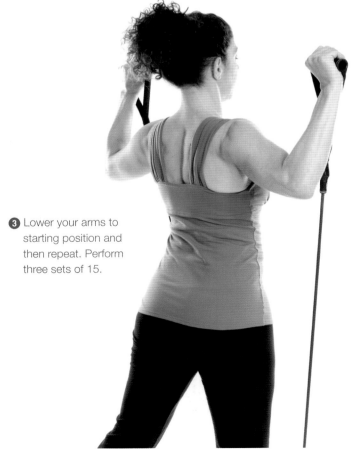

3 Lower your arms to starting position and then repeat. Perform three sets of 15.

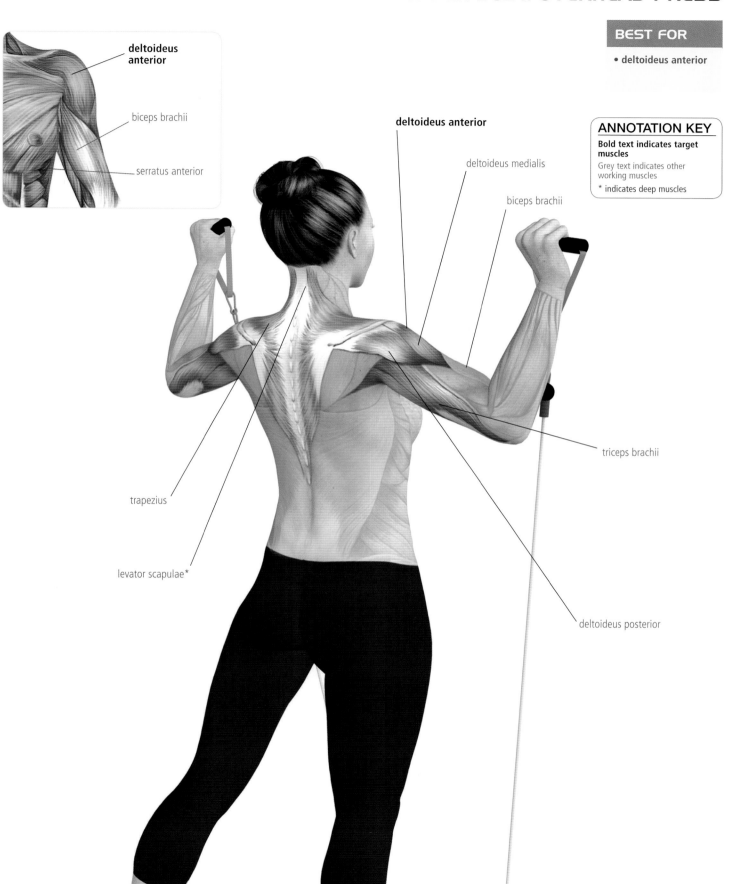

deltoideus anterior

biceps brachii

serratus anterior

• deltoideus anterior

deltoideus anterior

deltoideus medialis

biceps brachii

ANNOTATION KEY

Bold text indicates target muscles

Grey text indicates other working muscles

* indicates deep muscles

triceps brachii

trapezius

levator scapulae*

deltoideus posterior

ROTATION EXERCISES

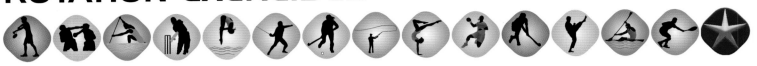

ROTATION STRETCH

1 Sit or stand, keeping your neck, shoulders, and torso straight. Place your right palm against your forehead.

2 Turn your head slowly to the right, moving gently until you feel a stretch in the left side of your neck. Hold for 10 seconds.

3 Move your head back to the forward position. Relax.

4 Place your left palm against your forehead, and turn your head slowly to the left, again moving gently until you feel a stretch in the right side of your neck. Hold for 10 seconds.

5 Move your head back to the forward position. Relax, and then repeat the entire sequence five times.

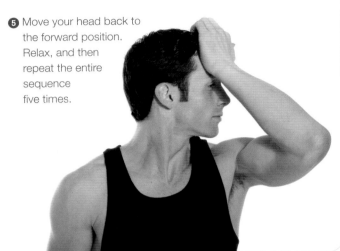

TARGETS
• Neck rotators

LEVEL
• Beginner

BENEFITS
• Improves range of motion
• Relieves neck pain

NOT ADVISABLE IF YOU HAVE . . .
• Numbness running down your arm or into your hand

DO IT RIGHT
• Relax your shoulder muscles.
• Keep your head in a neutral position.

AVOID
• Pushing too hard with your hand — this is a gentle stretch.
• Flexing or extending your head.

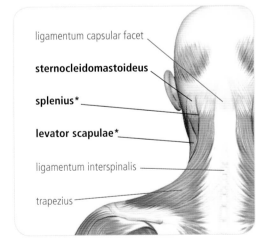

ligamentum capsular facet

sternocleidomastoideus

splenius*

levator scapulae*

ligamentum interspinalis

trapezius

BEST FOR
• splenius
• sternocleidomastoideus
• levator scapulae

ANNOTATION KEY
Bold text indicates target muscles
Grey text indicates other working muscles and ligaments
* indicates deep muscles

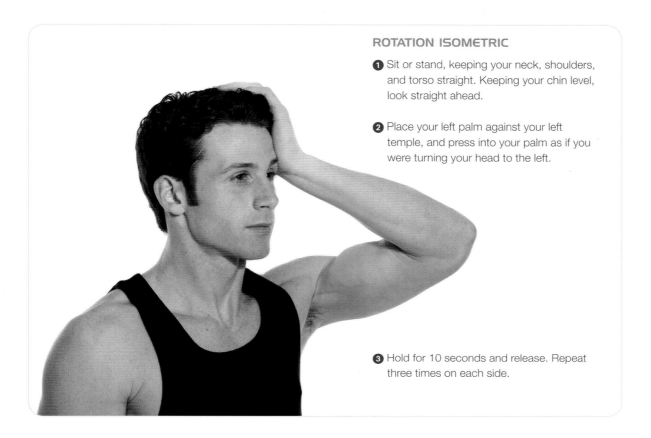

ROTATION ISOMETRIC

1 Sit or stand, keeping your neck, shoulders, and torso straight. Keeping your chin level, look straight ahead.

2 Place your left palm against your left temple, and press into your palm as if you were turning your head to the left.

3 Hold for 10 seconds and release. Repeat three times on each side.

DO IT RIGHT
- Apply a gentle pressure — overdoing it, especially when you first begin exercising, will make the neck muscles stiffer.

AVOID
- Any movement in the neck.

TARGETS
- Neck rotators

LEVEL
- Beginner

BENEFITS
- Strengthens the rotary muscles of the neck without irritating the ligaments, tendons or joints

NOT ADVISABLE IF YOU HAVE . . .
- Numbness running down your arm or into your hand

BEST FOR
- splenius
- sternocleidomastoideus
- levator scapulae
- trapezius

ANNOTATION KEY
Bold text indicates target muscles
Grey text indicates other working muscles
* indicates deep muscles

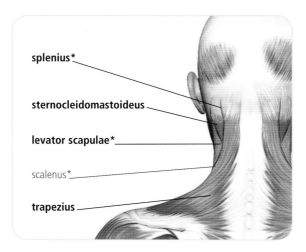

splenius*
sternocleidomastoideus
levator scapulae*
scalenus*
trapezius

EXTERNAL ROTATION WITH BAND

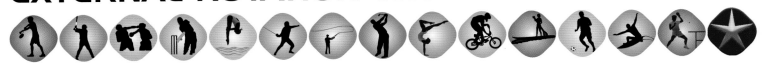

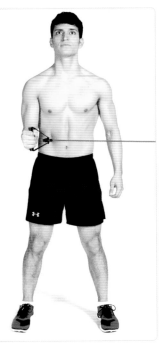

1 Fasten one end of a band around a post at elbow height. Grasp the other end with your right hand, keeping your upper arm pressed against your side and your forearm parallel to the ground.

TARGETS
- Deltoids

LEVEL
- Beginner

BENEFITS
- Builds strength in the shoulders

NOT ADVISABLE IF YOU HAVE . . .
- Elbow or wrist pain

DO IT RIGHT
- Keep your upper arm against your side.

AVOID
- Working at an excessively fast pace.

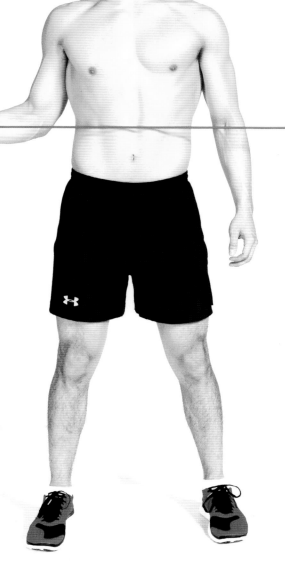

2 Keeping your upper arm in position, move your forearm as far out to the side as you can before returning to the starting position. Complete 12 to 15 repetitions, then switch to the other arm.

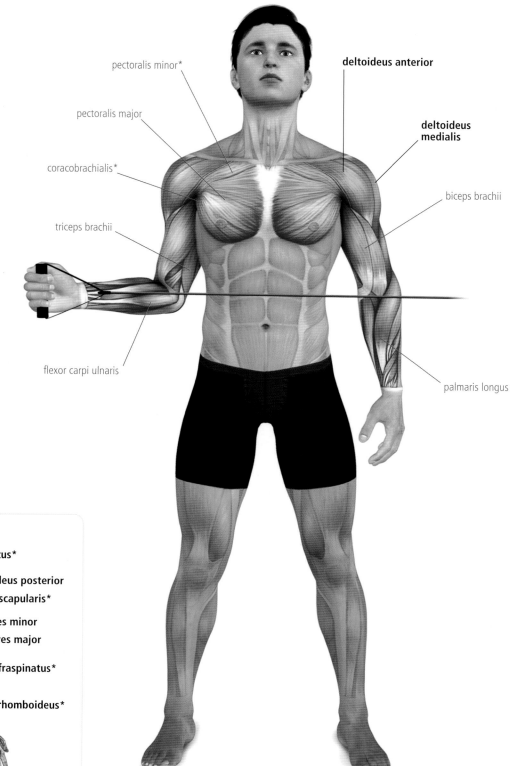

pectoralis minor*

pectoralis major

coracobrachialis*

triceps brachii

flexor carpi ulnaris

deltoideus anterior

deltoideus medialis

biceps brachii

palmaris longus

BEST FOR

- **supraspinatus**
- **infraspinatus**
- **deltoideus anterior**
- **deltoideus medialis**
- **deltoideus posterior**
- **teres major**
- **teres minor**
- **trapezius**
- **rhomboideus**
- **subscapularis**

ANNOTATION KEY

Bold text indicates target muscles

Grey text indicates other working muscles

* indicates deep muscles

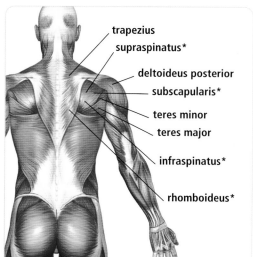

trapezius

supraspinatus*

deltoideus posterior

subscapularis*

teres minor

teres major

infraspinatus*

rhomboideus*

LATERAL RAISE

1 Stand upright with your arms at your sides and feet planted hip-width apart on top of your resistance band. Hold one handle in each hand, palms facing inward.

DO IT RIGHT
- Raise your arms directly out to the sides.
- Keep the movement slow, smooth and controlled.
- Keep your torso straight and look forward.

AVOID
- Rushing through the movement or jerking your arms.
- Lifting your arms above shoulder height.
- Moving your feet.

TARGETS
- Deltoids

LEVEL
- Intermediate

BENEFITS
- Strengthens and tones deltoids
- Sculpts triceps

NOT ADVISABLE IF YOU HAVE . . .
- Shoulder issues

2 Keeping your palms down, raise your arms out to your sides so that they are parallel to the floor.

3 Lower and repeat, completing three sets of 15.

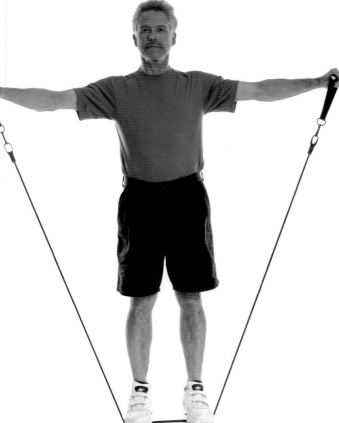

UPPER BODY: LATERAL RAISE

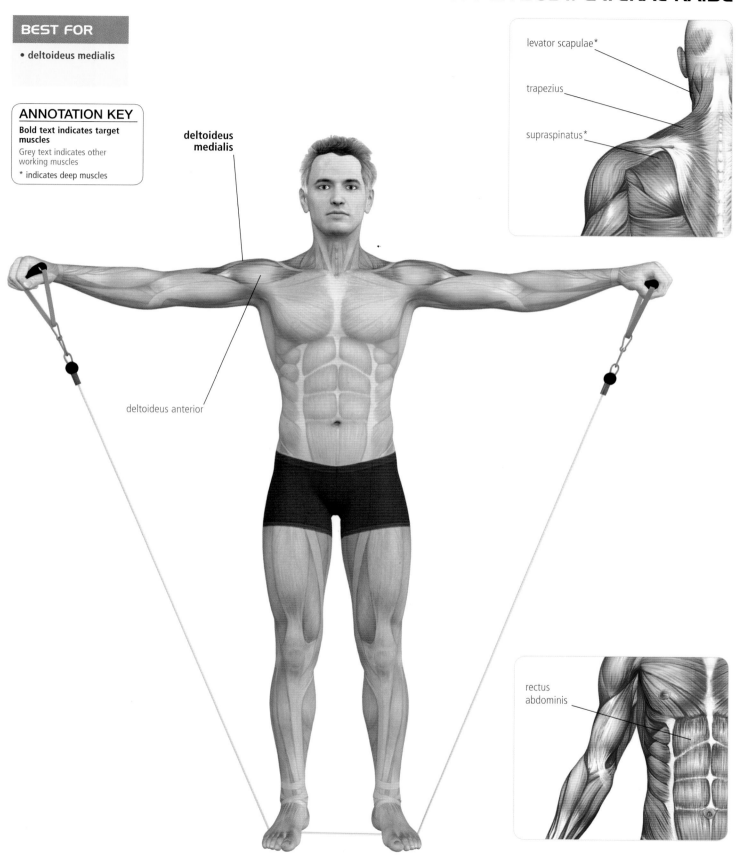

BEST FOR

• deltoideus medialis

ANNOTATION KEY

Bold text indicates target muscles

Grey text indicates other working muscles

* indicates deep muscles

deltoideus medialis

deltoideus anterior

levator scapulae*

trapezius

supraspinatus*

rectus abdominis

83

SHOULDER RAISE AND PULL

1 Holding a dumbbell or hand weight in each hand, stand with your legs and feet parallel and shoulder-width apart. Bend your knees very slightly and tuck your pelvis slightly forward, lift your chest and press your shoulders downward and back.

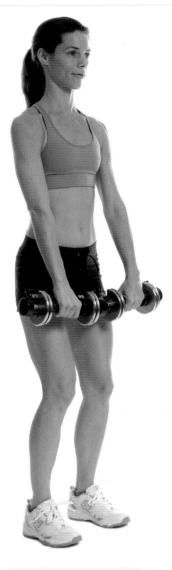

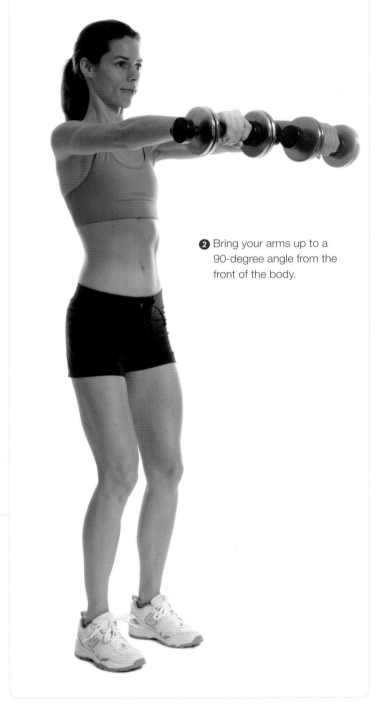

2 Bring your arms up to a 90-degree angle from the front of the body.

TARGETS
• Deltoids

LEVEL
• Beginner

BENEFITS
• Strengthens shoulders

NOT ADVISABLE IF YOU HAVE . . .
• Shoulder issues
• Rotator-cuff injury

DO IT RIGHT
• Keep a slight bend in your elbow as you lift upward to avoid stress on the joints.

AVOID
• Raising your elbows or the weight higher than your shoulders.

BEST FOR

- **deltoideus medialis**
- **pectoralis major**
- **serratus anterior**

ANNOTATION KEY

Bold text indicates target muscles

Grey text indicates other working muscles

* indicates deep muscles

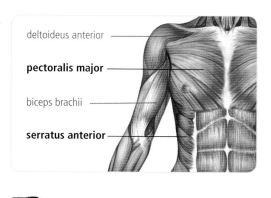

deltoideus anterior

pectoralis major

biceps brachii

serratus anterior

❸ Pull dumbbells to the front of your shoulder with elbows leading out to sides.

❹ Lower the weights back to the starting position, and repeat for two sets of 10.

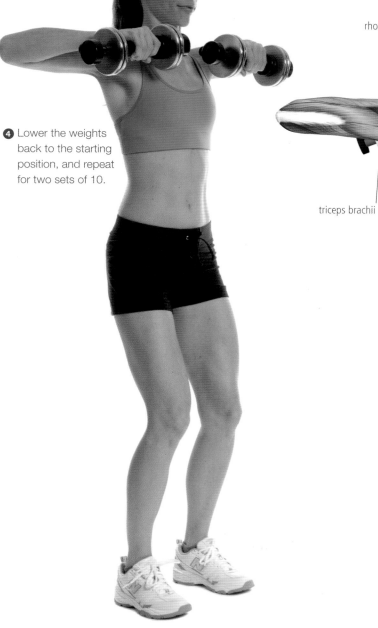

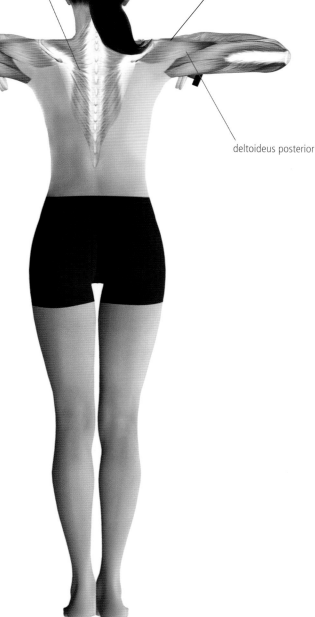

rhomboideus*

deltoideus medialis

triceps brachii

deltoideus posterior

BARBELL UPRIGHT ROW

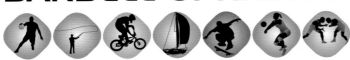

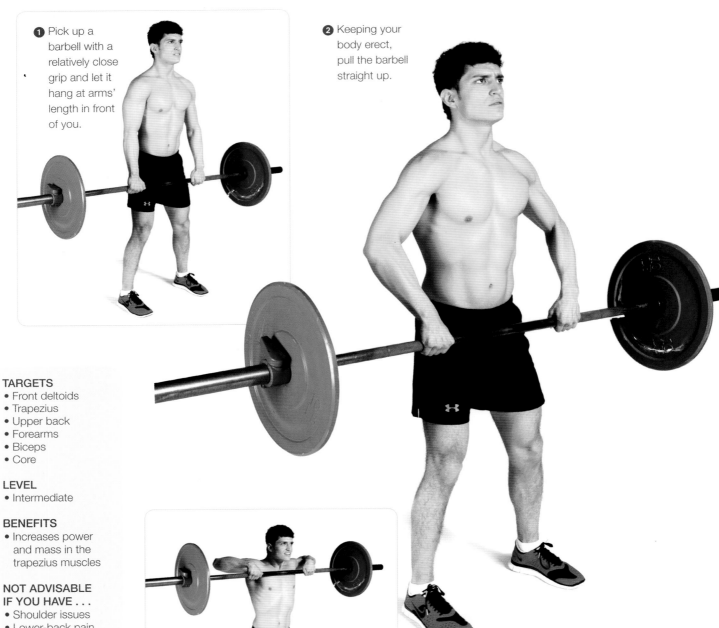

1 Pick up a barbell with a relatively close grip and let it hang at arms' length in front of you.

2 Keeping your body erect, pull the barbell straight up.

TARGETS
- Front deltoids
- Trapezius
- Upper back
- Forearms
- Biceps
- Core

LEVEL
- Intermediate

BENEFITS
- Increases power and mass in the trapezius muscles

NOT ADVISABLE IF YOU HAVE . . .
- Shoulder issues
- Lower-back pain

3 When the barbell is nearly touching your chin, lower it back to arms' length. Repeat 10 to 12 times.

DO IT RIGHT
- Always keep the barbell close to your body, and lead with your elbows.

AVOID
- Hitting your chin with the barbell.

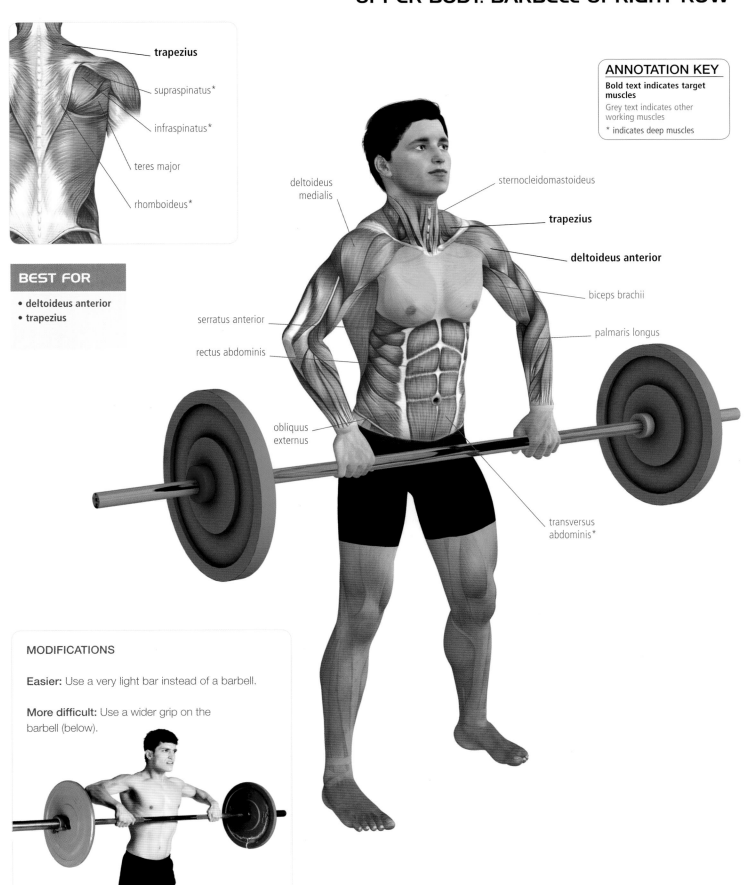

trapezius

supraspinatus*

infraspinatus*

teres major

rhomboideus*

ANNOTATION KEY

Bold text indicates target muscles

Grey text indicates other working muscles

* indicates deep muscles

deltoideus medialis

sternocleidomastoideus

trapezius

deltoideus anterior

biceps brachii

serratus anterior

palmaris longus

rectus abdominis

obliquus externus

transversus abdominis*

BEST FOR

• **deltoideus anterior**
• **trapezius**

MODIFICATIONS

Easier: Use a very light bar instead of a barbell.

More difficult: Use a wider grip on the barbell (below).

REVERSE FLY

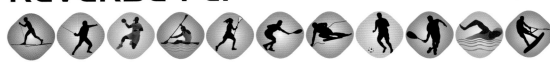

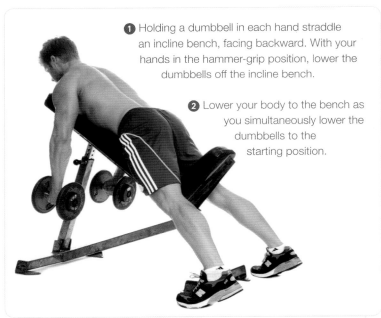

1 Holding a dumbbell in each hand straddle an incline bench, facing backward. With your hands in the hammer-grip position, lower the dumbbells off the incline bench.

2 Lower your body to the bench as you simultaneously lower the dumbbells to the starting position.

DO IT RIGHT
- Keep a steady, controlled movement during both the ascent and descent phases of the exercise.

AVOID
- Holding onto neck and jaw tension.
- Sliding down the bench while executing this exercise.

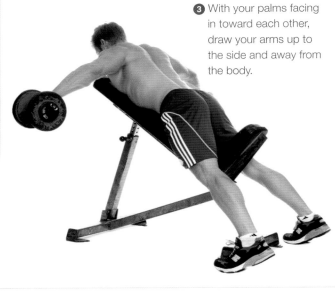

3 With your palms facing in toward each other, draw your arms up to the side and away from the body.

TARGETS
- Rear deltoids

LEVEL
- Intermediate

BENEFITS
- Increases power in shoulders and upper back

NOT ADVISABLE IF YOU HAVE . . .
- Shoulder or back issues

TRAINER'S TIPS
- Keep your feet firmly planted on floor.
- Keep your chest elevated while executing this exercise.
- Exhale as you lift the dumbbells up, and inhale as you bring them back to the starting position.

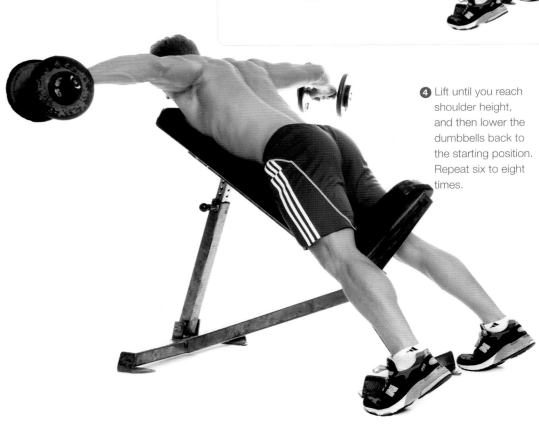

4 Lift until you reach shoulder height, and then lower the dumbbells back to the starting position. Repeat six to eight times.

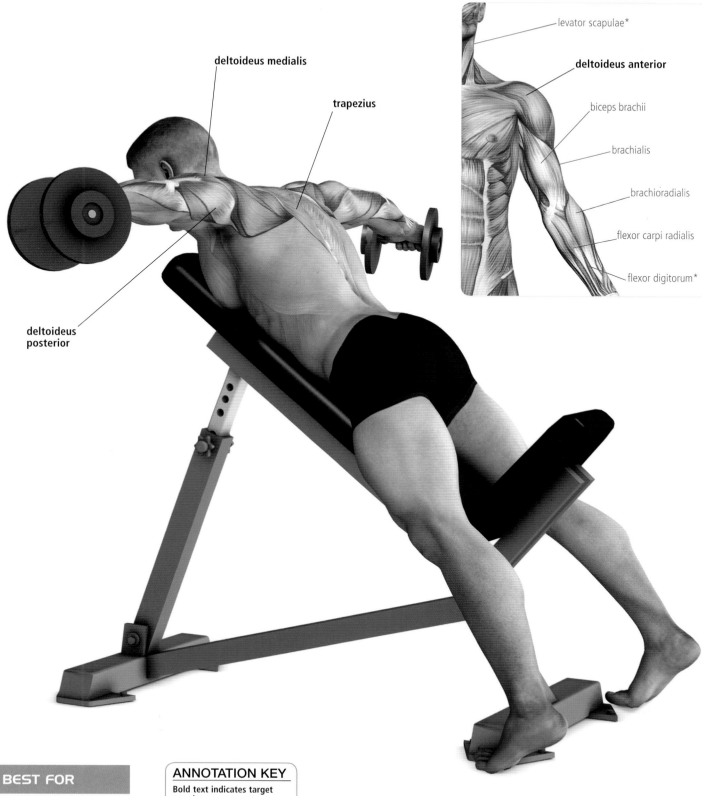

levator scapulae*

deltoideus anterior

biceps brachii

brachialis

brachioradialis

flexor carpi radialis

flexor digitorum*

deltoideus medialis

trapezius

deltoideus posterior

BEST FOR

- **deltoideus anterior**
- **deltoideus posterior**
- **deltoideus medialis**
- **trapezius**

ANNOTATION KEY

Bold text indicates target muscles

Grey text indicates other working muscles

* indicates deep muscles

SWISS BALL REVERSE FLY

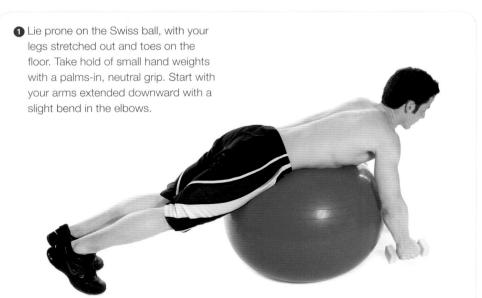

1 Lie prone on the Swiss ball, with your legs stretched out and toes on the floor. Take hold of small hand weights with a palms-in, neutral grip. Start with your arms extended downward with a slight bend in the elbows.

DO IT RIGHT
- Keep a slight bend in your elbows throughout the entire exercise.
- Raise your elbows as high as you can, so that they both reach the same height.

AVOID
- Moving your torso during the exercise.
- Allowing the weights to touch the floor.

2 Lift your elbows just past shoulder level, keeping your arms in a fixed position.

3 Hold for 5 seconds, and then lower your arms, returning the weights almost to the floor. Repeat 8 to 10 times.

TARGETS
- Back
- Quads
- Glutes
- Hamstrings
- Core
- Forearms
- Biceps

LEVEL
- Intermediate

BENEFITS
- Strengthens upper back and shoulders
- Stretches chest muscles

NOT ADVISABLE IF YOU HAVE . . .
- Neck issues
- Lower-back pain

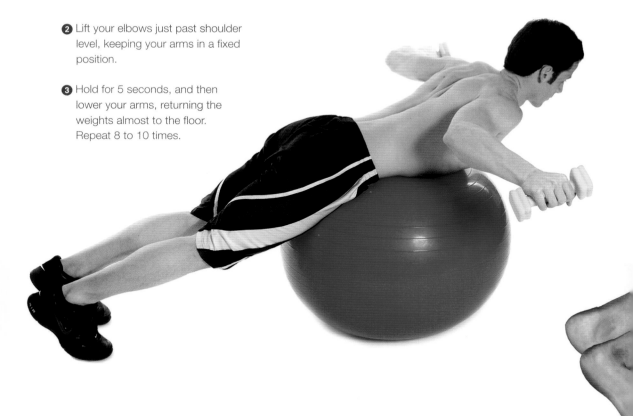

UPPER BODY: SWISS BALL REVERSE FLY

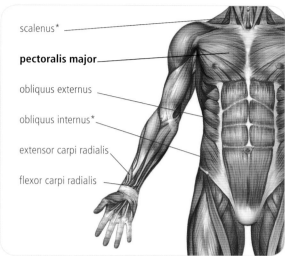

scalenus*

pectoralis major

obliquus externus

obliquus internus*

extensor carpi radialis

flexor carpi radialis

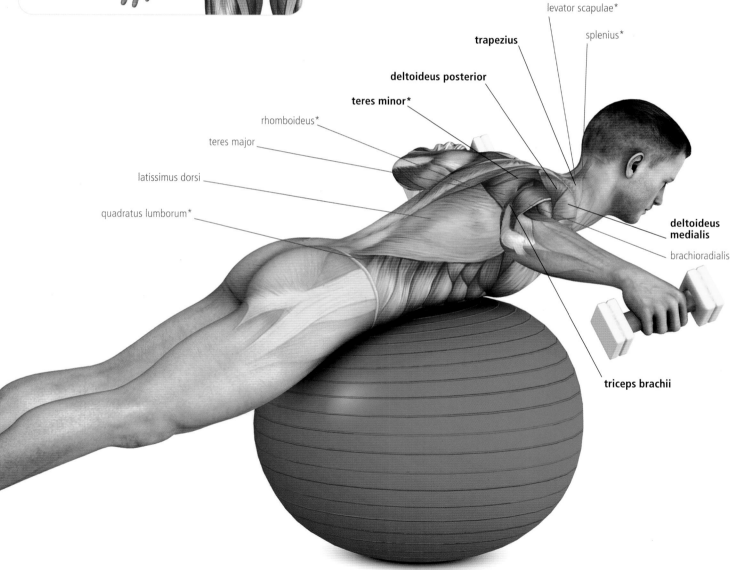

levator scapulae*

splenius*

trapezius

deltoideus posterior

teres minor*

rhomboideus*

teres major

latissimus dorsi

quadratus lumborum*

deltoideus medialis

brachioradialis

triceps brachii

FRONT-PLATE RAISE

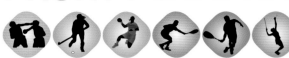

1. Holding onto a 45-pound (20 kg) plate with both hands in hammer-grip position in front of your hips, stand with your feet parallel and shoulder-width apart and your pelvis tucked in slightly.

2. Raise the plate to shoulder height.

3. Slowly lower the weight back to the starting position.

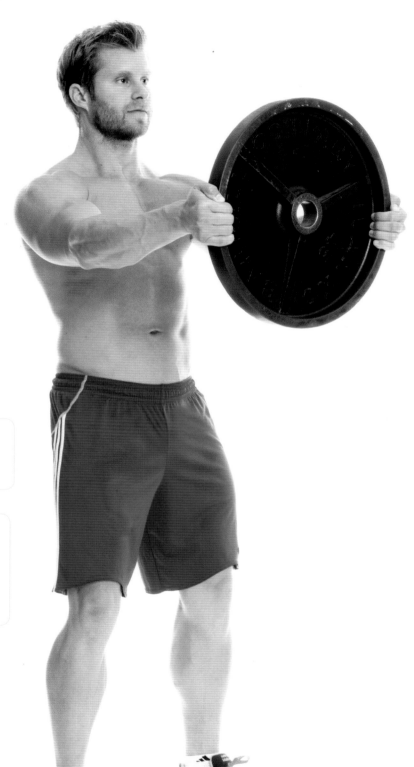

TARGETS
• Deltoids

LEVEL
• Intermediate

BENEFITS
• Increases power and definition in the shoulders

NOT ADVISABLE IF YOU HAVE . . .
• Shoulder or back issues

TRAINER'S TIPS
• Exhale as you lift the plate, and inhale as you lower the plate.
• Keep your posture erect while executing the exercise.
• Keep your shoulders down and back away from your ears.

DO IT RIGHT
• Maintain a steady, controlled movement.

AVOID
• Hyperextending your elbows while lifting the weight.
• Allowing your shoulders to rotate inward.

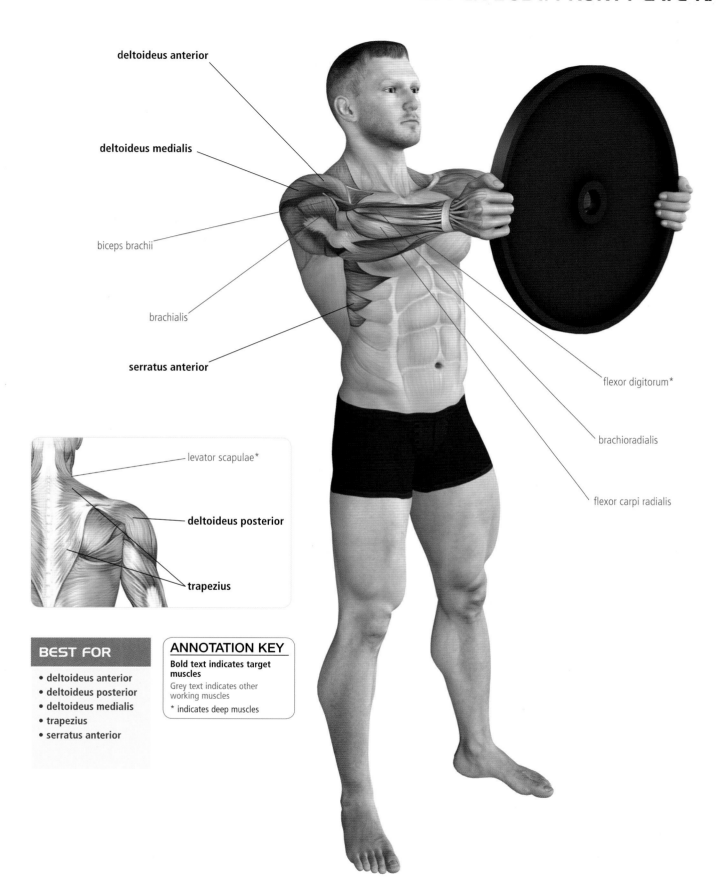

deltoideus anterior

deltoideus medialis

biceps brachii

brachialis

serratus anterior

flexor digitorum*

brachioradialis

flexor carpi radialis

levator scapulae*

deltoideus posterior

trapezius

BEST FOR

- deltoideus anterior
- deltoideus posterior
- deltoideus medialis
- trapezius
- serratus anterior

ANNOTATION KEY

Bold text indicates target muscles

Grey text indicates other working muscles

* indicates deep muscles

BARBELL SHOULDER SHRUG

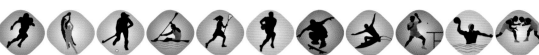

① Pick up a barbell and let it hang at arms' length in front of you.

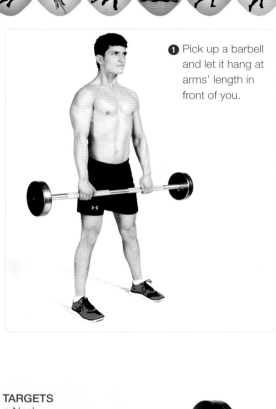

DO IT RIGHT
• Always shrug straight up and down.

AVOID
• Rolling your shoulders backward.

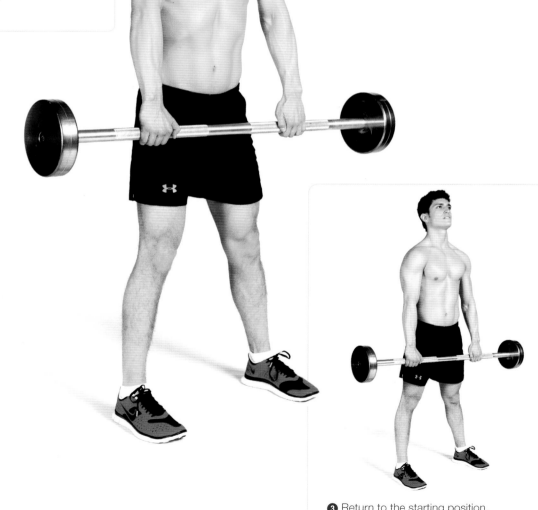

② Shrug your shoulders up, bringing them as close to your ears as possible.

TARGETS
• Neck
• Upper back
• Forearms
• Core

LEVEL
• Beginner

BENEFITS
• Increases power and mass in the trapezius muscles

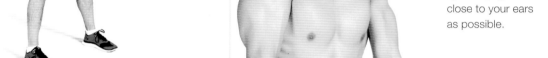

③ Return to the starting position. Complete 10 to 12 repetitions.

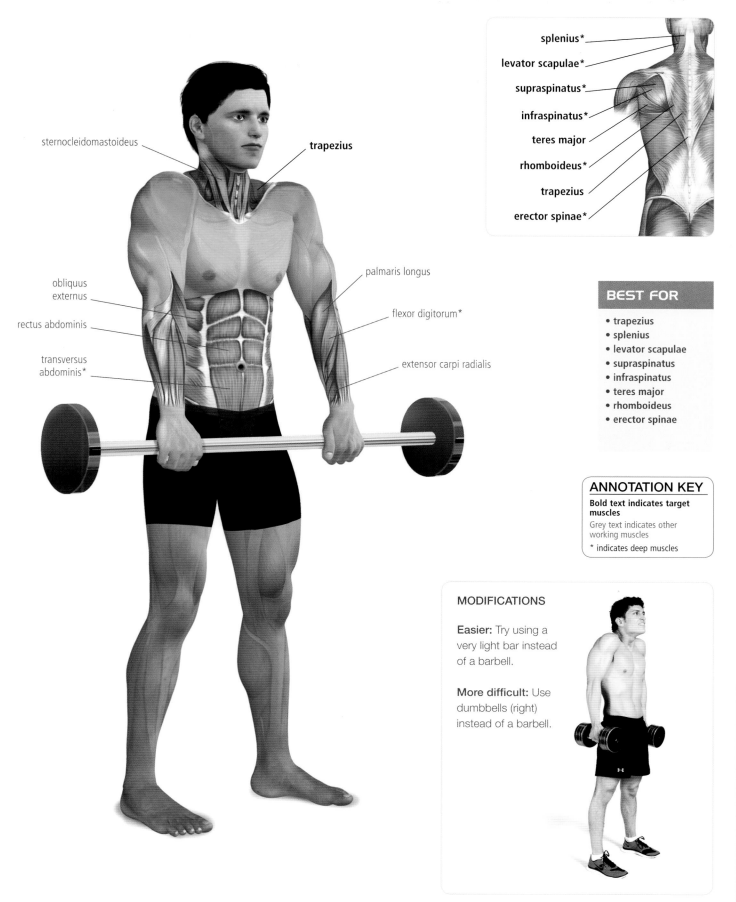

splenius*

levator scapulae*

supraspinatus*

infraspinatus*

teres major

rhomboideus*

trapezius

erector spinae*

sternocleidomastoideus

trapezius

obliquus externus

rectus abdominis

transversus abdominis*

palmaris longus

flexor digitorum*

extensor carpi radialis

BEST FOR

- trapezius
- splenius
- levator scapulae
- supraspinatus
- infraspinatus
- teres major
- rhomboideus
- erector spinae

ANNOTATION KEY

Bold text indicates target muscles

Grey text indicates other working muscles

* indicates deep muscles

MODIFICATIONS

Easier: Try using a very light bar instead of a barbell.

More difficult: Use dumbbells (right) instead of a barbell.

BICEPS CURL

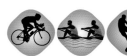

1 Stand upright with the resistance band beneath your feet. Your arms should be very slightly bent as you hold both handles of the resistance band in your hands, palms forward.

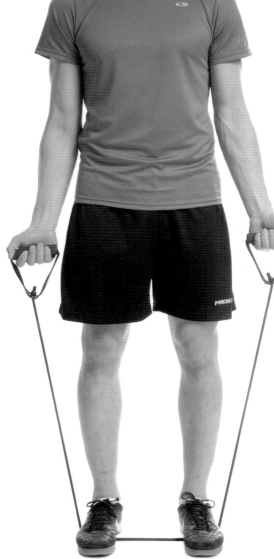

TARGETS
• Biceps

LEVEL
• Beginner

BENEFITS
• Strengthens and tones biceps

NOT ADVISABLE IF YOU HAVE . . .
• Wrist or elbow pain

DO IT RIGHT
• Keep your elbows at your sides.

AVOID
• Rushing through the exercise.

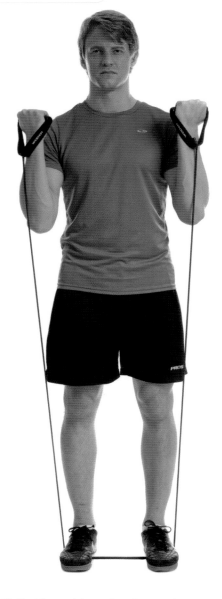

2 Curl the resistance band upward toward your shoulders.

3 Lower and repeat, completing three sets of 15.

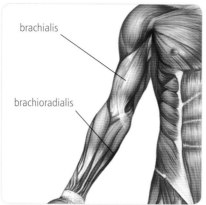

brachialis

brachioradialis

ANNOTATION KEY

Bold text indicates target muscles

Grey text indicates other working muscles

* indicates deep muscles

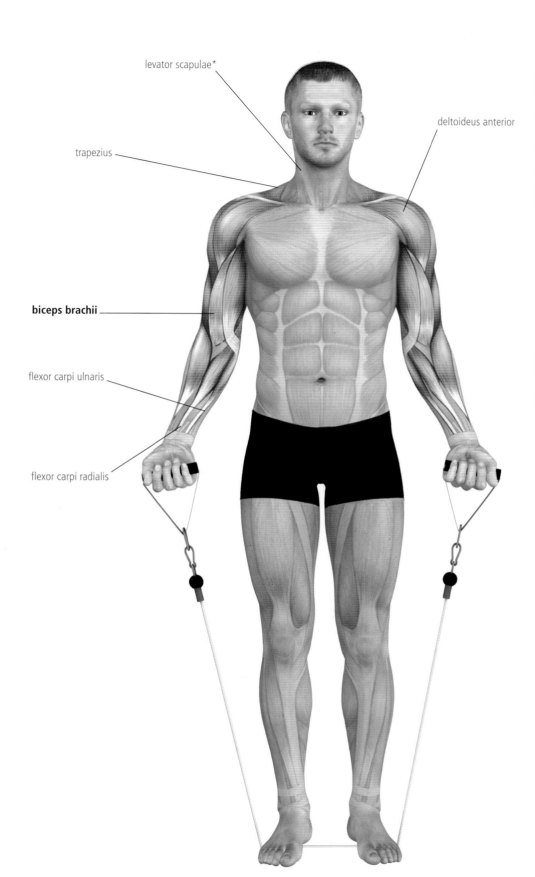

levator scapulae*

trapezius

deltoideus anterior

biceps brachii

flexor carpi ulnaris

flexor carpi radialis

ALTERNATING HAMMER CURL

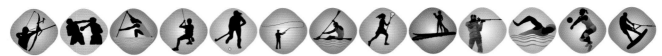

1 Stand with your feet parallel and shoulder-width apart, your knees slightly bent and your pelvis slightly tucked in.

2 Grasp a dumbbell in each hand, using hammer-grip position. Your elbows should be close to the torso.

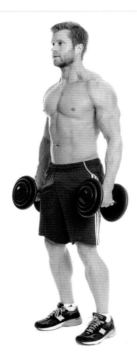

DO IT RIGHT
- Fully contract your biceps at the top range of the movement.

AVOID
- Using momentum to lift the weight — keep your torso upright and concentrate on isolating and engaging the biceps.
- Bending at the wrists — keep your wrists aligned with your forearms.

TARGETS
- Biceps

LEVEL
- Intermediate

BENEFITS
- Increases power and mass in the upper arms

NOT ADVISABLE IF YOU HAVE . . .
- Elbow issues

TRAINER'S TIPS
- Exhale as you lift the dumbbell up, and inhale as you lower it back to the starting position.
- If you find that you are swaying your back or leaning too far backward, use a lighter weight.

3 With your upper arms remaining stationary, curl the left dumbbell toward your upper chest.

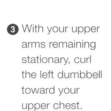

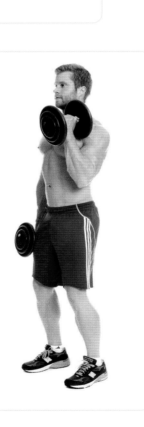

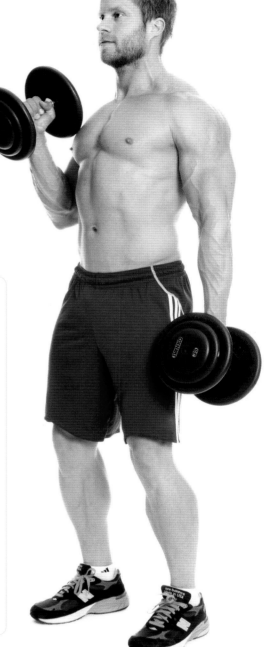

4 Slowly lower the weight back to the starting position, and repeat with the right dumbbell. Repeat 10 to 12 times, alternating sides.

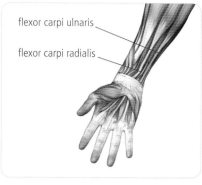

flexor carpi ulnaris

flexor carpi radialis

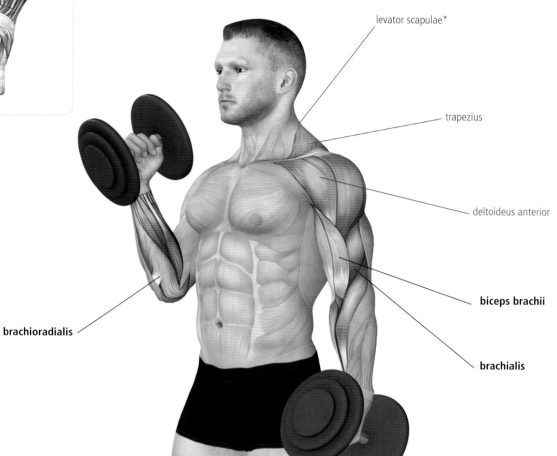

levator scapulae*

trapezius

deltoideus anterior

biceps brachii

brachialis

brachioradialis

BEST FOR

- **biceps brachii**
- **brachioradialis**
- **brachialis**

ANNOTATION KEY

Bold text indicates target muscles

Grey text indicates other working muscles

* indicates deep muscles

BARBELL CURL

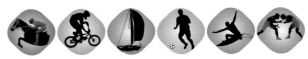

① Begin in a standing position, holding a barbell at arms' length, with an underhand grip shoulder-width apart.

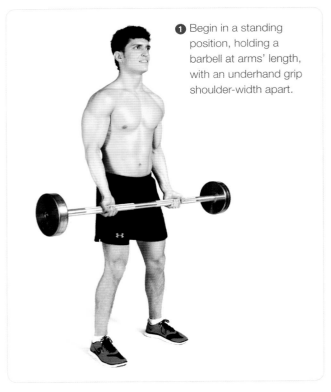

② Keeping your elbows in at your sides, bend the arms and bring the palms of your hands toward your chest.

TARGETS
• Biceps
• Forearms
• Core

LEVEL
• Intermediate

BENEFITS
• Increases both strength and mass in the biceps

NOT ADVISABLE IF YOU HAVE . . .
• Elbow issues

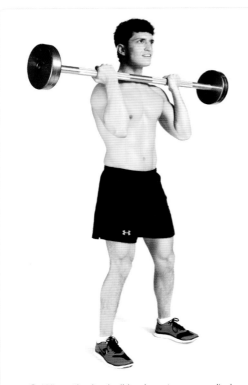

③ When the barbell is close to your collarbone, lower it. Repeat 8 to 10 times.

DO IT RIGHT
• Always employ a full range of motion.

AVOID
• Swinging the barbell up using your back.

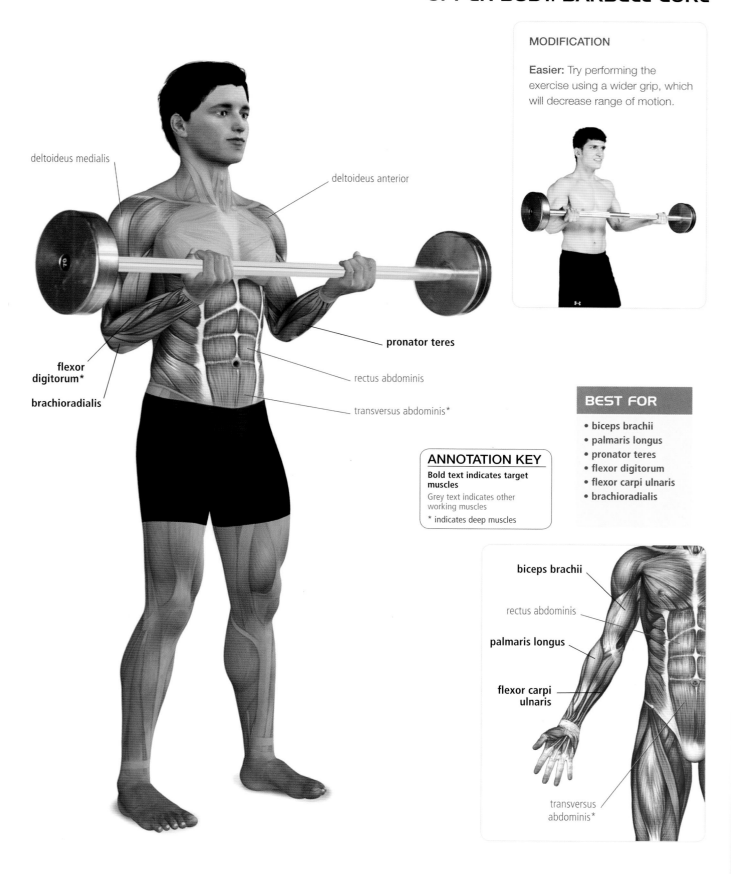

deltoideus medialis

deltoideus anterior

MODIFICATION

Easier: Try performing the exercise using a wider grip, which will decrease range of motion.

pronator teres

flexor digitorum*

rectus abdominis

brachioradialis

transversus abdominis*

ANNOTATION KEY

Bold text indicates target muscles

Grey text indicates other working muscles

* indicates deep muscles

BEST FOR

- biceps brachii
- palmaris longus
- pronator teres
- flexor digitorum
- flexor carpi ulnaris
- brachioradialis

biceps brachii

rectus abdominis

palmaris longus

flexor carpi ulnaris

transversus abdominis*

SINGLE-ARM CONCENTRATION CURL

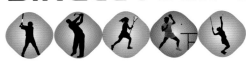

1 Sit facing forward on a flat bench with your legs spread generously outside of shoulder width. Hold a dumbbell in front of you between your legs.

2 Rest the back of your right upper arm on the top of your inner right thigh.

DO IT RIGHT
- The dumbbell should be a few inches from the floor when the arm is extended down in the starting position.

AVOID
- Swinging motions during this exercise.
- Bending your wrist — keep your wrist aligned with your forearm.
- Rolling your shoulder inward.

TARGETS
- Biceps

LEVEL
- Beginner

BENEFITS
- Increases power and mass in the upper arms

NOT ADVISABLE IF YOU HAVE . . .
- Knee pain

TRAINER'S TIPS
- Take a slight pause at the top range of the movement, concentrating on the contraction of the biceps.

3 With your right palm facing upward and your upper arm stationary, curl the dumbbell forward and up toward your face, stopping at shoulder height.

4 Slowly lower the weight back to the starting position and repeat.

5 Switch sides, and repeat all steps with your left hand holding the dumbbell.

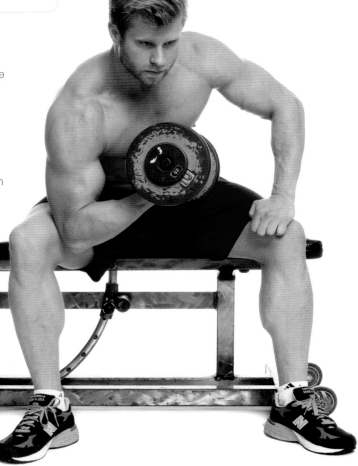

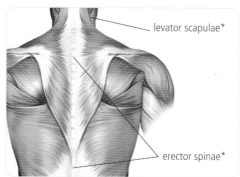

levator scapulae*

erector spinae*

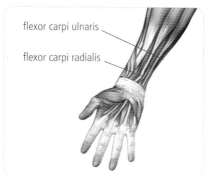

flexor carpi ulnaris

flexor carpi radialis

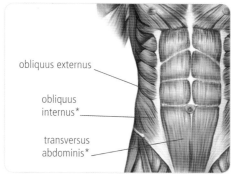

obliquus externus

obliquus internus*

transversus abdominis*

BEST FOR

- biceps brachii
- brachioradialis
- brachialis

ANNOTATION KEY

Bold text indicates target muscles

Grey text indicates other working muscles

* indicates deep muscles

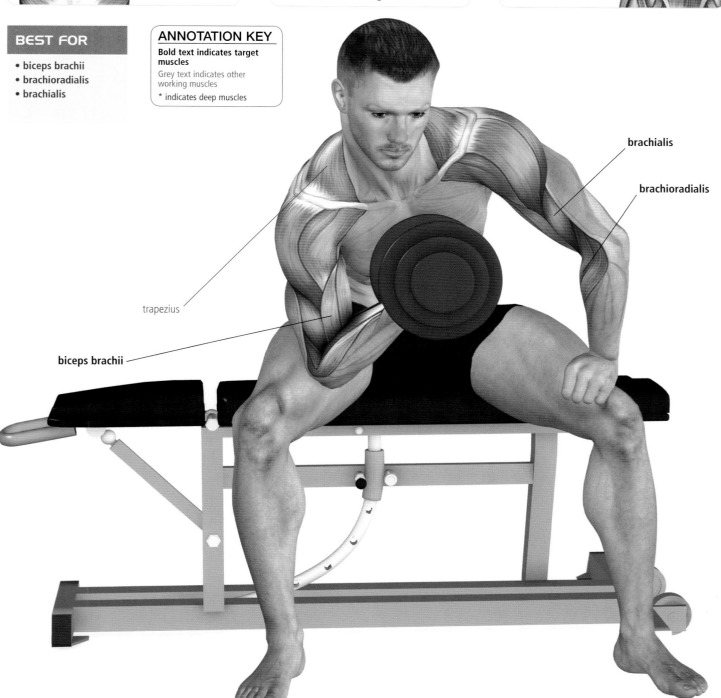

brachialis

brachioradialis

trapezius

biceps brachii

ROPE HAMMER CURL

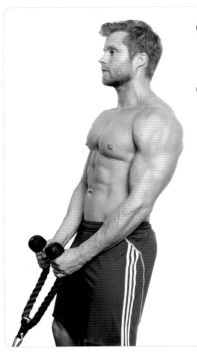

❶ Attach a rope attachment to the lowest setting of a cable machine.

❷ Stand about 1 foot (30 cm) from the cable upright with your feet parallel and shoulder-width apart, your knees slightly bent and your pelvis tucked in slightly. Grasp the rope with both hands in hammer-grip position, keeping your elbows tight to the sides of your body.

❸ Raise the cable weight toward your upper chest, keeping your upper arms stationary.

❹ Slowly lower the weight back to the starting position, and repeat.

DO IT RIGHT
- Keep your upper arms stationary throughout the exercise.
- Ensure your wrists stay in line with your forearms.

AVOID
- Tensing your neck or jaw during exercise.

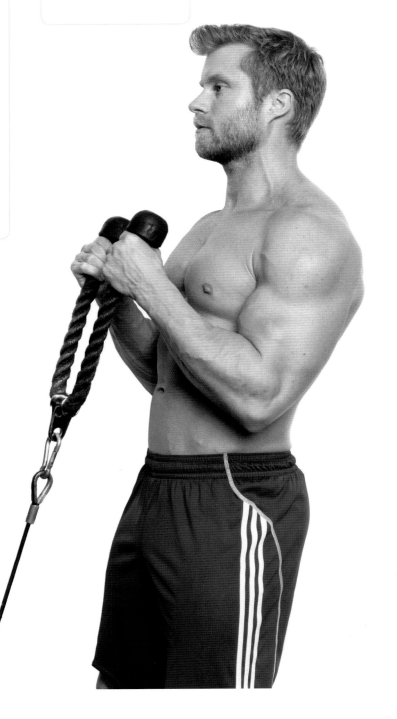

TARGETS
- Biceps

LEVEL
- Intermediate

BENEFITS
- Increases power and mass in the upper arm

NOT ADVISABLE IF YOU HAVE . . .
- Elbow pain

TRAINER'S TIPS
- For proper position, keep your neck back and your chin slightly up.
- Take a slight pause at the top range of the movement before lowering the cable weight back to the starting position.

BEST FOR

- biceps brachii
- brachialis
- brachioradialis

ANNOTATION KEY

Bold text indicates target muscles

Grey text indicates other working muscles

* indicates deep muscles

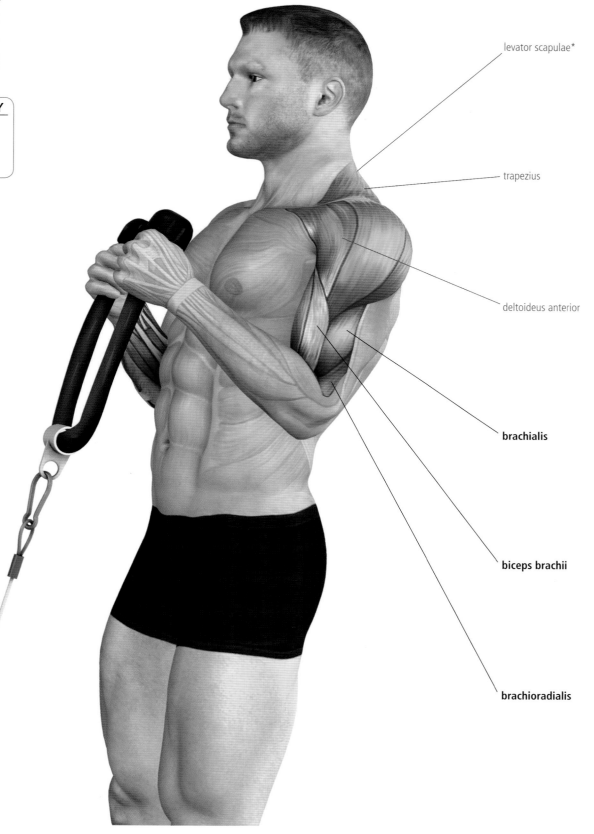

levator scapulae*

trapezius

deltoideus anterior

brachialis

biceps brachii

brachioradialis

ROPE PUSHDOWN

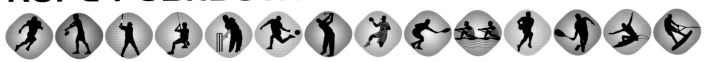

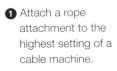

① Attach a rope attachment to the highest setting of a cable machine.

② Stand with your feet parallel and shoulder-width apart, your knees slightly bent and your pelvis tucked in slightly. Grasp the rope with both hands in hammer-grip position.

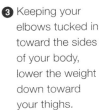

③ Keeping your elbows tucked in toward the sides of your body, lower the weight down toward your thighs.

④ Slowly raise the cable weight back to the starting position. Repeat 8 to 10 times.

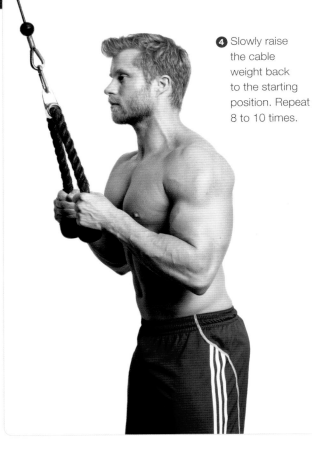

TARGETS
• Triceps

LEVEL
• Intermediate

BENEFITS
• Increases power and mass in the torso

NOT ADVISABLE IF YOU HAVE . . .
• Elbow or wrist pain

TRAINER'S TIPS
• For proper position, keep your neck, back and your chin slightly up.
• Exhale as you lower the cable weight, and inhale as you bring it back to the starting position.
• Take a slight pause at the lowest point of the movement.

DO IT RIGHT
• Keep your upper arms stationary throughout the exercise.
• Keep your wrists in line with your forearms.

AVOID
• Bending your wrists while lowering the weight.
• Using momentum to execute movement — concentrate on isolating and using the triceps muscle.

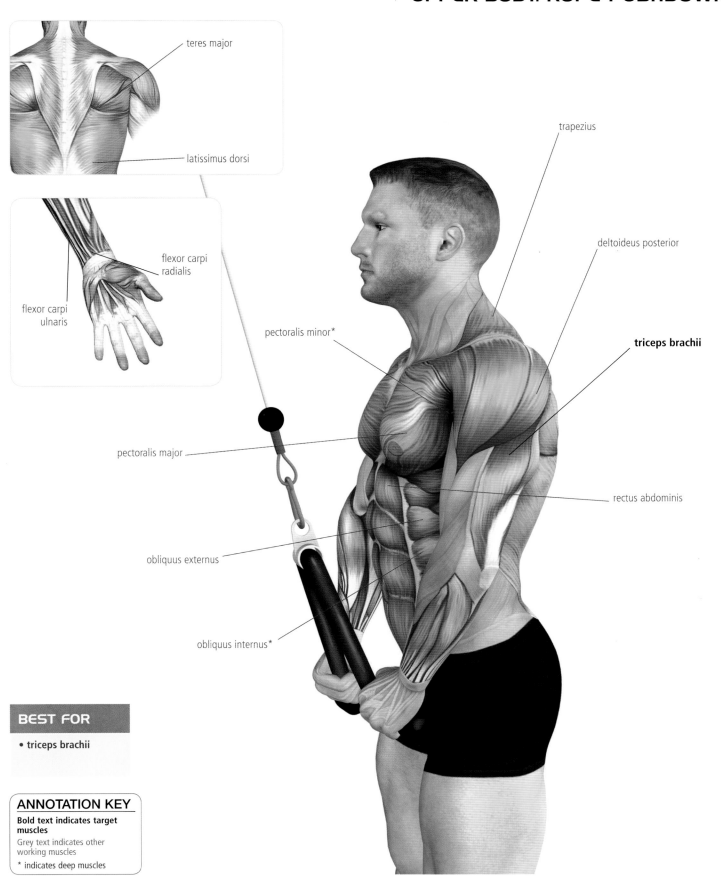

teres major

latissimus dorsi

flexor carpi radialis

flexor carpi ulnaris

trapezius

deltoideus posterior

triceps brachii

pectoralis minor*

pectoralis major

rectus abdominis

obliquus externus

obliquus internus*

BEST FOR

• **triceps brachii**

ANNOTATION KEY

Bold text indicates target muscles

Grey text indicates other working muscles

* indicates deep muscles

LYING TRICEPS EXTENSION

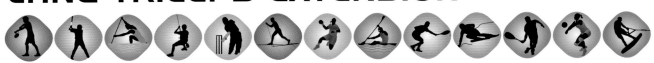

DO IT RIGHT
- Keep your forearms stable and your elbows over your shoulders.
- Keep your torso stable and feet planted throughout the exercise.
- Engage your abs.
- Keep your pelvis lifted so that your upper legs, torso and neck form a straight line.
- Move smoothly and with control.

AVOID
- Arching your back.
- Flaring your elbows outward.
- Swinging your weights — especially important as the weights are close to your head.

TARGETS
- Triceps

LEVEL
- Intermediate

BENEFITS
- Strengthens and tones triceps

AVOID IF YOU HAVE . . .
- Elbow pain

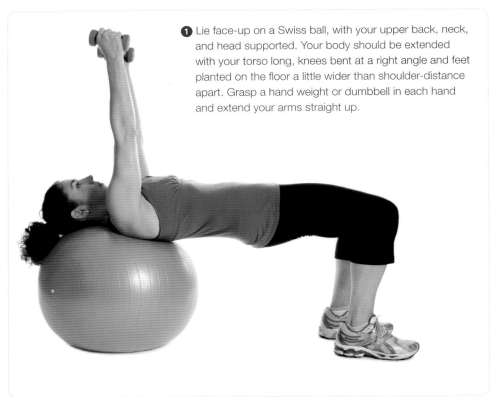

1 Lie face-up on a Swiss ball, with your upper back, neck, and head supported. Your body should be extended with your torso long, knees bent at a right angle and feet planted on the floor a little wider than shoulder-distance apart. Grasp a hand weight or dumbbell in each hand and extend your arms straight up.

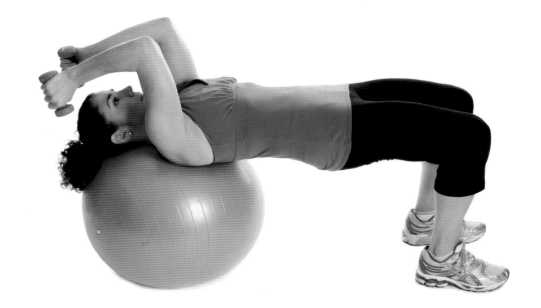

2 Bend your elbows as you lower the weights toward your head.

3 Straighten your arms upward to the starting position and then repeat. Perform three sets of 15 repetitions.

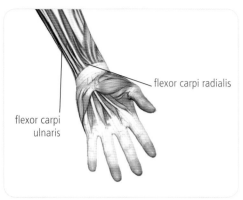

flexor carpi radialis

flexor carpi ulnaris

BEST FOR

• triceps brachii

ANNOTATION KEY

Bold text indicates target muscles

Grey text indicates other working muscles

* indicates deep muscles

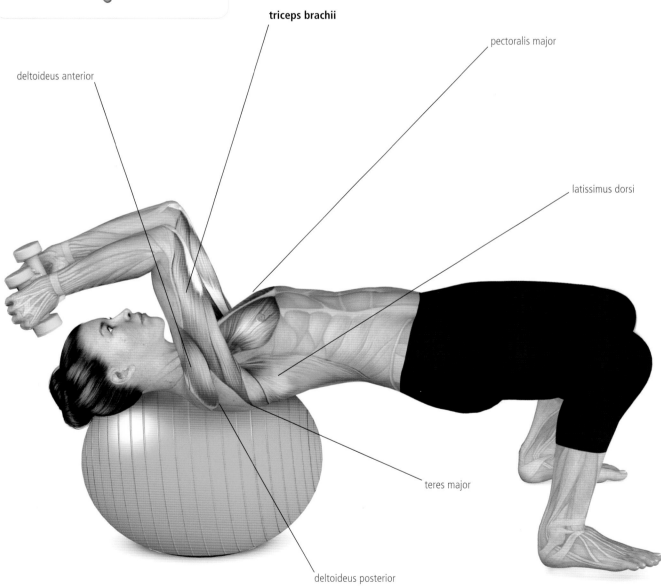

triceps brachii

pectoralis major

deltoideus anterior

latissimus dorsi

teres major

deltoideus posterior

109

TRICEPS ROLL-OUT

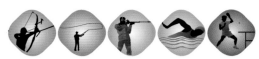

❶ Kneel on the floor, with the foam roller placed crosswise in front of you. Place your wrists on top of the roller, your fingers facing away from you.

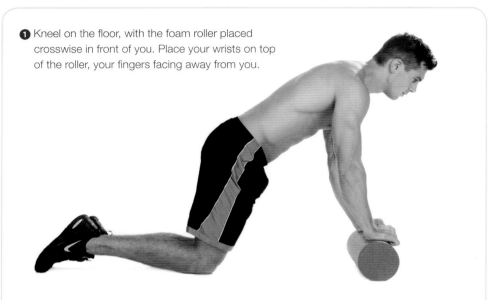

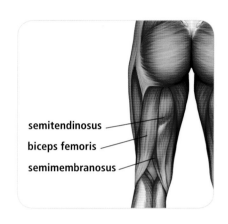

semitendinosus

biceps femoris

semimembranosus

DO IT RIGHT
- All movement should happen at the same time.
- Ensure your shoulders stay relaxed throughout the exercise.
- Press your feet firmly to the floor.

AVOID
- Allowing your shoulders to lift toward your ears.
- Allowing your hips and lower back to drop during the movement.
- Arching your back.

TARGETS
- Triceps
- Abdominals
- Trunk stabilizers

LEVEL
- Intermediate

BENEFITS
- Improves core and shoulder stability

NOT ADVISABLE IF YOU HAVE . . .
- Lower-back pain
- Shoulder pain

❷ Maintaining a neutral spine and making sure not to sink your neck into your shoulders, roll forward on your forearms.

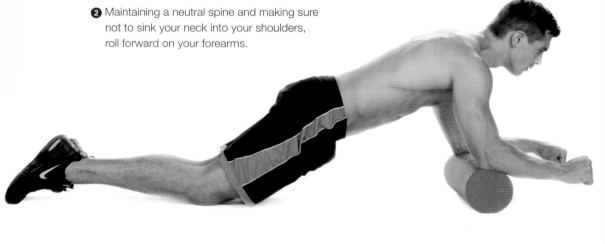

❸ Continue to roll forward until the roller reaches your elbows. Press into the roller, keeping your hips aligned, and roll back to the starting position. Repeat 15 times.

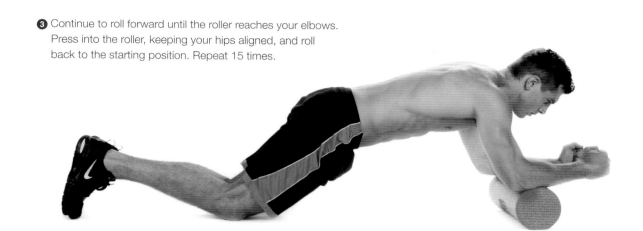

BEST FOR

- rectus abdominis
- triceps brachii
- gluteus maximus
- gluteus medius
- biceps femoris
- semitendinosus
- semimembranosus
- seratus anterior
- pectoralis major
- pectoralis minor

ANNOTATION KEY

Bold text indicates target muscles

Grey text indicates other working muscles

* indicates deep muscles

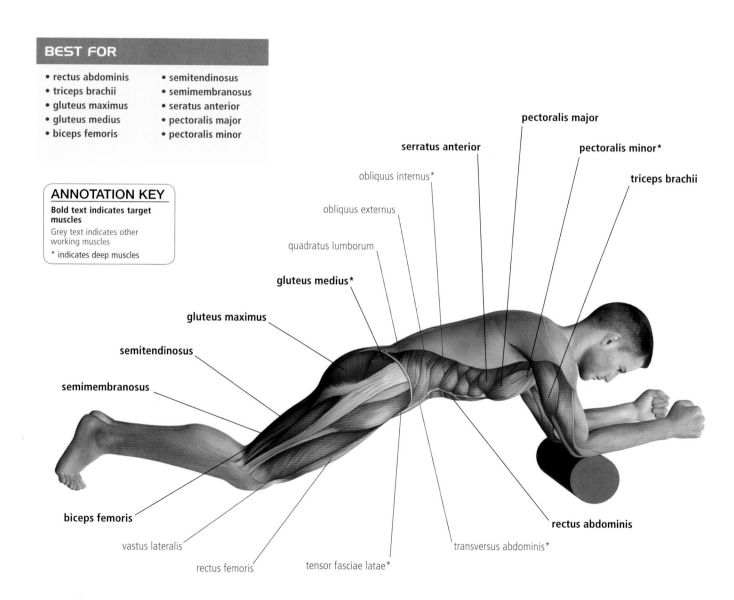

pectoralis major

serratus anterior

pectoralis minor*

obliquus internus*

triceps brachii

obliquus externus

quadratus lumborum

gluteus medius*

gluteus maximus

semitendinosus

semimembranosus

biceps femoris

rectus abdominis

vastus lateralis

transversus abdominis*

rectus femoris

tensor fasciae latae*

CHAIR DIP

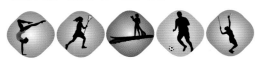

❶ Sit up tall near the front of a sturdy chair. Place your hands beside your hips, wrapping your fingers over the front edge of the chair.

❷ Extend your legs in front of you slightly, and place your feet flat on the floor.

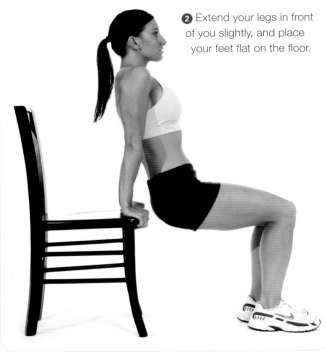

DO IT RIGHT
- Keep your body close to the chair.
- Your spine should remain neutral throughout the movement.

AVOID
- Allowing your shoulders to lift toward your ears.
- Moving your feet.
- Rounding your back at your hips.
- Pushing up only with your feet, rather than using your arm strength.

❸ Slide off the edge of the chair until your knees align directly above your feet and your torso is able to clear the chair as you dip down.

❹ Bending your elbows directly behind you, without splaying them out to the sides, lower your torso until your elbows make a 90-degree angle.

TARGET
- Triceps
- Deltoids
- Core

LEVEL
- Beginner

BENEFITS
- Strengthens the shoulder girdle
- Trains the torso to remain stable while the legs and arms are in motion

NOT ADVISABLE IF YOU HAVE
- Shoulder pain
- Wrist pain

❺ Press into the chair, raising your body back to the starting position. Repeat 15 times for two sets.

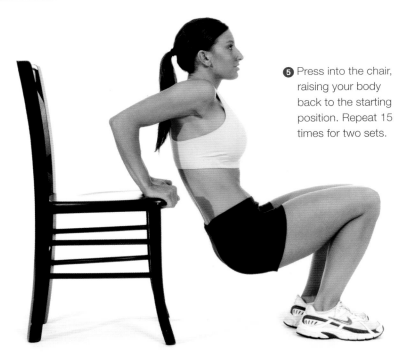

112

MODIFICATION

More difficult:
Keeping your knees squeezed together, perform the dips with one leg lifted straight out, parallel to the floor. Repeat 15 times on each side.

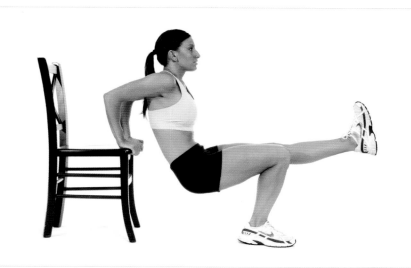

BEST FOR

- triceps brachii
- deltoideus
- pectoralis major
- pectoralis minor
- coracobrachialis

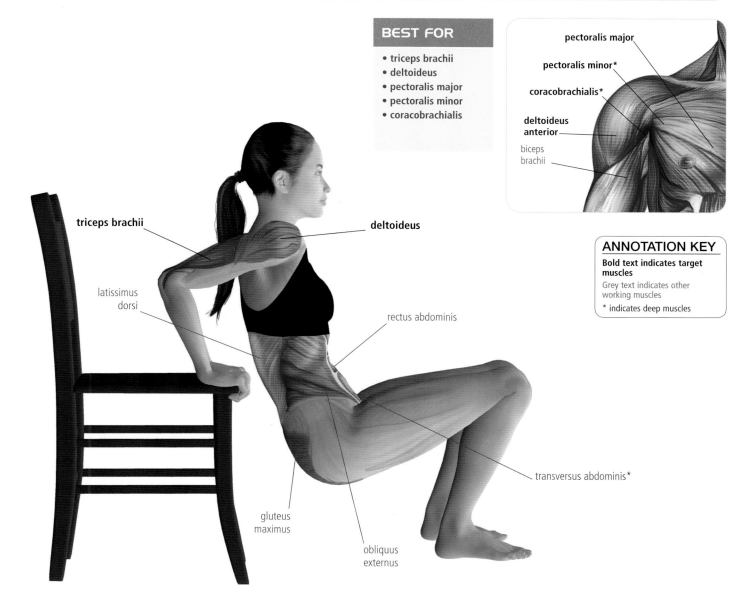

pectoralis major

pectoralis minor*

coracobrachialis*

deltoideus anterior

biceps brachii

triceps brachii

deltoideus

latissimus dorsi

rectus abdominis

transversus abdominis*

gluteus maximus

obliquus externus

ANNOTATION KEY

Bold text indicates target muscles

Grey text indicates other working muscles

* indicates deep muscles

ROPE OVERHEAD EXTENSION

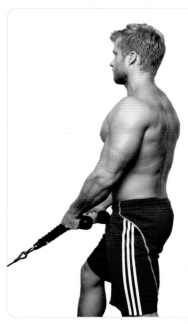

1 Attach a rope attachment to the lowest setting of a cable machine. Grasp the rope with both hands, keeping your elbows close to the body.

DO IT RIGHT
• Keep your upper arms stationary as you lower the weight behind your head.

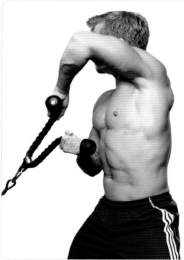

2 Maintaining a wide stance, begin to turn your torso as you pull upward on the rope.

TARGETS
• Triceps

LEVEL
• Intermediate

BENEFITS
• Increases power and mass in the shoulders and upper arms

NOT ADVISABLE IF YOU HAVE . . .
• Back, shoulder or elbow issues

TRAINER'S TIPS
• Take a short pause when your triceps are fully stretched at the bottom of the range of movement.
• When you are finished with this exercise, slowly and carefully lower the rope, keeping your elbows close to the body to avoid shoulder injury.

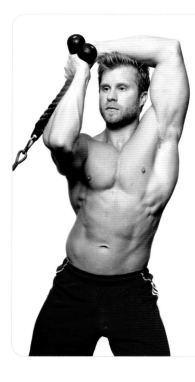

3 Continue to turn to face forward as you slide your hands up above your head.

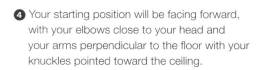

4 Your starting position will be facing forward, with your elbows close to your head and your arms perpendicular to the floor with your knuckles pointed toward the ceiling.

AVOID
• Using momentum to execute the movement — concentrate on isolating and using the triceps muscle.

114

UPPER BODY: ROPE OVERHEAD EXTENSION

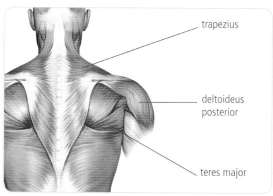

trapezius

deltoideus posterior

teres major

flexor carpi ulnaris

flexor carpi radialis

BEST FOR

• triceps brachii

ANNOTATION KEY

Bold text indicates target muscles

Grey text indicates other working muscles

* indicates deep muscles

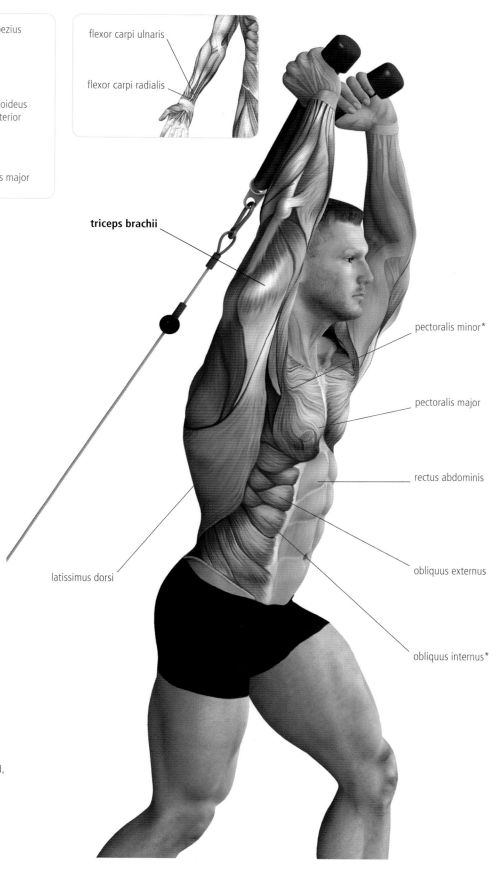

triceps brachii

pectoralis minor*

pectoralis major

rectus abdominis

obliquus externus

obliquus internus*

latissimus dorsi

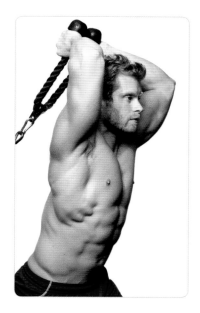

⑤ Slowly lower the weight behind your head, then raise the cable weight back to the starting position. Repeat 8 to 10 times.

WRIST FLEXION

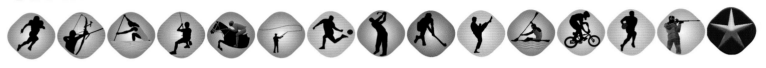

DO IT RIGHT
- Keep in mind that a flexing movement stretches the extensor muscles, and an extending movement stretches the flexors.
- Be sure to press your thumb into the meaty part of your palm, attached to the thumb, intensifying the stretch in your forearm and wrist.

AVOID
- Lifting or tensing your shoulders.

TARGETS
- Wrists
- Hands
- Forearms

TRAINER'S TIPS
- Perform these stretches after a long phone conversation or a stressful commute to release any tension in your hands and forearms, or if you often carry weight in your arms, such as when holding a child.

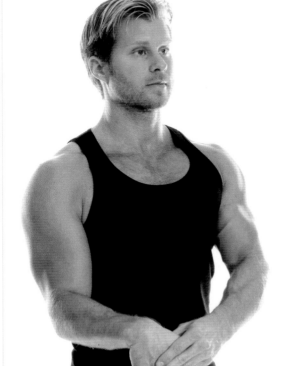

① Stand or sit with your arms at your sides.

② Bend your right forearm up from the elbow, creating a 90-degree bend. Your palm should be facing the floor.

③ Drop and flex your right wrist downward so that your palm faces inward.

④ Place your left fingers over the back of your right hand, and your left thumb on the palm of the hand, directly on the right thumb muscle.

⑤ Gently press your left fingers into the back of your right hand, bringing your right wrist to a 60- to 90-degree bend, while pressing your left thumb into the palm away from the body, creating a deeper stretch.

⑥ Release, switch hands, and repeat on the other side.

BEST FOR
- extensor carpi radialis
- extensor carpi ulnaris
- extensor digiti minimi
- extensor digitorum
- extensor indicis
- extensor pollicis

ANNOTATION KEY
Bold text indicates target muscles
Grey text indicates other working muscles
* indicates deep muscles

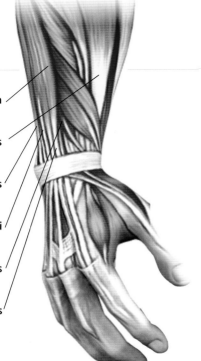

extensor digitorum

extensor carpi radialis

extensor carpi ulnaris

extensor digiti minimi

extensor pollicis

extensor indicis

WRIST EXTENSION

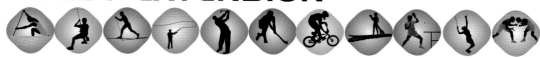

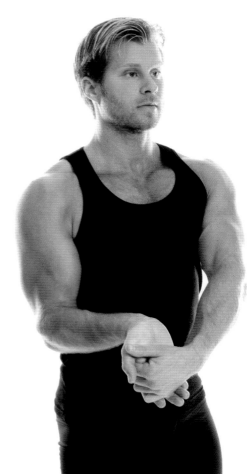

1. Stand or sit with your arms at your sides.

2. Bend your right forearm up from the elbow, creating a 90-degree bend. Your palm should be facing up toward the ceiling.

3. Drop and flex your right wrist downward so that your palm faces outward.

4. Place your left fingers over the back of your right hand, and your left thumb on the palm of the hand, directly on the right thumb muscle.

5. Using your left thumb and palm, gently press the right thumb and palm in toward your body. At the same time, use your left fingers to press in on the back of the right hand, thus flattening the right palm and creating a deeper stretch.

TRAINER'S TIPS

• Imagine that you are holding a pencil under each arm. Engage the muscles around your armpits to hold onto the imaginary pencil — keeping your shoulders perfectly positioned in the process. Use this technique for all stretches and resistance training that involve holding your elbows in toward your rib cage.

BEST FOR

• flexor carpi radialis
• flexor carpi ulnaris
• flexor digiti minimi
• flexor digitorum
• palmaris longus
• flexor pollicis

ANNOTATION KEY

Bold text indicates target muscles

Grey text indicates other working muscles

* indicates deep muscles

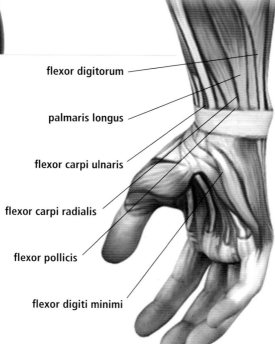

flexor digitorum

palmaris longus

flexor carpi ulnaris

flexor carpi radialis

flexor pollicis

flexor digiti minimi

CRUNCH

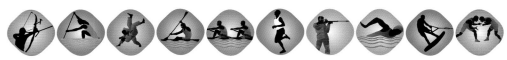

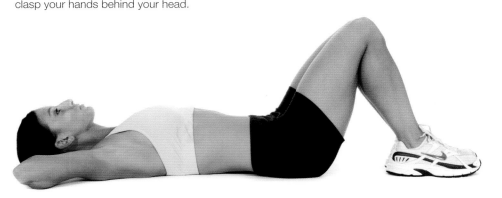

1 Lie supine on the floor with your knees bent, and clasp your hands behind your head.

DO IT RIGHT
- Use your shoulders and abdominals to initiate the movement.
- Ensure your pelvis remains in a neutral position during the crunching motion.
- Tuck in your chin slightly, directing your gaze toward the inner thighs.

AVOID
- Pulling from the neck.
- Tilting your hips toward the floor.

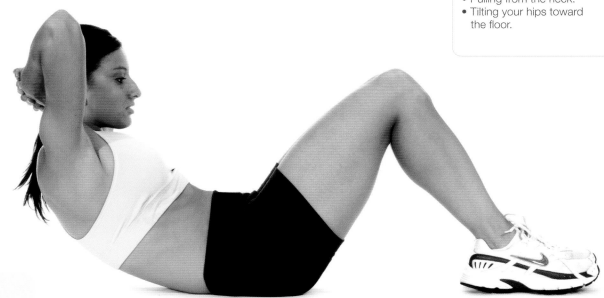

TARGETS
- Abdominals

LEVEL
- Beginner

BENEFITS
- Strengthens the torso
- Improves pelvic and core stability

NOT ADVISABLE IF YOU HAVE . . .
- Back pain
- Neck pain

2 Keeping your elbows wide, engage the abdominals, and lift your upper torso to achieve a crunching movement.

3 Slowly return to the starting position. Repeat 15 times for two sets.

MODIFICATION

More difficult: Begin by lying supine on the floor with your legs outstretched, and your arms over your head. Without lifting your legs, lift your arms and torso in a controlled movement. Continue to curl forward and grasp your feet.

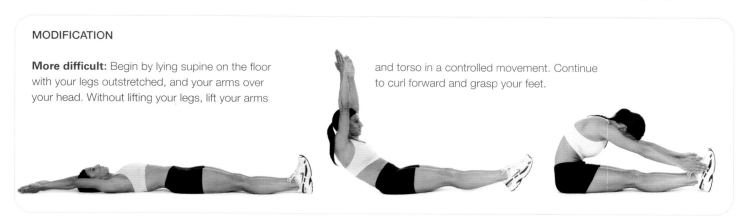

serratus anterior

rectus abdominis

transversus abdominis*

coracobrachialis

obliquus externus

latissimus dorsi

iliopsoas*

tensor fasciae latae

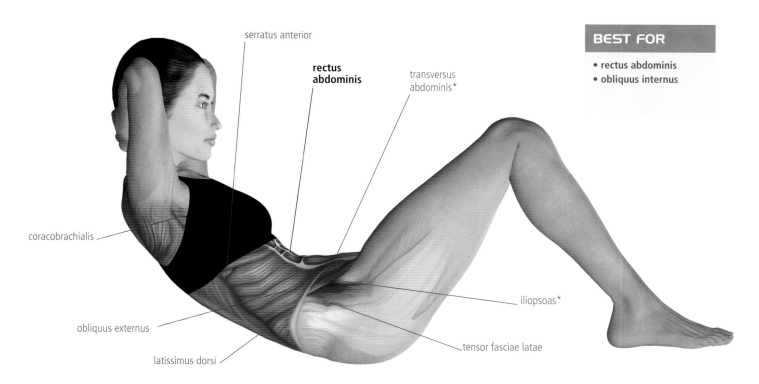

BEST FOR

• rectus abdominis
• obliquus internus

obliquus externus

obliquus internus*

transversus abdominis*

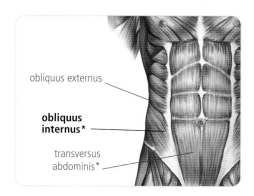

ANNOTATION KEY

Bold text indicates target muscles

Grey text indicates other working muscles

* indicates deep muscles

PLANK

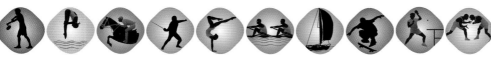

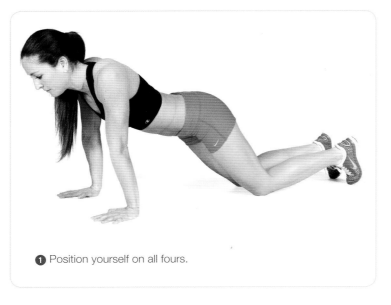

1 Position yourself on all fours.

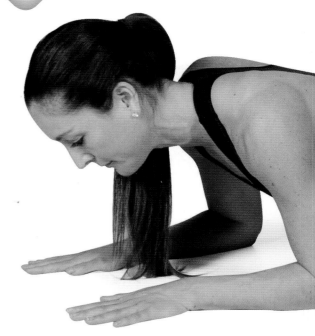

TARGETS
- Abdominals
- Back
- Obliques

LEVEL
- Beginner

BENEFITS
- Strengthens the entire core

NOT ADVISABLE IF YOU HAVE . . .
- Shoulder issues
- Back pain
- Elbow pain

MODIFICATION
- **More difficult:** Lift one foot off the floor for a greater challenge.

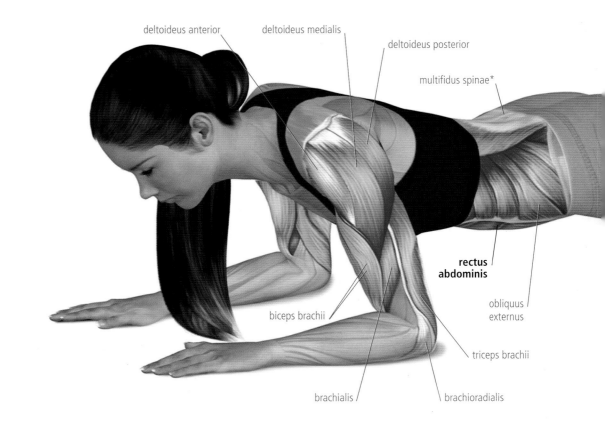

deltoideus anterior

deltoideus medialis

deltoideus posterior

multifidus spinae*

rectus abdominis

obliquus externus

triceps brachii

biceps brachii

brachialis

brachioradialis

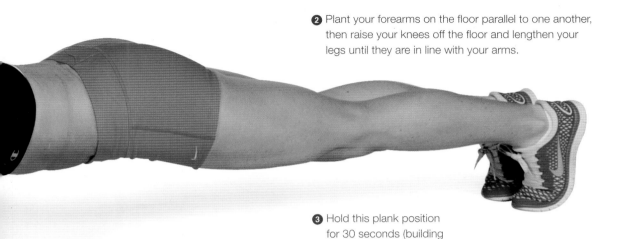

② Plant your forearms on the floor parallel to one another, then raise your knees off the floor and lengthen your legs until they are in line with your arms.

③ Hold this plank position for 30 seconds (building up to 120 seconds).

DO IT RIGHT
• Keep your abdominal muscles tight and your body in a straight line.

AVOID
• Bridging too high, since this can take stress off working muscles.

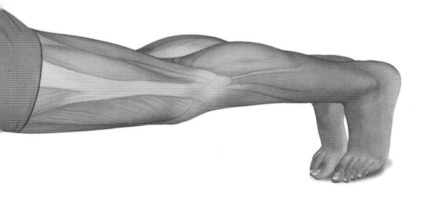

BEST FOR

• **rectus abdominis**
• **erector spinae**

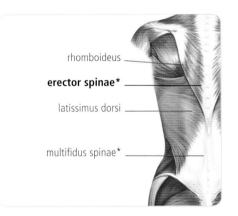

rhomboideus

erector spinae*

latissimus dorsi

multifidus spinae***

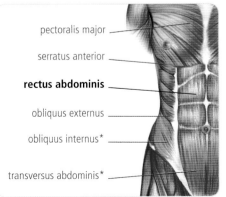

pectoralis major

serratus anterior

rectus abdominis

obliquus externus

obliquus internus***

transversus abdominis***

ANNOTATION KEY

Bold text indicates target muscles

Grey text indicates other working muscles

* indicates deep muscles

SIDE PLANK

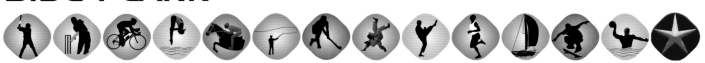

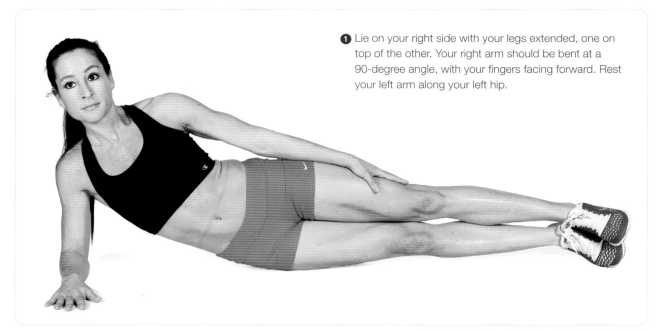

1 Lie on your right side with your legs extended, one on top of the other. Your right arm should be bent at a 90-degree angle, with your fingers facing forward. Rest your left arm along your left hip.

TARGETS
• Lower abdominals
• Back
• Deltoids

LEVEL
• Intermediate

BENEFITS
• Strengthens the abdominals, lower back and shoulders

NOT ADVISABLE IF YOU HAVE . . .
• Shoulder issues
• Back pain
• Elbow pain

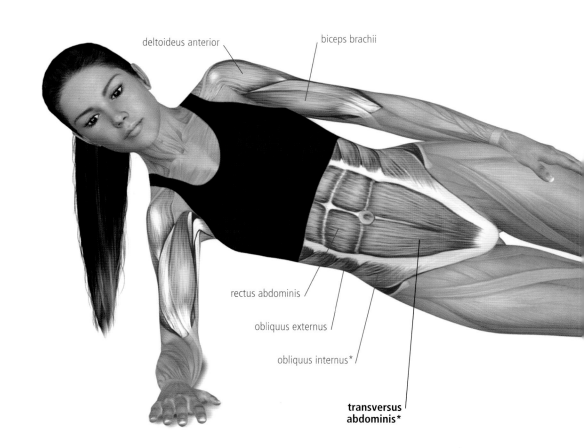

deltoideus anterior

biceps brachii

rectus abdominis

obliquus externus

obliquus internus*

transversus abdominis*

MODIFICATIONS

Easier: Use your resting arm as an anchor, assisting with the lift.

More difficult: Open your legs slightly while in hold (right).

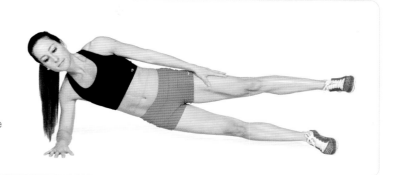

DO IT RIGHT
• Push evenly from both your forearm and hips.

AVOID
• Placing too much strain on your shoulders.

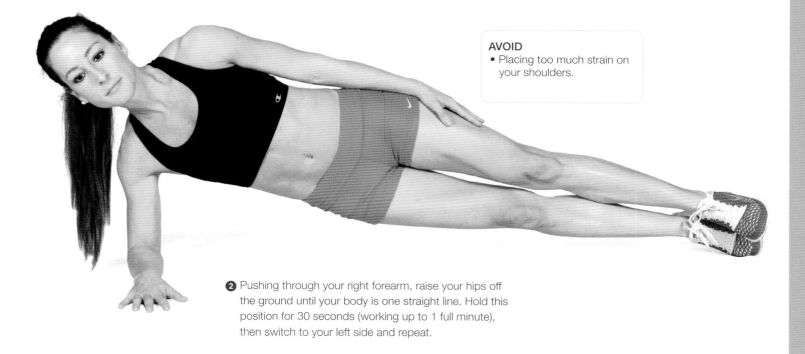

❷ Pushing through your right forearm, raise your hips off the ground until your body is one straight line. Hold this position for 30 seconds (working up to 1 full minute), then switch to your left side and repeat.

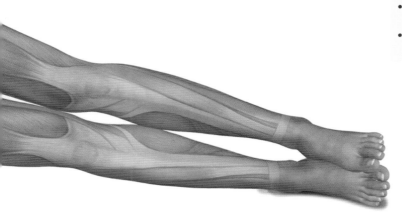

BEST FOR
• **transversus abdominis**
• **erector spinae**

ANNOTATION KEY
Bold text indicates target muscles
Grey text indicates other working muscles
* indicates deep muscles

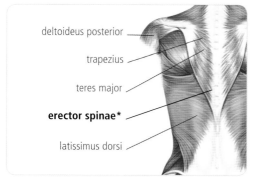

deltoideus posterior

trapezius

teres major

erector spinae*

latissimus dorsi

T-STABILIZATION

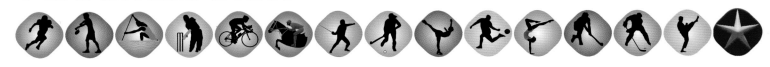

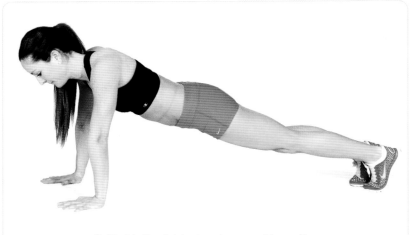

DO IT RIGHT
• Keep your body in one straight line.

AVOID
• Arching or bridging your back.

❶ Start in the finished push-up position, with your arms extended to full lockout and your palms facing forward, supporting yourself on your toes.

TARGETS
• Abdominals
• Hips
• Lower back
• Obliques

LEVEL
• Intermediate

BENEFITS
• Strengthens the abdominals, hips, lower back and obliques

NOT ADVISABLE IF YOU HAVE . . .
• Shoulder issues
• Back pain
• Elbow pain

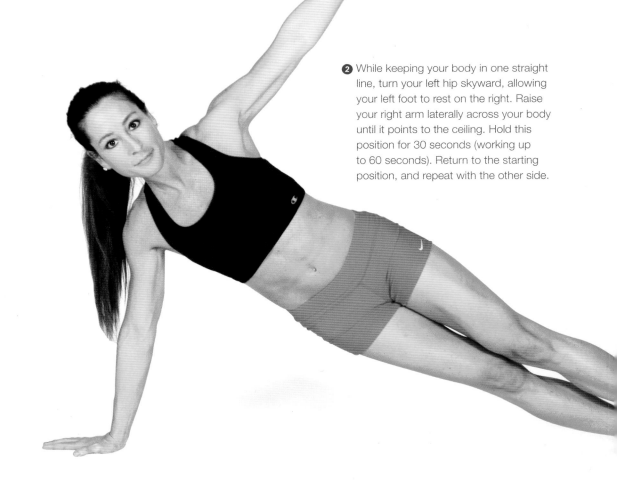

❷ While keeping your body in one straight line, turn your left hip skyward, allowing your left foot to rest on the right. Raise your right arm laterally across your body until it points to the ceiling. Hold this position for 30 seconds (working up to 60 seconds). Return to the starting position, and repeat with the other side.

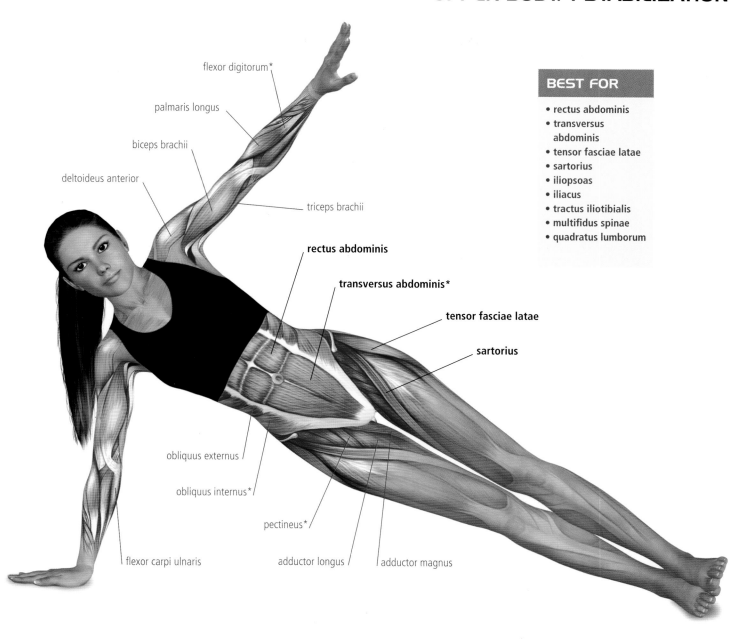

flexor digitorum*

palmaris longus

biceps brachii

deltoideus anterior

triceps brachii

rectus abdominis

transversus abdominis*

tensor fasciae latae

sartorius

obliquus externus

obliquus internus*

pectineus*

flexor carpi ulnaris

adductor longus

adductor magnus

BEST FOR

- rectus abdominis
- transversus abdominis
- tensor fasciae latae
- sartorius
- iliopsoas
- iliacus
- tractus iliotibialis
- multifidus spinae
- quadratus lumborum

ANNOTATION KEY

Bold text indicates target muscles

Grey text indicates other working muscles

* indicates deep muscles

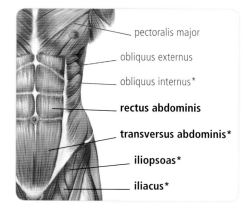

pectoralis major

obliquus externus

obliquus internus*

rectus abdominis

transversus abdominis*

iliopsoas*

iliacus*

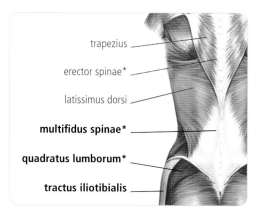

trapezius

erector spinae*

latissimus dorsi

multifidus spinae*

quadratus lumborum*

tractus iliotibialis

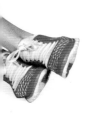

SWISS BALL WALK-AROUND

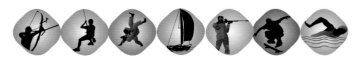

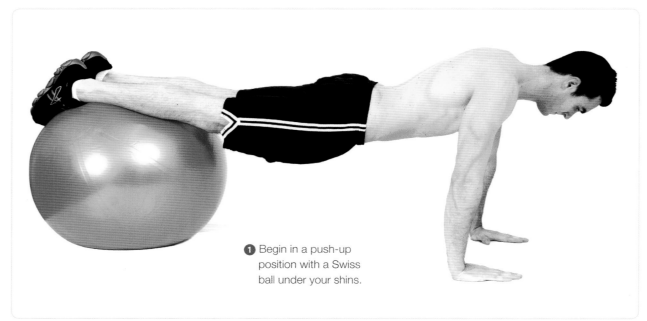

1 Begin in a push-up position with a Swiss ball under your shins.

TARGETS
- Triceps
- Abdominals
- Trunk stabilizers

LEVEL
- Intermediate

BENEFITS
- Helps keep the upper body stabilized and working cohesively

NOT ADVISABLE IF YOU HAVE . . .
- Lower-back pain
- Shoulder pain

DO IT RIGHT
- Keep the Swiss ball as still and centered as possible.

AVOID
- Placing excessive strain on the wrists.

2 "Walk" one hand at a time toward the right, turning the body with it until you have completed a semicircle. Then hand-walk to the left, returning to your starting position. Complete three semicircles in each direction.

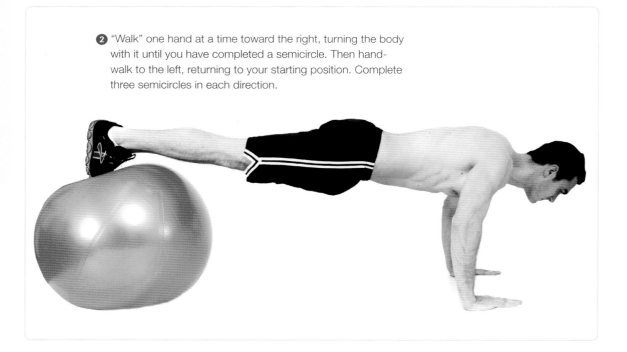

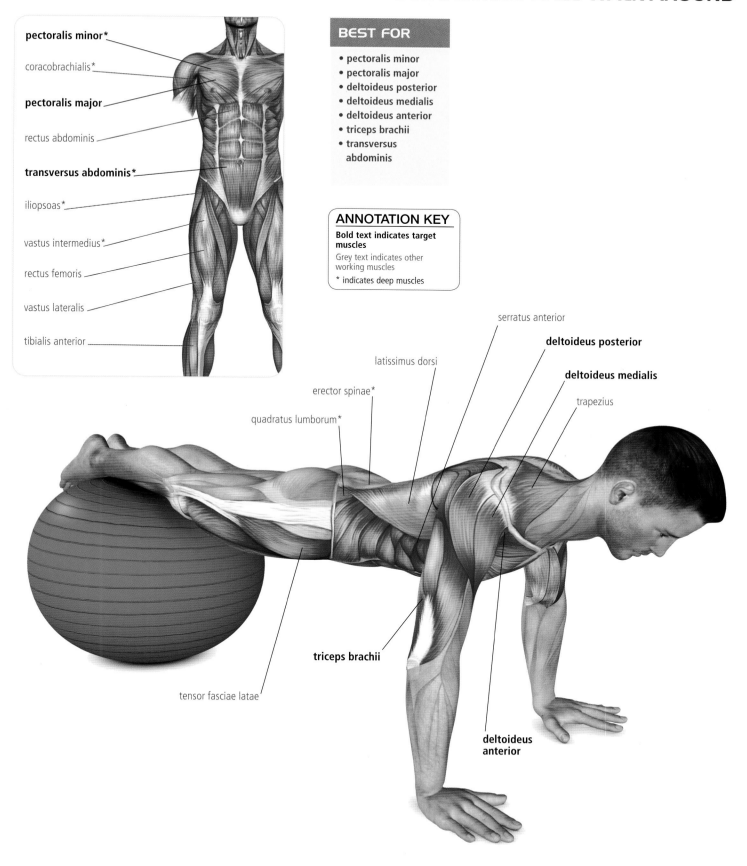

pectoralis minor*

coracobrachialis*

pectoralis major

rectus abdominis

transversus abdominis*

iliopsoas*

vastus intermedius*

rectus femoris

vastus lateralis

tibialis anterior

BEST FOR

- pectoralis minor
- pectoralis major
- deltoideus posterior
- deltoideus medialis
- deltoideus anterior
- triceps brachii
- transversus abdominis

ANNOTATION KEY

Bold text indicates target muscles

Grey text indicates other working muscles

* indicates deep muscles

serratus anterior

deltoideus posterior

deltoideus medialis

trapezius

latissimus dorsi

erector spinae*

quadratus lumborum*

triceps brachii

tensor fasciae latae

deltoideus anterior

SWISS BALL JACKKNIFE

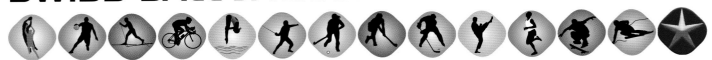

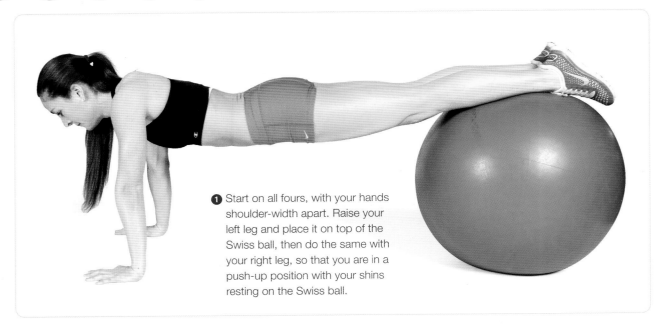

1 Start on all fours, with your hands shoulder-width apart. Raise your left leg and place it on top of the Swiss ball, then do the same with your right leg, so that you are in a push-up position with your shins resting on the Swiss ball.

TARGETS
- Hip flexors
- Abdominals
- Erectors
- Obliques

LEVEL
- Intermediate

BENEFITS
- Strengthens your hip flexors, as well as your abdominals and erectors

NOT ADVISABLE IF YOU HAVE . . .
- Lower-back pain
- Shoulder pain

MODIFICATION
- **More difficult:** Try taking one leg off the ball for added resistance.

DO IT RIGHT
- Brace your core.

AVOID
- Rounding your back.

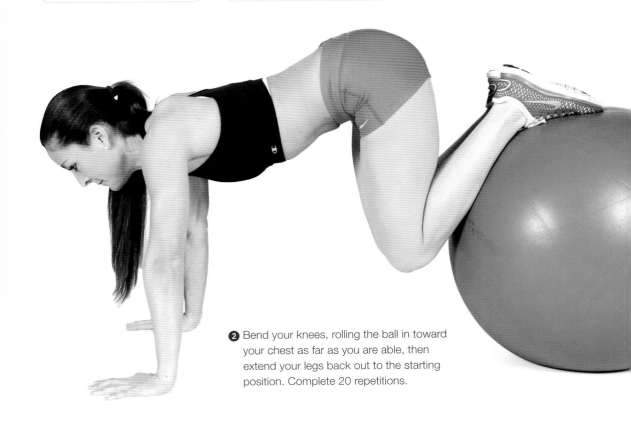

2 Bend your knees, rolling the ball in toward your chest as far as you are able, then extend your legs back out to the starting position. Complete 20 repetitions.

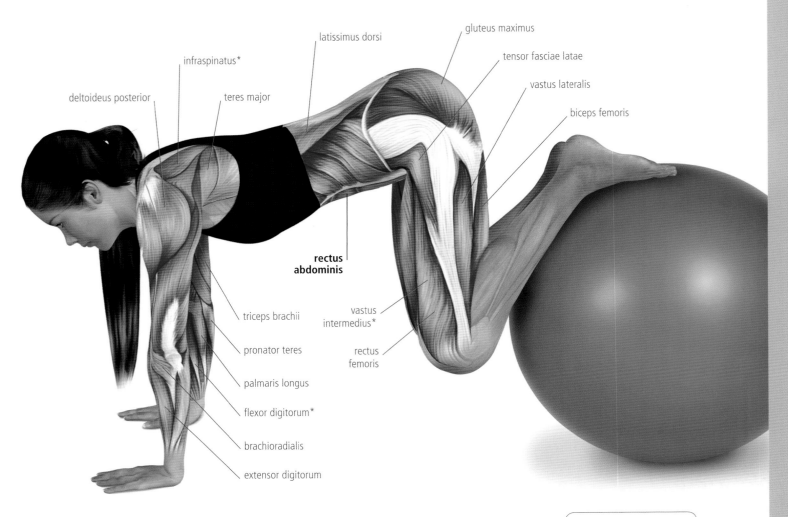

latissimus dorsi

gluteus maximus

infraspinatus*

tensor fasciae latae

vastus lateralis

deltoideus posterior

teres major

biceps femoris

rectus abdominis

triceps brachii

vastus intermedius*

pronator teres

rectus femoris

palmaris longus

flexor digitorum*

brachioradialis

extensor digitorum

ANNOTATION KEY

Bold text indicates target muscles

Grey text indicates other working muscles

* indicates deep muscles

BEST FOR

- sartorius
- iliopsoas
- iliacus
- rectus abdominis
- erector spinae

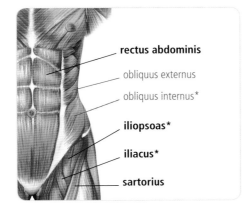

rectus abdominis

obliquus externus

obliquus internus*

iliopsoas*

iliacus*

sartorius

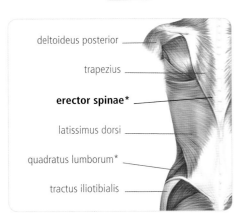

deltoideus posterior

trapezius

erector spinae*

latissimus dorsi

quadratus lumborum*

tractus iliotibialis

MEDICINE BALL WOOD CHOP

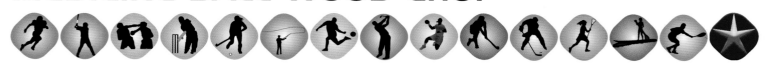

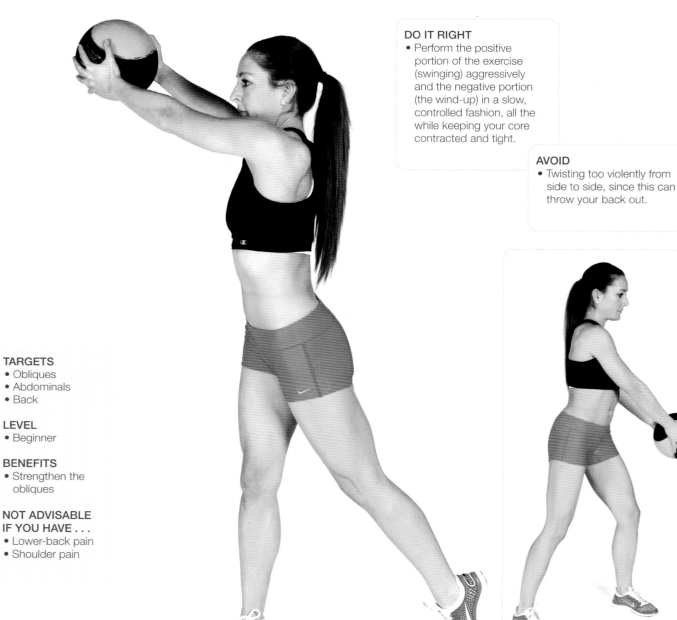

DO IT RIGHT
- Perform the positive portion of the exercise (swinging) aggressively and the negative portion (the wind-up) in a slow, controlled fashion, all the while keeping your core contracted and tight.

AVOID
- Twisting too violently from side to side, since this can throw your back out.

TARGETS
- Obliques
- Abdominals
- Back

LEVEL
- Beginner

BENEFITS
- Strengthen the obliques

NOT ADVISABLE IF YOU HAVE . . .
- Lower-back pain
- Shoulder pain

❶ Stand upright, with your feet shoulder-width apart, holding a medicine ball with both hands to the right side of your head.

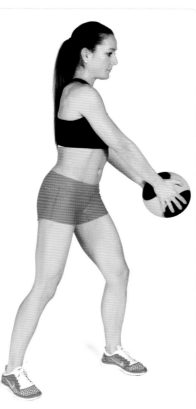

❷ Twist your core toward the left while lowering the medicine ball to the outside of your left leg, then return to the starting position. Repeat 20 times, then switch to the other side.

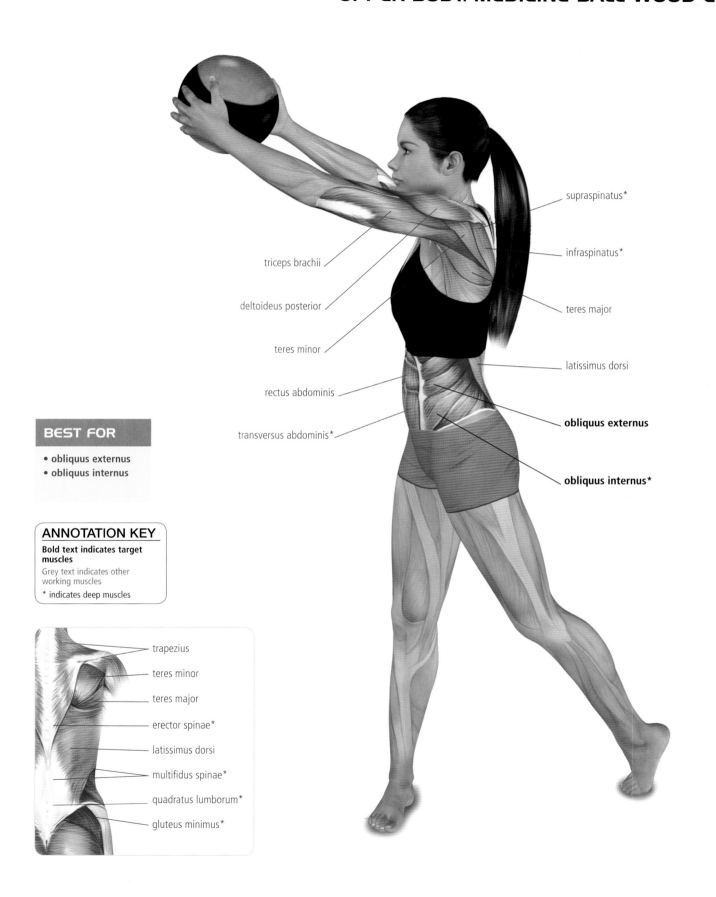

supraspinatus*

infraspinatus*

triceps brachii

teres major

deltoideus posterior

teres minor

latissimus dorsi

rectus abdominis

obliquus externus

transversus abdominis*

obliquus internus*

BEST FOR

- **obliquus externus**
- **obliquus internus**

ANNOTATION KEY

Bold text indicates target muscles

Grey text indicates other working muscles

* indicates deep muscles

trapezius

teres minor

teres major

erector spinae*

latissimus dorsi

multifidus spinae*

quadratus lumborum*

gluteus minimus*

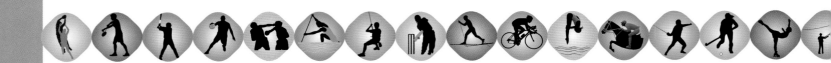

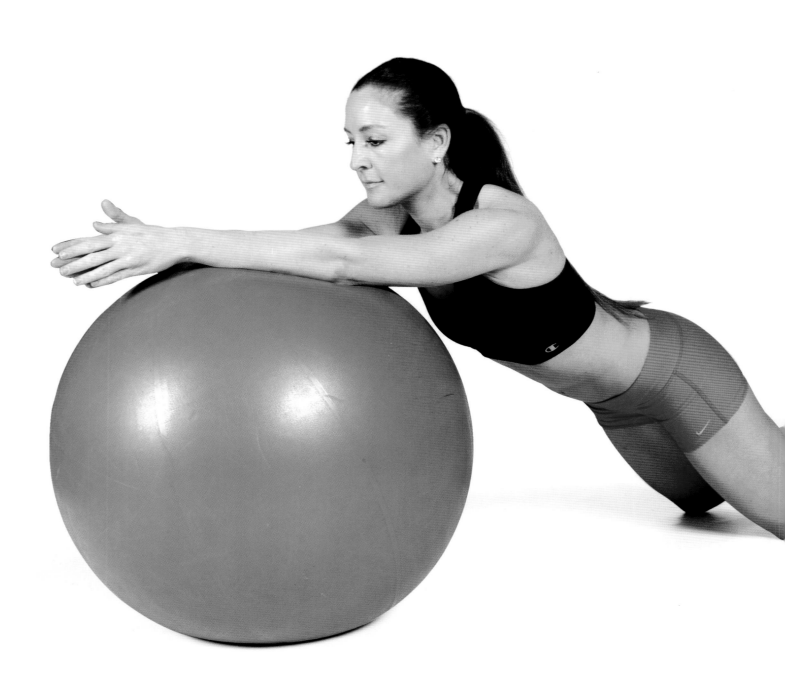

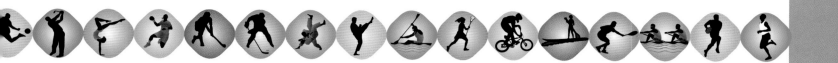

LOWER-BODY EXERCISES

The lower-body exercises provided here represent some of the most effective movements that have been proven to enhance your performance in a given sport or activity. All exercises are clearly defined and have complete step-by-step instructions. This section includes exercises aimed at strengthening and toning all the muscle groups of the legs, the hips, and the backside. The routines provided later in the book use these exercises in the most effective combinations for specific sports or activities. However, feel free to dip into these pages and enjoy the individual exercises at any time to introduce variety into your workout. As always, it is important to pay strict to attention to form to be sure to fire from the intended muscle rather than rely on ancillary help. All levels of experience are represented with plenty of variety. Enjoy!

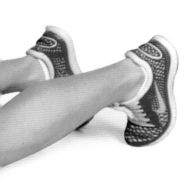

SWISS BALL WALL SIT

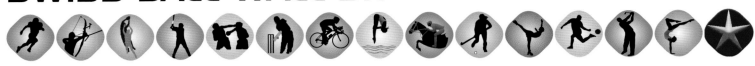

1 Place a Swiss ball against a wall and stand with your back to it so that your back and shoulders are pinning it to the wall. Your feet should be about hip-width apart, but slightly ahead of your hips.

DO IT RIGHT
- Place your feet ahead of your hips by half the length of your thigh.
- Keep your body firm throughout the exercise.
- Relax your shoulders and neck.

AVOID
- Sitting below 90 degrees.
- Shifting from side to side as you begin to fatigue.

2 Raise your arms straight in front of you and relax the upper torso. Keeping the ball pinned against the wall, slowly bend your hips and knees as you lower to a sitting position, rolling the ball down the wall with you as you sit.

3 Hold for a count of 10 and then press back to the starting position, rolling the ball up the wall with your shoulders as you rise. Repeat for a second set of 10.

TARGETS
- Quadriceps
- Glutes

LEVEL
- Intermediate

BENEFITS
- Strengthens quadriceps and gluteal muscles
- Trains the body to place weight evenly between the legs

NOT ADVISABLE IF YOU HAVE . . .
- Knee pain

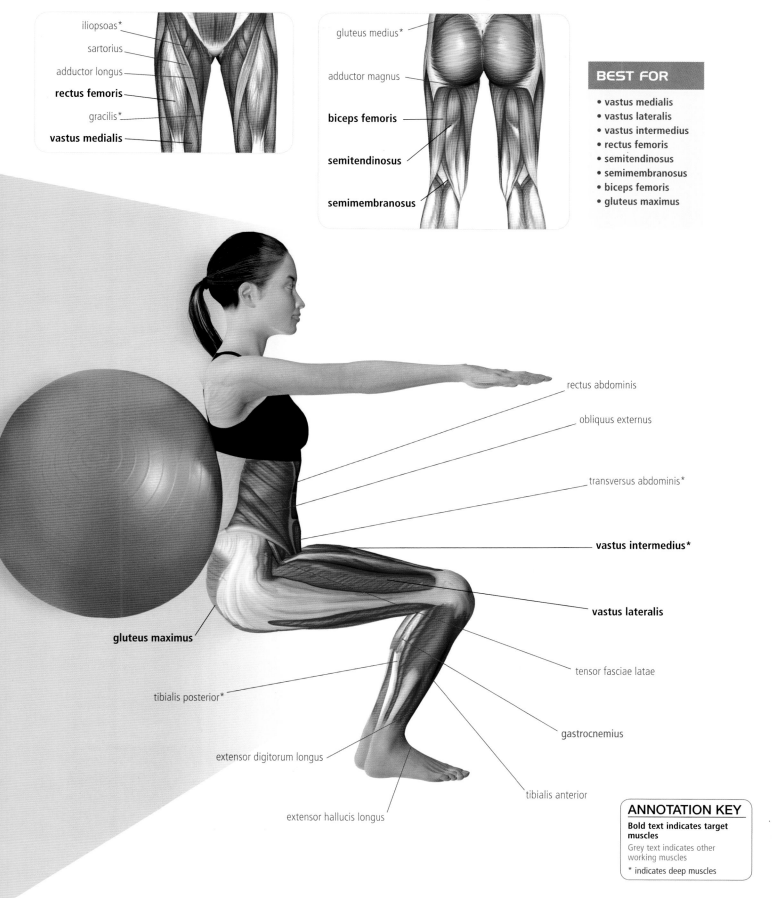

iliopsoas*
sartorius
adductor longus
rectus femoris
gracilis*
vastus medialis

gluteus medius*
adductor magnus
biceps femoris
semitendinosus
semimembranosus

BEST FOR

• vastus medialis
• vastus lateralis
• vastus intermedius
• rectus femoris
• semitendinosus
• semimembranosus
• biceps femoris
• gluteus maximus

rectus abdominis
obliquus externus
transversus abdominis*
vastus intermedius*
vastus lateralis
tensor fasciae latae
gastrocnemius
tibialis anterior

gluteus maximus
tibialis posterior*
extensor digitorum longus
extensor hallucis longus

ANNOTATION KEY

Bold text indicates target muscles

Grey text indicates other working muscles

* indicates deep muscles

BARBELL SQUAT

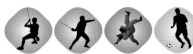

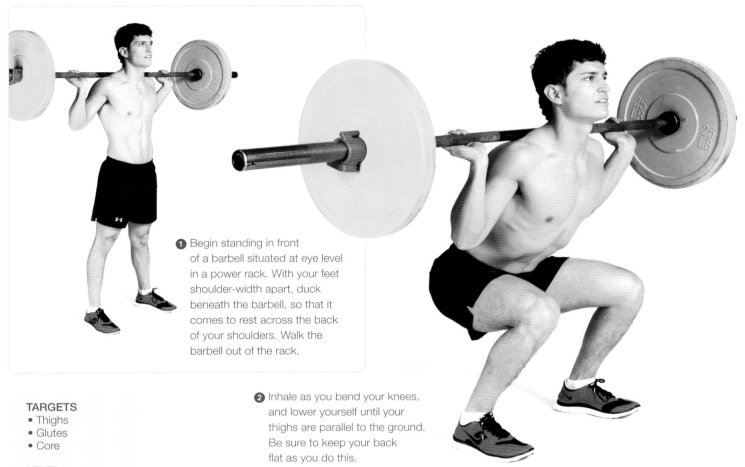

1 Begin standing in front of a barbell situated at eye level in a power rack. With your feet shoulder-width apart, duck beneath the barbell, so that it comes to rest across the back of your shoulders. Walk the barbell out of the rack.

2 Inhale as you bend your knees, and lower yourself until your thighs are parallel to the ground. Be sure to keep your back flat as you do this.

TARGETS
- Thighs
- Glutes
- Core

LEVEL
- Intermediate

BENEFITS
- Increases power and mass in the thighs

NOT ADVISABLE IF YOU HAVE . . .
- Knee pain

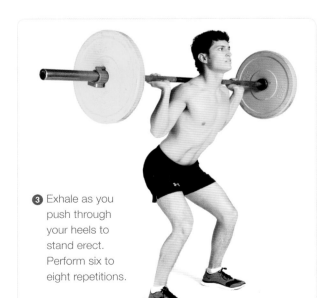

3 Exhale as you push through your heels to stand erect. Perform six to eight repetitions.

DO IT RIGHT
- Squat deep while keeping your thighs parallel to the ground.

AVOID
- Hyperextending your knees past your toes.

BEST FOR

- vastus intermedius
- vastus lateralis
- vastus medialis
- rectus femoris
- semitendinosus
- biceps femoris
- semimembranosus
- gluteus maximus
- gluteus medius
- gluteus minimus

ANNOTATION KEY

Bold text indicates target muscles

Grey text indicates other working muscles

* indicates deep muscles

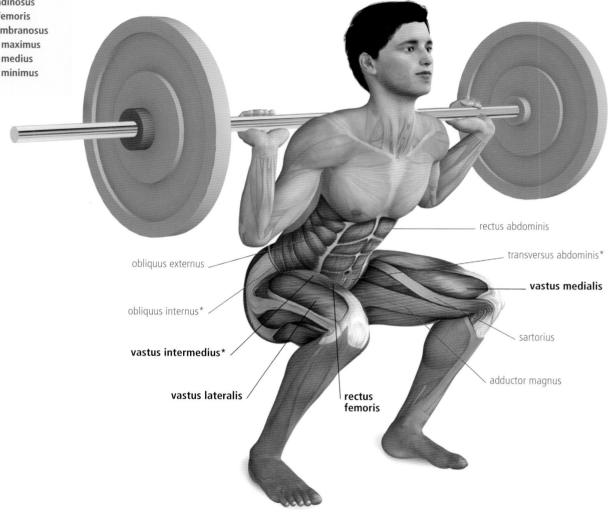

rectus abdominis

transversus abdominis*

vastus medialis

obliquus externus

obliquus internus*

sartorius

adductor magnus

vastus intermedius*

vastus lateralis

rectus femoris

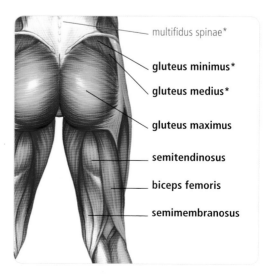

multifidus spinae*

gluteus minimus*

gluteus medius*

gluteus maximus

semitendinosus

biceps femoris

semimembranosus

MODIFICATIONS

Easier: Complete the exercise as in the steps illustrated, but using your own body weight (right) instead of a barbell.

More difficult: Vary your foot stance. Bringing your feet closer together tends to increase the range of motion required, making the exercise more difficult.

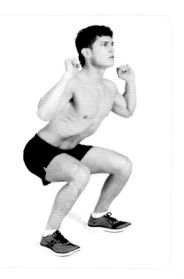

DUMBBELL LUNGE

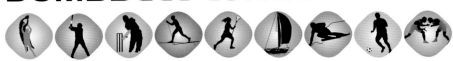

1 Stand with your feet planted about shoulder-width apart, with your arms at your sides and a hand weight or dumbbell in each hand.

2 Keeping your head up and your spine neutral, take a big step forward.

DO IT RIGHT
- Keep your body facing forward as you step one leg in front of you.
- Stand upright.
- Gaze forward.
- Ease into the lunge.
- Make sure that your front knee is facing forward.

AVOID
- Turning your body to one side.
- Allowing your knee to extend past your foot.
- Arching your back.

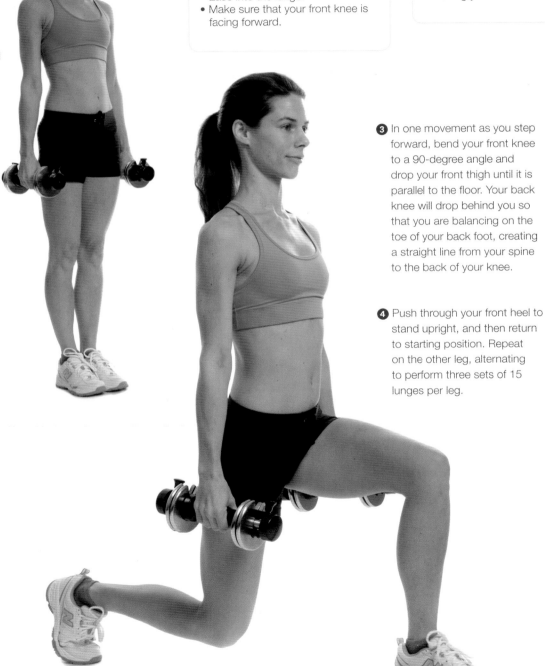

3 In one movement as you step forward, bend your front knee to a 90-degree angle and drop your front thigh until it is parallel to the floor. Your back knee will drop behind you so that you are balancing on the toe of your back foot, creating a straight line from your spine to the back of your knee.

4 Push through your front heel to stand upright, and then return to starting position. Repeat on the other leg, alternating to perform three sets of 15 lunges per leg.

TARGETS
- Glutes
- Quadriceps

LEVEL
- Beginner

BENEFITS
- Strengthens and tones quadriceps and glutes

NOT ADVISABLE IF YOU HAVE . . .
- Knee issues

BEST FOR

- gluteus maximus
- rectus femoris
- vastus lateralis
- vastus intermedius
- vastus medialis

ANNOTATION KEY

Bold text indicates target muscles

Grey text indicates other working muscles

* indicates deep muscles

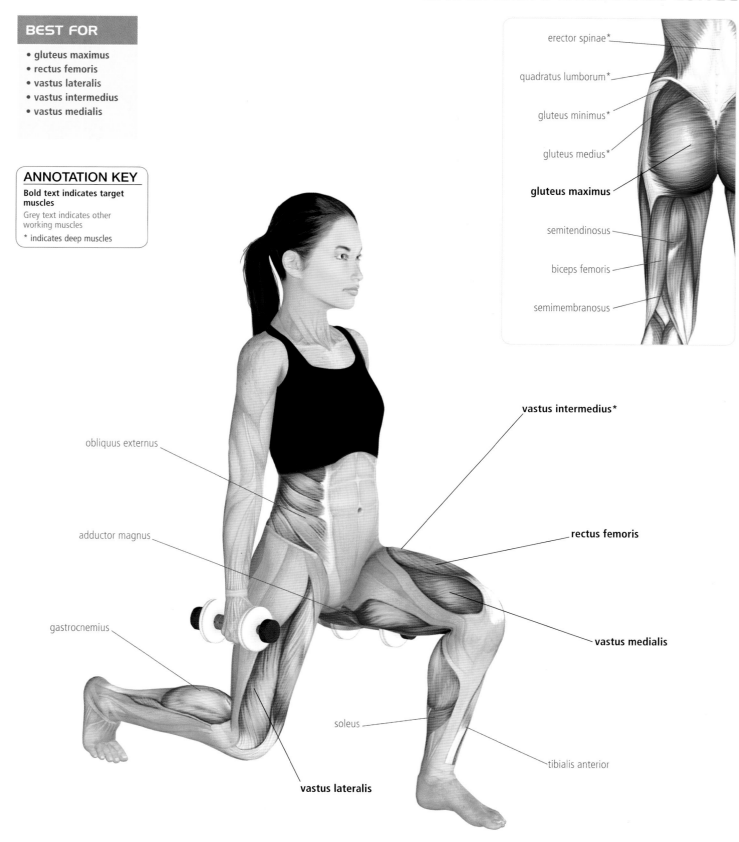

erector spinae*

quadratus lumborum*

gluteus minimus*

gluteus medius*

gluteus maximus

semitendinosus

biceps femoris

semimembranosus

vastus intermedius*

obliquus externus

rectus femoris

adductor magnus

vastus medialis

gastrocnemius

soleus

tibialis anterior

vastus lateralis

REVERSE LUNGE

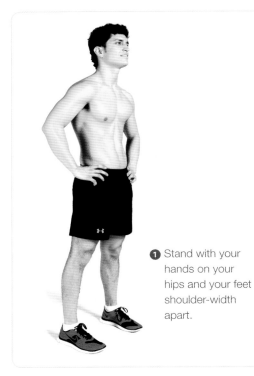

1 Stand with your hands on your hips and your feet shoulder-width apart.

2 Take a big step backward, bending your knees as you do so.

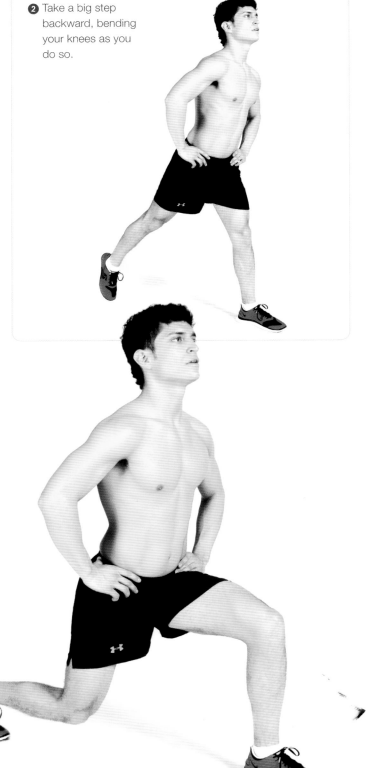

TARGETS
- Quadriceps
- Glutes
- Hamstrings

LEVEL
- Beginner

BENEFITS
- Strengthens the quadriceps and glutes
- Improves balance

NOT ADVISABLE IF YOU HAVE . . .
- Knee issues

DO IT RIGHT
- Maintain an erect posture throughout the movement.

AVOID
- Hyperextending your knee past your toes when lunging.

3 When the front thigh is roughly parallel to the ground, push through your front heel to return to the starting position. Perform 15 repetitions per leg.

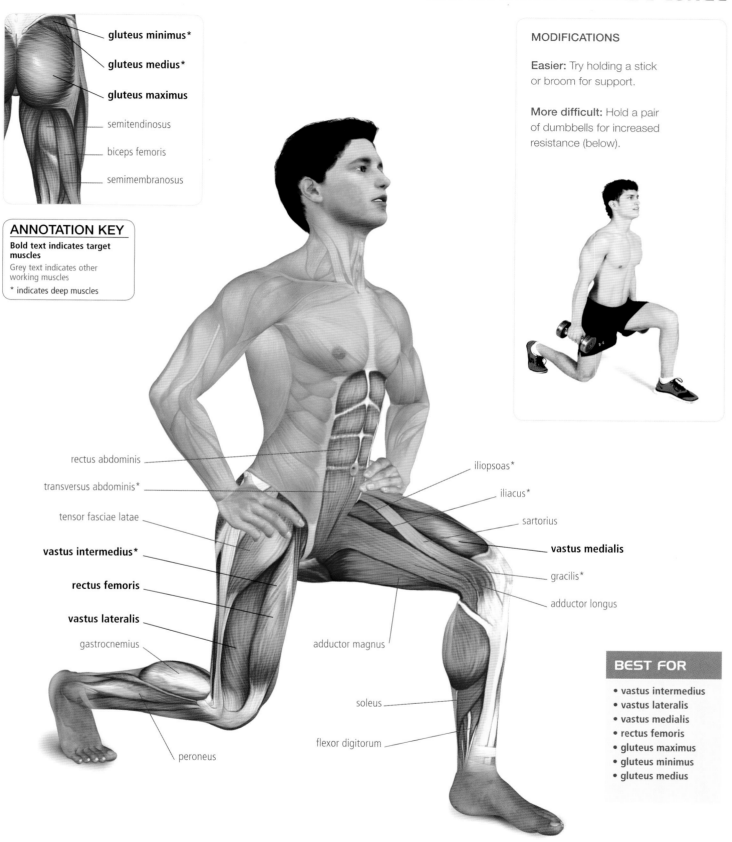

gluteus minimus*

gluteus medius*

gluteus maximus

semitendinosus

biceps femoris

semimembranosus

ANNOTATION KEY

Bold text indicates target muscles

Grey text indicates other working muscles

* indicates deep muscles

MODIFICATIONS

Easier: Try holding a stick or broom for support.

More difficult: Hold a pair of dumbbells for increased resistance (below).

rectus abdominis

transversus abdominis*

tensor fasciae latae

vastus intermedius*

rectus femoris

vastus lateralis

gastrocnemius

peroneus

adductor magnus

soleus

flexor digitorum

iliopsoas*

iliacus*

sartorius

vastus medialis

gracilis*

adductor longus

BEST FOR

- **vastus intermedius**
- **vastus lateralis**
- **vastus medialis**
- **rectus femoris**
- **gluteus maximus**
- **gluteus minimus**
- **gluteus medius**

LATERAL LOW LUNGE

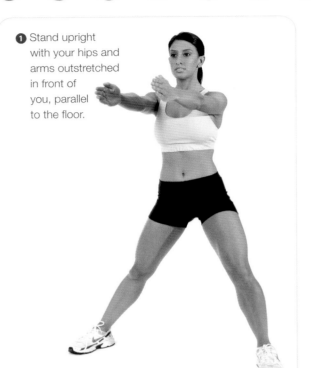

1 Stand upright with your hips and arms outstretched in front of you, parallel to the floor.

DO IT RIGHT
- Your spine should remain neutral as you bend your hips.
- Keep your shoulders and neck relaxed.
- Align your knee with the toe of your bent leg.
- Keep the gluteal muscles tight as you bend.

AVOID
- Craning your neck as you perform the movement.
- Lifting your feet off the floor.
- Arching or extending your back.

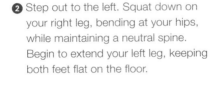

2 Step out to the left. Squat down on your right leg, bending at your hips, while maintaining a neutral spine. Begin to extend your left leg, keeping both feet flat on the floor.

3 Bend your right knee until your thigh is parallel to the floor, and your left leg is fully extended.

4 Keeping your arms parallel to the ground, squeeze your buttocks and press off your right leg to return to the starting position, and repeat. Repeat sequence 10 times on each side.

TARGETS
- Glutes
- Quadriceps

LEVEL
- Beginner

BENEFITS
- Strengthens the pelvic, trunk and knee stabilizers

NOT ADVISABLE IF YOU HAVE . . .
- Sharp knee pain
- Back pain
- Trouble bearing weight on one leg

BEST FOR

- adductor longus
- adductor magnus
- sartorius
- vastus lateralis
- rectus femoris
- transversus abdominis
- trapezius
- rhombodieus

ANNOTATION KEY

Bold text indicates target muscles

Grey text indicates other working muscles

* indicates deep muscles

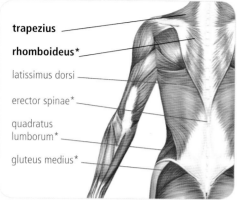

trapezius

rhomboideus*

latissimus dorsi

erector spinae*

quadratus lumborum*

gluteus medius*

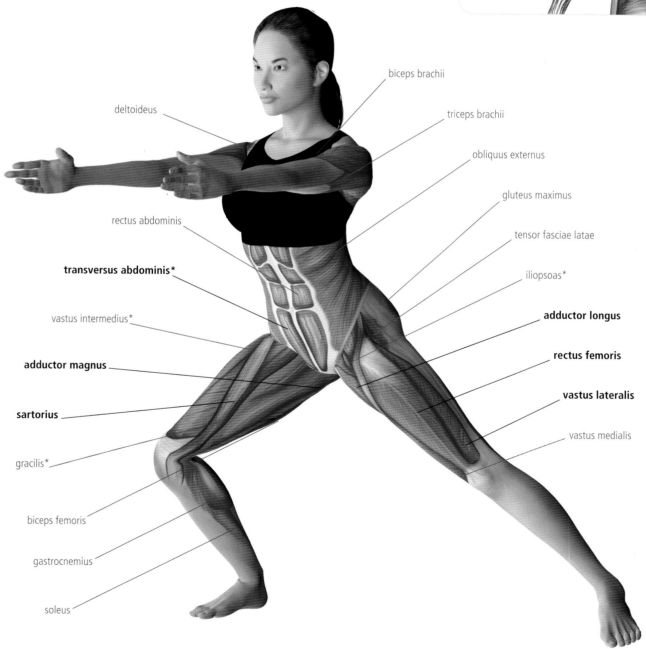

deltoideus

biceps brachii

triceps brachii

obliquus externus

gluteus maximus

rectus abdominis

tensor fasciae latae

transversus abdominis*

iliopsoas*

adductor longus

vastus intermedius*

rectus femoris

adductor magnus

vastus lateralis

sartorius

vastus medialis

gracilis*

biceps femoris

gastrocnemius

soleus

DUMBBELL WALKING LUNGE

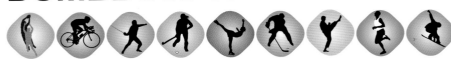

1 Stand with your feet parallel and slightly narrower than shoulder-width apart, holding a dumbbell in each hand in hammer-grip position, palms facing each other. Keep your arms close to the sides of your body.

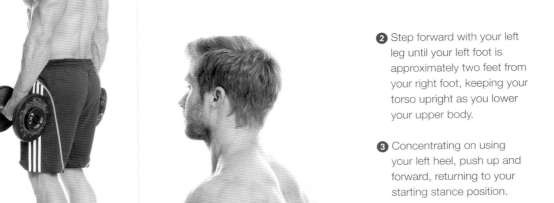

DO IT RIGHT
- Keep your front shin perpendicular to the ground.
- Keep your torso upright for the duration of this exercise.

AVOID
- Allowing the stepping knee to go forward beyond your toes as you lower down — this could stress the knee joint and cause possible injury.

2 Step forward with your left leg until your left foot is approximately two feet from your right foot, keeping your torso upright as you lower your upper body.

3 Concentrating on using your left heel, push up and forward, returning to your starting stance position.

4 Repeat steps 2 and 3 starting with right leg.

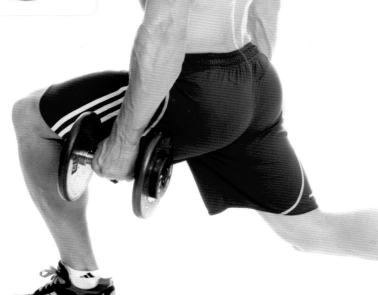

TARGETS
- Quadriceps
- Glutes

LEVEL
- Advanced

BENEFITS
- Increases power and mass in the quads and glutes

NOT ADVISABLE IF YOU HAVE . . .
- Knee pain

TRAINER'S TIPS
- Think of this exercise as an etiquette class in which you must balance a book on the top of your head. This will ensure that you attain proper upper-body posture while executing your lunge.

BEST FOR

- rectus femoris
- vastus lateralis
- vastus intermedius
- adductor magnus
- gluteus maximus
- soleus

ANNOTATION KEY

Bold text indicates target muscles

Grey text indicates other working muscles

* indicates deep muscles

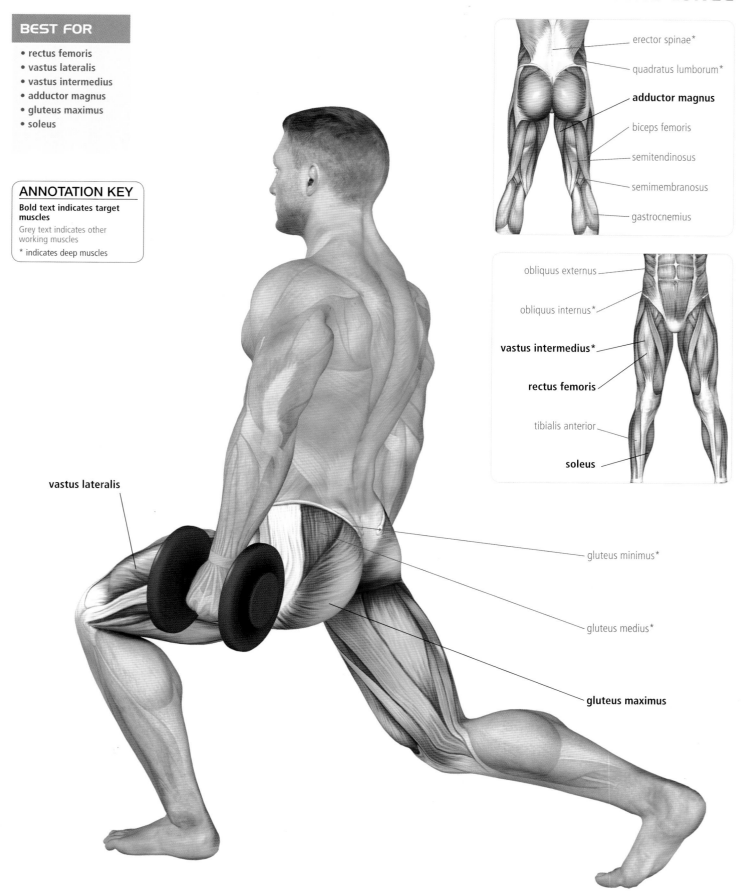

erector spinae*

quadratus lumborum*

adductor magnus

biceps femoris

semitendinosus

semimembranosus

gastrocnemius

obliquus externus

obliquus internus*

vastus intermedius*

rectus femoris

tibialis anterior

soleus

vastus lateralis

gluteus minimus*

gluteus medius*

gluteus maximus

HIGH LUNGE

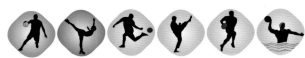

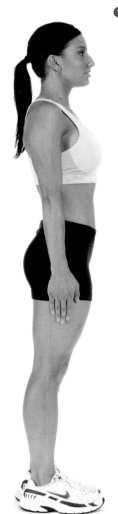

1 Standing tall, move your right foot forward and bend at the hips, bringing your hands down to either side of your foot.

DO IT RIGHT
• Lengthen your spine by maintaining the proper position of your shoulders and whole upper body.

AVOID
• Dropping your back-extended knee to the floor.

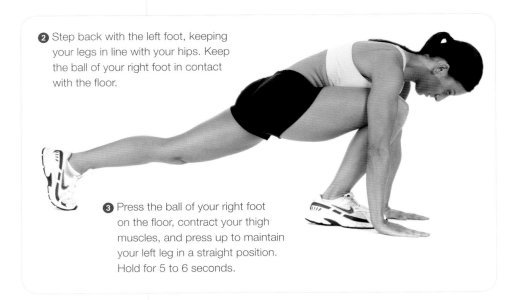

2 Step back with the left foot, keeping your legs in line with your hips. Keep the ball of your right foot in contact with the floor.

3 Press the ball of your right foot on the floor, contract your thigh muscles, and press up to maintain your left leg in a straight position. Hold for 5 to 6 seconds.

TARGETS
• Legs
• Abdominals

LEVEL
• Beginner

BENEFITS
• Stretches groins
• Strengthens legs and abdominals

NOT ADVISABLE IF YOU HAVE . . .
• Hip injury
• High or low blood pressure

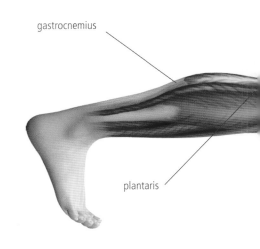

gastrocnemius

plantaris

4 Slowly return to standing position, and then repeat on the right side. Repeat 10 times on each side.

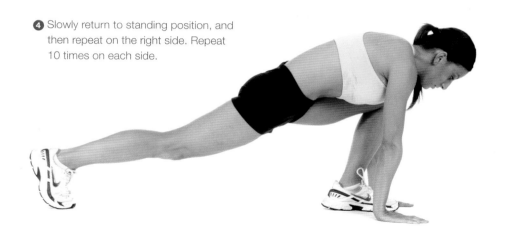

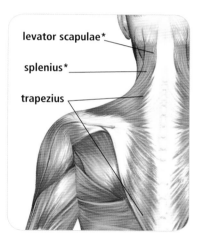

levator scapulae*

splenius*

trapezius

BEST FOR

- gluteus medius
- gluteus maximus
- adductor magnus
- vastus lateralis
- semimembranosus
- rectus femoris
- levator scapulae
- splenius
- trapezius

ANNOTATION KEY

Bold text indicates target muscles

Grey text indicates other working muscles

* indicates deep muscles

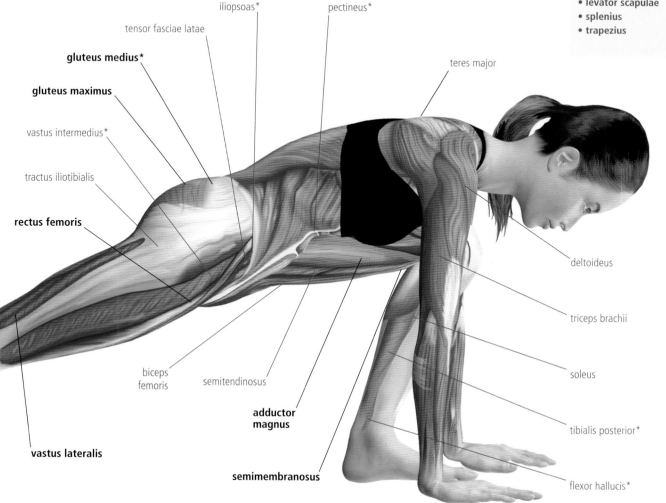

iliopsoas*

tensor fasciae latae

pectineus*

gluteus medius*

teres major

gluteus maximus

vastus intermedius*

tractus iliotibialis

rectus femoris

deltoideus

triceps brachii

biceps femoris

semitendinosus

soleus

adductor magnus

tibialis posterior*

vastus lateralis

semimembranosus

flexor hallucis*

147

CROSSOVER STEP

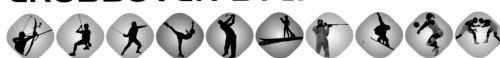

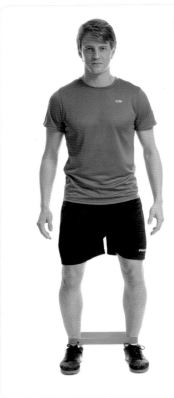

1 Stand with your feet shoulder-width apart, with a resistance loop or a resistance band tied around your ankles. Tuck your pelvis slightly forward, lift your chest and press your shoulders downward and back.

DO IT RIGHT
- Flex the toes of the moving foot toward your shin.
- Keep your hips square and pointed forward.
- Move at a pace that allows you to keep tension in the resistance band.

AVOID
- Rotating your torso.
- Hunching your shoulders.

TARGETS
- Hip adductors

LEVEL
- Beginner

BENEFITS
- Strengthens hips

NOT ADVISABLE IF YOU HAVE . . .
- Acute hip pain

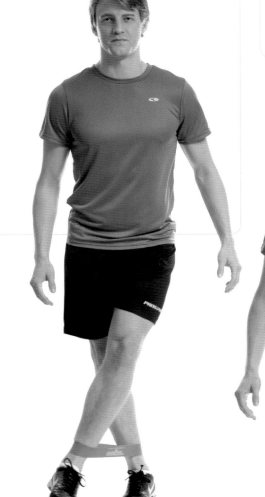

2 Step out with your left foot until you feel moderate tension in the band, and then cross your left foot over your right.

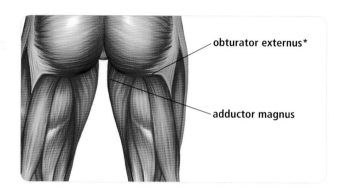

obturator externus*

adductor magnus

BEST FOR

- adductor longus
- adductor magnus
- adductor brevis
- gracilis
- pectineus
- obturator externus

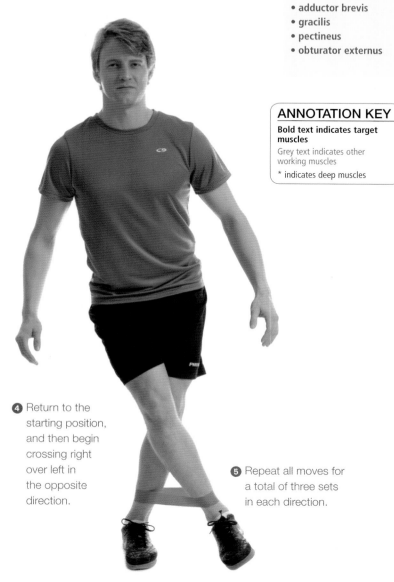

ANNOTATION KEY

Bold text indicates target muscles

Grey text indicates other working muscles

* indicates deep muscles

③ Next, step your right foot in front of your left, and then step your left foot out, for a total of three steps with both feet to the left.

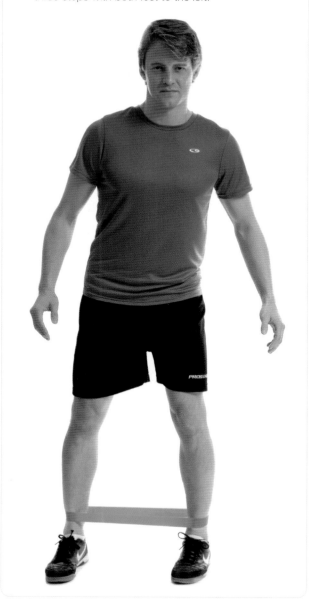

④ Return to the starting position, and then begin crossing right over left in the opposite direction.

⑤ Repeat all moves for a total of three sets in each direction.

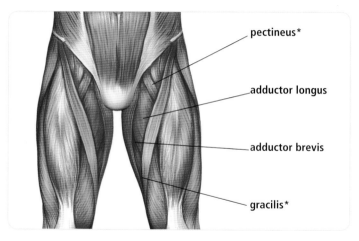

pectineus*

adductor longus

adductor brevis

gracilis*

GOBLET SQUAT

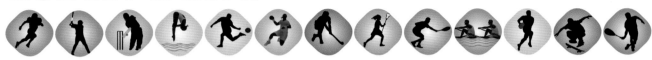

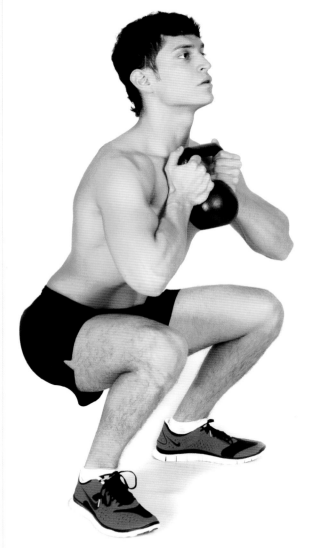

DO IT RIGHT
- Always employ a full range of motion.

AVOID
- Hyperextending your knees past your toes.

TARGETS
- Quadriceps
- Calves
- Glutes
- Hamstrings
- Shoulders

LEVEL
- Beginner

BENEFITS
- Helps build strength in the quadriceps

NOT ADVISABLE IF YOU HAVE . . .
- Acute hip pain

MODIFICATIONS
- **Easier:** A wider stance will reduce range of motion.
- **More difficult:** A closer stance will increase range of motion.

❶ While in a standing position, hold a kettlebell with both hands close to your chest. Your legs should be a little more than shoulder-width apart, with your toes pointing slightly outward.

❷ Squat down until your thighs are parallel to the floor, bringing your elbows to your thighs.

❸ Keep your back flat as you push through your heels back to the standing position. Complete 8 to 10 repetitions.

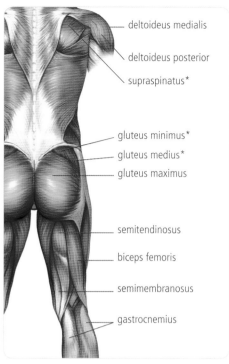

deltoideus medialis

deltoideus posterior

supraspinatus*

gluteus minimus*

gluteus medius*

gluteus maximus

semitendinosus

biceps femoris

semimembranosus

gastrocnemius

ANNOTATION KEY

Bold text indicates target muscles

Grey text indicates other working muscles

* indicates deep muscles

BEST FOR

- **vastus intermedius**
- **vastus lateralis**
- **vastus medialis**
- **rectus femoris**

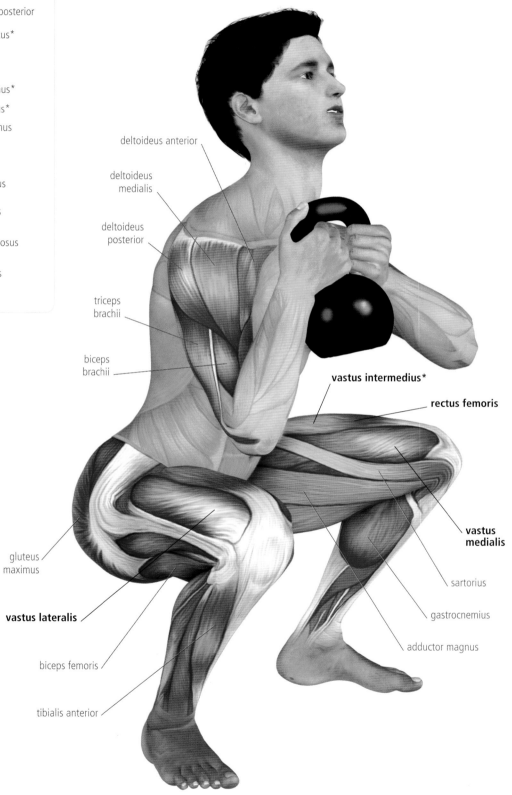

deltoideus anterior

deltoideus medialis

deltoideus posterior

triceps brachii

biceps brachii

vastus intermedius*

rectus femoris

vastus medialis

gluteus maximus

sartorius

gastrocnemius

adductor magnus

vastus lateralis

biceps femoris

tibialis anterior

151

ONE-LEGGED STEP-DOWN

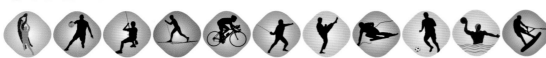

1 Stand facing forward on a step.

DO IT RIGHT
• Move slowly and with control.
• Focus on maintaining good form.

TARGETS
• Quadriceps
• Glutes

LEVEL
Intermediate

BENEFITS
• Strengthens pelvic and knee stabilizers

**NOT ADVISABLE
IF YOU HAVE . . .**
• Knee issues

TRAINER'S TIPS
• Hold onto a wall if it helps you maintain balance and good form when you first try this exercise.

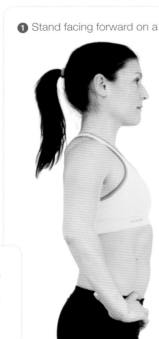
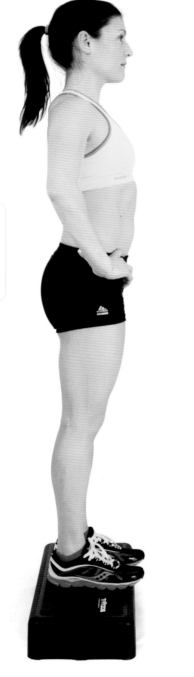

2 Step down to the floor with your left leg, Lift your right heel so that only your right toe is on the step; you should be balancing on the ball of your foot. As you step, bend your arms and raise your hands to shoulder height.

3 Gradually straighten your supporting leg and return to the starting position. Switch legs and repeat, completing 20 repetitions.

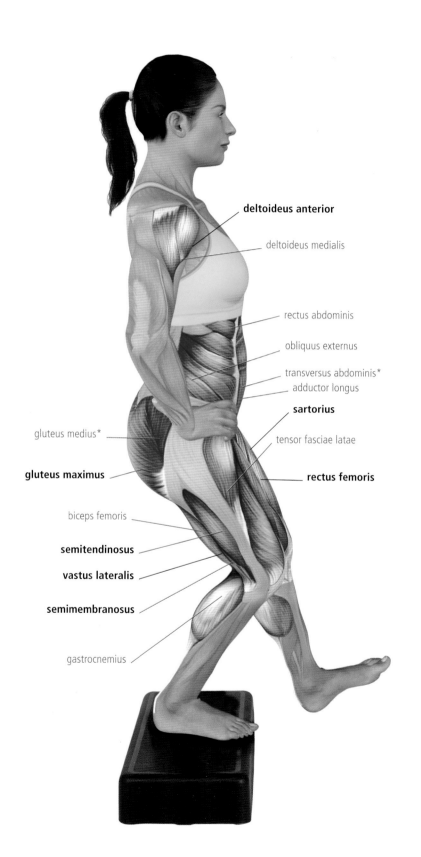

deltoideus anterior

deltoideus medialis

rectus abdominis

obliquus externus

transversus abdominis*
adductor longus

sartorius

tensor fasciae latae

rectus femoris

gluteus medius*

gluteus maximus

biceps femoris

semitendinosus

vastus lateralis

semimembranosus

gastrocnemius

BEST FOR

- **deltoideus anterior**
- **quadratus lumborum**
- **vastus lateralis**
- **vastus intermedius**
- **vastus medialis**
- **sartorius**
- **rectus femoris**
- **gluteus maximus**
- **semitendinosus**
- **semimembranosus**
- **gluteus minimus**

ANNOTATION KEY

Bold text indicates target muscles

Grey text indicates other working muscles

* indicates deep muscles

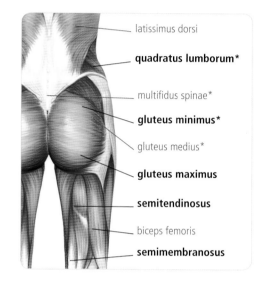

latissimus dorsi

quadratus lumborum*

multifidus spinae*

gluteus minimus*

gluteus medius*

gluteus maximus

semitendinosus

biceps femoris

semimembranosus

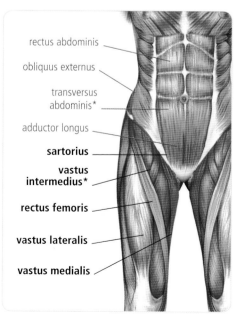

rectus abdominis

obliquus externus

transversus abdominis*

adductor longus

sartorius

vastus intermedius*

rectus femoris

vastus lateralis

vastus medialis

153

KNEE EXTENSION WITH ROTATION

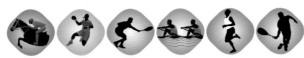

1. Sit upright on a chair, with your feet planted on the floor, your hands on your knees, and your gaze forward.

2. Slowly extend and raise one leg as high as you can, or until it is parallel to the floor, with your foot flexed. Rotate it outward, pausing at the top of the circle, and then rotate your foot inward.

3. Lower your foot, and repeat on the other side. Continue to alternate, performing two sets of 10 per side

TARGETS
• Inner and outer thighs

LEVEL
• Beginner

BENEFITS
• Strengthens the lateral muscles of the thigh during external rotation phase of exercise
• Strengthens the medial muscles of the thigh during internal rotation phase of exercise

NOT ADVISABLE IF YOU HAVE . . .
• Knee pain
• Ankle pain

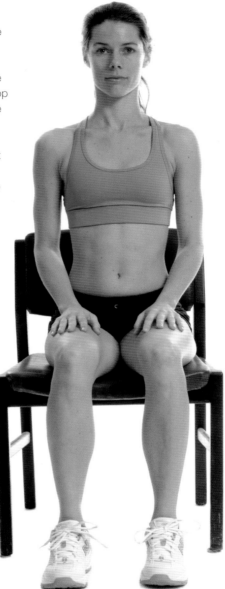

DO IT RIGHT
• Keep the thigh of the moving leg stabilized on the chair.

AVOID
• Lifting your knee.

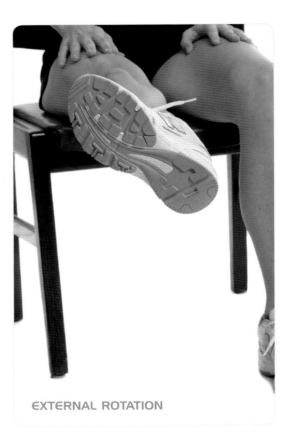

EXTERNAL ROTATION

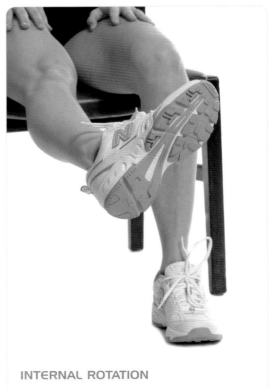

INTERNAL ROTATION

MODIFICATION

Harder: Wrap one end of an resistance band loop around a chair leg, the other around your ankle, and then follow steps 2 and 3.

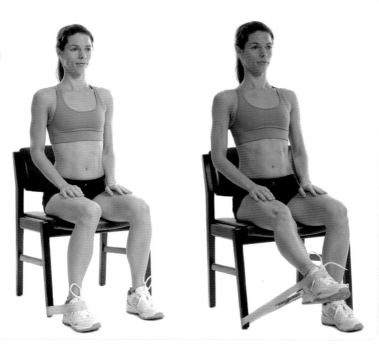

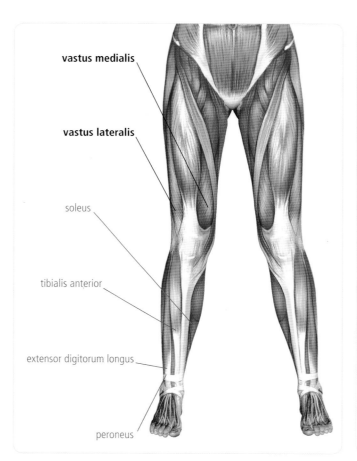

vastus medialis

vastus lateralis

soleus

tibialis anterior

extensor digitorum longus

peroneus

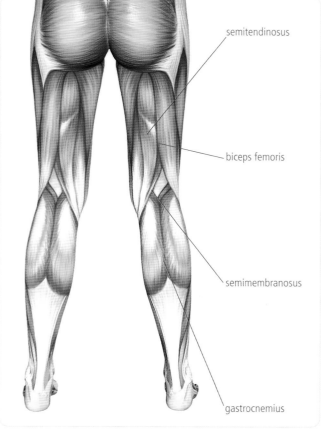

semitendinosus

biceps femoris

semimembranosus

gastrocnemius

STAR JUMP

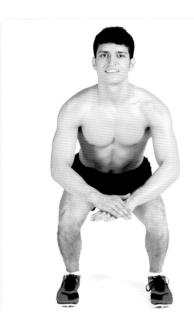

1 Start by crouching down in a half-squat position, with your arms slightly bent in front of you and your hands crossed over each other.

TARGETS
- Quadriceps
- Hamstrings
- Glutes
- Calves

LEVEL
- Beginner

BENEFITS
- Produces explosive power in your lower body

NOT ADVISABLE IF YOU HAVE . . .
- Knee issues

MODIFICATIONS
- **Easier:** Jump at a very low height.
- **More difficult:** Add a higher jump.

DO IT RIGHT
- Be sure to keep a tight core throughout the movement.

AVOID
- Landing excessively hard.

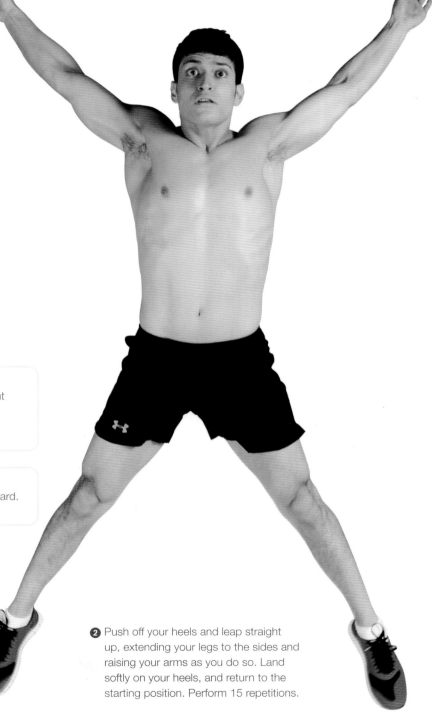

2 Push off your heels and leap straight up, extending your legs to the sides and raising your arms as you do so. Land softly on your heels, and return to the starting position. Perform 15 repetitions.

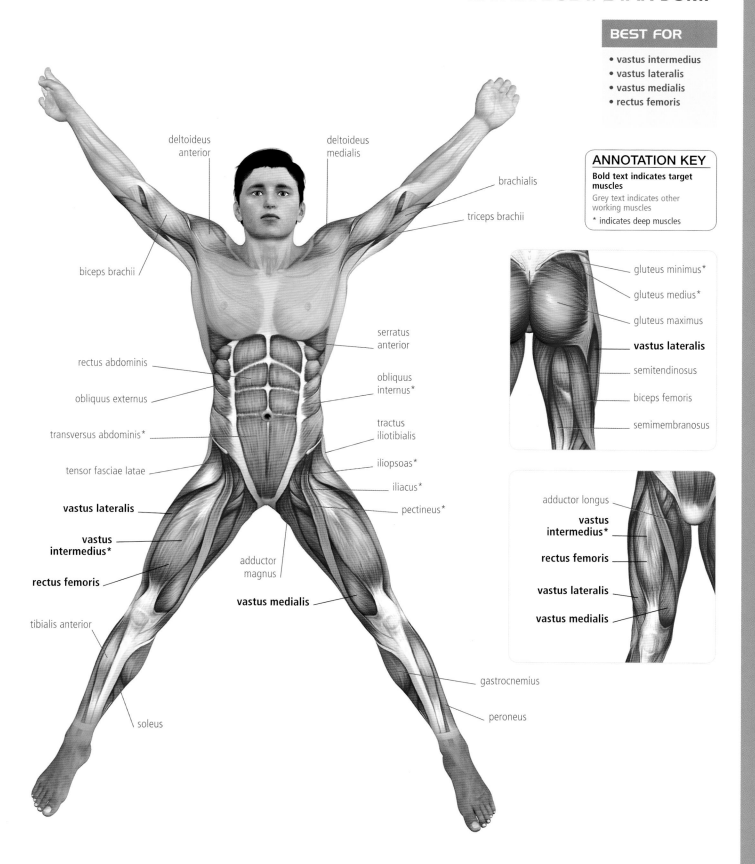

BEST FOR
- vastus intermedius
- vastus lateralis
- vastus medialis
- rectus femoris

ANNOTATION KEY

Bold text indicates target muscles

Grey text indicates other working muscles

* indicates deep muscles

deltoideus anterior

deltoideus medialis

brachialis

triceps brachii

biceps brachii

serratus anterior

rectus abdominis

obliquus internus*

obliquus externus

tractus iliotibialis

transversus abdominis*

iliopsoas*

tensor fasciae latae

iliacus*

pectineus*

vastus lateralis

vastus intermedius*

adductor magnus

rectus femoris

vastus medialis

tibialis anterior

gastrocnemius

peroneus

soleus

gluteus minimus*

gluteus medius*

gluteus maximus

vastus lateralis

semitendinosus

biceps femoris

semimembranosus

adductor longus

vastus intermedius*

rectus femoris

vastus lateralis

vastus medialis

MOUNTAIN CLIMBER

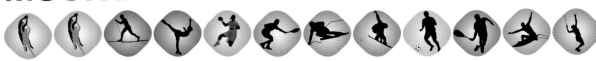

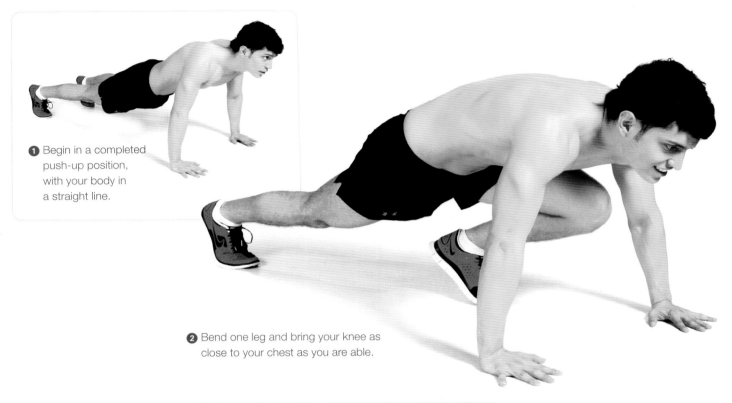

① Begin in a completed push-up position, with your body in a straight line.

② Bend one leg and bring your knee as close to your chest as you are able.

TARGETS
- Quadriceps
- Glutes
- Hamstrings
- Calves
- Core

LEVEL
- Beginner

BENEFITS
- Increases cardiovascular ability and power in the legs

NOT ADVISABLE IF YOU HAVE . . .
- Knee issues

MODIFICATION
- **More difficult:** Wear ankle weights for increased resistance.

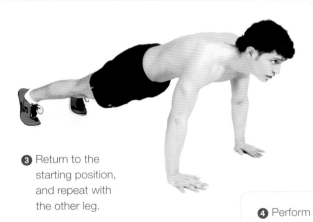

③ Return to the starting position, and repeat with the other leg.

DO IT RIGHT
- Keep your back flat throughout the movement.

AVOID
- Excessively swinging your hips throughout the motion.

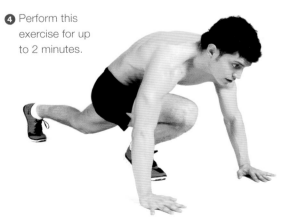

④ Perform this exercise for up to 2 minutes.

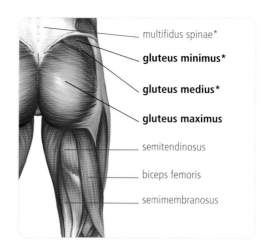

multifidus spinae*

gluteus minimus*

gluteus medius*

gluteus maximus

semitendinosus

biceps femoris

semimembranosus

ANNOTATION KEY

Bold text indicates target muscles

Grey text indicates other working muscles

* indicates deep muscles

BEST FOR

- **vastus intermedius**
- **vastus lateralis**
- **vastus medialis**
- **rectus femoris**
- **gluteus maximus**
- **gluteus minimus**
- **gluteus medius**

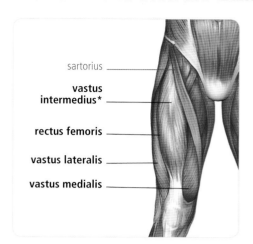

sartorius

vastus intermedius*

rectus femoris

vastus lateralis

vastus medialis

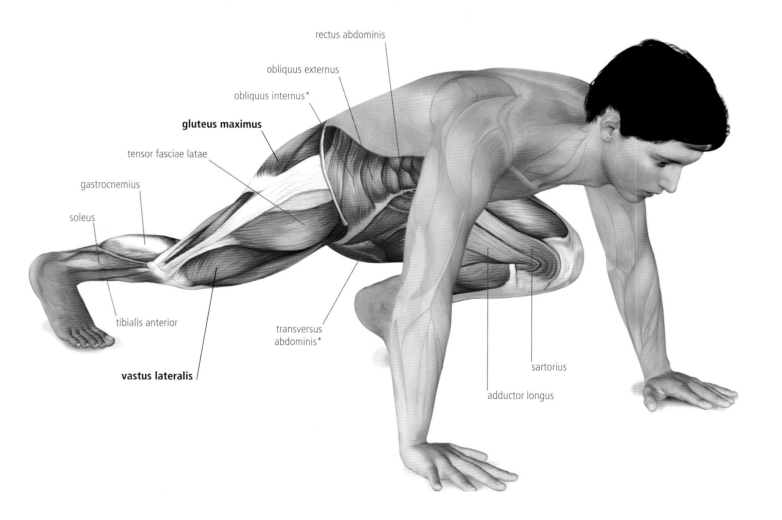

rectus abdominis

obliquus externus

obliquus internus*

gluteus maximus

tensor fasciae latae

gastrocnemius

soleus

tibialis anterior

transversus abdominis*

vastus lateralis

sartorius

adductor longus

BURPEE

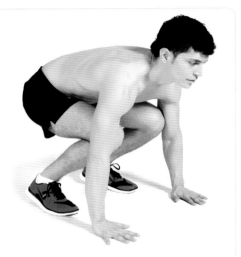

1 Start in a squat position, with your hands firmly planted on the floor, shoulder-width apart.

DO IT RIGHT
- Be sure to keep a tight core throughout the movement.

AVOID
- Landing excessively hard.

TARGETS
- Glutes
- Quadriceps
- Hamstrings
- Back
- Calves

LEVEL
- Intermediate

BENEFITS
- Increases both muscular strength and endurance

NOT ADVISABLE IF YOU HAVE . . .
- Knee issues

MODIFICATIONS
- **Easier:** Jump at a very low height.
- **More difficult:** Add a push-up to the routine.

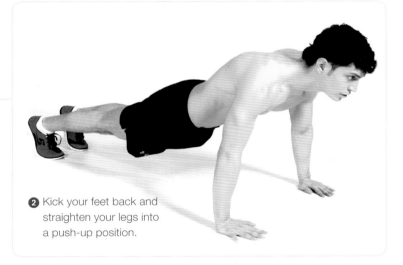

2 Kick your feet back and straighten your legs into a push-up position.

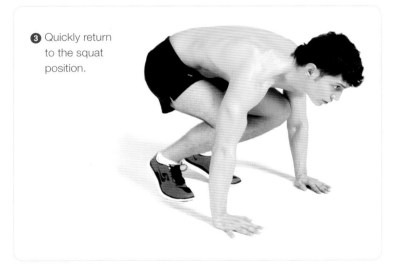

3 Quickly return to the squat position.

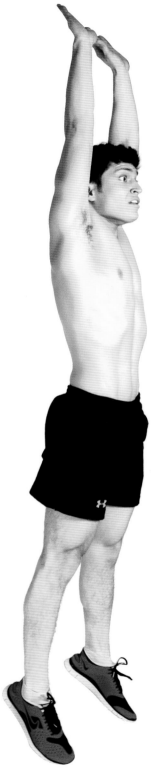

4 Leap vertically from the squat position as high as possible, raising your arms as you jump. Complete 15 repetitions.

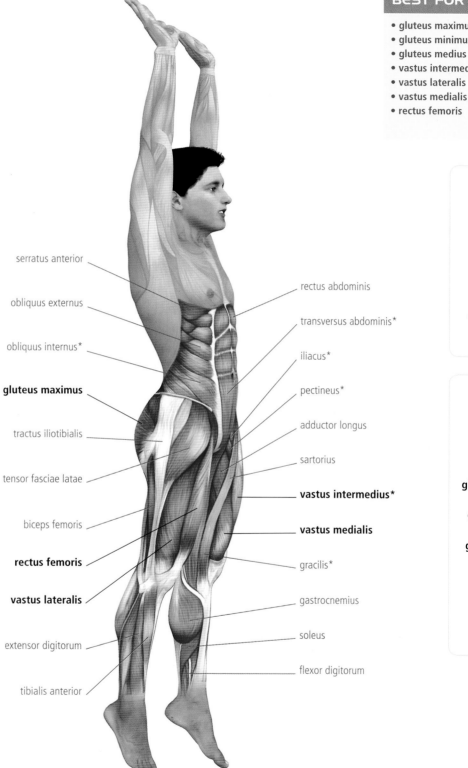

BEST FOR

- gluteus maximus
- gluteus minimus
- gluteus medius
- vastus intermedius
- vastus lateralis
- vastus medialis
- rectus femoris

ANNOTATION KEY

Bold text indicates target muscles

Grey text indicates other working muscles

* indicates deep muscles

serratus anterior

obliquus externus

obliquus internus*

gluteus maximus

tractus iliotibialis

tensor fasciae latae

biceps femoris

rectus femoris

vastus lateralis

extensor digitorum

tibialis anterior

rectus abdominis

transversus abdominis*

iliacus*

pectineus*

adductor longus

sartorius

vastus intermedius*

vastus medialis

gracilis*

gastrocnemius

soleus

flexor digitorum

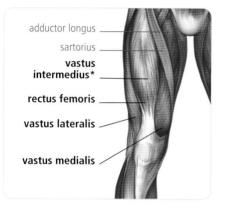

adductor longus

sartorius

vastus intermedius*

rectus femoris

vastus lateralis

vastus medialis

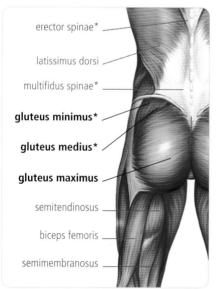

erector spinae*

latissimus dorsi

multifidus spinae*

gluteus minimus*

gluteus medius*

gluteus maximus

semitendinosus

biceps femoris

semimembranosus

ADDUCTOR EXTENSION

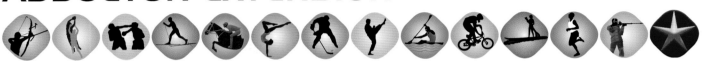

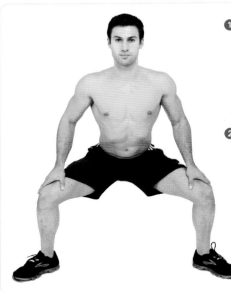

1 Standing, separate your feet wider than hip width, so that you are in a straddle position. Bend your knees.

2 Place your hands on your knees and bend at your hips, keeping your spine in neutral and your shoulders slightly forward.

3 Keeping your torso in the same position and your hips behind your heels, shift your weight to one side, bending your knee while extending your opposite leg. Hold for 10 seconds and repeat on the other side.

DO IT RIGHT
- Keep your trunk aligned as you move from side to side.
- Maintain your hand placement on your thighs to assist your posture.
- Keep your neck and shoulders relaxed.

BEST FOR
- **adductor longus**
- **adductor magnus**
- **peroneus**
- **biceps femoris**
- **semitendinosus**
- **semimembranosus**
- **piriformis**

ANNOTATION KEY
Bold text indicates target muscles
Grey text indicates other working muscles
* indicates deep muscles

AVOID
- Rounding your spine.
- Allowing your feet to shift or lift off the floor.
- Allowing your knees to extend over your toes while bending.

TARGETS
- Hip adductors
- Hamstrings
- Glutes

LEVEL
- Intermediate

BENEFITS
- Stretches hips, hamstrings, and gluteal muscles

NOT ADVISABLE IF YOU HAVE
- Hip injury
- Knee injury

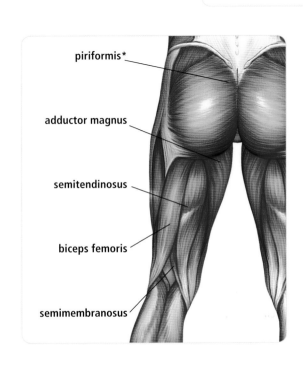

piriformis*

adductor magnus

semitendinosus

biceps femoris

semimembranosus

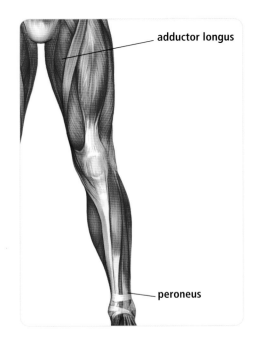

adductor longus

peroneus

HAMSTRING ABDUCTOR

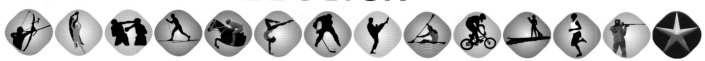

1. Stand with your feet planted well beyond shoulder-width apart, so that you are in a straddle position. Bend your knees.

2. Place both hands on your left knee, keeping your spine in neutral position and your shoulders slightly forward.

3. Keeping your torso in the same position and your hips behind your heels, shift your weight to the left, bending your left knee while extending your right leg. Hold for 10 seconds and repeat on other side.

DO IT RIGHT
- Keep your hips squared and facing forward.

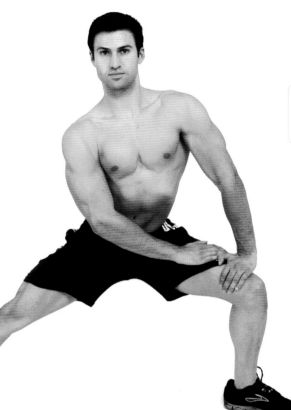

AVOID
- Arching your back, or hunching it forward.

BEST FOR
- abductor longus
- abductor magnus
- peroneus
- biceps femoris
- semitendinosus
- semimembranosus
- piriformis

ANNOTATION KEY

Bold text indicates target muscles

Grey text indicates other working muscles

* indicates deep muscles

TARGETS
- Hamstrings
- Inner thighs

LEVEL
- Intermediate

BENEFITS
- Stretches hamstrings, gluteal muscles, and abductors

NOT ADVISABLE IF YOU HAVE
- Knee injury

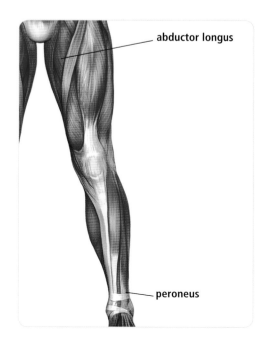

abductor longus

peroneus

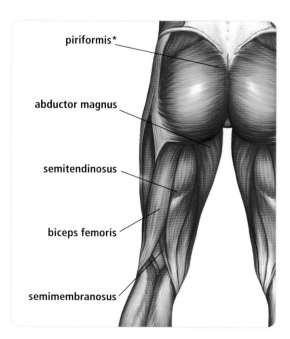

piriformis*

abductor magnus

semitendinosus

biceps femoris

semimembranosus

SWISS BALL HAMSTRING CURL

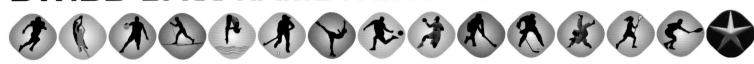

① Lie on your back with your arms along your sides, angled slightly away from your body. Extend your legs and rest your lower legs and ankles on top of a Swiss ball.

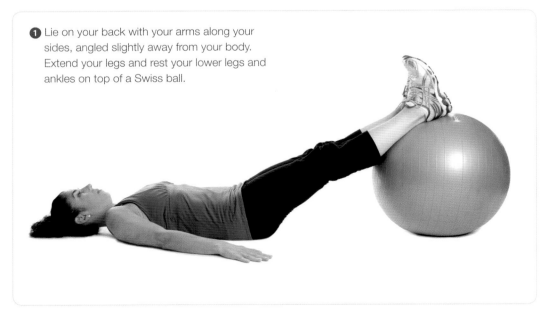

DO IT RIGHT
- Position your legs on the ball to form a 45-degree angle with the rest of your body before you curl.
- Move smoothly, maintaining control of the ball.
- Keep your arms anchored to the floor.
- Engage your abs, and squeeze your glutes.

AVOID
- Rushing through the movement.
- Arching your back in the curl position; instead, keep it as straight as possible.

TARGETS
- Glutes
- Hamstrings

LEVEL
- Intermediate

BENEFITS
- Strengthens and tones hamstrings and glutes

AVOID IF YOU HAVE . . .
- Lower-back issues
- Shoulder issues
- Neck issues

② Pressing downward with your feet, bend your knees as you roll the ball toward you. Curl your pelvis, and raise your lower body off the floor. Hold for 5 seconds.

③ With control, return to starting position and then repeat, working up to three sets of 15 repetitions.

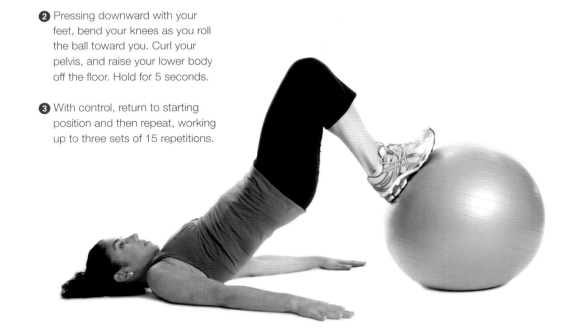

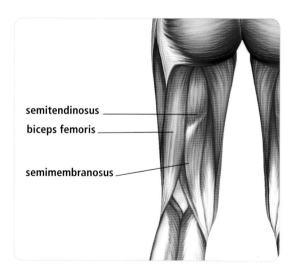

semitendinosus

biceps femoris

semimembranosus

BEST FOR

- biceps femoris
- semitendinosus
- semimembranosus

ANNOTATION KEY

Bold text indicates target muscles

Grey text indicates other working muscles

* indicates deep muscles

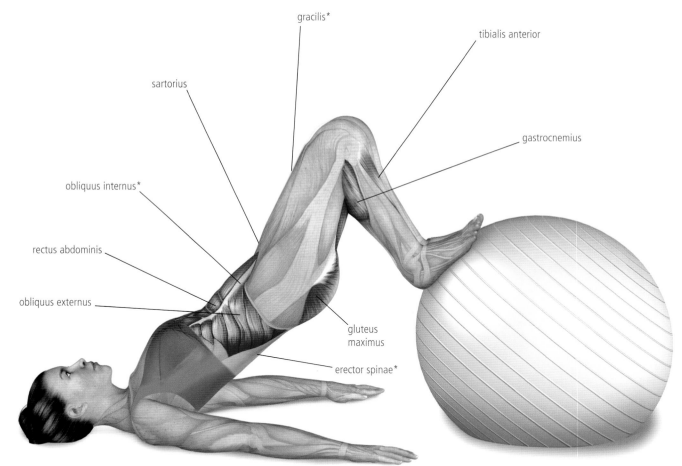

gracilis*

tibialis anterior

sartorius

gastrocnemius

obliquus internus*

rectus abdominis

obliquus externus

gluteus maximus

erector spinae*

INVERTED HAMSTRING

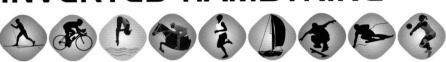

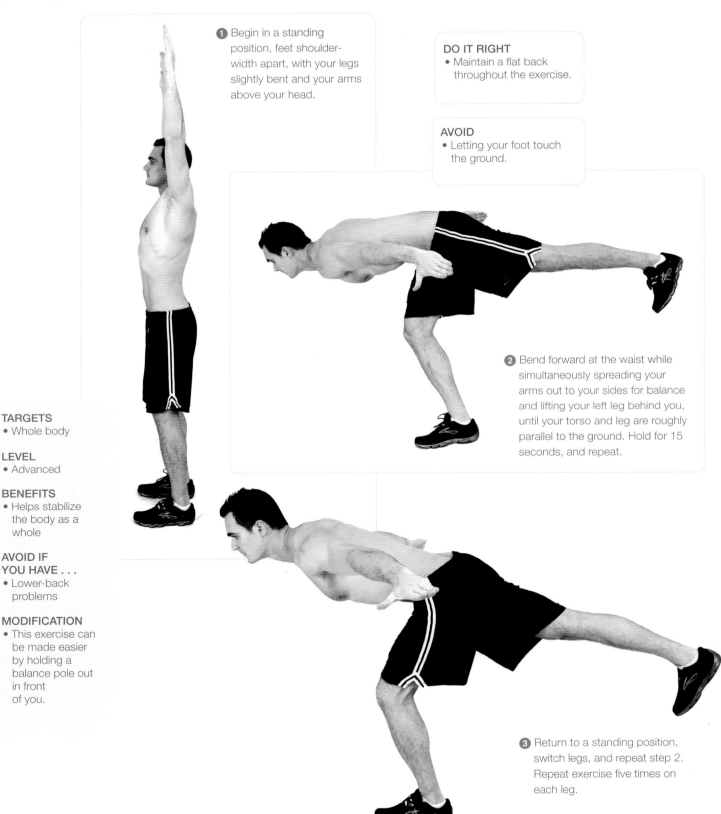

1 Begin in a standing position, feet shoulder-width apart, with your legs slightly bent and your arms above your head.

DO IT RIGHT
• Maintain a flat back throughout the exercise.

AVOID
• Letting your foot touch the ground.

2 Bend forward at the waist while simultaneously spreading your arms out to your sides for balance and lifting your left leg behind you, until your torso and leg are roughly parallel to the ground. Hold for 15 seconds, and repeat.

TARGETS
• Whole body

LEVEL
• Advanced

BENEFITS
• Helps stabilize the body as a whole

AVOID IF YOU HAVE . . .
• Lower-back problems

MODIFICATION
• This exercise can be made easier by holding a balance pole out in front of you.

3 Return to a standing position, switch legs, and repeat step 2. Repeat exercise five times on each leg.

LOWER BODY: INVERTED HAMSTRING

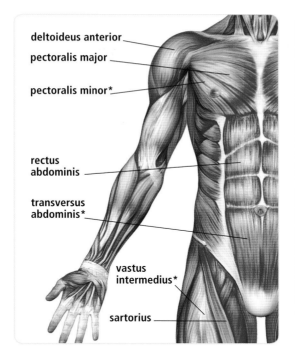

deltoideus anterior
pectoralis major
pectoralis minor*
rectus abdominis
transversus abdominis*
vastus intermedius*
sartorius

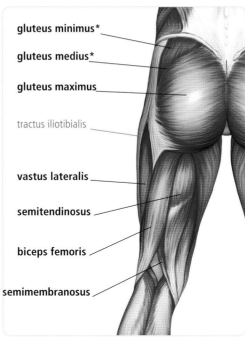

gluteus minimus*
gluteus medius*
gluteus maximus
tractus iliotibialis
vastus lateralis
semitendinosus
biceps femoris
semimembranosus

ANNOTATION KEY

Bold text indicates target muscles

Grey text indicates other working muscles

* indicates deep muscles

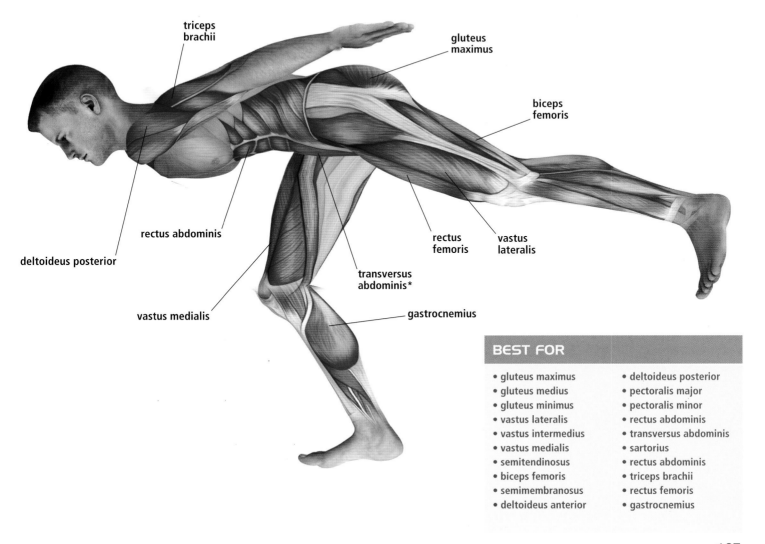

triceps brachii
gluteus maximus
biceps femoris
rectus abdominis
deltoideus posterior
rectus femoris
vastus lateralis
transversus abdominis*
vastus medialis
gastrocnemius

BEST FOR

- gluteus maximus
- gluteus medius
- gluteus minimus
- vastus lateralis
- vastus intermedius
- vastus medialis
- semitendinosus
- biceps femoris
- semimembranosus
- deltoideus anterior
- deltoideus posterior
- pectoralis major
- pectoralis minor
- rectus abdominis
- transversus abdominis
- sartorius
- rectus abdominis
- triceps brachii
- rectus femoris
- gastrocnemius

STIFF-LEGGED BARBELL DEADLIFT

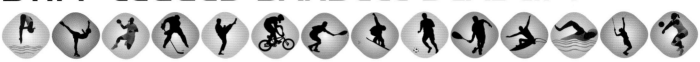

1 Stand with your feet parallel and shoulder-width apart, with a barbell in front of you on the ground. Keeping your back as straight as possible, bend forward and grasp the bar with an overhand grip, palms facing downward.

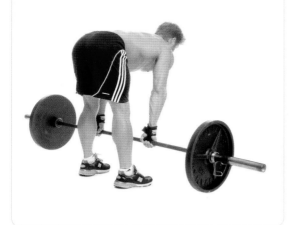

2 With your knees straight or only very slightly bent and shins kept vertical, hips back, and back straight, use your hips to lift the bar.

TARGETS
• Hamstrings
• Glutes
• Lower back

LEVEL
• Advanced

BENEFITS
• Increases power in the hamstrings and glutes

NOT ADVISABLE IF YOU HAVE . . .
• Lower-back issues

TRAINER'S TIPS
• If you find holding onto the bar difficult, wrist straps will secure the bar and allow you to lift a heavier weight.
• This exercise can also be performed using dumbbells in each hand.

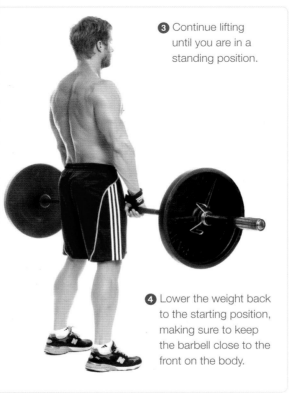

3 Continue lifting until you are in a standing position.

4 Lower the weight back to the starting position, making sure to keep the barbell close to the front on the body.

DO IT RIGHT
• Use a slightly faster movement than with other exercises.
• Maintain a steady but controlled movement — safety and proper form is necessary.

AVOID
• Rounding the back forward when you perform this exercise.
• Using momentum to raise and lower the barbell.

LOWER BODY: STIFF-LEGGED BARBELL DEADLIFT

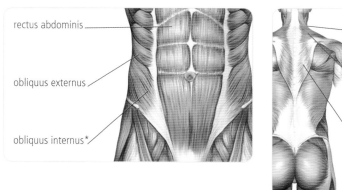

rectus abdominis

obliquus externus

obliquus internus*

levator scapulae*

trapezius

rhomboideus*

semimembranosus

BEST FOR

- **biceps femoris**
- **semitendinosus**
- **semimembranosus**
- **gluteus maximus**
- **erector spinae**

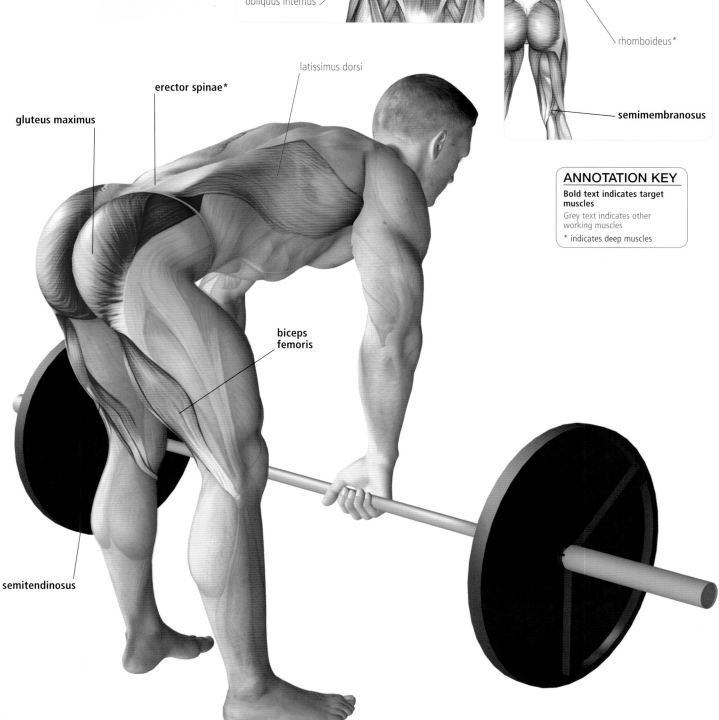

latissimus dorsi

erector spinae*

gluteus maximus

biceps femoris

semitendinosus

ANNOTATION KEY

Bold text indicates target muscles

Grey text indicates other working muscles

* indicates deep muscles

HAMSTRING PULL-IN

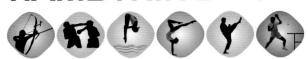

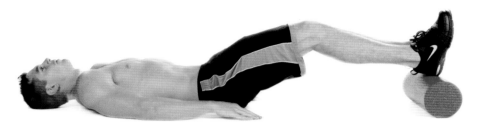

1 Lie supine on the floor, your knees bent and the roller under your feet.

DO IT RIGHT
• Your shoulders should remain relaxed throughout the exercise.
• Your body should form a straight line from shoulder to knee.

2 Pull your legs inward, rolling the bridge of your foot onto the top of the roller.

TARGETS
• Hamstrings
• Glutes

LEVEL
• Intermediate

BENEFITS
• Increases hamstring strength and endurance
• Strengthens gluteal muscles and pelvic stabilizers

NOT ADVISABLE IF YOU HAVE . . .
• Hamstring injury
• Lower-back pain
• Ankle pain

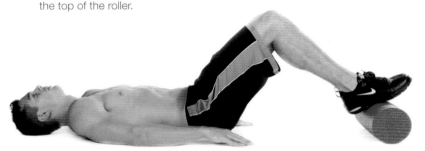

3 Bridge up, lifting your hips so that they align with the shoulders in a neutral position.

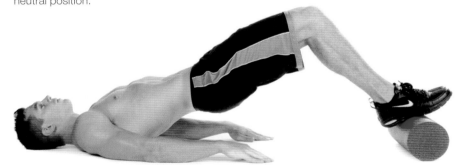

AVOID
• Allowing your hips and lower back to drop as movement is performed.
• Arching your back.

4 Squeeze your buttocks, and pull your calves in and out as you roll the roller under your feet. Repeat 15 times for two sets.

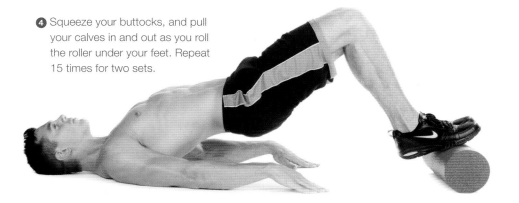

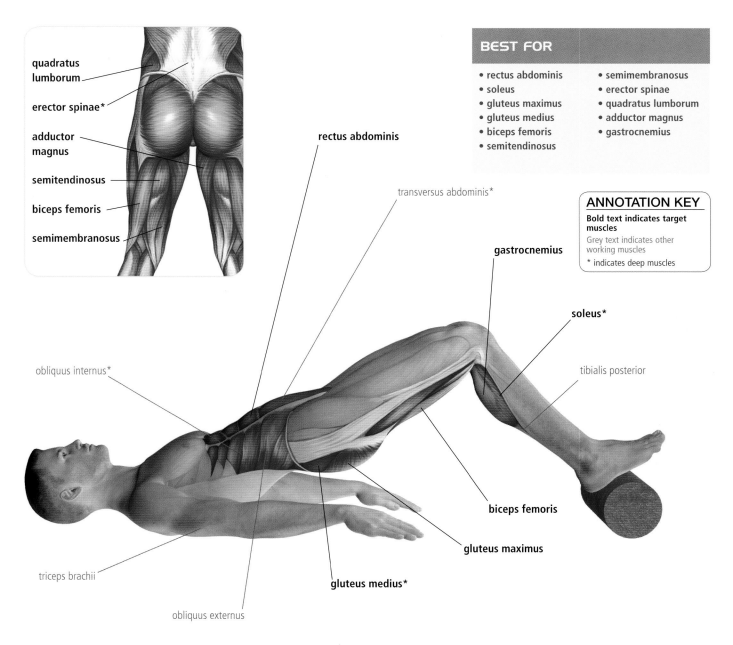

quadratus lumborum

erector spinae*

adductor magnus

semitendinosus

biceps femoris

semimembranosus

rectus abdominis

transversus abdominis*

gastrocnemius

soleus*

tibialis posterior

obliquus internus*

biceps femoris

gluteus maximus

triceps brachii

gluteus medius*

obliquus externus

BEST FOR

- rectus abdominis
- soleus
- gluteus maximus
- gluteus medius
- biceps femoris
- semitendinosus
- semimembranosus
- erector spinae
- quadratus lumborum
- adductor magnus
- gastrocnemius

ANNOTATION KEY

Bold text indicates target muscles

Grey text indicates other working muscles

* indicates deep muscles

SUMO SQUAT

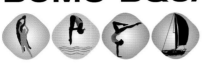

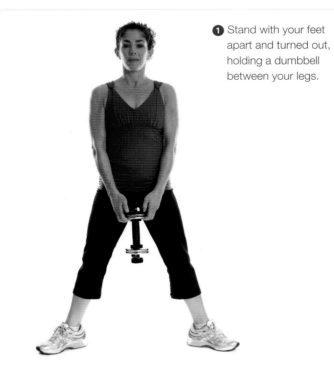

1 Stand with your feet apart and turned out, holding a dumbbell between your legs.

DO IT RIGHT
- Gaze forward.
- Keep your chest lifted and your shoulders down.
- Engage your core.

AVOID
- Allowing your knees to extend past your feet.
- Arching your back or slumping forward.
- Hunching your shoulders.
- Twisting your torso.

TARGETS
- Glutes
- Thighs

LEVEL
- Beginner

BENEFITS
- Tones glutes and thighs

NOT ADVISABLE IF YOU HAVE . . .
- Lower-back issues

2 Keeping your torso upright, bend your knees as you lower into a squat position.

3 Push through your heels as you rise back into an upright position. Repeat, completing three sets of 15.

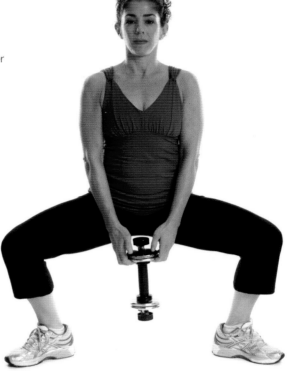

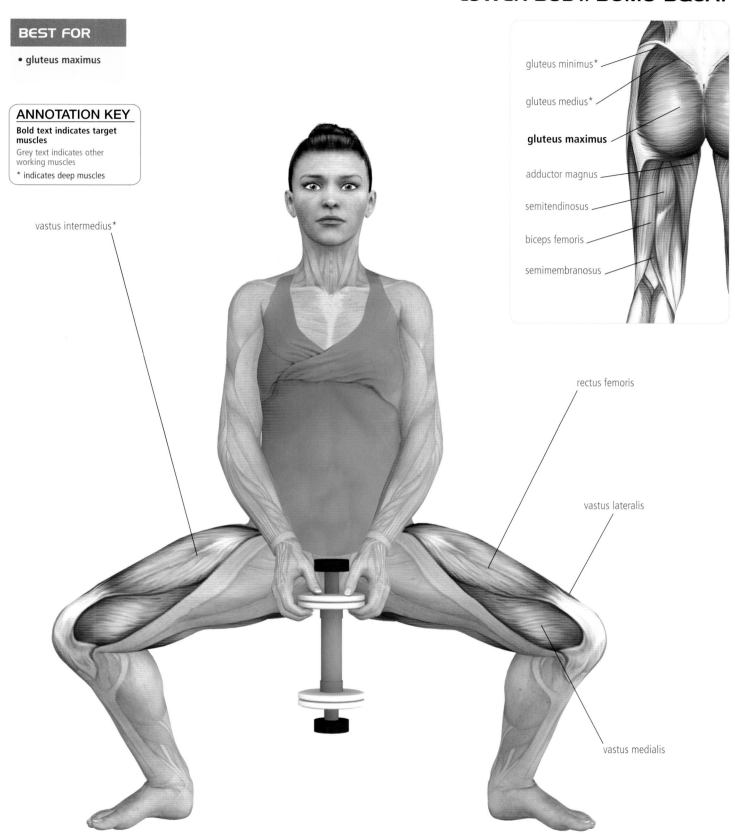

BEST FOR

• **gluteus maximus**

ANNOTATION KEY

Bold text indicates target muscles

Grey text indicates other working muscles

* indicates deep muscles

gluteus minimus*

gluteus medius*

gluteus maximus

adductor magnus

semitendinosus

biceps femoris

semimembranosus

vastus intermedius*

rectus femoris

vastus lateralis

vastus medialis

173

STIFF-LEGGED DEADLIFT

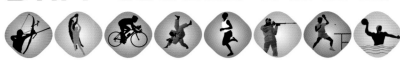

1 Stand upright, feet planted about shoulder-width apart, with your arms slightly in front of your thighs with a hand weight or dumbbell in each hand. Your knees should be slightly bent and your rear pushed slightly outward.

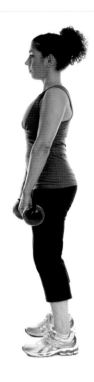

DO IT RIGHT
- Maintain the straight line of your back.
- Keep your torso stable.
- Keep your neck straight.
- Keep your arms extended.

AVOID
- Allowing your lower back to sag or arch.
- Arching your neck, straining to look forward while you are bent over.

TARGETS
- Back
- Glutes
- Hamstrings

LEVEL
- Intermediate

BENEFITS
- Improves flexibility and stabilization throughout lower body

NOT ADVISABLE IF YOU HAVE . . .
- Lower-back issues

2 Keeping your back flat, hinge at the hips and bend forward as you lower the dumbbells toward the floor. You should feel a stretch in the backs of your legs.

3 With control, raise your upper body back to starting position. Repeat, completing three sets of 15.

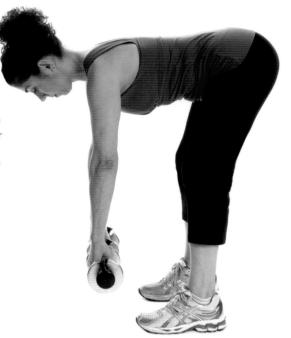

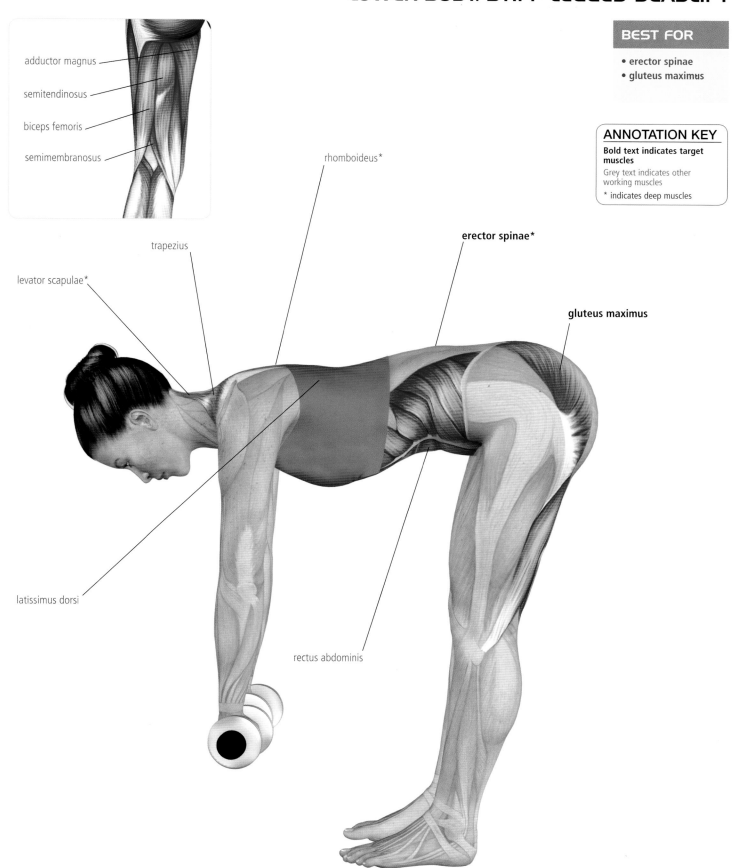

adductor magnus

semitendinosus

biceps femoris

semimembranosus

ANNOTATION KEY

Bold text indicates target muscles

Grey text indicates other working muscles

* indicates deep muscles

rhomboideus*

trapezius

erector spinae*

levator scapulae*

gluteus maximus

latissimus dorsi

rectus abdominis

175

SINGLE-LEG CALF PRESS

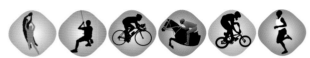

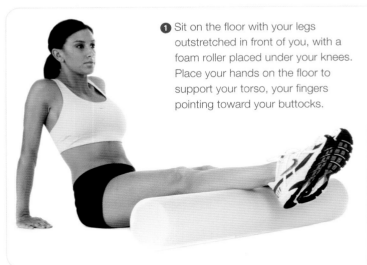

1 Sit on the floor with your legs outstretched in front of you, with a foam roller placed under your knees. Place your hands on the floor to support your torso, your fingers pointing toward your buttocks.

2 Press into the floor to lift your hips, keeping your legs firm.

DO IT RIGHT
- Make sure your raised leg forms a long, straight line.
- Keep your hips elevated throughout the exercise.

AVOID
- Allowing your shoulders to lift toward your ears.
- Bending your knees.
- Bending your elbows.

TARGET
- Triceps
- Shoulder stabilizers
- Abdominals
- Hamstrings

LEVEL
- Intermediate

BENEFITS
- Improves core, pelvic and shoulder stability

NOT ADVISABLE IF YOU HAVE . . .
- Wrist pain
- Shoulder pain
- Discomfort in the back of the knee

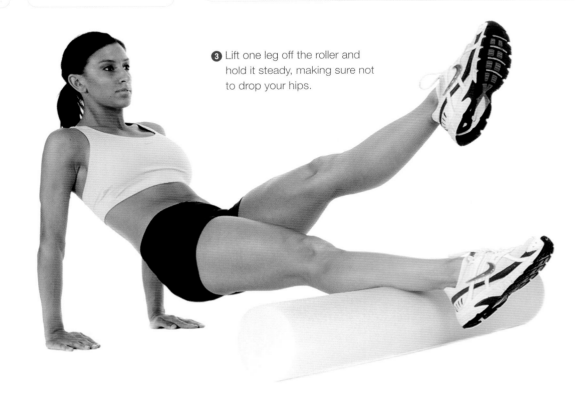

3 Lift one leg off the roller and hold it steady, making sure not to drop your hips.

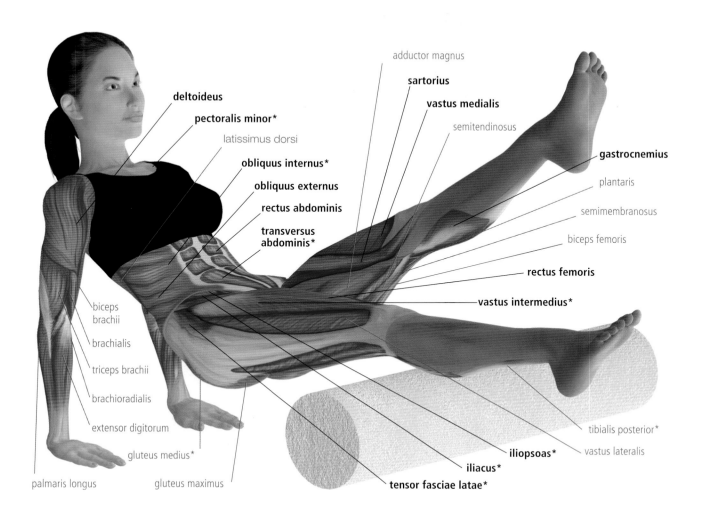

adductor magnus

sartorius

vastus medialis

semitendinosus

gastrocnemius

plantaris

semimembranosus

biceps femoris

rectus femoris

vastus intermedius*

deltoideus

pectoralis minor*

latissimus dorsi

obliquus internus*

obliquus externus

rectus abdominis

transversus abdominis*

biceps brachii

brachialis

triceps brachii

brachioradialis

extensor digitorum

gluteus medius*

palmaris longus

gluteus maximus

tensor fasciae latae*

iliacus*

iliopsoas*

tibialis posterior*

vastus lateralis

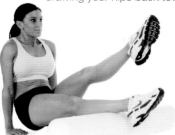

4 Keep the leg lifted, and press your opposite leg into the roller, drawing your hips back toward your hands.

5 Return to the starting position, rolling your calf muscle along the roller and keeping your lifted leg straight in the air. Repeat 15 times on each leg.

BEST FOR

- rectus abdominis
- transversus abdominis
- deltoideus
- pectoralis minor
- rectus femoris
- obliquus externus
- obliquus internus
- sartorius
- vastus medialis
- vastus internedius
- tensor fasciae latae
- iliacus
- iliopsoas
- gastrocnemius

ANNOTATION KEY

Bold text indicates target muscles

Grey text indicates other working muscles

* indicates deep muscles

DUMBBELL CALF RAISE

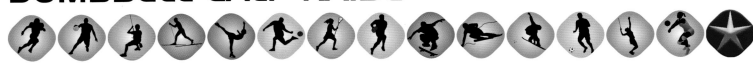

① Stand with your arms at your sides, holding a hand weight or dumbbell in each hand with palms facing inward.

DO IT RIGHT
• Keep your legs straight.
• Concentrate on the contraction in your calves as you balance on the balls of your feet; to feel a greater contraction, rise higher.
• Keep your core stable and your back straight.
• Gaze forward.
• Try to balance on the balls of your feet.

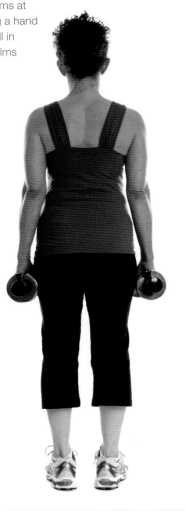

TARGETS
• Calves

LEVEL
• Intermediate

BENEFITS
• Strengthens calf muscles

NOT ADVISABLE IF YOU HAVE . . .
• Ankle issues

AVOID
• Bending your knees.
• Rushing through the movement.
• Arching your back or slumping forward.
• "Sickling," or rolling onto your smaller toes, in the raised position.

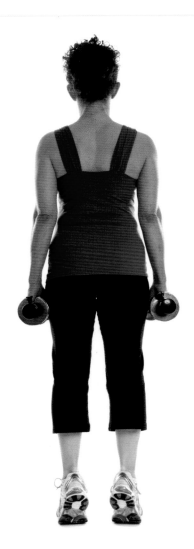

② Keeping the rest of your body steady, slowly raise your heels off the floor to balance on the balls of your feet.

③ Hold for 10 seconds, lower, and repeat, performing three sets of 15.

BEST FOR

- gastrocnemius

ANNOTATION KEY

Bold text indicates target muscles

Grey text indicates other working muscles

* indicates deep muscles

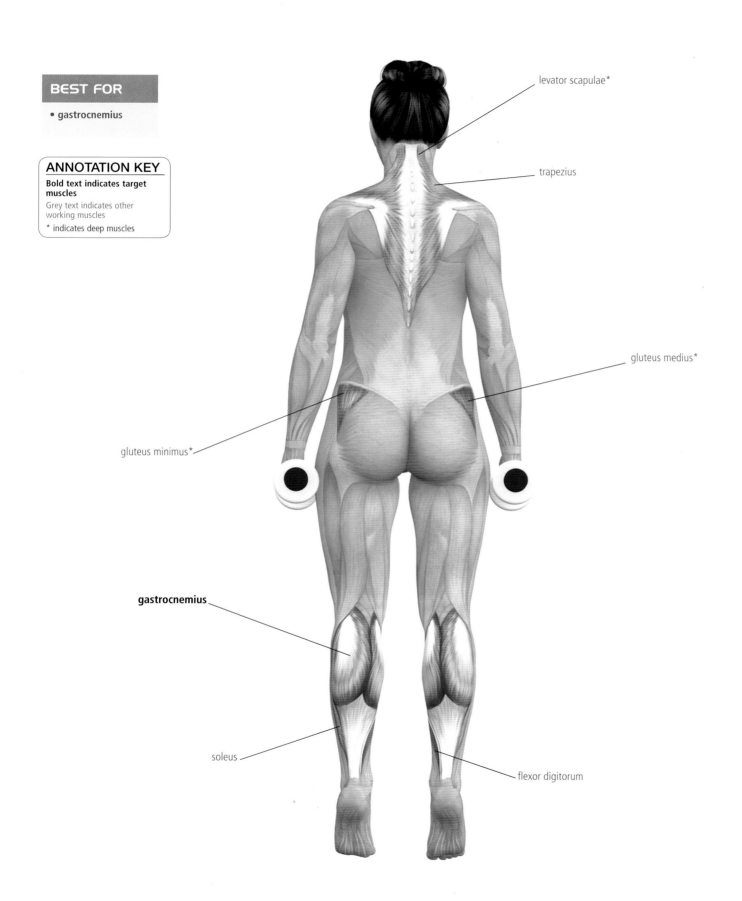

levator scapulae*

trapezius

gluteus medius*

gluteus minimus*

gastrocnemius

soleus

flexor digitorum

DUMBBELL SHIN RAISE

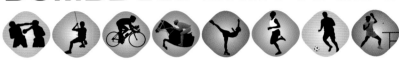

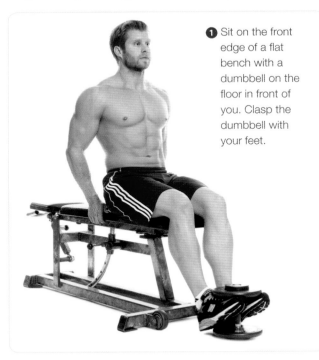

1 Sit on the front edge of a flat bench with a dumbbell on the floor in front of you. Clasp the dumbbell with your feet.

2 Shimmy back onto the bench so that only your feet hang off the bench. Keeping your legs straight and torso sitting up straight, point the feet slowly.

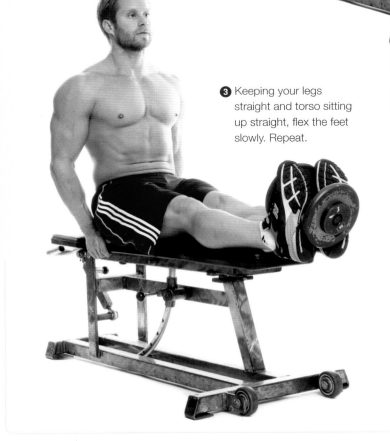

3 Keeping your legs straight and torso sitting up straight, flex the feet slowly. Repeat.

TARGETS
• Shins

LEVEL
• Intermediate

BENEFITS
• Increases strength in the legs

NOT ADVISABLE IF YOU HAVE . . .
• Knee pain

TRAINER'S TIPS
• When you are finished with this exercise, carefully lower the dumbbell to the floor.

DO IT RIGHT
• Maintain a full range of movement while pointing and flexing the feet.
• Keep your neck and jaw relaxed throughout the exercise.

AVOID
• Bending the knees while performing this exercise.

LOWER BODY: DUMBBELL SHIN RAISE

ANNOTATION KEY

Bold text indicates target muscles

Grey text indicates other working muscles

* indicates deep muscles

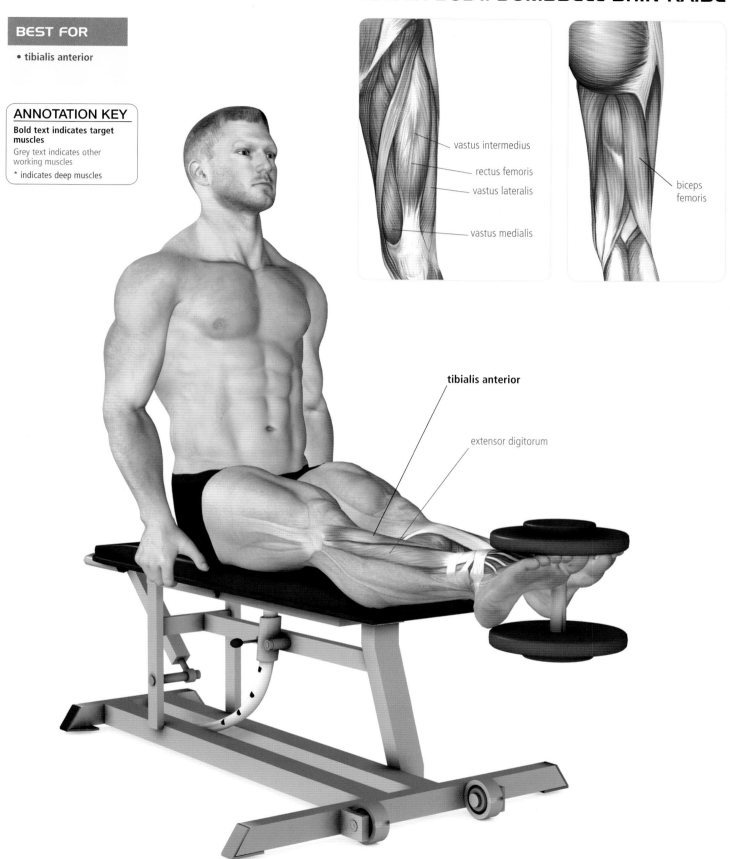

vastus intermedius

rectus femoris

vastus lateralis

vastus medialis

biceps femoris

tibialis anterior

extensor digitorum

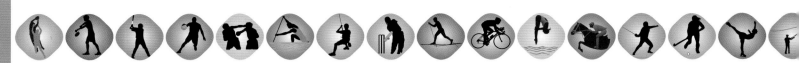

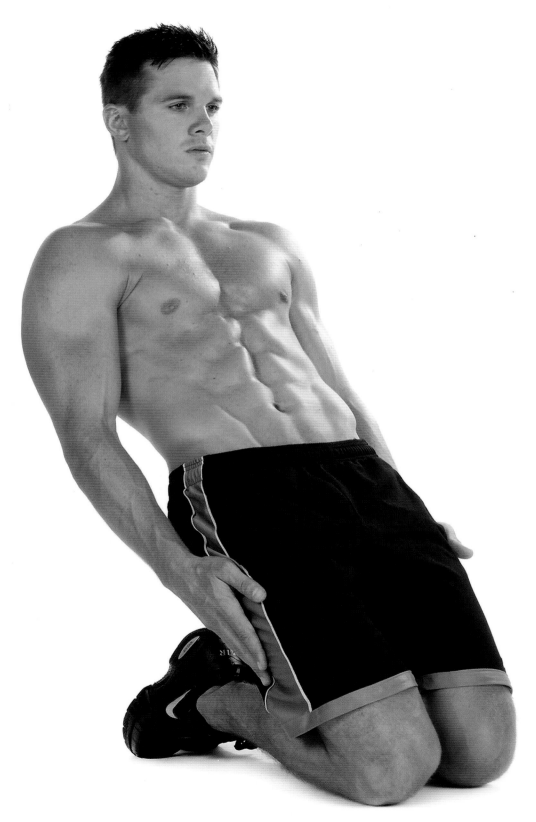

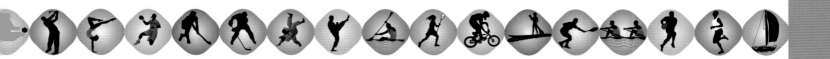

CORE EXERCISES

The core exercises provided here represent some of the most effective movements that have been proven to enhance your performance in a given sport or activity. All exercises are clearly defined and are complete with step-by-step instructions. This section includes exercise aimed at strengthening and toning all the "core" muscles, including the abdominals, obliques and extensors. The routines provided later in the book use these exercises in the most effective combinations for specific sports or activities. However, feel free to dip into these pages and enjoy the individual exercises at any time to introduce variety into your workout. As always, it is important to pay strict attention to form to be sure that you fire from the intended muscle rather than rely on ancillary help. All levels of experience are represented with plenty of variety. Enjoy!

ABDOMINAL KICK

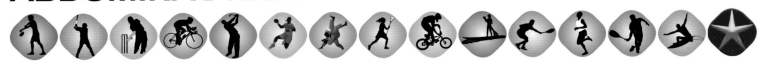

① Pull your right knee toward your chest and straighten your left leg, raising it about 45 degrees from the floor.

② Place your right hand on your right ankle, and your left hand on your right knee (this maintains proper alignment of leg).

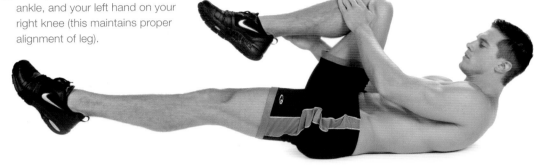

DO IT RIGHT
- Place your outside hand on the ankle of your bent leg, and your inside hand on your bent knee.
- Lift the top of your sternum forward.

AVOID
- Allowing your lower back to rise up off the floor; use your abdominals to stabilize core while switching legs.

③ Switch your legs two times, switching your hand placement simultaneously.

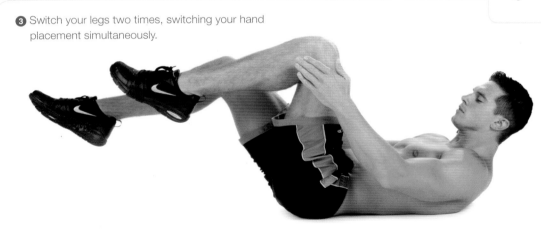

TARGETS
- Abdominals

LEVEL
- Intermediate

BENEFITS
- Stabilizes core while extremities are in motion
- Strengthens abdominals

NOT ADVISABLE IF YOU HAVE . . .
- Neck issues
- Lower-back pain

④ Switch your legs two more times, keeping your hands in their proper placement.

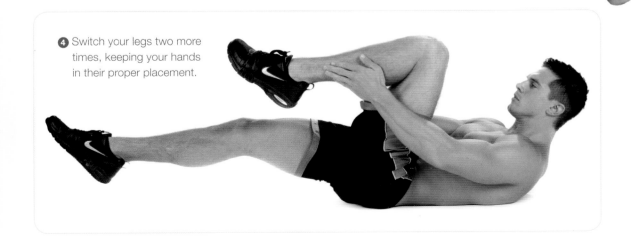

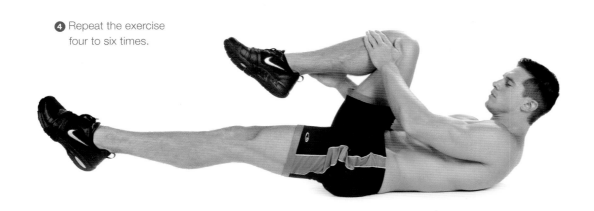

4 Repeat the exercise four to six times.

BEST FOR

- rectus abdominis
- transversus abdominis
- obliquus internus
- biceps femoris
- triceps brachii
- biceps brachii
- tibialis anterior
- tensor fasciae latae
- rectus femoris

ANNOTATION KEY

Bold text indicates target muscles
Grey text indicates other working muscles
* indicates deep muscles

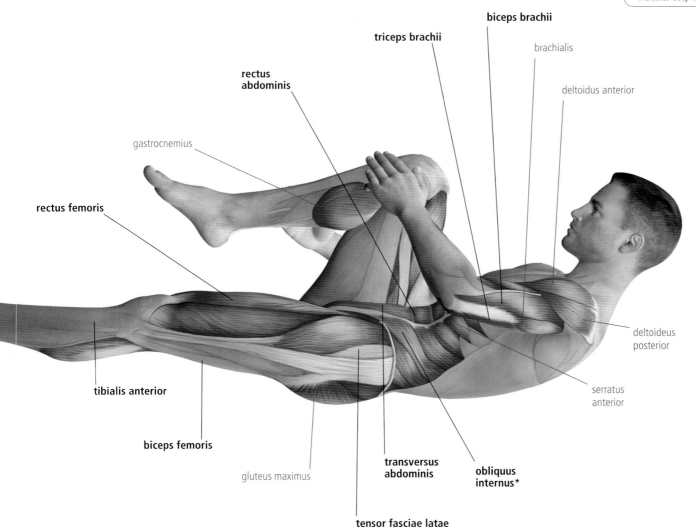

biceps brachii

triceps brachii

brachialis

rectus abdominis

deltoidus anterior

gastrocnemius

rectus femoris

deltoideus posterior

serratus anterior

tibialis anterior

biceps femoris

gluteus maximus

transversus abdominis

obliquus internus*

tensor fasciae latae

ABDOMINAL HIP LIFT

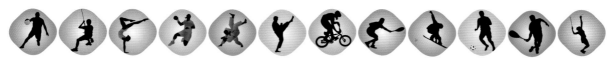

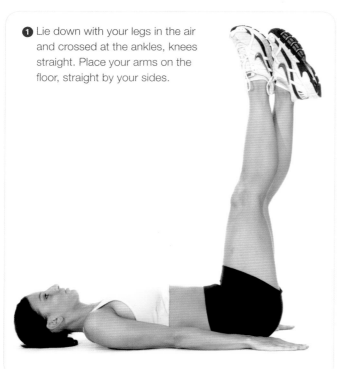

1 Lie down with your legs in the air and crossed at the ankles, knees straight. Place your arms on the floor, straight by your sides.

DO IT RIGHT
- Keep your legs straight and firm throughout the exercise.
- Relax your neck and shoulders as you lift the hips.

AVOID
- Jerking your movements or using momentum to lift the hips.

TARGETS
- Abdominals
- Triceps

LEVEL
- Intermediate

BENEFITS
- Strengthens core and pelvic stabilizers
- Firms and tones lower abdominals

NOT ADVISABLE IF YOU HAVE . . .
- Back pain
- Neck pain
- Shoulder pain

2 Pinching your legs together and squeezing your buttocks, press into the back of your arms to lift your hips upward.

3 Slowly return your hips to the floor. Repeat 10 times, then switch with the opposite leg crossed in the front.

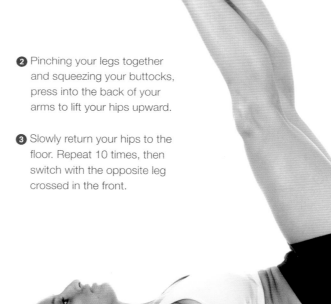

MODIFICATION

More difficult: Keeping your hips on the floor, raise your arms toward the ceiling. Reach toward your toes as you lift your shoulders off the floor.

quadratus lumborum*

gluteus medius*

piriformis*

gluteus maximus

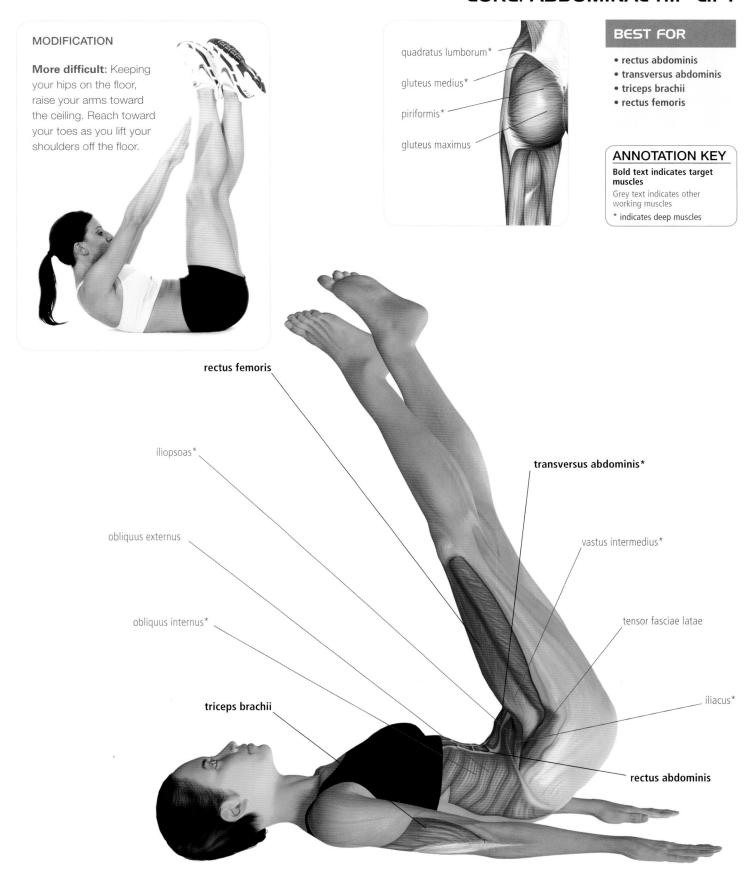

rectus femoris

iliopsoas*

transversus abdominis*

vastus intermedius*

obliquus externus

tensor fasciae latae

obliquus internus*

iliacus*

triceps brachii

rectus abdominis

TURKISH GET-UP

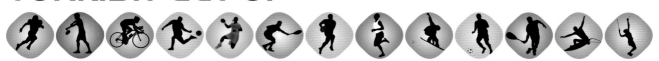

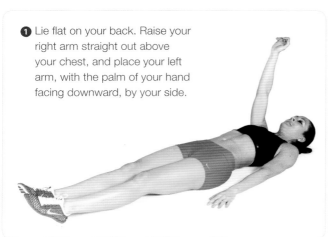

1 Lie flat on your back. Raise your right arm straight out above your chest, and place your left arm, with the palm of your hand facing downward, by your side.

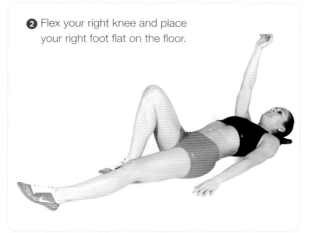

2 Flex your right knee and place your right foot flat on the floor.

DO IT RIGHT
• Keep a tight core throughout the movement.

AVOID
• Performing the exercise at excessive speed.

TARGETS
• Shoulders
• Core
• Thighs
• Glutes
• Upper back
• Triceps

LEVEL
• Intermediate

BENEFITS
• Increases stability in the hips and aids balance throughout the body

NOT ADVISABLE IF YOU HAVE . . .
• Wrist pain
• Shoulder pain
• Discomfort in the back of the knee

3 Rotate your core slightly to the left and lift your shoulders off the floor, supporting your weight on your left forearm. Next, plant your left hand on the floor and lift yourself up to a sitting position.

4 Lift your hips skyward and tuck your left leg under your body to support yourself on your left knee.

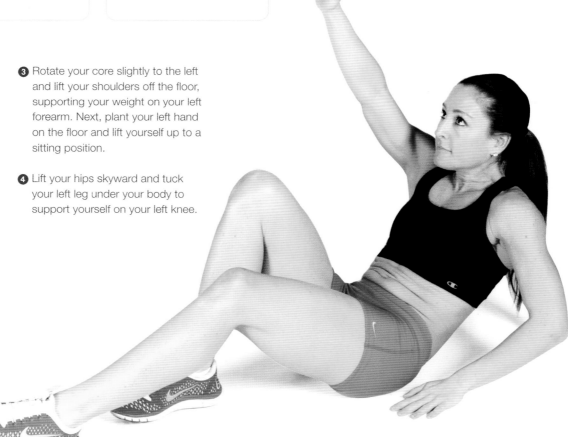

⑤ Lift your left hand off the floor and push through your right foot to a standing position, keeping your right arm stretched over your head throughout the exercise.

⑥ Return to the starting position. Perform 10 repetitions per arm.

- deltoideus anterior
- deltoideus posterior
- deltoideus medialis
- rectus abdominis
- transversus abdominis
- obliquus externus
- obliquus internus
- multifidus spinae
- vastus intermedius
- vastus lateralis
- vastus medialis
- rectus femoris
- semitendinosus
- biceps femoris
- semimembranosus
- gluteus minimus
- gluteus medius
- gluteus maximus

ANNOTATION KEY

Bold text indicates target muscles
Grey text indicates other working muscles
* indicates deep muscles

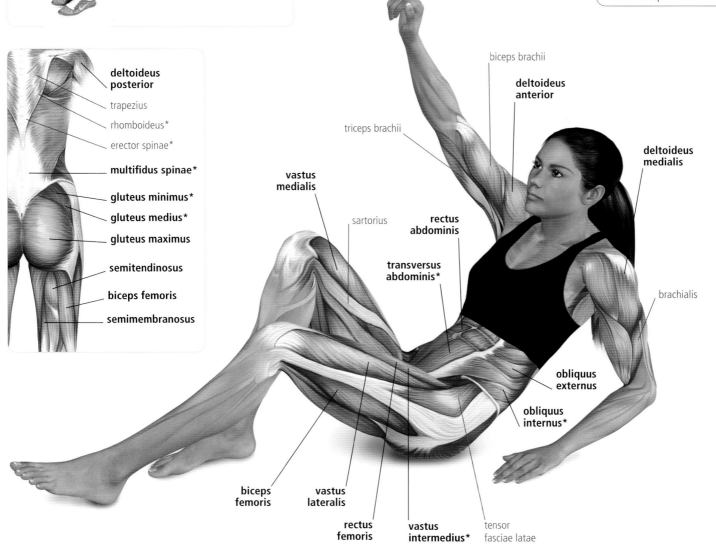

deltoideus posterior
trapezius
rhomboideus*
erector spinae*
multifidus spinae*
gluteus minimus*
gluteus medius*
gluteus maximus
semitendinosus
biceps femoris
semimembranosus

biceps brachii
deltoideus anterior
triceps brachii
deltoideus medialis
vastus medialis
sartorius
rectus abdominis
transversus abdominis*
brachialis
biceps femoris
vastus lateralis
rectus femoris
vastus intermedius*
tensor fasciae latae
obliquus externus
obliquus internus*

BICYCLE CRUNCH

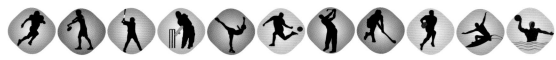

1 Lie supine on the floor with your knees bent. Bring your hands behind your head, lifting your legs off the floor.

2 Roll up with your torso, reaching your left elbow to your right knee while extending the left leg in front of you. Imagine pulling your shoulder blades off the floor and twisting from your ribs and oblique muscles.

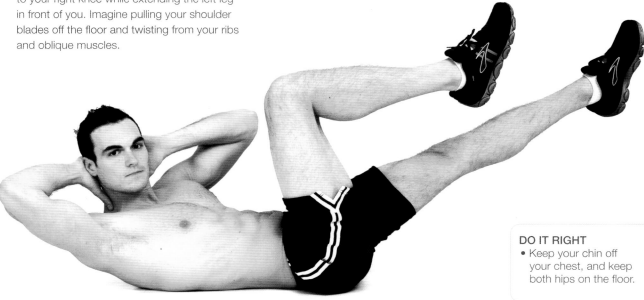

DO IT RIGHT
• Keep your chin off your chest, and keep both hips on the floor.

AVOID
• Pulling with your hands or arching your back.

TARGETS
• Core
• Thighs
• Glutes

LEVEL
• Advanced

BENEFITS
• Stabilizes the core and strengthens the abdominals

NOT ADVISABLE IF YOU HAVE . . .
• Lower-back or neck problems

3 Switch sides. Complete the movement six times on each side.

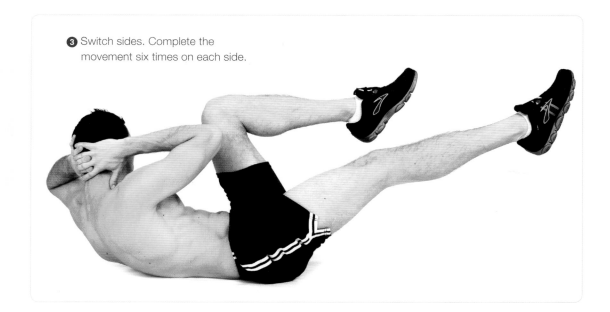

BEST FOR

- transversus abdominis
- rectus abdominis
- obliquus internus
- obliquus externus

ANNOTATION KEY

Bold text indicates target muscles

Grey text indicates other working muscles

* indicates deep muscles

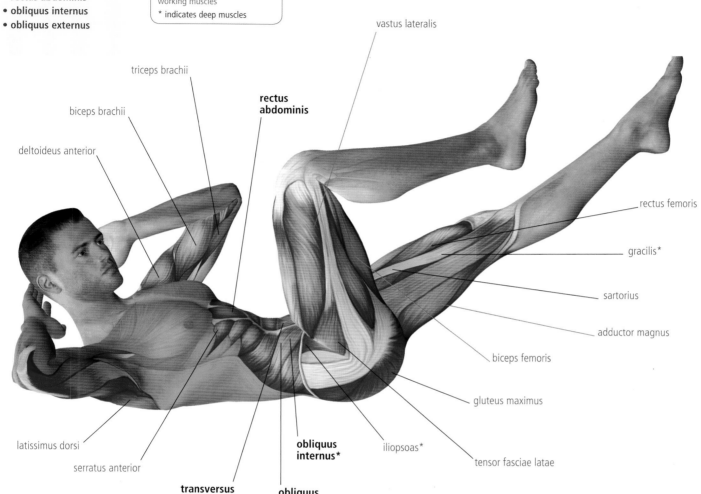

vastus lateralis

triceps brachii

biceps brachii

rectus abdominis

deltoideus anterior

rectus femoris

gracilis*

sartorius

adductor magnus

biceps femoris

gluteus maximus

latissimus dorsi

obliquus internus*

iliopsoas*

tensor fasciae latae

serratus anterior

transversus abdominis*

obliquus externus

MODIFICATION

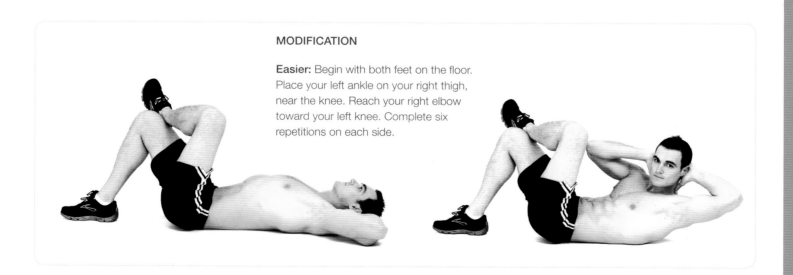

Easier: Begin with both feet on the floor. Place your left ankle on your right thigh, near the knee. Reach your right elbow toward your left knee. Complete six repetitions on each side.

REVERSE CRUNCH

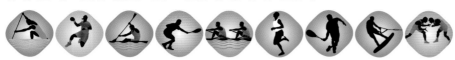

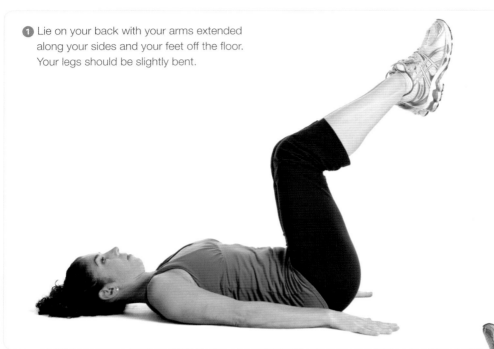

1 Lie on your back with your arms extended along your sides and your feet off the floor. Your legs should be slightly bent.

DO IT RIGHT
• Use your abdominals to drive your lower body's movement.
• Keep your arms flat on the floor.

AVOID
• Lifting with your lower back or neck.
• Relying on momentum to help you perform the movement.

TARGETS
• Upper abdominals

LEVEL
• Intermediate

BENEFITS
• Strengthens and helps to define abdominals

NOT ADVISABLE IF YOU HAVE . . .
• Hip instability
• Lower-back issues

2 Tuck your legs in toward your body as you lift your glutes, and then lower back a few inches off the floor.

3 Lower in a controlled manner, returning your feet to their original position. Repeat, performing three sets of 20.

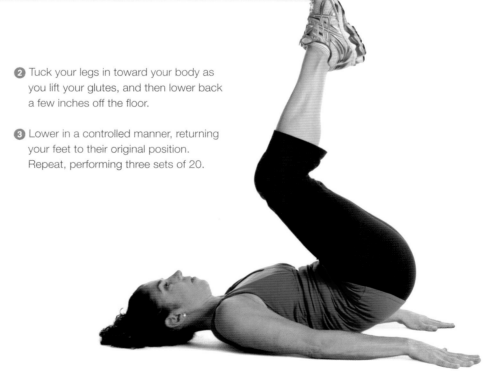

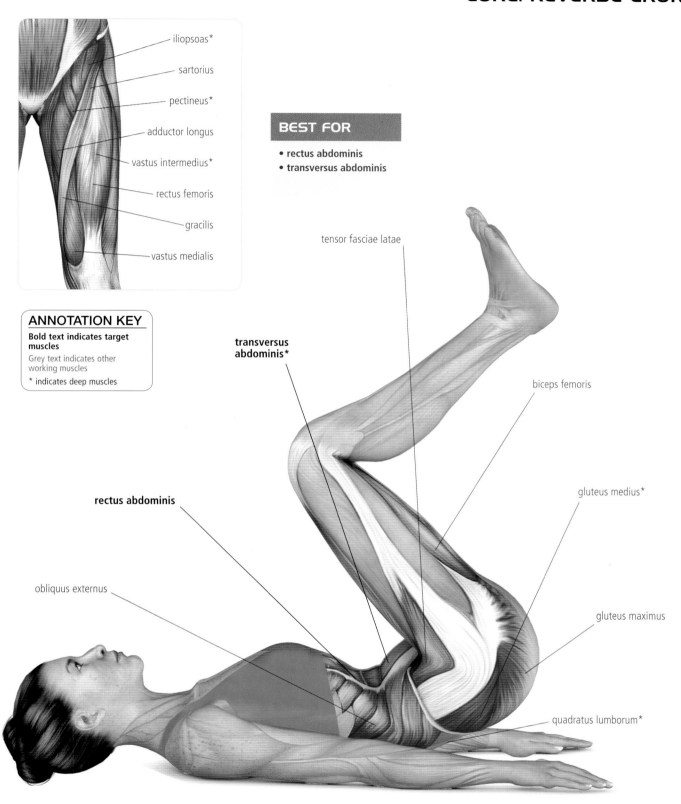

iliopsoas*

sartorius

pectineus*

adductor longus

vastus intermedius*

rectus femoris

gracilis

vastus medialis

BEST FOR

- **rectus abdominis**
- **transversus abdominis**

ANNOTATION KEY

Bold text indicates target muscles

Grey text indicates other working muscles

* indicates deep muscles

tensor fasciae latae

transversus abdominis*

biceps femoris

gluteus medius*

rectus abdominis

gluteus maximus

obliquus externus

quadratus lumborum*

COBRA STRETCH

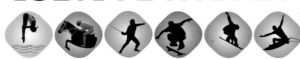

1 Lie facedown, legs extended behind you with toes pointed. Position the palms of your hands on the floor slightly above your shoulders, and rest your elbows on the floor.

DO IT RIGHT
- You should feel a slight pressure between your hips and the floor.
- Keep your shoulders relaxed, pressed down and away from your ears.

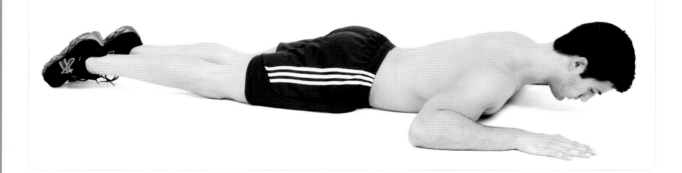

TARGETS
- Spinal joints

LEVEL
- Intermediate

BENEFITS
- Strengthens spine
- Stretches chest, abdominals and shoulders

NOT ADVISABLE IF YOU HAVE . . .
- Lower-back injury

2 Push down into the floor, and slowly lift through the top of your chest as you straighten your arms.

3 Pull your tailbone down toward your pubis as you push your shoulders down and back.

4 Elongate your neck and gaze forward.

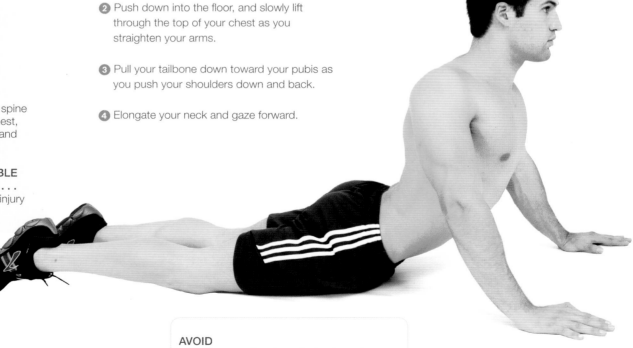

AVOID
- Tipping your head too far backward.
- Overdoing this stretch — it can lead to excessive pressure on your lower back.

194

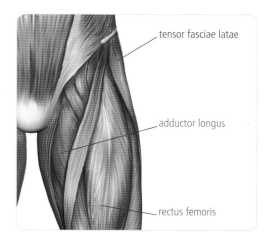

tensor fasciae latae

adductor longus

rectus femoris

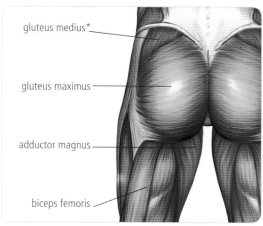

gluteus medius*

gluteus maximus

adductor magnus

biceps femoris

BEST FOR

- **rectus abdominis**
- **transversus abdominis**
- **obliquus externus**
- **obliquus internus**

ANNOTATION KEY

Bold text indicates target muscles

Grey text indicates other working muscles

* indicates deep muscles

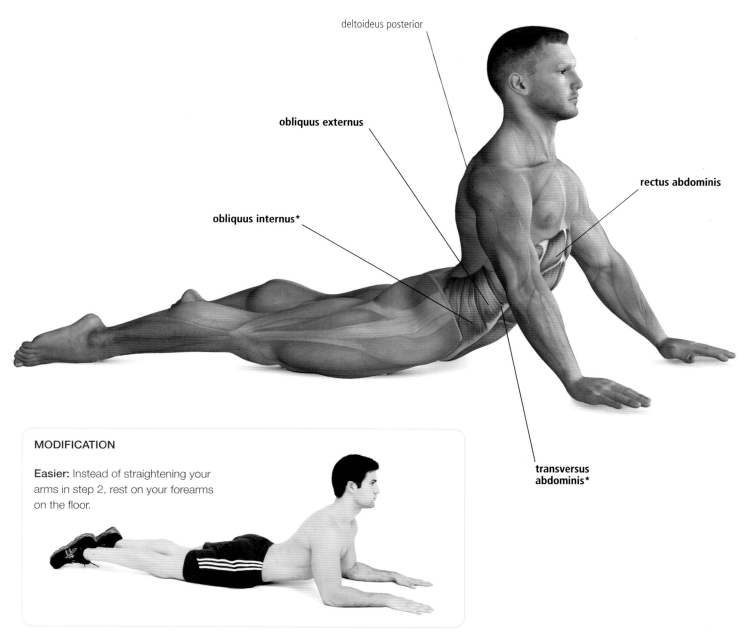

deltoideus posterior

obliquus externus

rectus abdominis

obliquus internus*

transversus abdominis*

MODIFICATION

Easier: Instead of straightening your arms in step 2, rest on your forearms on the floor.

SWISS BALL PELVIC TILT

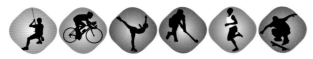

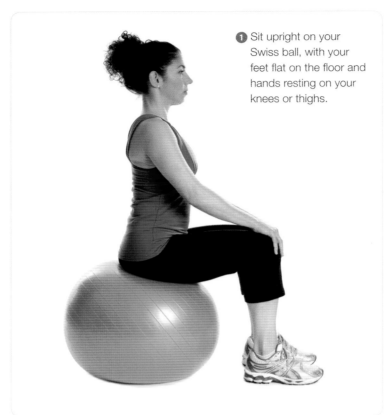

1 Sit upright on your Swiss ball, with your feet flat on the floor and hands resting on your knees or thighs.

DO IT RIGHT
- Position your hips over the center of the ball so that you are fully supported.
- Exhale while contracting.

AVOID
- Rushing through the movement.

TARGETS
- Lower back
- Abdominals
- Glutes

LEVEL
- Beginner

BENEFITS
- Improves posture
- Relieves mild-to-moderate lower-back pain

NOT ADVISABLE IF YOU HAVE . . .
- Severe lower-back pain

2 Tilt your pelvis forward, using the motion of the ball to assist you. Contract your abdominals, and hold for 5 seconds.

3 Return to starting position, and contract again. Repeat the back-and-forth motion, holding each position for 5 seconds for 10 reps.

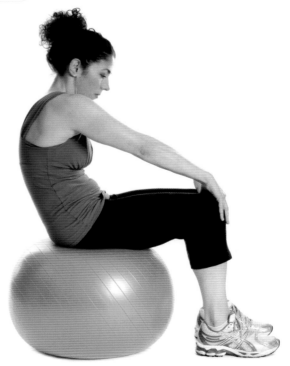

BEST FOR

- rectus abdominis
- transversus abdominis
- gluteus maximus
- gluteus minimus
- gluteus medius
- erector spinae

ANNOTATION KEY

Bold text indicates target muscles

Grey text indicates other working muscles

* indicates deep muscles

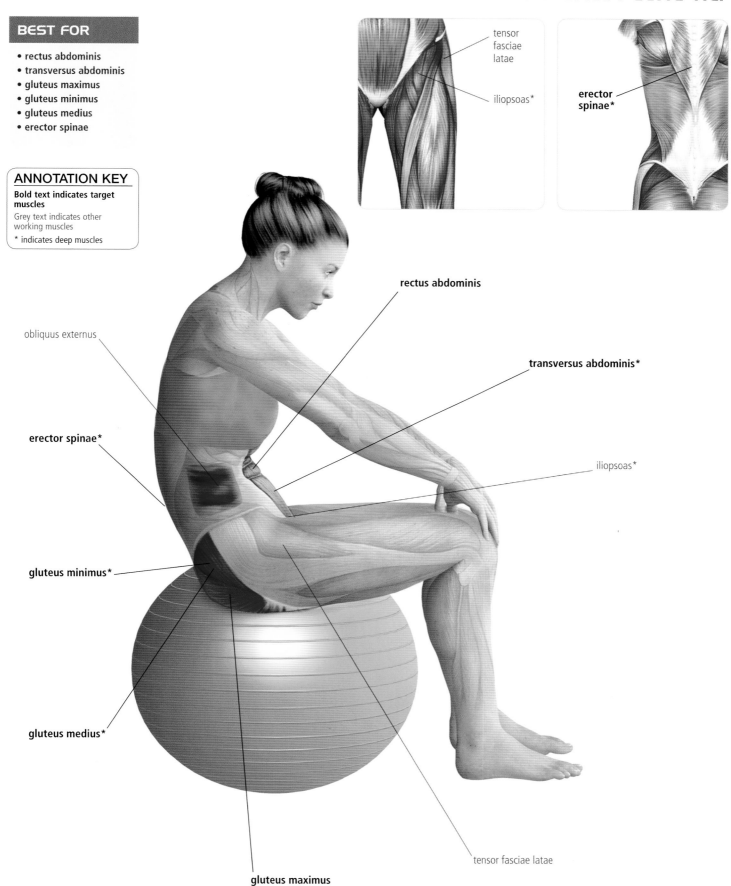

tensor fasciae latae

iliopsoas*

erector spinae*

obliquus externus

rectus abdominis

transversus abdominis*

erector spinae*

iliopsoas*

gluteus minimus*

gluteus medius*

tensor fasciae latae

gluteus maximus

PLANK PRESS-UP

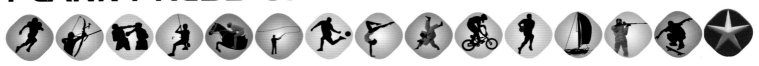

1 Lying on the mat with your forearms underneath your chest, press your body up into a plank position, lengthening through your heels.

DO IT RIGHT
• Lengthen through your neck without looking forward.

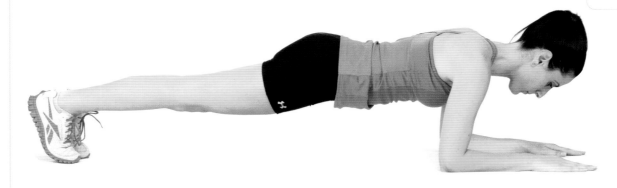

AVOID
• Allowing your back to sag.
• Allowing your shoulders to collapse into your shoulder joints.

2 Push through your forearms to bring your shoulders up toward the ceiling. With control, lower your shoulders until you feel them coming together in your back.

TARGETS
• Deltoids
• Core stabilizers

LEVEL
• Intermediate

BENEFITS
• Strengthens core muscles
• Improves core stability
• Strengthens triceps
• Improves posture

NOT ADVISABLE IF YOU HAVE . . .
• Shoulder injury
• Intense back pain

3 Repeat five times.

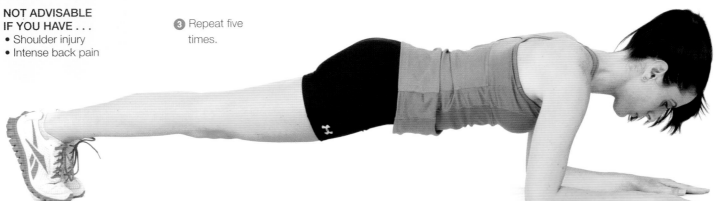

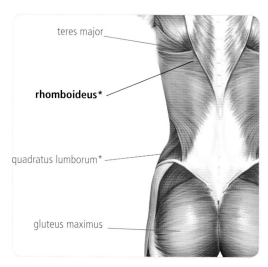

teres major

rhomboideus*

quadratus lumborum*

gluteus maximus

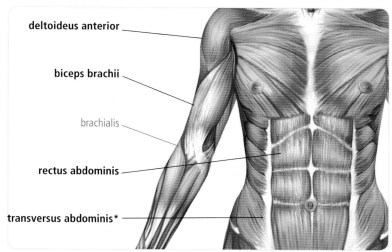

deltoideus anterior

biceps brachii

brachialis

rectus abdominis

transversus abdominis*

BEST FOR

- deltoideus anterior
- deltoideus posterior
- rhomboideus
- rectus abdominis
- biceps brachii
- triceps brachii
- tensor fasciae latae
- rectus femoris
- transversus abdominis
- obliquus internus
- serratus anterior
- tibialis anterior

ANNOTATION KEY

Bold text indicates target muscles

Grey text indicates other working muscles

* indicates deep muscles

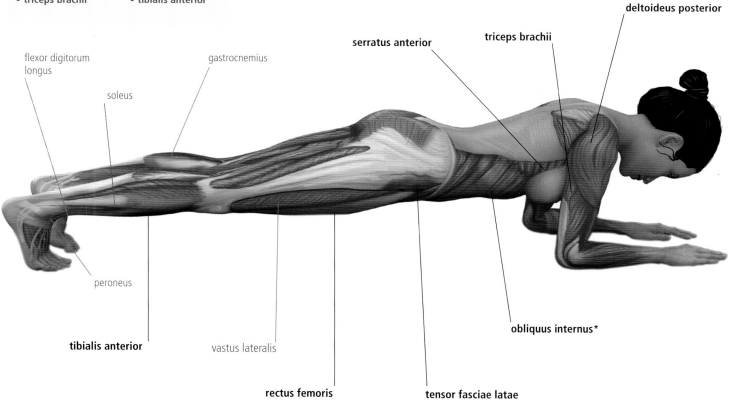

flexor digitorum longus

gastrocnemius

soleus

serratus anterior

triceps brachii

deltoideus posterior

tibialis anterior

vastus lateralis

peroneus

obliquus internus*

rectus femoris

tensor fasciae latae

SEATED RUSSIAN TWIST

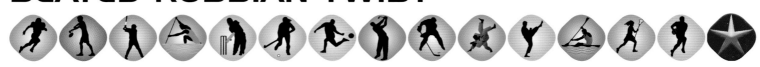

1 Sit upright with your legs bent, feet flat on the floor. Extend your arms straight ahead, and lean back slightly to activate your core.

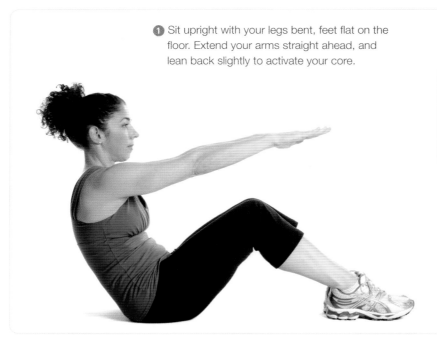

DO IT RIGHT
- Twist smoothly and with control.
- Keep your back flat as you twist.
- Keep your feet on the floor.
- Keep your arms straight.

AVOID
- Rushing through the twist.
- Shift your feet or knees to the side as you twist.

TARGETS
- Back
- Obliques
- Upper abdominals

LEVEL
- Intermediate

BENEFITS
- Stabilizes and strengthens core

NOT ADVISABLE IF YOU HAVE . . .
- Lower-back issues

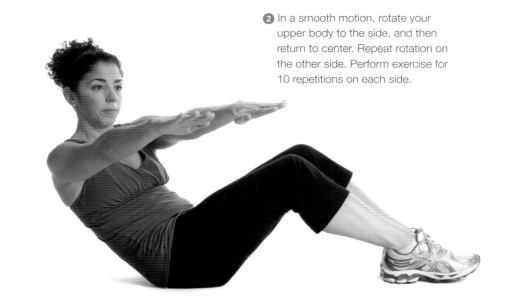

2 In a smooth motion, rotate your upper body to the side, and then return to center. Repeat rotation on the other side. Perform exercise for 10 repetitions on each side.

3 Return to center, and repeat the full twist, performing three sets of 20.

MODIFICATION

More difficult:
Perform twists holding a medicine ball.

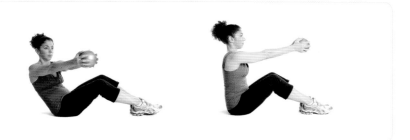

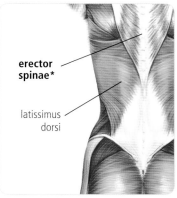

erector spinae*

latissimus dorsi

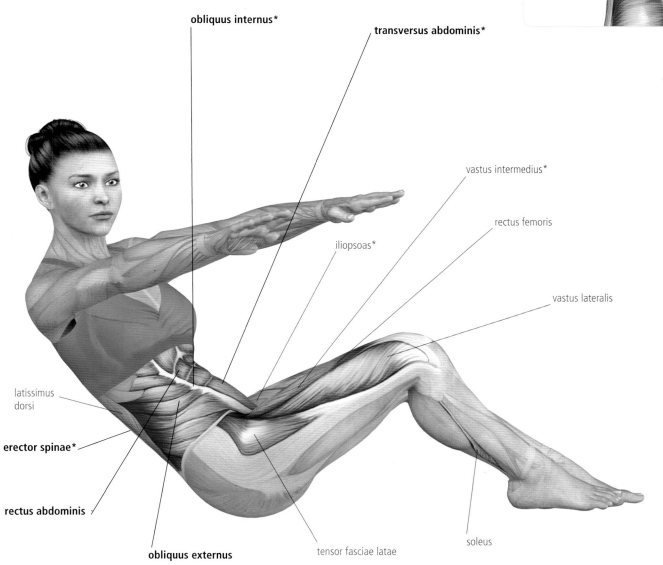

obliquus internus*

transversus abdominis*

vastus intermedius*

rectus femoris

iliopsoas*

vastus lateralis

latissimus dorsi

erector spinae*

rectus abdominis

obliquus externus

tensor fasciae latae

soleus

BEST FOR

- **rectus abdominis**
- **obliquus externus**
- **obliquus internus**
- **erector spinae**
- **transversus abdominis**

ANNOTATION KEY

Bold text indicates target muscles

Grey text indicates other working muscles

* indicates deep muscles

WOOD CHOP WITH RESISTANCE BAND

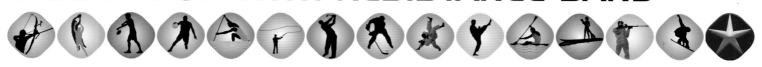

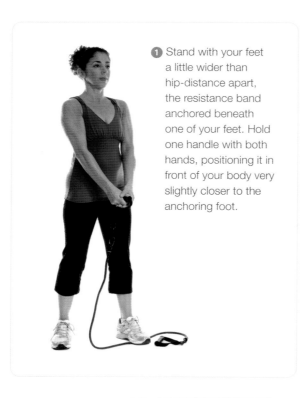

1 Stand with your feet a little wider than hip-distance apart, the resistance band anchored beneath one of your feet. Hold one handle with both hands, positioning it in front of your body very slightly closer to the anchoring foot.

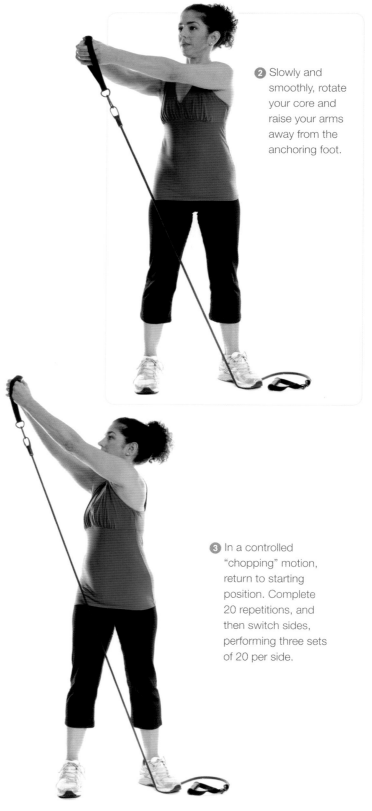

2 Slowly and smoothly, rotate your core and raise your arms away from the anchoring foot.

3 In a controlled "chopping" motion, return to starting position. Complete 20 repetitions, and then switch sides, performing three sets of 20 per side.

TARGETS
• Obliques

LEVEL
• Beginner

BENEFITS
• Improves core strength and support
• Strengthens and tones obliques

NOT ADVISABLE IF YOU HAVE . . .
• Lower-back issues
• Shoulder issues

DO IT RIGHT
• Keep your arms straight.
• Follow your arms with your gaze as you raise and lower them.
• Keep your core contracted and your abs engaged.

AVOID
• Twisting too jerkily from side to side.
• Raising your arms so high that you lose control of your core and/or arch your back.
• Hunching your shoulders.

CORE: WOOD CHOP WITH RESISTANCE BAND

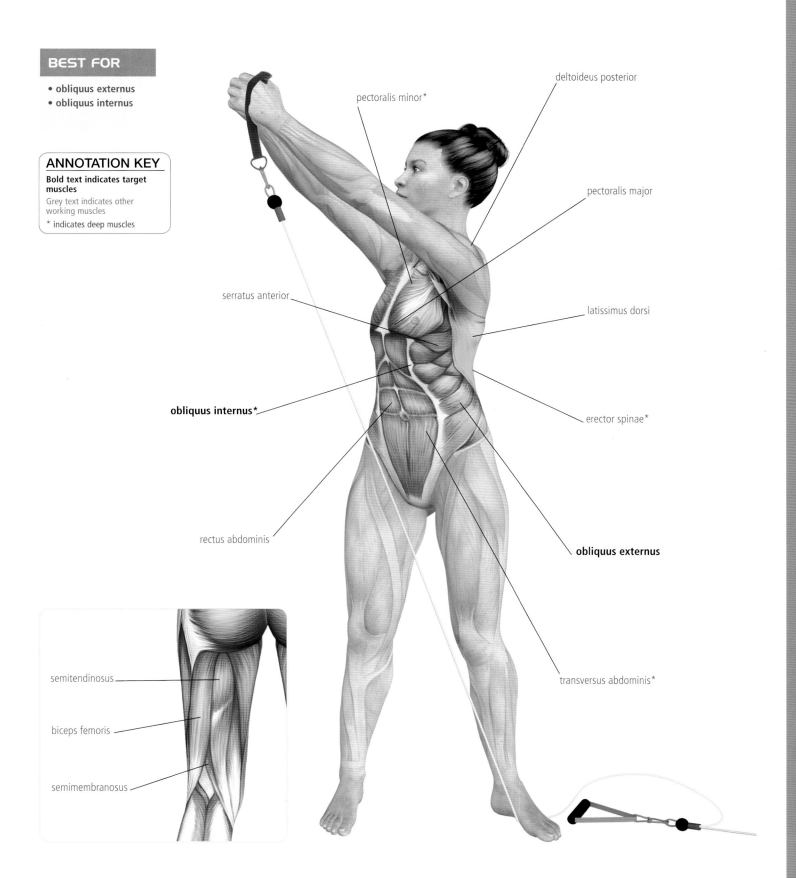

BEST FOR

- obliquus externus
- obliquus internus

ANNOTATION KEY

Bold text indicates target muscles

Grey text indicates other working muscles

* indicates deep muscles

pectoralis minor*

deltoideus posterior

pectoralis major

serratus anterior

latissimus dorsi

obliquus internus*

erector spinae*

rectus abdominis

obliquus externus

transversus abdominis*

semitendinosus

biceps femoris

semimembranosus

HIP ABDUCTION AND ADDUCTION

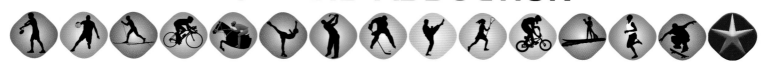

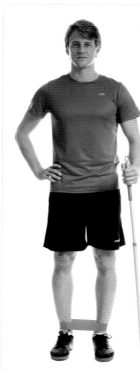

1 Stand with your feet shoulder-width apart, with a resistance loop or a resistance band tied around your ankles. Tuck your pelvis slightly forward, lift your chest and press your shoulders downward and back. With your left hand, hold onto a support such as a mop handle or chair back.

2 Keeping your back and knee straight and foot facing forward, move your right foot directly to the right, moving away from your body. Hold for 2 seconds and repeat 10 times.

3 Return to starting position.

TARGETS
• Hip abductors
• Hip adductors

LEVEL
• Beginner

BENEFITS
• Strengthens hips

NOT ADVISABLE IF YOU HAVE . . .
• Balance issues

DO IT RIGHT
• Tighten the muscles at the side of your thigh and hip as you move your leg.

AVOID
• Touching your moving foot to the floor as you move your foot sideways and inward.
• Leaning your torso to one side.

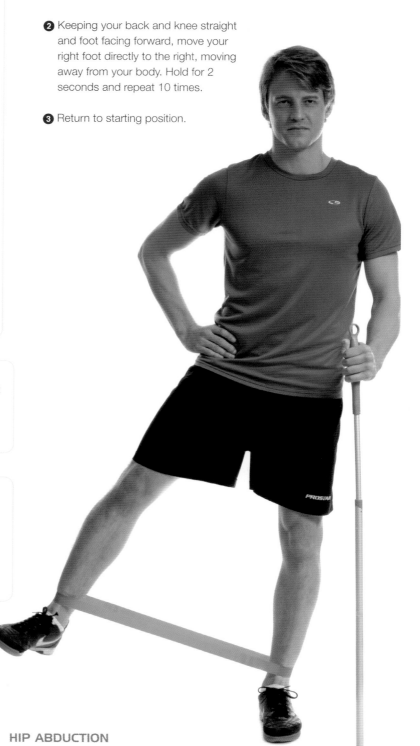

HIP ABDUCTION

CORE: HIP ABDUCTION AND ADDUCTION

4 Keeping your back and knee straight and foot facing forward, move your left foot directly to the right, moving it toward and across your body. Hold for 2 seconds and repeat 10 times.

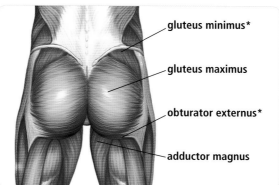

gluteus minimus*

gluteus maximus

obturator externus*

adductor magnus

BEST FOR

- adductor longus
- adductor magnus
- adductor brevis
- gracilis
- pectineus
- obturator externus
- gluteus minimus
- tensor fasciae latae
- gluteus maximus

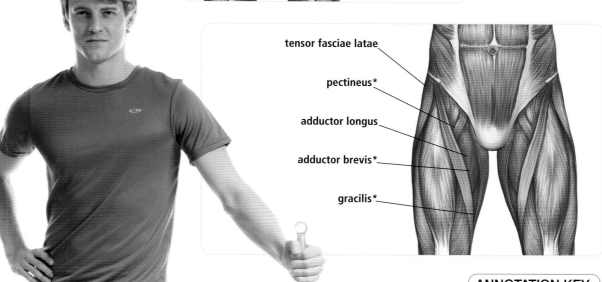

tensor fasciae latae

pectineus*

adductor longus

adductor brevis*

gracilis*

ANNOTATION KEY

Bold text indicates target muscles

Grey text indicates other working muscles

* indicates deep muscles

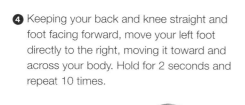

5 Return to starting position, and repeat the entire sequence on the opposite side.

HIP ADDUCTION

SWISS BALL ROLL-OUT

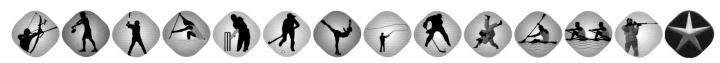

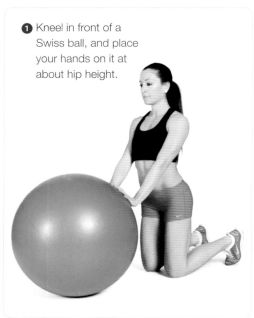

❶ Kneel in front of a Swiss ball, and place your hands on it at about hip height.

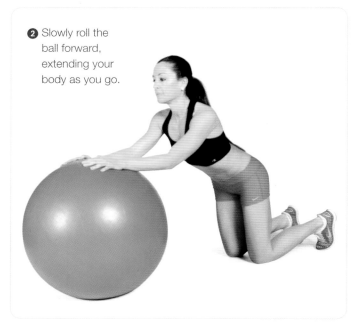

❷ Slowly roll the ball forward, extending your body as you go.

TARGETS
• Abdominals
• Lower back
• Obliques

LEVEL
• Intermediate

BENEFITS
• Helps stabilize the core

NOT ADVISABLE IF YOU HAVE . . .
• Lower-back issues
• Knee issues

MODIFICATION
• **Easier:** Plant your feet against a solid surface for extra support.

❸ Keep rolling forward until you are completely stretched out while keeping a flat back and remaining anchored on your knees. Then, using your abdominals and lower-back muscles, roll back to the starting position. Perform 15 to 20 repetitions.

DO IT RIGHT
• Keep your body elongated throughout the movement.

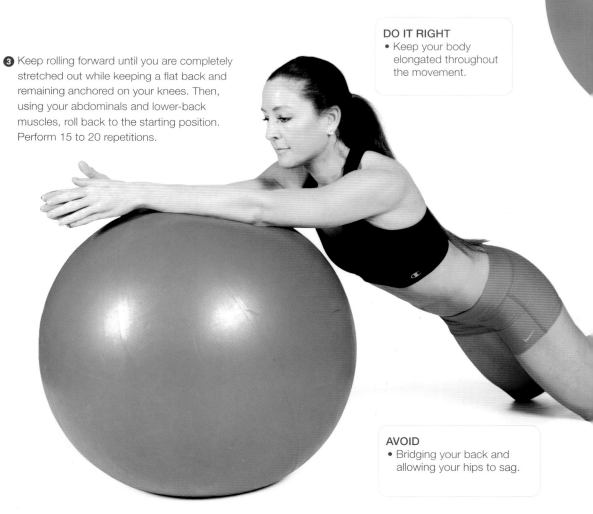

AVOID
• Bridging your back and allowing your hips to sag.

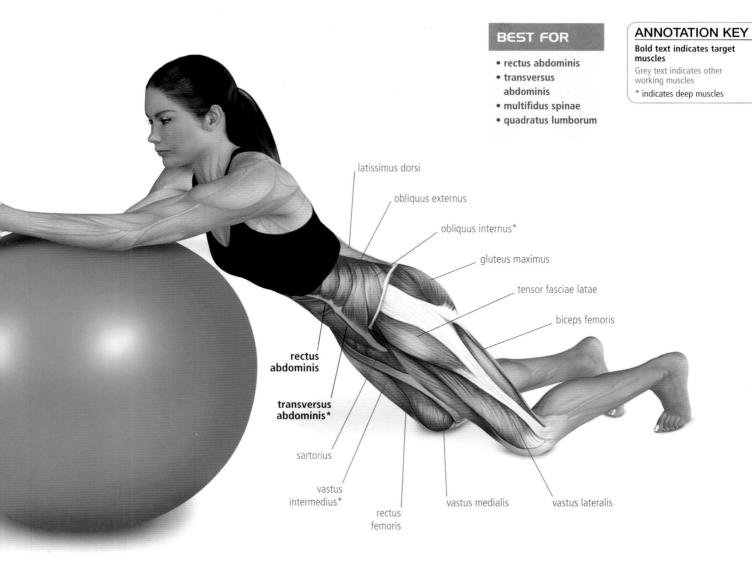

- rectus abdominis
- transversus abdominis
- multifidus spinae
- quadratus lumborum

ANNOTATION KEY

Bold text indicates target muscles

Grey text indicates other working muscles

* indicates deep muscles

latissimus dorsi

obliquus externus

obliquus internus*

gluteus maximus

tensor fasciae latae

biceps femoris

rectus abdominis

transversus abdominis*

sartorius

vastus intermedius*

rectus femoris

vastus medialis

vastus lateralis

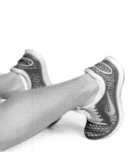

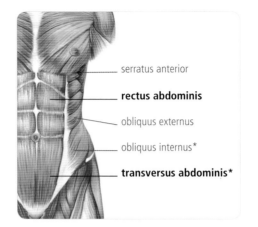

serratus anterior

rectus abdominis

obliquus externus

obliquus internus*

transversus abdominis*

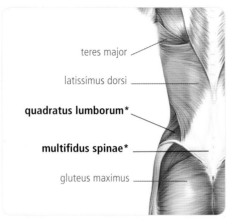

teres major

latissimus dorsi

quadratus lumborum*

multifidus spinae*

gluteus maximus

THIGH ROCK-BACK

① Kneel with your back straight and your knees hip-width apart on the floor, your arms by your sides. Pull in your abdominals, drawing your navel toward your spine.

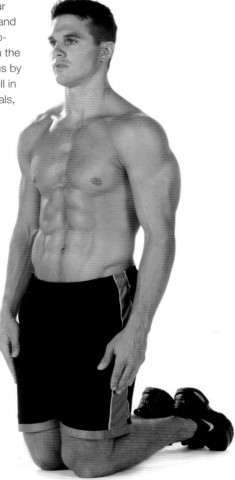

DO IT RIGHT
- Form a straight line between your shoulders and your knees.
- Work your abdominals to control the movement.
- Keep your buttocks tight.

② Lean back, keeping your hips open and aligned with your shoulders, stretching the front of your thighs.

③ Once you have leaned back as far as you can, squeeze your buttocks and slowly bring your body back to the upright position. Repeat four to five times.

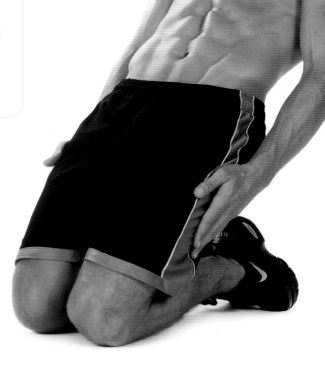

TARGETS
- Quadriceps
- Abdominals

LEVEL
- Intermediate

BENEFITS
- Stretches thighs
- Strengthens abdominals
- Increases range of motion of anterior ankle

NOT ADVISABLE IF YOU HAVE . . .
- Lower-back issues
- Ankle issues

AVOID
- Rocking so far back that you cannot return to the starting position.
- Bending in your hips.

ANNOTATION KEY

Bold text indicates target muscles

Grey text indicates other working muscles

* indicates deep muscles

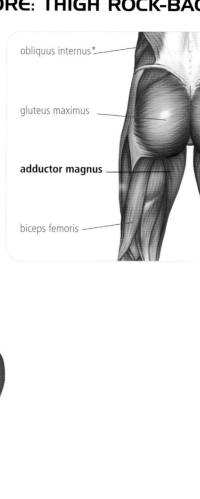

obliquus internus*

gluteus maximus

adductor magnus

biceps femoris

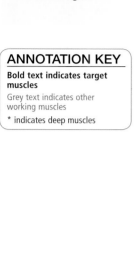

rectus abdominis

transversus abdominis*

tensor fasciae latae

sartorius

vastus intermedius*

rectus femoris

vastus lateralis

vastus medialis

SWISS BALL HIP CROSSOVER

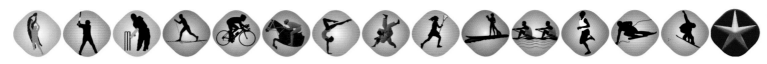

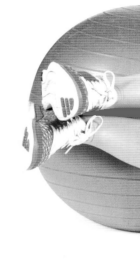

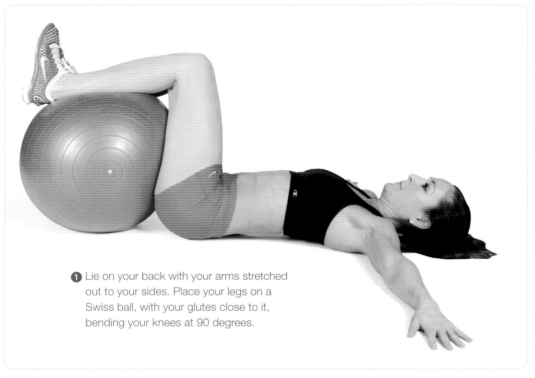

1 Lie on your back with your arms stretched out to your sides. Place your legs on a Swiss ball, with your glutes close to it, bending your knees at 90 degrees.

TARGETS
• Lower back
• Obliques
• Abdominals

LEVEL
• Intermediate

BENEFITS
• Strengthens the lower back and obliques

NOT ADVISABLE IF YOU HAVE . . .
• Lower-back issues

MODIFICATION
• **More difficult:** Try holding a medicine ball between your thighs for added resistance.

DO IT RIGHT
• Keep your core centered.

AVOID
• Swinging your legs excessively.

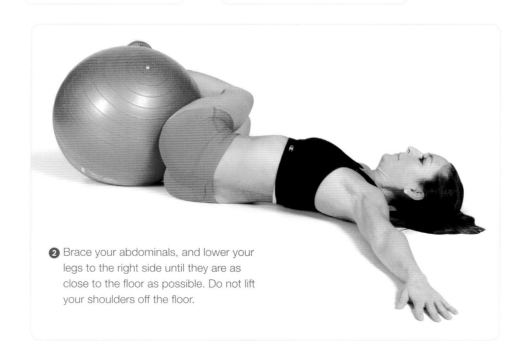

2 Brace your abdominals, and lower your legs to the right side until they are as close to the floor as possible. Do not lift your shoulders off the floor.

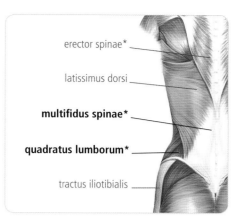

erector spinae*

latissimus dorsi

multifidus spinae*

quadratus lumborum*

tractus iliotibialis

3 Return to the starting position, then rotate your legs to the other side. Complete 15 repetitions per side.

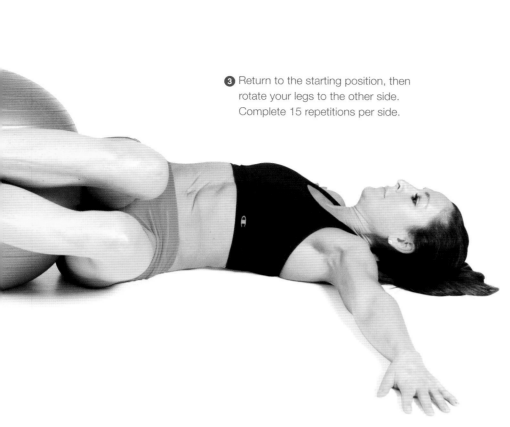

BEST FOR

- multifidus spinae
- quadratus lumborum
- obliquus externus
- obliquus internus

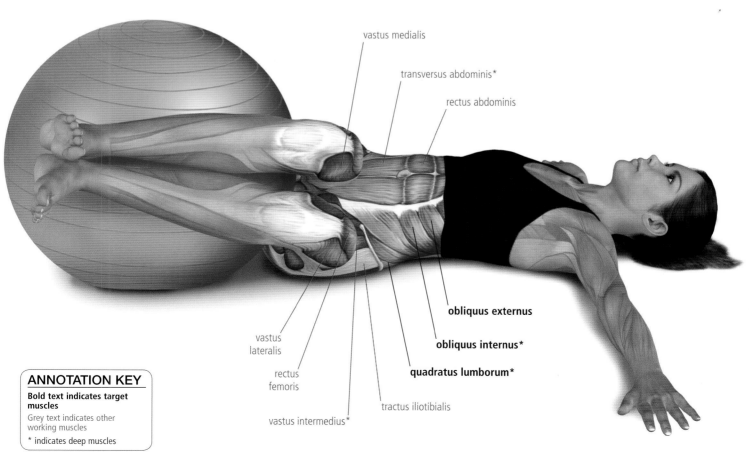

vastus medialis

transversus abdominis*

rectus abdominis

obliquus externus

obliquus internus*

quadratus lumborum*

vastus lateralis

rectus femoris

tractus iliotibialis

vastus intermedius*

ANNOTATION KEY

Bold text indicates target muscles

Grey text indicates other working muscles

* indicates deep muscles

V-UP

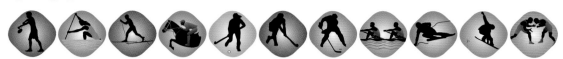

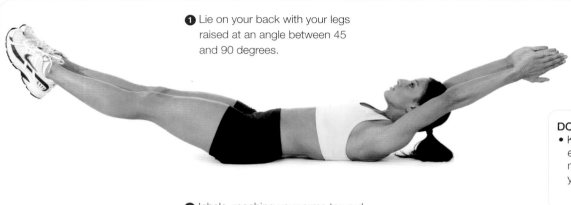

1 Lie on your back with your legs raised at an angle between 45 and 90 degrees.

2 Inhale, reaching your arms toward the ceiling as you lift your head and shoulders off the floor.

DO IT RIGHT
- Keep your neck elongated but relaxed, minimizing the tension in your upper spine.

AVOID
- Using momentum to carry you through the exercise. Use your abdominal muscles to lift your legs and torso.

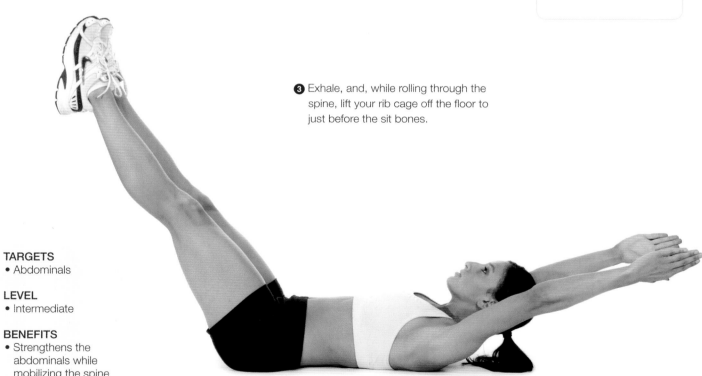

3 Exhale, and, while rolling through the spine, lift your rib cage off the floor to just before the sit bones.

TARGETS
- Abdominals

LEVEL
- Intermediate

BENEFITS
- Strengthens the abdominals while mobilizing the spine

NOT ADVISABLE IF YOU HAVE . . .
- Lower-back pain

❹ Inhale, and reach your arms toward your toes while maintaining a C curve in your back. Exhale, and roll down the spine by articulating one vertebra at a time. Return to the starting position.

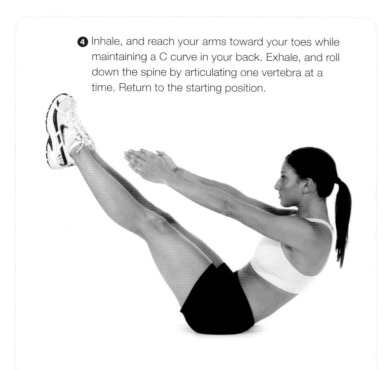

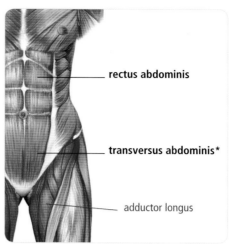

rectus abdominis

transversus abdominis*

adductor longus

BEST FOR

- rectus abdominis
- rectus femoris
- brachialis
- transversus abdominis

ANNOTATION KEY

Bold text indicates target muscles

Grey text indicates other working muscles

* indicates deep muscles

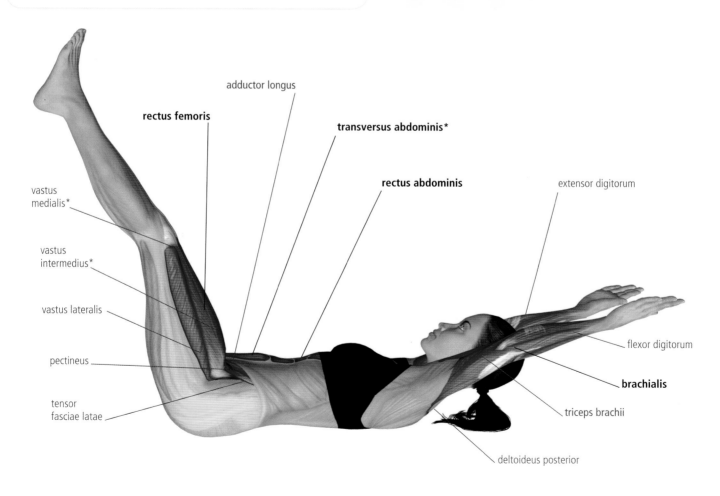

adductor longus

rectus femoris

transversus abdominis*

rectus abdominis

extensor digitorum

vastus medialis*

vastus intermedius*

vastus lateralis

flexor digitorum

pectineus

brachialis

tensor fasciae latae

triceps brachii

deltoideus posterior

MEDICINE BALL SLAM

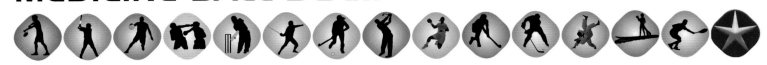

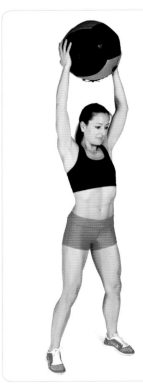

1 Stand upright with your feet shoulder-width apart and knees slightly bent, holding a medicine ball above your head with arms outstretched.

DO IT RIGHT
- Keep your torso straight on throughout the movement.

AVOID
- Rounding your back excessively.

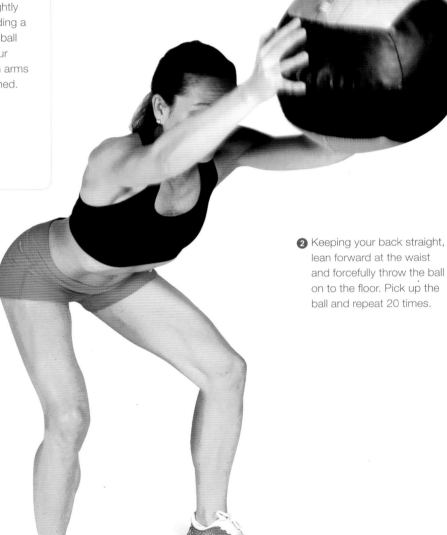

2 Keeping your back straight, lean forward at the waist and forcefully throw the ball on to the floor. Pick up the ball and repeat 20 times.

TARGETS
- Abdominals
- Deltoids
- Upper back

LEVEL
- Intermediate

BENEFITS
- Is effective for engaging and readying the frontal core

NOT ADVISABLE IF YOU HAVE . . .
- Lower-back issues
- Shoulder issues

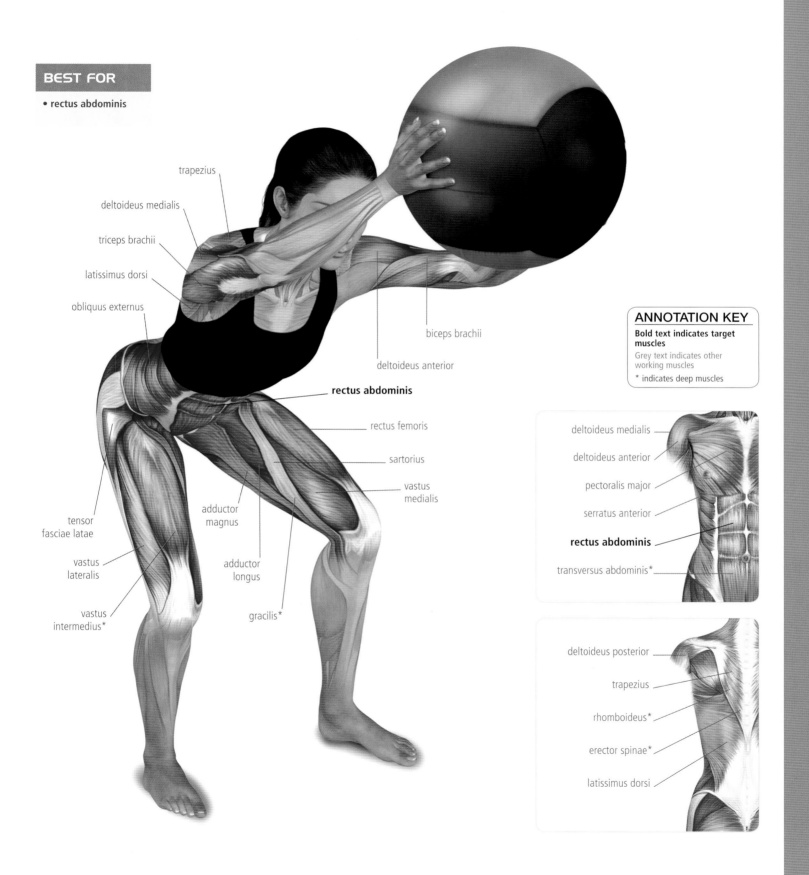

BEST FOR

• rectus abdominis

trapezius

deltoideus medialis

triceps brachii

latissimus dorsi

obliquus externus

biceps brachii

deltoideus anterior

rectus abdominis

rectus femoris

sartorius

vastus medialis

tensor fasciae latae

vastus lateralis

adductor magnus

adductor longus

vastus intermedius*

gracilis*

ANNOTATION KEY

Bold text indicates target muscles

Grey text indicates other working muscles

* indicates deep muscles

deltoideus medialis

deltoideus anterior

pectoralis major

serratus anterior

rectus abdominis

transversus abdominis*

deltoideus posterior

trapezius

rhomboideus*

erector spinae*

latissimus dorsi

THE WINDMILL

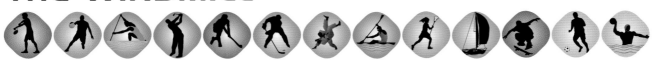

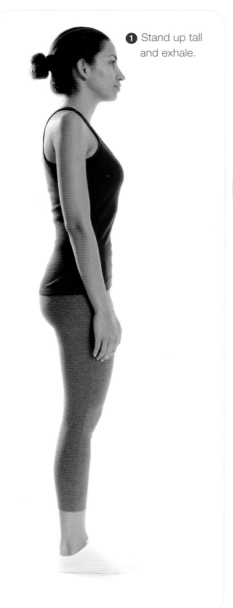

1 Stand up tall and exhale.

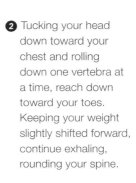

2 Tucking your head down toward your chest and rolling down one vertebra at a time, reach down toward your toes. Keeping your weight slightly shifted forward, continue exhaling, rounding your spine.

TARGETS
• Back

LEVEL
• Intermediate

BENEFITS
• Stretches the spine and hamstrings
• Refines spinal stacking skills

NOT ADVISABLE IF YOU HAVE . . .
• Lower-back pain

DO IT RIGHT
• Stack your spine one vertebra at a time.
• Connect the stretch in your back with the stretch in your hamstrings.

AVOID
• Facing forward as you stretch down.

levator scapulae*

rhomboideus*

teres minor

teres major

trapezius

erector spinae*

quadratus
lumborum*

gluteus
medius*

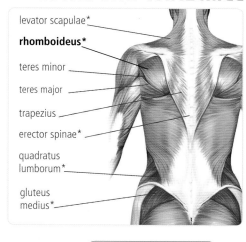

quadratus
lumborum*

latissimus dorsi

rhomboideus*

trapezius

gluteus
maximus

biceps
femoris

ANNOTATION KEY

**Bold text indicates target
muscles**

Grey text indicates other
working muscles

* indicates deep muscles

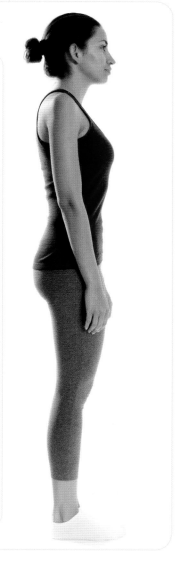

❸ When you are completely folded over,
inhale and begin uncurling your spine,
stacking the spine from your hips up to
your shoulders. Roll your shoulders back
and stand up tall. Repeat three times.

BEST FOR

• latissimus dorsi
• rhomboideus
• quadratus lumborum
• biceps femoris

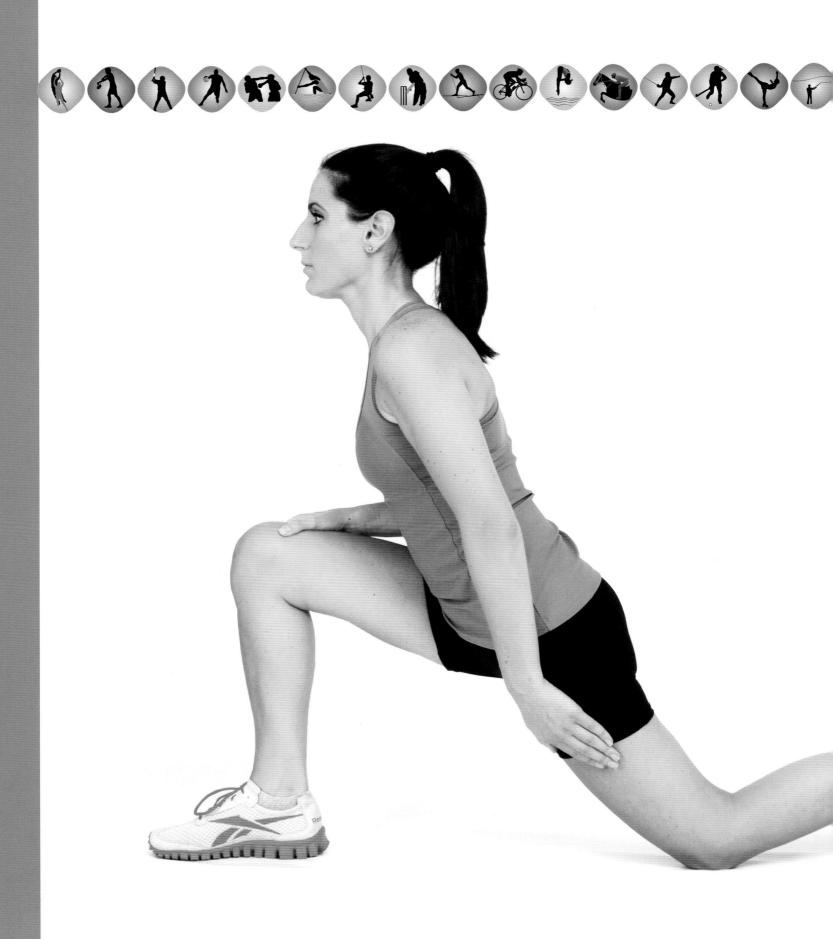

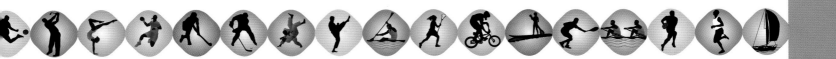

STRETCHES

Stretching is absolutely essential not only for your athletic achievement in the gym, but also for keeping the muscles and connective tissue strong and pliable. A muscle that is flexible has a full range of motion that is both elastic and sturdy. The better your range of motion, the more lean muscle tissue you can develop, which will bring with it an improvement in strength and performance. Stretching can be performed both during and after exercise, when the muscles are warm and have been activated through their respective ranges of motion. In addition, regular stretching brings a host of other benefits, including improving the blood supply to joint structures, helping to relieve pain, increasing energy levels, improving posture and relieving stress.

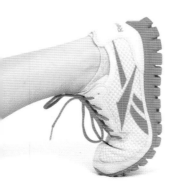

CHEST STRETCH

1 Stand with your hands behind your head, with fingers interlocked. Your elbows should be pointing outward.

2 Draw your elbows back as you feel the stretch in your chest. Hold for 30 seconds.

3 Bring your elbows back to the starting position, and repeat. Perform three 30-second holds.

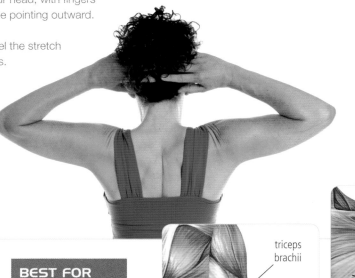

DO IT RIGHT
- Keep your elbows pointed outward.
- Gaze straight ahead.

AVOID
- Hunching your shoulders.
- Arching your back or neck.

TARGETS
- Chest

LEVEL
- Beginner

BENEFITS
- Helps to keep chest muscles flexible

NOT ADVISABLE IF YOU HAVE . . .
- Shoulder issues

BEST FOR
- pectoralis major
- pectoralis minor

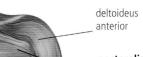

triceps brachii

deltoideus anterior

pectoralis minor*

pectoralis major

ANNOTATION KEY
Bold text indicates target muscles
Grey text indicates other working muscles
* indicates deep muscles

SHOULDER STRETCH

1 Stand up straight, with your right arm drawn across your body at chest height. With your left hand, apply pressure to your right elbow.

2 Hold for 15 seconds, release, and repeat three times. Repeat three times on your left arm.

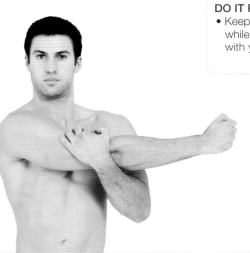

DO IT RIGHT
- Keep your elbow straight while you apply pressure with your hand.

AVOID
- Allowing your shoulders to lift toward your ears.

BEST FOR
- deltoideus posterior
- triceps brachii
- obliquus externus
- teres minor
- infraspinatus

TARGETS
- Shoulders

LEVEL
- Beginner

BENEFITS
- Stretches shoulders, preventing stiffness

NOT ADVISABLE IF YOU HAVE . . .
- Shoulder injury

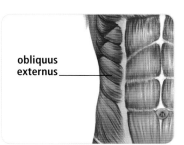

obliquus externus

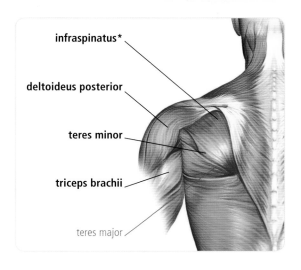

infraspinatus*

deltoideus posterior

teres minor

triceps brachii

teres major

TRICEPS STRETCH

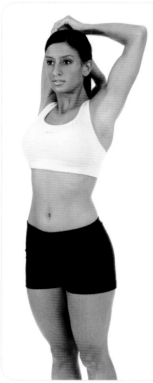

1 While standing, raise your right arm and bend it behind your head.

2 Keeping your shoulders relaxed, gently pull on the raised elbow with your left hand.

3 Continue to pull your elbow back until you feel the stretch on the underside of your arm. Hold for 15 seconds, and repeat three times on each arm.

DO IT RIGHT
- Keep your stretching arm bent at the elbow.

AVOID
- Releasing your grip on the elbow of your stretching arm.
- Pulling too hard on your stretching arm.
- Hunching your shoulders.

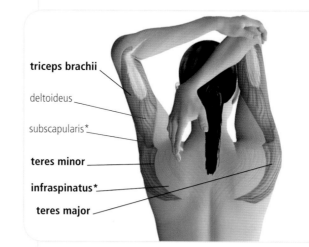

triceps brachii

deltoideus

subscapularis*

teres minor

infraspinatus*

teres major

TARGETS
- Fronts of shoulders

LEVEL
- Beginner

BENEFITS
- Helps to keep shoulders flexible

NOT ADVISABLE IF YOU HAVE . . .
- Shoulder issues

STANDING BICEPS STRETCH

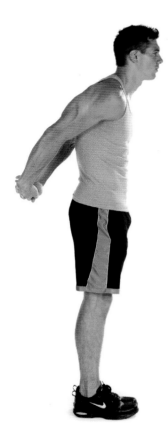

1 Stand with your hands behind your back, clasping them together with fingers interlaced.

2 Lift your arms a few inches away from your body, allowing your fingers to stretch. Hold for 30 seconds.

3 Relax and repeat, performing three 30-second holds.

DO IT RIGHT
- Keep your shoulders down.
- Keep your torso still.

AVOID
- Allowing your hands to unclasp.
- Arching your back.
- Hunching your shoulders.
- Lifting your arms uncomfortably high.

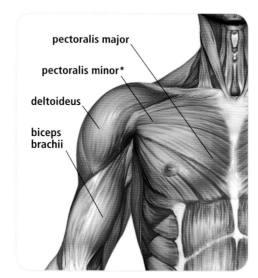

pectoralis major

pectoralis minor*

deltoideus

biceps brachii

ANNOTATION KEY

Bold text indicates target muscles

Grey text indicates other working muscles

* indicates deep muscles

BEST FOR
- biceps brachii
- pectoralis major
- pectoralis minor
- deltoideus

TARGETS
- Biceps

LEVEL
- Beginner

BENEFITS
- Helps to keep biceps flexible

NOT ADVISABLE IF YOU HAVE. . . .
- Shoulder issues

LATISSIMUS DORSI STRETCH

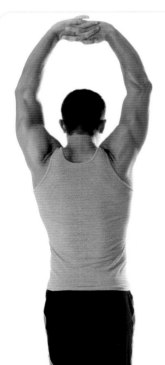

1 Clasp your hands together above your head, your palms turned upward toward the ceiling.

2 Reach your hands outward as you make a circular pattern with your torso.

3 Slowly make a full circle. Repeat the sequence three times in each direction.

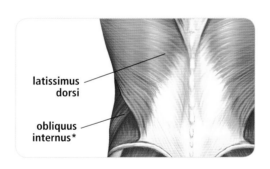

latissimus dorsi

obliquus internus*

BEST FOR

• latissimus dorsi
• obliquus internus

ANNOTATION KEY

Bold text indicates target muscles

Grey text indicates other working muscles

* indicates deep muscles

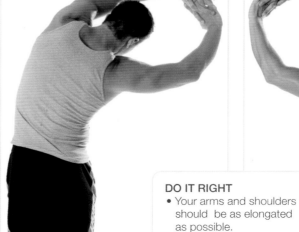

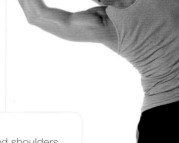

DO IT RIGHT
• Your arms and shoulders should be as elongated as possible.

AVOID
• Leaning back as you come to the top of the circle.

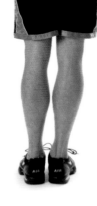

TARGETS
• Back

LEVEL
• Beginner

BENEFITS
• Increases suppleness in the shoulders and back

NOT ADVISABLE IF YOU HAVE . . .
• Back problems

SPINE STRETCH

1 Lie on your back with your left leg straight and the right leg bent, placing your right foot on your left shin.

DO IT RIGHT
• Make sure your lower back remains relaxed.

AVOID
• Allowing your shoulders to lift off the floor.

2 Keeping both shoulders on the floor, slowly bring your right leg across your body until you feel the stretch in the area between your lower back and hips. Stretch only as far as your shoulders will allow without one of them rising from the floor.

3 Hold for 15 seconds. Repeat the sequence three times on each side.

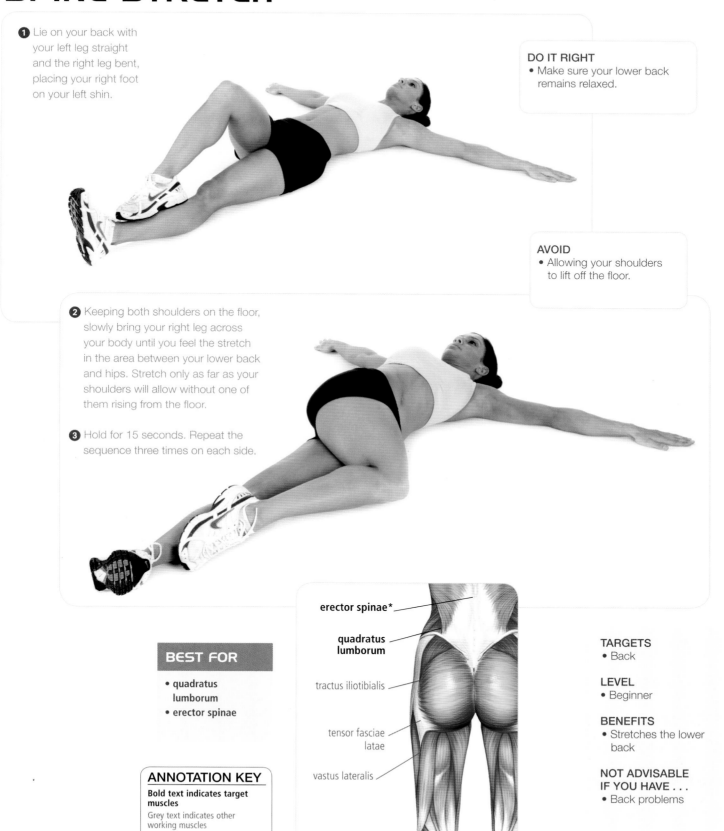

erector spinae*

quadratus
lumborum

tractus iliotibialis

tensor fasciae
latae

vastus lateralis

BEST FOR

• quadratus
  lumborum
• erector spinae

ANNOTATION KEY
**Bold text indicates target
muscles**
Grey text indicates other
working muscles
* indicates deep muscles

TARGETS
• Back

LEVEL
• Beginner

BENEFITS
• Stretches the lower
  back

**NOT ADVISABLE
IF YOU HAVE . . .**
• Back problems

SUPINE LOWER BACK STRETCH

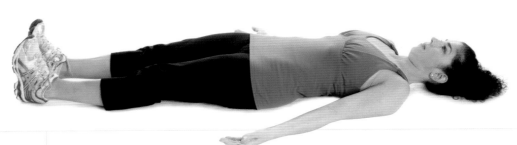

1 Lie on your back with your arms and legs extended, arms angled slightly away from your body.

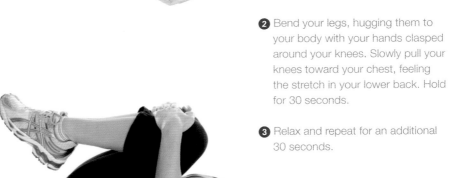

2 Bend your legs, hugging them to your body with your hands clasped around your knees. Slowly pull your knees toward your chest, feeling the stretch in your lower back. Hold for 30 seconds.

3 Relax and repeat for an additional 30 seconds.

DO IT RIGHT
• Keep your knees and feet together.

AVOID
• Raising your head off the floor.

TARGETS
• Glutes
• Lower back

LEVEL
• Beginner

BENEFITS
• Helps to keep lower-back and gluteal muscles flexible

NOT ADVISABLE IF YOU HAVE . . .
• Severe back pain
• Numbness or tingling in the lower extremities

BEST FOR

• erector spinae

ANNOTATION KEY
Bold text indicates target muscles
Grey text indicates other working muscles
* indicates deep muscles

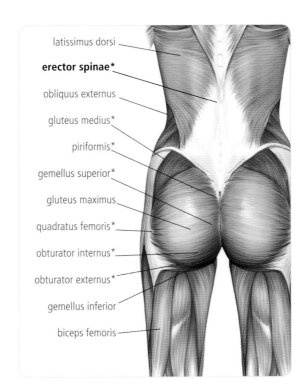

latissimus dorsi

erector spinae*

obliquus externus

gluteus medius*

piriformis*

gemellus superior*

gluteus maximus

quadratus femoris*

obturator internus*

obturator externus*

gemellus inferior

biceps femoris

KNEELING SWISS BALL LAT STRETCH

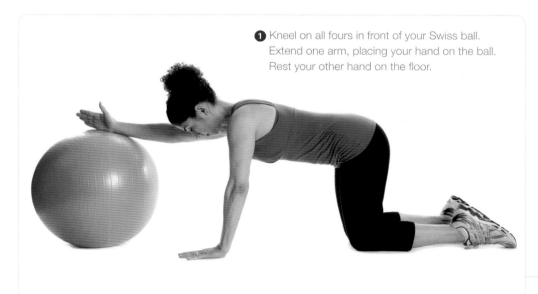

1 Kneel on all fours in front of your Swiss ball. Extend one arm, placing your hand on the ball. Rest your other hand on the floor.

DO IT RIGHT
- Keep your arm fully extended on the ball.
- Face the floor throughout the stretch.

AVOID
- Allowing your torso to twist.
- Arching your neck.

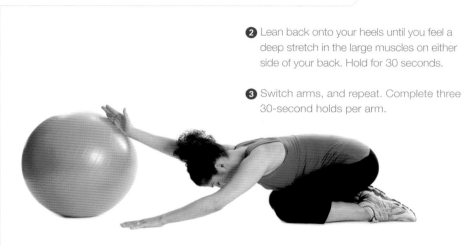

2 Lean back onto your heels until you feel a deep stretch in the large muscles on either side of your back. Hold for 30 seconds.

3 Switch arms, and repeat. Complete three 30-second holds per arm.

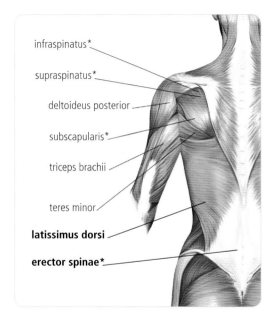

infraspinatus*

supraspinatus*

deltoideus posterior

subscapularis*

triceps brachii

teres minor

latissimus dorsi

erector spinae*

BEST FOR
- **latissimus dorsi**
- **erector spinae**

ANNOTATION KEY
Bold text indicates target muscles
Grey text indicates other working muscles
* indicates deep muscles

TARGETS
- Back

LEVEL
- Beginner

BENEFITS
- Helps to keep back muscles flexible

NOT ADVISABLE IF YOU HAVE . . .
- Lower-back issues

ILIOTIBIAL BAND STRETCH

1 Standing, cross your left leg in front of your right.

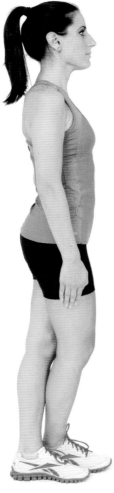

2 Bend at the waist while keeping both knees straight, and reach your hands toward the floor.

3 Hold for 15 seconds. Repeat sequence three times on each leg.

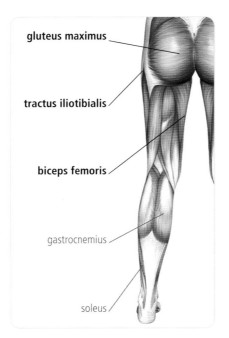

DO IT RIGHT
• Keep your arms and legs relatively straight.

AVOID
• Arching your back at any point.
• Forcing your hands to reach the floor.

TARGETS
• Knees
• Outer thighs

LEVEL
• Beginner

BENEFITS
• Stretches iliotibial band, calves, hamstrings and glutes

NOT ADVISABLE IF YOU HAVE . . .
• Back injury

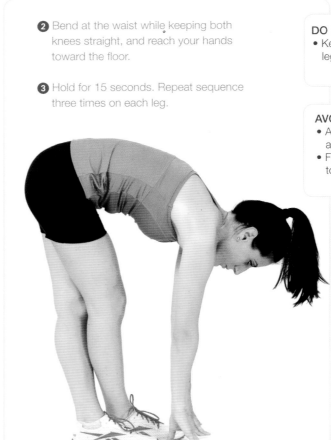

gluteus maximus

tractus iliotibialis

biceps femoris

gastrocnemius

soleus

rectus femoris

vastus lateralis

BEST FOR
• tractus iliotibialis
• biceps femoris
• gluteus maximus
• vastus lateralis

ANNOTATION KEY
Bold text indicates target muscles
Grey text indicates other working muscles
* indicates deep muscles

HIP-TO-THIGH STRETCH

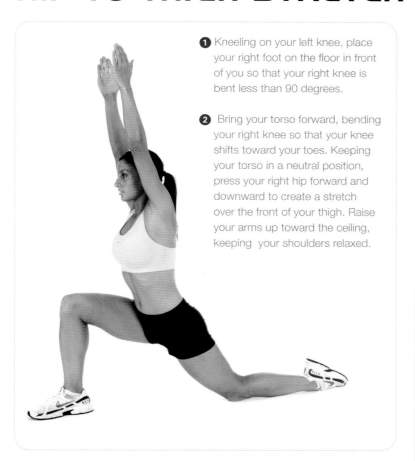

1 Kneeling on your left knee, place your right foot on the floor in front of you so that your right knee is bent less than 90 degrees.

2 Bring your torso forward, bending your right knee so that your knee shifts toward your toes. Keeping your torso in a neutral position, press your right hip forward and downward to create a stretch over the front of your thigh. Raise your arms up toward the ceiling, keeping your shoulders relaxed.

DO IT RIGHT
- Ensure your shoulders and neck remain relaxed.
- Move your entire body as a single unit as you go into the stretch.

AVOID
- Extending your knee too far over the planted foot.
- Rotating your hips.
- Shifting the knee of the back leg outward.

3 Bring your arms down and move your hips backward. Straighten your right leg, and bring your torso forward. Place your hands on either side of your straight leg for support.

4 Hold for 10 seconds, and repeat the forward and backward movement five times on each leg.

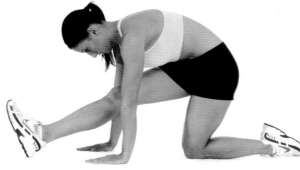

MODIFICATION
More difficult: During the backward movement, raise your back knee off the floor and straighten your back leg. Keep your hands on the floor.

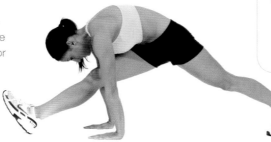

tensor fasciae latae

pectineus*

psoas minor*

iliopsoas*

psoas major*

iliacus*

adductor longus

rectus femoris

gracilis*

ANNOTATION KEY
Bold text indicates target muscles
Grey text indicates other working muscles
* indicates deep muscles

TARGETS
- Hips
- Thighs

LEVEL
- Beginner

BENEFITS
- Stretches front and back of the thighs

NOT ADVISABLE IF YOU HAVE . . .
- Back problems

STANDING HAMSTRING STRETCH

1 Stand with one leg bent and the other extended in front of you with the heel on the floor.

2 Lean over your extended leg, resting both hands above your knee. Place the majority of your body weight on your front heel while feeling the stretch in the back of your thigh. Hold for 30 seconds.

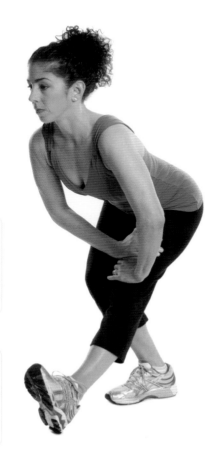

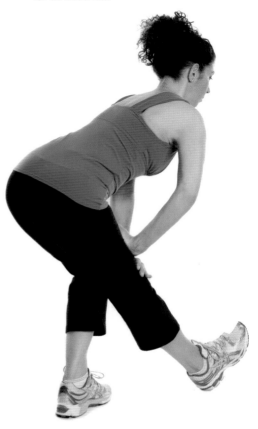

DO IT RIGHT
• Keep your front leg straight.
• Flex the foot of your front leg as you stretch.

AVOID
• Allowing your back to arch or round forward.
• Hunching your shoulders.

3 Switch sides and repeat. Complete three 30-second holds on each leg.

TARGETS
• Hamstrings

LEVEL
• Beginner

BENEFITS
• Helps to keep hamstring muscles flexible

NOT ADVISABLE IF YOU HAVE . . .
• Lower-back issues
• Knee issues

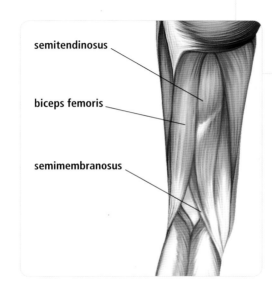

semitendinosus

biceps femoris

semimembranosus

BEST FOR
• biceps femoris
• semitendinosus
• semimembranosus

ANNOTATION KEY
Bold text indicates target muscles
Grey text indicates other working muscles
* indicates deep muscles

LYING HAMSTRING STRETCH

1 Lie on your back with both knees bent and your feet flat on the floor.

2 Grasp your right leg behind the knee, and draw your knee in toward your chest.

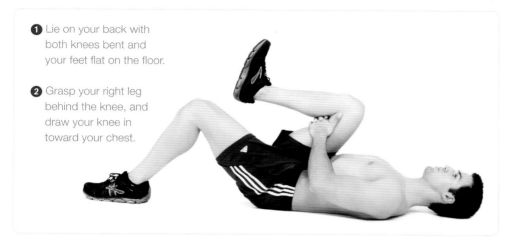

DO IT RIGHT
- Make sure your neck and shoulders remain relaxed.
- Keep your knee pulled in toward the chest throughout the movement.
- Remember to flex your toes.

3 Keeping your knee pulled into your chest, flex your toes and contract your quadriceps, so that you begin to straighten your leg.

4 Release your leg into the stretch, and pull it closer toward your chest. Repeat 10 times on each leg.

AVOID
- Rounding your shoulders and lifting your head.
- Rolling your stabilizing leg out of neutral position.

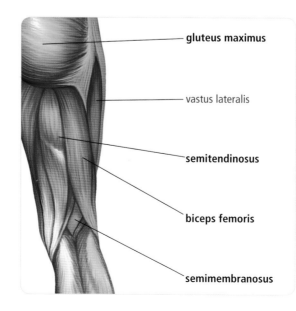

BEST FOR
- semitendinosus
- semimembranosus
- biceps femoris
- gluteus maximus

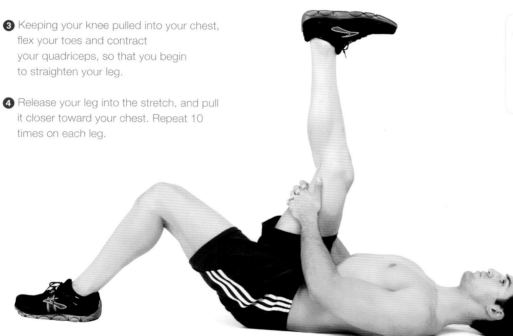

gluteus maximus

vastus lateralis

semitendinosus

biceps femoris

semimembranosus

ANNOTATION KEY
Bold text indicates target muscles
Grey text indicates other working muscles
* indicates deep muscles

TARGETS
- Hamstrings
- Glutes

LEVEL
- Beginner

BENEFITS
- Stretches hamstrings and gluteal muscles

NOT ADVISABLE IF YOU HAVE . . .
- Hip injury
- Knee injury

PIRIFORMIS STRETCH

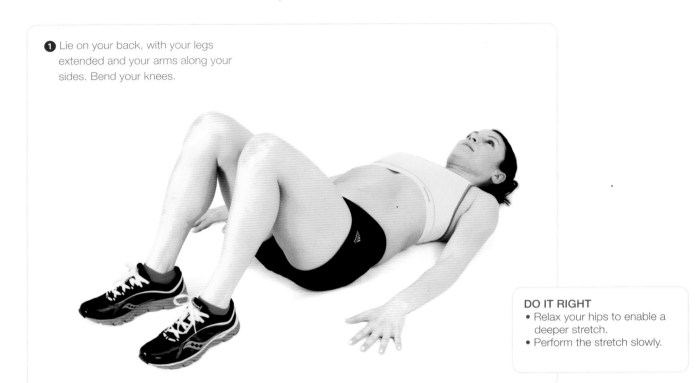

① Lie on your back, with your legs extended and your arms along your sides. Bend your knees.

DO IT RIGHT
- Relax your hips to enable a deeper stretch.
- Perform the stretch slowly.

② Keeping your arms and torso in place, lift both feet off the ground. Bring your right ankle over your left knee, resting it on the thigh. Grasp your left thigh with both hands.

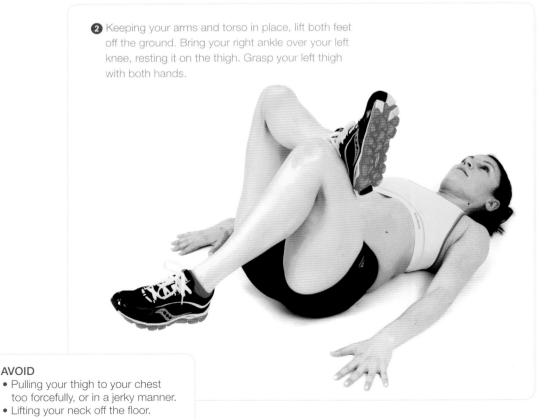

TARGETS
- Lower back
- Glutes

LEVEL
- Beginner

BENEFITS
- Releases stiffness in hips, piriformis and lower back

NOT ADVISABLE IF YOU HAVE . . .
- Lower-back issues
- Knee issues

AVOID
- Pulling your thigh to your chest too forcefully, or in a jerky manner.
- Lifting your neck off the floor.

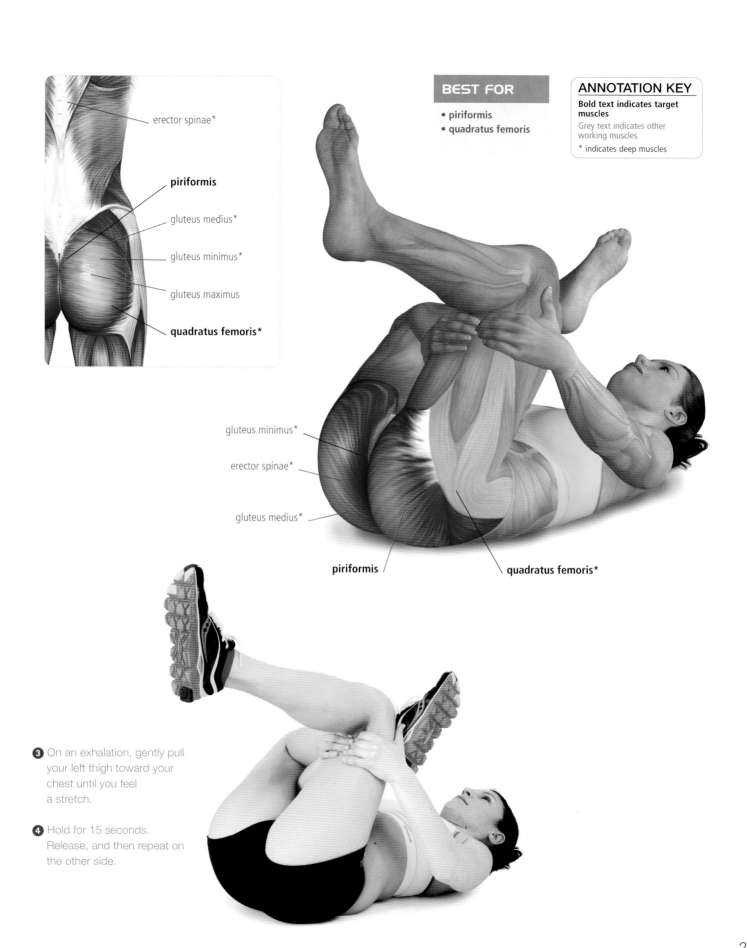

erector spinae*

piriformis

gluteus medius*

gluteus minimus*

gluteus maximus

quadratus femoris*

BEST FOR

- piriformis
- quadratus femoris

ANNOTATION KEY
Bold text indicates target muscles
Grey text indicates other working muscles
* indicates deep muscles

gluteus minimus*

erector spinae*

gluteus medius*

piriformis

quadratus femoris*

❸ On an exhalation, gently pull your left thigh toward your chest until you feel a stretch.

❹ Hold for 15 seconds. Release, and then repeat on the other side.

CALF STRETCH

DO IT RIGHT
• Keep your foot strongly flexed.
• To enhance the stretch, bend your knee more deeply and lower your body further.

AVOID
• Tensing your shoulders.

BEST FOR
• gastrocnemius

ANNOTATION KEY
Bold text indicates target muscles
Grey text indicates other working muscles
* indicates deep muscles

TARGETS
• Lower legs
• Calves

LEVEL
• Beginner

BENEFITS
• Stretches the calves and releases the Achilles tendons.

NOT ADVISABLE IF YOU HAVE . . .
• Lower-back issues
• Achilles tendon problemss
• Knee issues

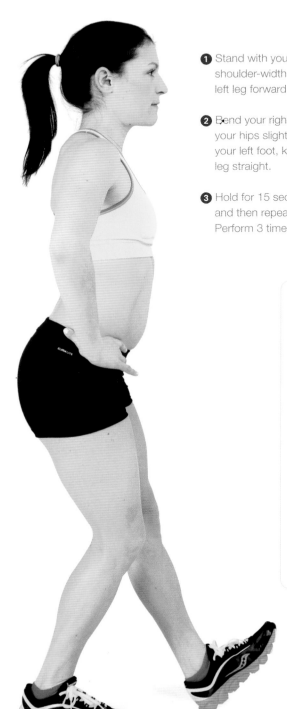

1 Stand with your feet parallel and shoulder-width apart. Extend your left leg forward.

2 Bend your right knee as you tip your hips slightly forward. Flex your left foot, keeping the left leg straight.

3 Hold for 15 seconds. Release, and then repeat on the other side. Perform 3 times on each leg.

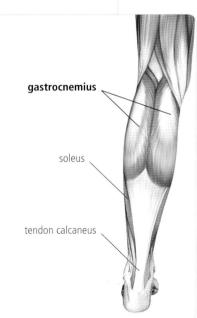

gastrocnemius

soleus

tendon calcaneus

SHIN RELEASE

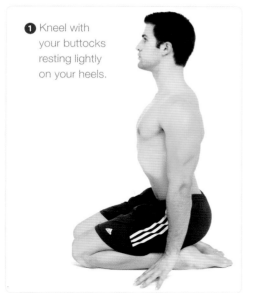

1 Kneel with your buttocks resting lightly on your heels.

DO IT RIGHT
- Make sure your gluteal muscles are contracted and engaged to avoid a curve in your lumbar spine.
- Keep a space between the heels and the glutes.

AVOID
- Arching your back.

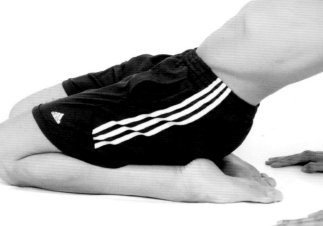

2 Place your hands flat on the floor behind you, with your fingers pointing forward. Keep a slight bend in your elbows.

3 Lean back slightly to increase the intensity of the stretch.

BEST FOR

- gastrocnemius
- soleus
- rectus femoris
- vastus lateralis
- vastus intermedius
- vastus medialis
- tibialis anterior

ANNOTATION KEY

Bold text indicates target muscles

Grey text indicates other working muscles

* indicates deep muscles

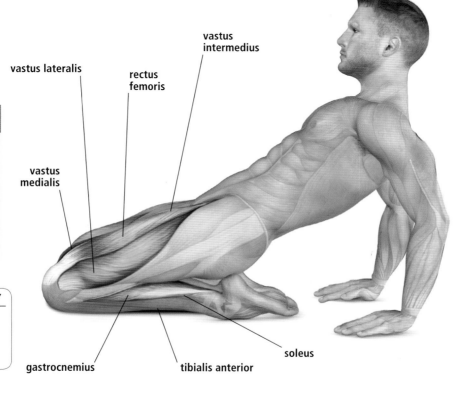

vastus lateralis

rectus femoris

vastus intermedius

vastus medialis

gastrocnemius

tibialis anterior

soleus

TARGETS
- Shins
- Quadriceps

LEVEL
- Beginner

BENEFITS
- Stretches shins and quadriceps

NOT ADVISABLE IF YOU HAVE . . .
- Lower-back pain

STANDING QUADRICEPS STRETCH

1 Stand with your feet together. Bend your right leg behind you, and grasp your foot with your right hand. Pull your heel toward your buttocks until you feel a stretch in the front of your thigh. Keep both knees together and aligned.

2 Hold for 15 seconds. Repeat sequence three times on each leg.

DO IT RIGHT
• Keep both knees pressed together.
• With the arm opposite your bent leg, lean against a wall or other stable object to aid your balance.

AVOID
• Leaning forward with your chest.
• Bringing your foot closer to your buttocks than you can reach with a comfortable stretch — this can compress the knee joint.

TARGETS
• Thighs

LEVEL
• Beginner

BENEFITS
• Helps to keep thigh muscles flexible

NOT ADVISABLE IF YOU HAVE . . .
• Knee issues

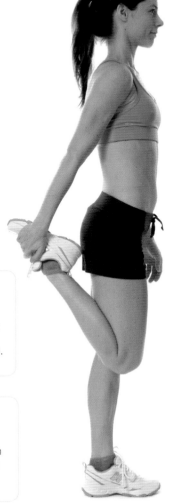

MODIFICATION
Easier: Wrap a resistance band or small towel around your ankle and grasp both ends to aid in raising your foot.

BEST FOR
• rectus femoris
• vastus lateralis
• vastus medialis
• vastus intermedius

ANNOTATION KEY
Bold text indicates target muscles
Grey text indicates other working muscles
* indicates deep muscles

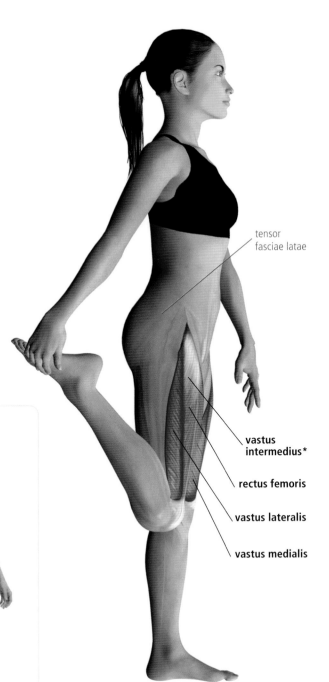

tensor fasciae latae

vastus intermedius*

rectus femoris

vastus lateralis

vastus medialis

BUTTERFLY

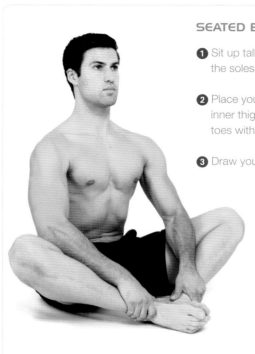

SEATED BUTTERFLY

1 Sit up tall on the floor or a mat, with the soles of your feet pressed together.

2 Place your forearms or elbows on your inner thighs, and grab your feet and toes with your hands.

3 Draw your heels in toward your core.

DO IT RIGHT
• Exhale as you drop your chest toward the floor.

AVOID
• Slouching.
• Holding your breath.
• Rocking backward, off your hip bones; instead, feel them anchored on the floor.

FOLDED BUTTERFLY

1 From the seated butterfly position, place your forearms or elbows on your inner thighs, and grab your feet and toes with your hands. Keep your heels a comfortable distance from your core.

2 Fold your upper body forward until you feel a stretch in your groin and in your upper inner thighs.

3 Slowly roll up, and repeat if desired.

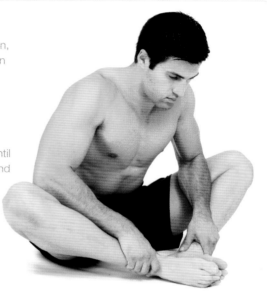

BEST FOR

• adductor longus
• adductor brevis
• gracilis
• pectineus

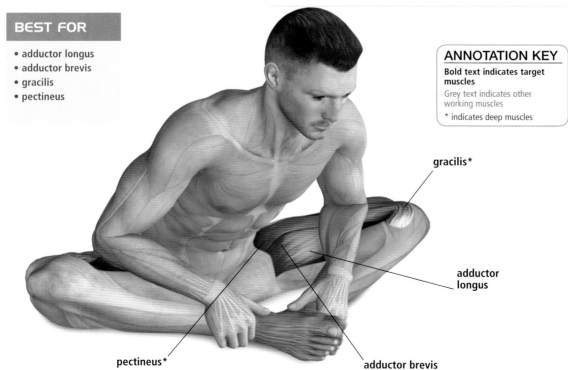

ANNOTATION KEY
Bold text indicates target muscles
Grey text indicates other working muscles
* indicates deep muscles

gracilis*

adductor longus

pectineus*

adductor brevis

TARGETS
• Hips and thighs
• Lower back
• Trunk and core

LEVEL
• Beginner

BENEFITS
• Stretches hips and lower back
• Prevents and counteracts soreness caused by long bike rides

NOT ADVISABLE IF YOU HAVE . . .
• Hip issues
• Lower-back issues (Folded position)

TOE TOUCH

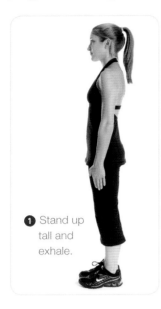

1 Stand up tall and exhale.

2 Tucking your head down toward your chest and rolling down one vertebra at a time, reach down toward your toes. Keeping your weight slightly shifted forward, continue exhaling, rounding your spine.

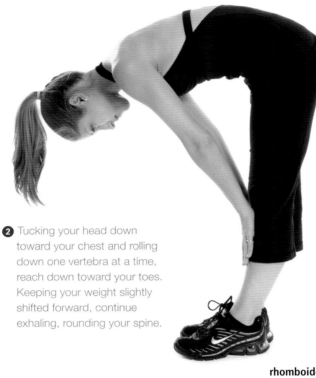

3 When you are completely folded over, inhale and begin uncurling your spine, stacking the spine from your hips up to your shoulders. Roll your shoulders back and stand up tall. Repeat three times.

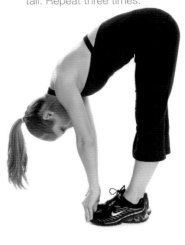

DO IT RIGHT
- Stack your spine one vertebra at a time.
- Connect the stretch in your back with the stretch in your hamstrings.
- Make the stretch long and smooth.

AVOID
- Tensing your neck muscles.
- Bouncing as you try to reach your hands to your toes—reach down only as far as you can comfortably extend.

TARGETS
- Spine

LEVEL
- Beginner

BENEFITS
- Stretches the spine and hamstrings
- Refines spinal stacking skills

NOT ADVISABLE IF YOU HAVE . . .
- Lower-back pain that radiates down the leg

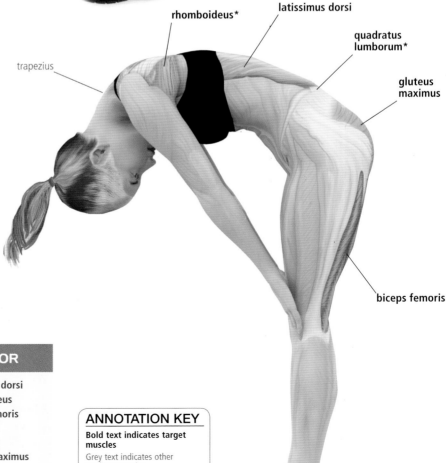

rhomboideus*

latissimus dorsi

quadratus lumborum*

gluteus maximus

trapezius

biceps femoris

BEST FOR
- **latissimus dorsi**
- **rhomboideus**
- **biceps femoris**
- **quadratus lumborum**
- **gluteus maximus**

ANNOTATION KEY
Bold text indicates target muscles
Grey text indicates other working muscles
* indicates deep muscles

CHILD'S STRETCH

1 Kneel on a mat with your hips aligned over your knees. Bring your legs together so that your big toes are touching.

2 Sit back, resting your buttocks on your heels. Separate your knees about hip-width apart.

DO IT RIGHT
• Round your back to create a dome shape.

AVOID
• Rushing the pose. It can take a few minutes to allow your body to deepen into the full stretch.
• Compressing the back of your neck.

3 Lower your chest onto your thighs as you extend your hands in front of your head, elongating your neck and spine as you stretch your tailbone toward the mat.

4 Place your forehead on the mat, and hold this position for 30 seconds to 3 minutes.

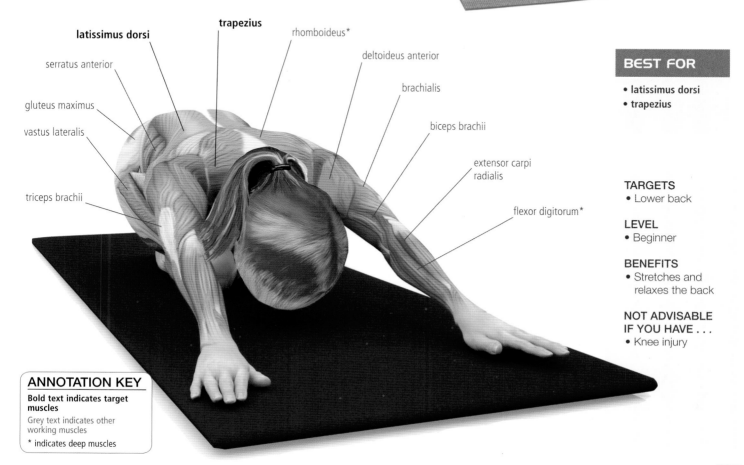

latissimus dorsi

trapezius

serratus anterior

rhomboideus*

deltoideus anterior

brachialis

gluteus maximus

biceps brachii

vastus lateralis

extensor carpi radialis

triceps brachii

flexor digitorum*

ANNOTATION KEY
Bold text indicates target muscles
Grey text indicates other working muscles
* indicates deep muscles

BEST FOR
• **latissimus dorsi**
• **trapezius**

TARGETS
• Lower back

LEVEL
• Beginner

BENEFITS
• Stretches and relaxes the back

NOT ADVISABLE IF YOU HAVE . . .
• Knee injury

237

UNILATERAL SEATED FORWARD BEND

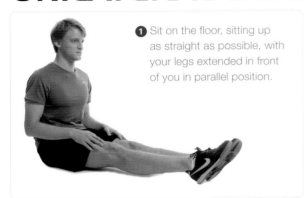

1 Sit on the floor, sitting up as straight as possible, with your legs extended in front of you in parallel position.

2 Bend your right leg until it is turned out, with the bottom of your right foot resting at your left inner thigh just above the kneecap. Rest your hands on your knee.

3 Bend from your waist, and lean forward over your left leg. Place your forearms above your left kneecap.

4 Switch legs, and repeat on the other side.

MODIFICATION

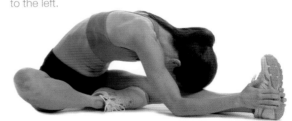

Harder: Follow steps 1 through 3, then exhale and stretch your sternum forward as you fold your torso over your left leg. Grasp the inside of your left foot with your right hand. Use your left hand to guide your torso to the left.

DO IT RIGHT
- Drop your head to benefit your rhomboids, and for a more intense overall stretch.

AVOID
- Allowing the foot of your bent leg to shift beneath your straight leg.
- Straining your back—if yours is tight, try performing this stretch with a support, such as a sofa, behind you. Be sure to position your lower back as close to the support as possible.

TARGETS
- Hamstrings

LEVEL
- Beginner

BENEFITS
- Stretches and flexes hamstrings, groins and spine

NOT ADVISABLE IF YOU HAVE . . .
- Knee injury
- Lower-back injury

BEST FOR
- biceps femoris
- semitendinosus
- semimembranosus
- multifidus spinae
- erector spinae
- gastrocnemius
- soleus
- rhomboideus

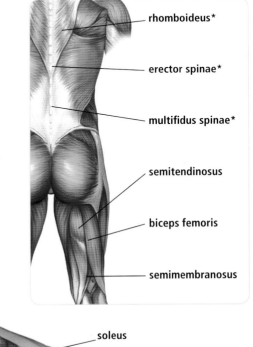

rhomboideus*

erector spinae*

multifidus spinae*

semitendinosus

biceps femoris

semimembranosus

soleus

gastrocnemius

ANNOTATION KEY
Bold text indicates target muscles

Grey text indicates other working muscles

* indicates deep muscles

BILATERAL SEATED FORWARD BEND

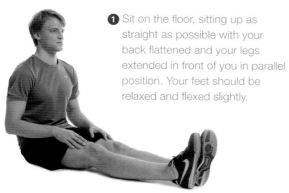

1 Sit on the floor, sitting up as straight as possible with your back flattened and your legs extended in front of you in parallel position. Your feet should be relaxed and flexed slightly.

DO IT RIGHT
- Bend at the hips and keep your spine straight as you stretch.
- Extend your torso as far forward over your legs as possible.

AVOID
- Holding your breath.
- Tensing your jaw or clenching your teeth while performing any stretch: relaxing your mouth will help you breathe evenly.

MODIFICATION
Harder: For a deeper stretch in your hamstrings, place an elastic exercise band around the balls of your feet, using both hands to draw the band toward you.

2 Lean forward, lowering your abdominals over your thighs, forearms resting above your kneecaps as you stretch.

3 Slowly roll up, and repeat if desired.

BEST FOR
- biceps femoris
- semitendinosus
- semimembranosus
- multifidus spinae
- erector spinae
- gastrocnemius
- soleus
- rhomboideus

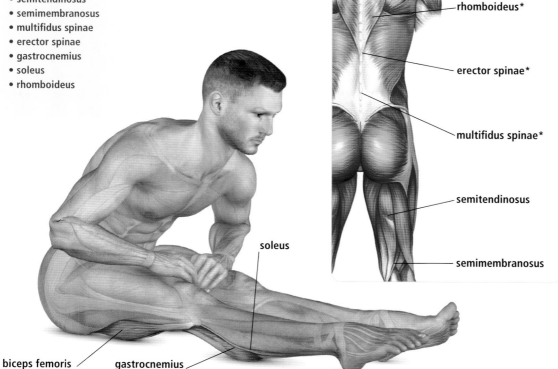

rhomboideus*

erector spinae*

multifidus spinae*

semitendinosus

semimembranosus

soleus

biceps femoris   gastrocnemius

ANNOTATION KEY
Bold text indicates target muscles
Grey text indicates other working muscles
* indicates deep muscles

TARGETS
- Hamstrings

LEVEL
- Beginner

BENEFITS
- Stretches and flexes hamstrings, groins and spine

NOT ADVISABLE IF YOU HAVE . . .
- Knee injury
- Lower-back injury

SEATED HIP AND SPINE STRETCH

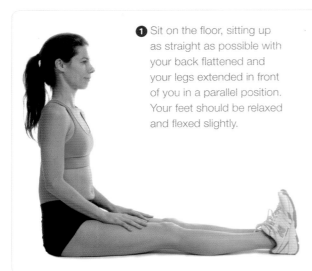

1 Sit on the floor, sitting up as straight as possible with your back flattened and your legs extended in front of you in a parallel position. Your feet should be relaxed and flexed slightly.

2 Extend your left leg straight in front of you, and bend your right knee. Cross your bent knee over the straight leg, and keep your foot flat on the floor.

3 Wrap your left arm around the bent knee so that you are able to apply pressure to your leg to rotate your torso.

DO IT RIGHT
- Keep your neck and shoulders relaxed.
- Apply even pressure to your leg with your active hand.
- Keep your torso upright as you pull your knee and torso together.

AVOID
- Rounding your torso.
- Lifting the foot of your bent leg off the floor.
- Straining your neck as you rotate.

4 Keeping your hips aligned, rotate your upper spine as you pull your chest in toward your knee.

5 Hold for 30 seconds. Slowly release, and repeat three times on each side.

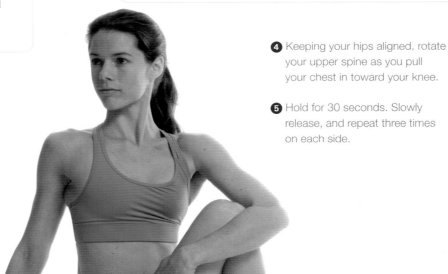

TARGETS
- Back
- Hips
- Glutes

LEVEL
- Beginner

BENEFITS
- Stretches hips, glutes and spine

NOT ADVISABLE IF YOU HAVE . . .
- Back issues
- Hip problems

BEST FOR

- adductor longus
- iliopsoas
- rhomboideus
- sternocleidomastoideus
- latissimus dorsi
- obliquus internus
- obliquus externus
- quadratus lumborum
- erector spinae
- multifidus spinae
- tractus iliotibialis
- gluteus maximus
- gluteus medius
- piriformis

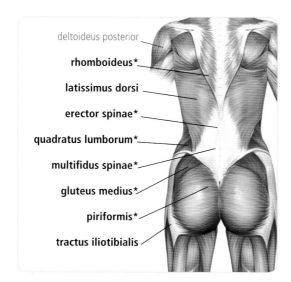

deltoideus posterior
rhomboideus*
latissimus dorsi
erector spinae*
quadratus lumborum*
multifidus spinae*
gluteus medius*
piriformis*
tractus iliotibialis

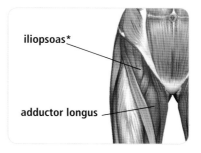

iliopsoas*
adductor longus

ANNOTATION KEY

Bold text indicates target muscles

Grey text indicates other working muscles

* indicates deep muscles

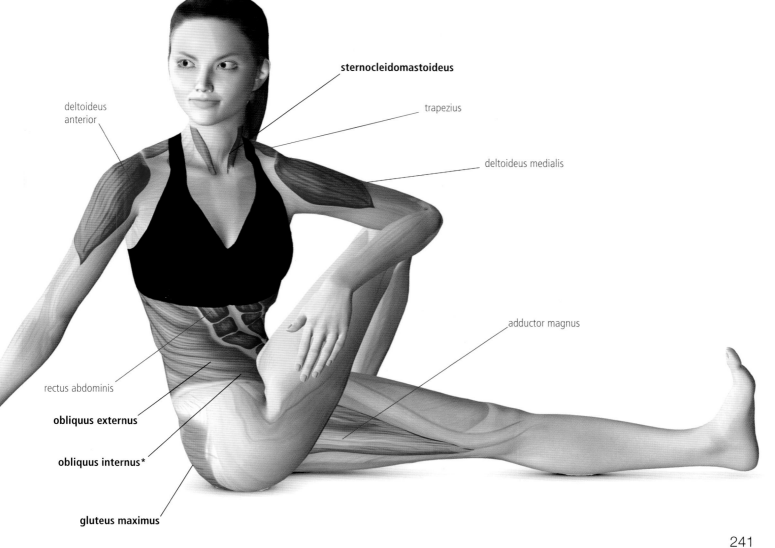

deltoideus anterior

sternocleidomastoideus

trapezius

deltoideus medialis

rectus abdominis

adductor magnus

obliquus externus

obliquus internus*

gluteus maximus

PRETZEL (SPINAL ROTATION) STRETCH

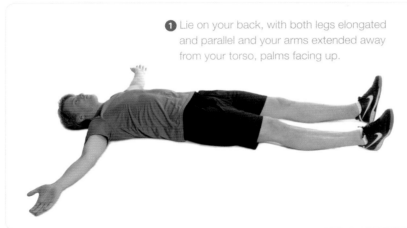

❶ Lie on your back, with both legs elongated and parallel and your arms extended away from your torso, palms facing up.

DO IT RIGHT
- Keep your elbows and wrists lower than your shoulders, protecting your rotator cuff from strain.
- Before you cross one leg over the other, ensure that your body is in a straight line from your head to toe.

AVOID
- Lifting your shoulders; try to keep both shoulder blades in contact with the floor throughout the stretch.

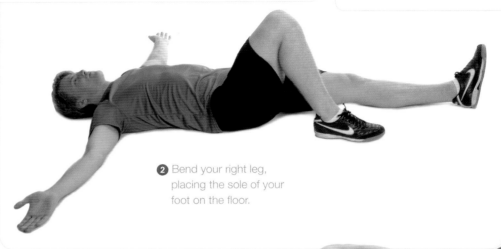

❷ Bend your right leg, placing the sole of your foot on the floor.

TARGETS
- Lumbar spine
- Glutes
- Chest

LEVEL
- Intermediate

BENEFITS
- Stretches lower back

NOT ADVISABLE IF YOU HAVE . . .
- Severe lower-back pain

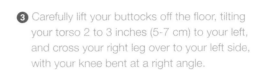

❸ Carefully lift your buttocks off the floor, tilting your torso 2 to 3 inches (5-7 cm) to your left, and cross your right leg over to your left side, with your knee bent at a right angle.

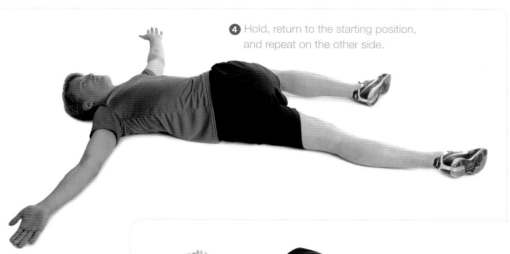

④ Hold, return to the starting position, and repeat on the other side.

MODIFICATION

Harder: Place the palm of your right hand on your left quadriceps, and exert gentle downward pressure while your left leg is crossed over your right, and vice versa.

BEST FOR

- gemellus inferior
- gemellus superior
- gluteus medius
- gluteus minimus
- piriformis
- obturator externus
- obturator internus
- pectoralis major
- pectoralis minor
- quadratus femoris
- gluteus maximus

ANNOTATION KEY

Bold text indicates target muscles

Grey text indicates other working muscles

* indicates deep muscles

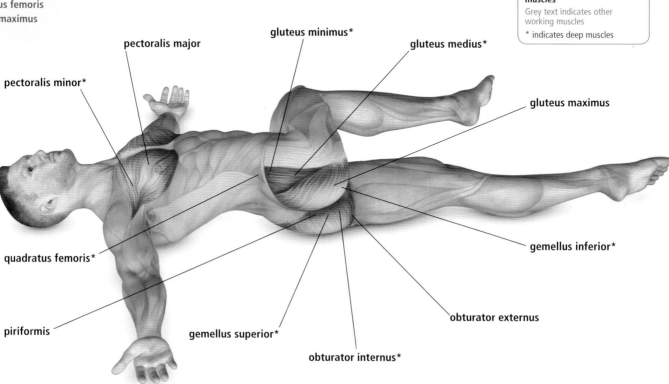

pectoralis minor*

pectoralis major

gluteus minimus*

gluteus medius*

gluteus maximus

quadratus femoris*

gemellus inferior*

piriformis

gemellus superior*

obturator internus*

obturator externus

KNEE-TO-CHEST FLEX

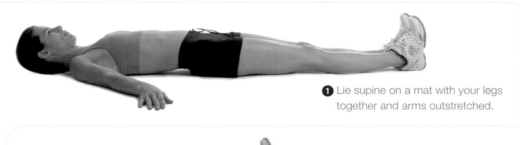

1 Lie supine on a mat with your legs together and arms outstretched.

DO IT RIGHT
- Keep your spine in a neutral position.

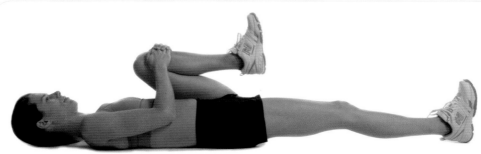

2 Bend your left knee and bring your foot to your body's midline while clasping your hands together to hold your knee. Hold the stretch for 15 seconds.

3 Return to the start position.

AVOID
- Lifting your buttocks off the floor.

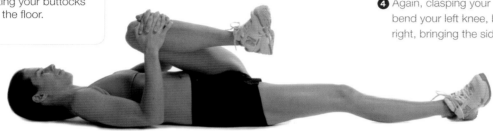

4 Again, clasping your hands together to hold your knee, bend your left knee, but this time rotate the left leg to the right, bringing the side of your leg against your chest.

5 Hold the stretch for 15 seconds, and then return to the start position. Repeat the entire sequence with the right leg bent.

ANNOTATION KEY

Bold text indicates target muscles

Grey text indicates other working muscles

* indicates deep muscles

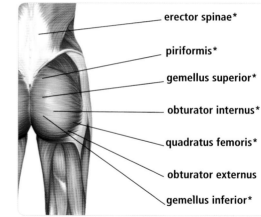

biceps femoris

obliquus externus

latissimus dorsi

gluteus minimus*

gluteus maximus

erector spinae*

piriformis*

gemellus superior*

obturator internus*

quadratus femoris*

obturator externus

gemellus inferior*

TARGETS
- Lower back
- Hips

LEVEL
- Beginner

BENEFITS
- Stretches lower back, hip extensors and hip rotators

NOT ADVISABLE IF YOU HAVE . . .
- Advanced degenerative joint disease

BEST FOR

- **erector spinae**
- **latissimus dorsi**
- **gluteus maximus**
- **gluteus minimus**
- **piriformis**
- **gemellus superior**
- **gemellus inferior**
- **obturator externus**
- **obturator internus**
- **quadratus femoris**

WIDE-LEGGED FORWARD BEND

1 Stand with your feet parallel and wide apart. Bend your knees slightly and tuck your pelvis slightly forward, lift your chest and press your shoulders downward and back.

DO IT RIGHT
• Contract your leg muscles.
• Keep your feet firmly on the ground throughout.
• Keep your chest elevated.

2 Exhale, and bend forward from your hips, keeping your back flat. Draw your sternum forward as you lower your torso, gazing straight ahead. With your elbows straight, place your fingertips or palms on the floor.

3 With another exhalation, move your hands to the floor between your feet, and lower your torso into a full forward bend. Lengthen your spine by drawing your head to the floor. If possible, bend your elbows and place your forehead on the floor.

4 Hold for 30 seconds to 1 minute. To return to the start position, straighten your elbows and raise your torso while keeping your back flat.

AVOID
• Bending forward from your waist.
• Compressing the back of your neck as you look forward.
• Tensing your shoulders.

ANNOTATION KEY
Bold text indicates target muscles
working muscles
* indicates deep muscles

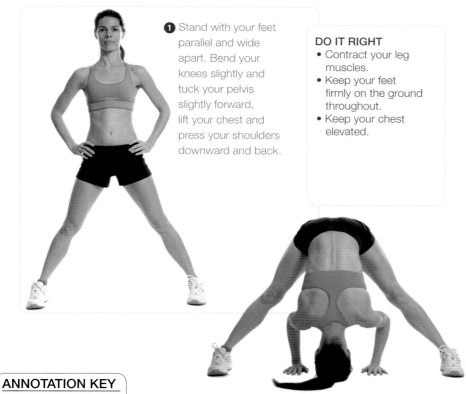

gluteus maximus

gluteus medius*

erector spinae*

rectus femoris

latissimus dorsi

vastus lateralis

peroneus

vastus medialis

soleus

piriformis*

quadratus lumborum*

multifidus spinae*

vastus intermedius*

gastrocnemius

adductor longus

tibialis anterior

BEST FOR
• gluteus maximus
• gluteus medius
• rectus abdominis
• transversus abdominis
• erector spinae
• gastrocnemius
• soleus

TARGETS
• Hamstrings
• Lower back
• Glutes
• Calves

LEVEL
• Advanced

BENEFITS
• Stretches and strengthens hamstrings, groins and spine

NOT ADVISABLE IF YOU HAVE . . .
• Lower-back issues

PREGNANCY STRETCHES

SHOULD YOU BEGIN OR CONTINUE A STRETCHING PROGRAM IF YOU ARE PREGNANT? THE ANSWER IS A RESOUNDING YES.

To prepare for childbirth, a woman's body undergoes a host of changes, including an alteration in your center of gravity, realigning your posture and loosening some of your joints, ligaments and muscles. Many of these changes can result in aches and pains and a general feeling of immobility or estrangement from your own body. Regular stretching helps you stay in touch with your body, and it can help relieve some of the discomfort, while keeping you supple.

YOUR CHANGING BODY

Among the most noticeable changes is the change in your center of gravity. To compensate, the muscles in your chest, lower back and hips tighten. Stretches that focus on posture and balance are an excellent way to combat this tightness. During pregnancy, levels of the hormone relaxin rise in a woman's body. This hormone, which is believed to soften the pubic symphysis in the pelvis and facilitate labor, may be produced up to 3 months after childbirth. It relaxes ligaments, as well as muscles, and makes pregnant women and new mothers vulnerable to overstretching. Relaxin levels may also remain high after a miscarriage. This means that all stretches must be done with great care before and after childbirth.

STRETCHING DURING PREGNANCY

For most healthy women experiencing normal pregnancies, the benefits of stretching include:

- It relaxes the body and prepares it for delivery.
- It allows you to practice breathing.
- It helps to ease stress.

AFTER PREGNANCY

After your baby is born, your body will again undergo changes. Adhering to a regular stretching program can help you adjust. Stretching also helps ease the aches or stiffness that often accompany caring for an infant. For instance, holding your newborn and breast-feeding can make your upper body and shoulders feel stiff, which regular stretches can relieve. While allowing you time to focus on your own needs, post-pregnancy, stretching rebalances your muscles, helps you to avoid injury, reduces stress and rebuilds your body image.

THE "BABY BOUNCE-BACK"

You can regain the body you had prior to pregnancy — and even improve it — by following a few simple dietary guidelines.

• Eat a nutrient-rich diet. Eating healthy is not always easy with a baby, so plan ahead and have nutritious snacks readily available.

• Eat high-protein foods. The protein will help you build necessary muscle to make your workouts more intense and powerful. This, in turn, speeds up your metabolism, which aids in weight loss.

• Eat fiber-rich foods. Foods high in fiber help make you feel full sooner. Fiber also helps fat pass through the digestive system.

Once you have had the all-clear from your doctor, you can begin building up to a full workout program that includes stretching exercises, along with toning exercises and cardiovascular exercises. Although you can do the exercises outlined in this book, you should also focus on high-intensity activities, such as cycling, skipping, swimming and running.

STRETCHING SAFELY BEFORE AND AFTER CHILDBIRTH

Always consult your doctor prior to engaging in any type of workout program. Even though you will derive enormous benefits from stretching, you must also proceed carefully.

• Never "bounce" with these stretches; this can cause serious injury. Keep the stretches soft and small; never extend even slightly beyond what feels completely comfortable.

• During your third trimester, consult your doctor before attempting and performing any stretches that require you to lie on your back. This may cause shortness of breath and dizziness.

• Avoid stretches that require the legs to be wide apart for up to three months after giving birth. When possible, keep your knees together. This is to avoid overstretching of the softened ligaments and to allow your body to recover from the rigours of childbirth

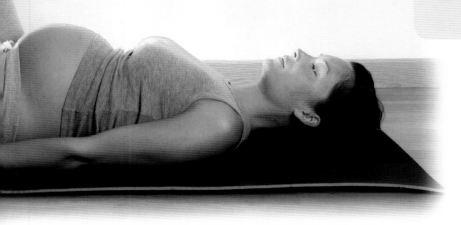

Regular and gentle stretching exercises are beneficial both during and after pregnancy.

TORSO ROTATION

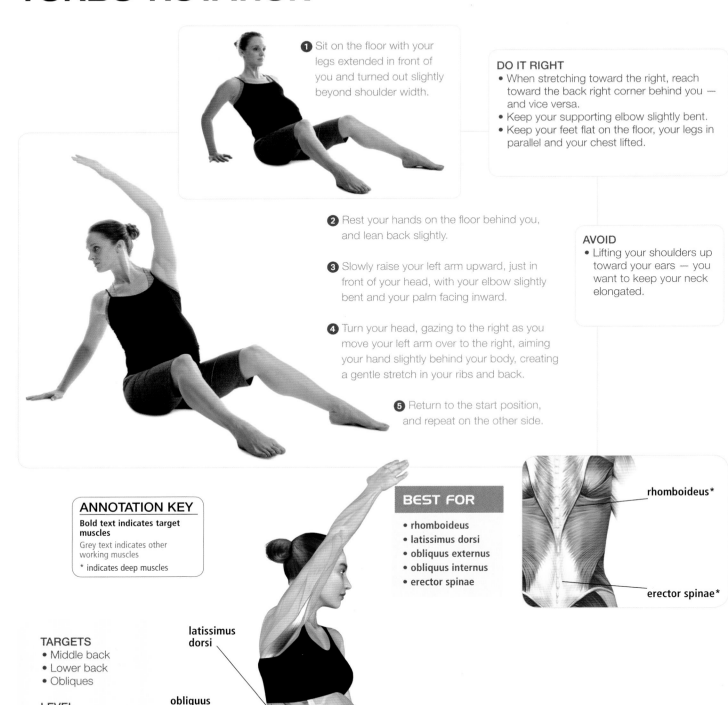

1 Sit on the floor with your legs extended in front of you and turned out slightly beyond shoulder width.

DO IT RIGHT
- When stretching toward the right, reach toward the back right corner behind you — and vice versa.
- Keep your supporting elbow slightly bent.
- Keep your feet flat on the floor, your legs in parallel and your chest lifted.

2 Rest your hands on the floor behind you, and lean back slightly.

3 Slowly raise your left arm upward, just in front of your head, with your elbow slightly bent and your palm facing inward.

AVOID
- Lifting your shoulders up toward your ears — you want to keep your neck elongated.

4 Turn your head, gazing to the right as you move your left arm over to the right, aiming your hand slightly behind your body, creating a gentle stretch in your ribs and back.

5 Return to the start position, and repeat on the other side.

ANNOTATION KEY
Bold text indicates target muscles
Grey text indicates other working muscles
* indicates deep muscles

BEST FOR
- **rhomboideus**
- **latissimus dorsi**
- **obliquus externus**
- **obliquus internus**
- **erector spinae**

rhomboideus*

erector spinae*

latissimus dorsi

obliquus externus

obliquus internus*

TARGETS
- Middle back
- Lower back
- Obliques

LEVEL
- Beginner

BENEFITS
- Stretches lower back and obliques

NOT ADVISABLE IF YOU HAVE . . .
- Back problems

HAND-ON-KNEE STRETCH

1. Sit on the floor with your legs extended in front of you, your feet relaxed and flexed slightly. Bend your right leg, and rest the sole of your foot on your left inner thigh.

2. Place the palms of your hands on top of your left thigh, just above your kneecap.

3. Gently lean over your left leg until you feel a comfortable stretch in your hamstring.

4. Return to the start position, and repeat on the other side.

DO IT RIGHT
- Keep your chest lifted.
- Aim to decrease the space under the kneecap of your extended leg.
- Keep your shoulders pressed slightly and gently downward, away from your ears. Place one hand on your lower back to guard against strain, if necessary.

AVOID
- Lifting and holding tension in your bent knee.

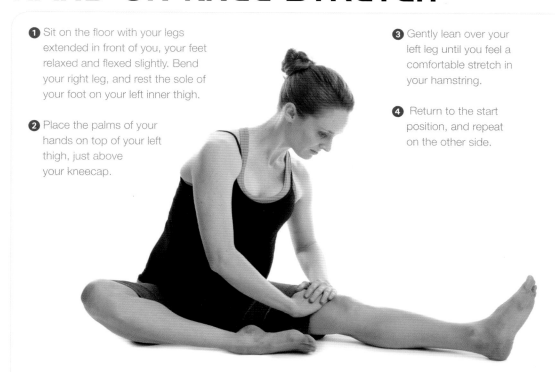

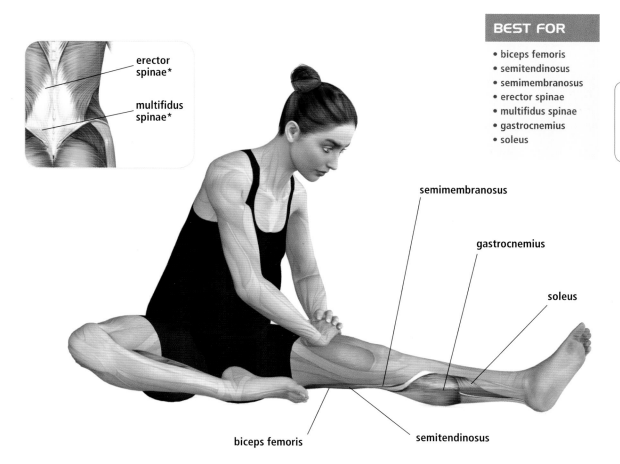

erector spinae*

multifidus spinae*

semimembranosus

gastrocnemius

soleus

biceps femoris

semitendinosus

BEST FOR
- **biceps femoris**
- **semitendinosus**
- **semimembranosus**
- **erector spinae**
- **multifidus spinae**
- **gastrocnemius**
- **soleus**

ANNOTATION KEY
Bold text indicates target muscles
Grey text indicates other working muscles
* indicates deep muscles

TARGETS
- Lower back
- Hamstrings
- Calves

LEVEL
- Beginner

BENEFITS
- Stretches lower back and legs

NOT ADVISABLE IF YOU HAVE . . .
- Hip problems
- Lower back problems

LYING PELVIC TILT

1 Lie on your back with your knees bent. Your feet should be flat on the floor and your legs in parallel.

2 Place your hands comfortably on your belly.

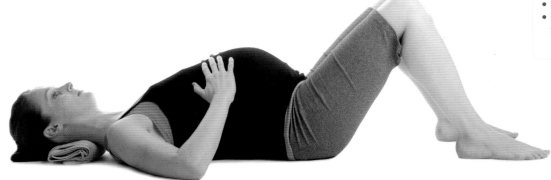

DO
Keep your chest slightly elevated.
• Relax your jaw.
• Breathe normally throughout the exercise.

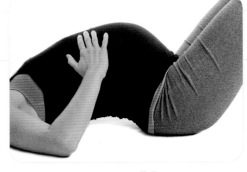

3 Slightly and carefully arch your lower back.

4 Rotate your pelvis forward, which will flatten your lower back onto the floor.

5 Return to the start position, and repeat if desired.

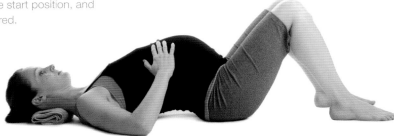

AVOID
• Performing this stretch during your third trimester. During your first and second trimesters, proceed with caution and stop immediately if you feel any discomfort.

TARGETS
• Lower back

LEVEL
• Beginner

BENEFITS
• Stretches and eases lower back

NOT ADVISABLE IF YOU HAVE . . .
• Back problems

BEST FOR

• erector spinae
• multifidus spinae

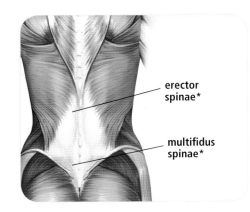

erector spinae*

multifidus spinae*

ANNOTATION KEY
Bold text indicates target muscles
Grey text indicates other working muscles
* indicates deep muscles

UNILATERAL GOOD MORNING STRETCH

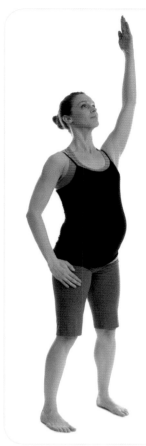

1 Stand with your legs and feet parallel and shoulder-width apart. Bend your knees very slightly. Your pelvis should be slightly tucked, your chest lifted, and your shoulders pressed gently downward away from your ears.

2 Place your right hand on your upper thigh. With your left arm, reach up toward the ceiling, palm inward.

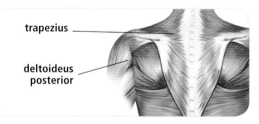

3 Carefully lean to the right.

4 Return to the start position, and repeat on the other side.

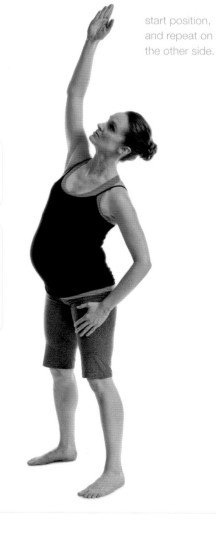

DO IT RIGHT
- Align your head with your spine by lifting your chin.

AVOID
- Moving your lower body.
- Holding your breath.
- Forcing your body too far over; keep the stretch high and soft.

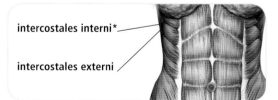

trapezius

deltoideus posterior

intercostales interni*

intercostales externi

BEST FOR
- **trapezius**
- **intercostales externi**
- **intercostales interni**
- **deltoideus posterior**

TARGETS
- Neck and shoulders

LEVEL
- Beginner

BENEFITS
- Loosens shoulders

NOT ADVISABLE IF YOU HAVE . . .
- Back trouble

CAT STRETCH

1 Kneel on all fours, with your hands at shoulder width and your knees 2 to 3 inches (5-7 cm) apart.

2 Round your spine upward as you draw your navel in toward your spine, keeping your hips lifted and your shoulders stable.

3 Hold the stretch at the top, and release.

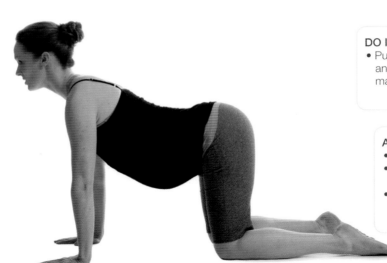

DO IT RIGHT
• Push down with your hands and knees to achieve maximum contraction.

AVOID
• Tensing your neck and shoulders.
• Hyperextending your lower back or arms.
• Holding your breath.

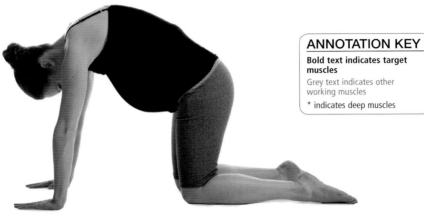

ANNOTATION KEY
Bold text indicates target muscles

Grey text indicates other working muscles

* indicates deep muscles

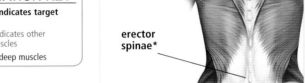

erector spinae*

BEST FOR

• erector spinae

TARGETS
• Back
• Hips

LEVEL
• Beginner

BENEFITS
• Stretches back and glutes.

NOT ADVISABLE IF YOU HAVE . . .
• Back or hip issues

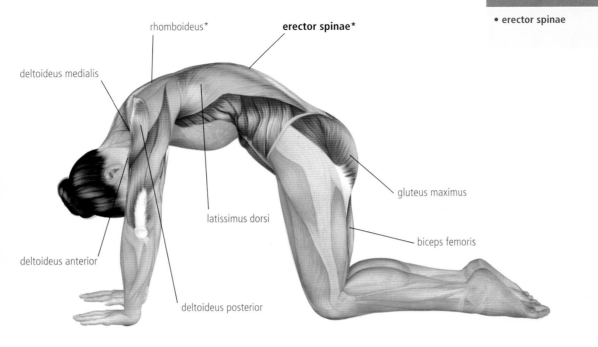

rhomboideus*

erector spinae*

deltoideus medialis

gluteus maximus

latissimus dorsi

biceps femoris

deltoideus anterior

deltoideus posterior

DOWNWARD-FACING DOG

1 Stand with your legs and feet parallel and shoulder-width apart. Bend your knees very slightly and carefully fold forward to touch your fingertips to the floor.

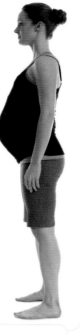

2 Bend your knees slightly, and tuck your pelvis slightly forward, lift your chest, and press your shoulders downward and back.

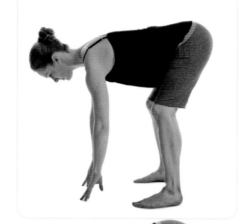

3 Slowly "walk" your hands forward as you lift your tailbone up toward the ceiling.

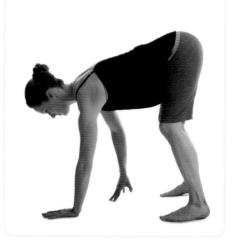

DO IT RIGHT
- Engage your entire hand fully into the floor at all times to avoid excess strain on your wrist joint.
- Keep your head in line with your spine.
- Keep your back flat and your chest elevated.

AVOID
- Holding your breath: relax your jaw slightly and breathe normally.

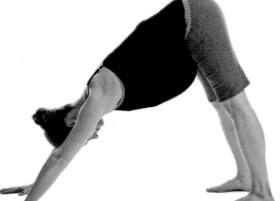

4 Press your heels toward the floor and contract your thighs as you straighten your legs to form a V shape with your body. Broaden your chest and shoulders and position your head between your arms.

ANNOTATION KEY
Bold text indicates target muscles
Grey text indicates other working muscles
* indicates deep muscles

BEST FOR
- pectoralis major
- pectoralis minor
- serratus anterior
- triceps brachii
- deltoideus posterior
- intercostales interni
- intercostales externi
- biceps femoris
- semitendinosus
- semimembranosus
- erector spinae
- gastrocnemius
- soleus
- gluteus maximus

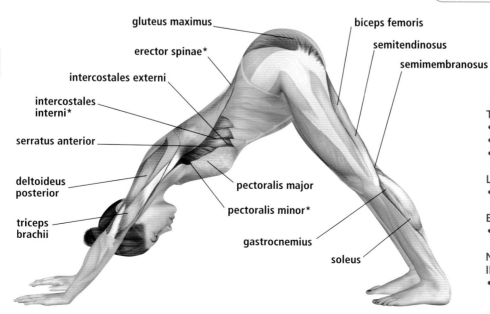

gluteus maximus

erector spinae*

intercostales externi

intercostales interni*

serratus anterior

deltoideus posterior

triceps brachii

biceps femoris

semitendinosus

semimembranosus

pectoralis major

pectoralis minor*

gastrocnemius

soleus

TARGETS
- Back of the legs
- Back
- Upper arms

LEVEL
- Intermediate

BENEFITS
- Stretches

NOT ADVISABLE IF YOU HAVE . . .
- Back or shoulder problems

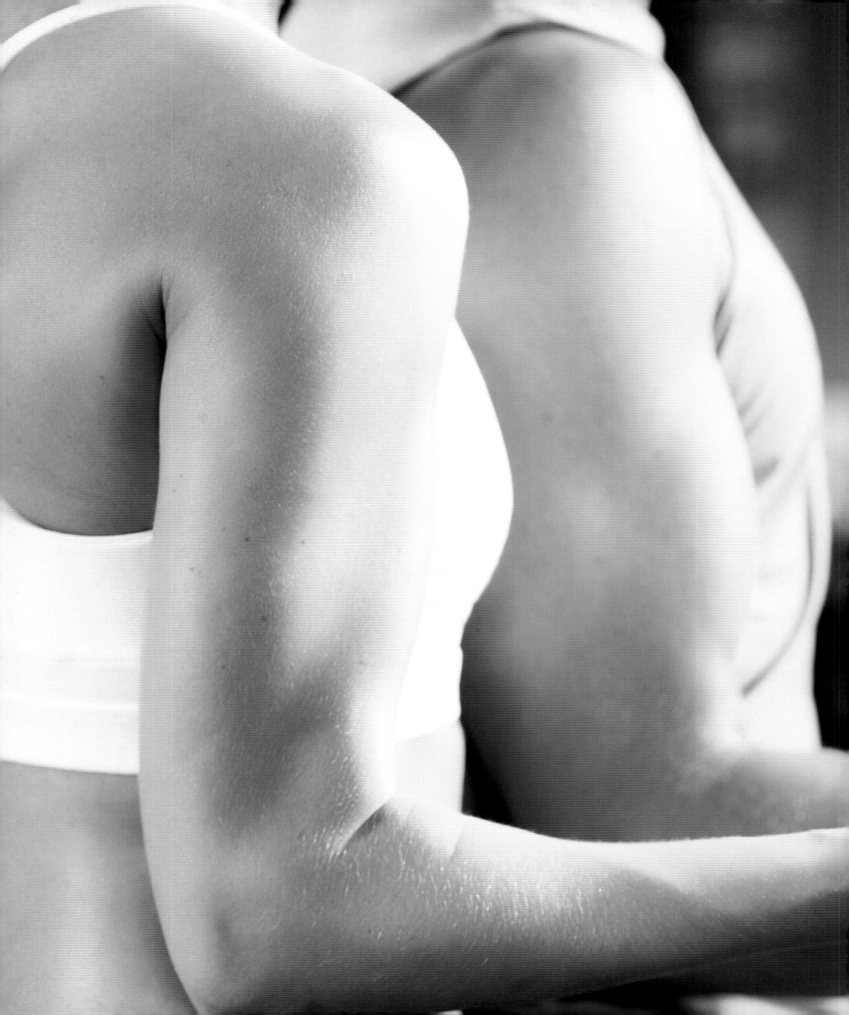

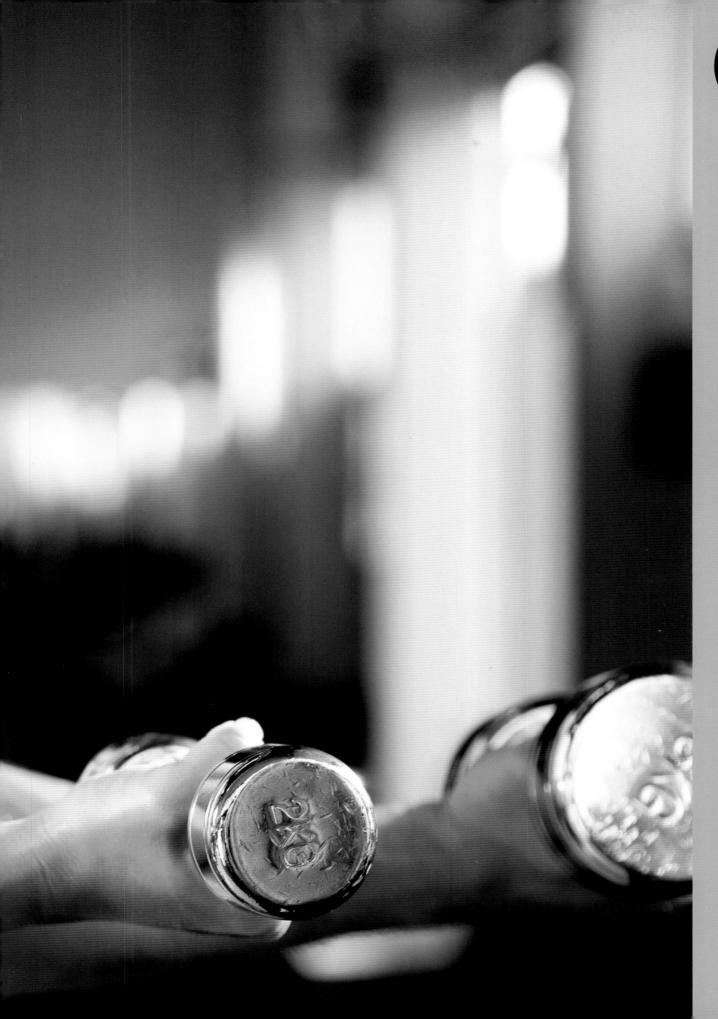

Part 3

Workouts

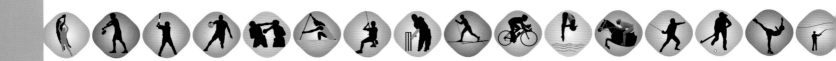
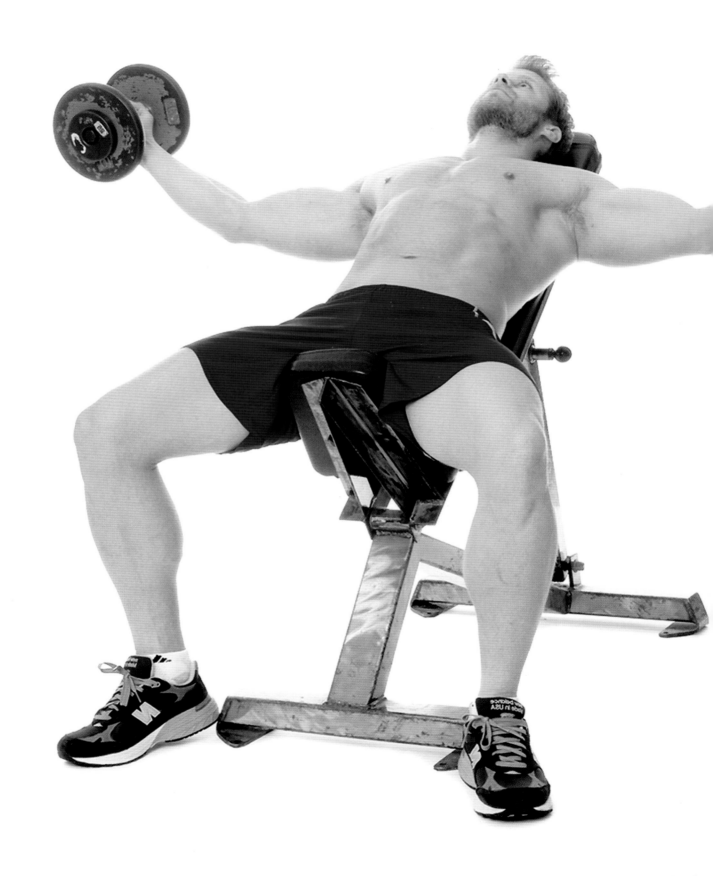

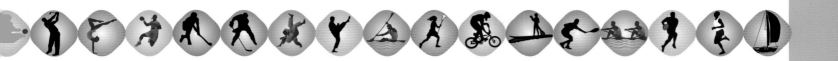

SPORT-SPECIFIC WORKOUTS

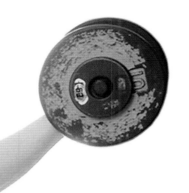

The following routines have been designed especially to improve performance in your chosen sport, increasing your strength, stamina and flexibility. The programs are organized into two levels, each with three stages that you can work through as your fitness improves. Remember, no matter how fit you feel, if you're working with a new and unfamiliar exercise, start slow and focus on form. If you're new to the sport, start with the beginner program, alternating the first and second workouts each week to maintain an overall balance. At first, you will need to refer back to the individual exercises to remind yourself of the correct procedure (and at-a-glance images and page references are provided for each exercise). And it goes without saying that any exercise shown for one side of the body should be repeated on the other side so your muscles develop evenly. Most importantly, have fun! Stick with the program and you'll soon find that the sport you already love will become even more rewarding!

AMERICAN FOOTBALL

A lot of football play is reliant on the legs for running, speed and agility. The powerful chest and triceps muscles are needed for pushing and tackling and especially well-developed shoulders are assets for their padding and protection when blocking or tackling. The back will help to keep the athlete upright and balanced, as will the core, which provides further full-body support.

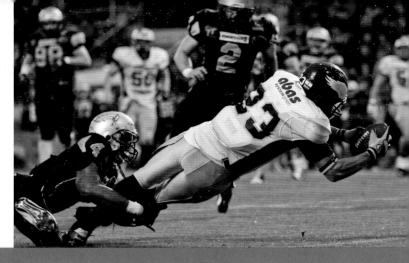

WORKOUT LEVEL 1

BEGINNER ROUTINE 1

Day One:
A 3 sets 6–8
D 3 sets 8–10
G 3 sets 10–12
J 3 sets 10–12
M 3 sets 10–12
Q 15

Day Two:
Rest

Day Three:
A 3 sets 6–8
D 3 sets 8–10
G 3 sets 10–12
J 3 sets 10–12
M 3 sets 10–12
Q 15

Day Four:
Rest

Day Five:
A 3 sets 6–8
D 3 sets 8–10
G 3 sets 10–12
J 3 sets 10–12
M 3 sets 10–12
Q 15

Day Six:
Cardio 30–45 minutes

Day Seven:
Rest

INTERMEDIATE ROUTINE 1

Day One:
A 3 sets 6–8
B 3 sets of 8–10
D 3 sets 8–10
E 3 sets of 8–10
G 3 sets 10–12
J 3 sets 10–12
M 3 sets 10–12
Q 15

Day Two:
Cardio 30–45 minutes

Day Three:
A 3 sets 6–8
B 3 sets of 8–10
D 3 sets 8–10
E 3 sets of 8–10
G 3 sets 10–12
J 3 sets 10–12
M 3 sets 10–12
Q 15

Day Four:
Rest

Day Five:
A 3 sets 6–8
B 3 sets of 8–10
D 3 sets 8–10
E 3 sets of 8–10
G 3 sets 10–12
J 3 sets 10–12
M 3 sets 10–12
Q 15

Day Six:
Cardio 30–45 minutes

Day Seven:
Rest

ADVANCED ROUTINE 1

Day One:
A 3 sets 6–8
B 3 sets of 8–10
D 3 sets 8–10
E 3 sets of 8–10
G 3 sets 10–12
J 3 sets 10–12
M 3 sets 10–12
N 3 sets 12–15
Q 15
S 20 per side

Day Two:
Cardio 30–45 minutes

Day Three:
A 3 sets 6–8
B 3 sets of 8–10
D 3 sets 8–10
E 3 sets of 8–10
G 3 sets 10–12
J 3 sets 10–12
M 3 sets 10–12
N 3 sets 12–15
Q 15
S 20 per side

Day Four:
Cardio 30–45 minutes

Day Five:
A 3 sets 6–8
B 3 sets of 8–10
D 3 sets 8–10
E 3 sets of 8–10
G 3 sets 10–12
J 3 sets 10–12
M 3 sets 10–12
N 3 sets 12–15
Q 15
S 20 per side

Day Six:
Cardio 30–45 minutes

Day Seven:
Rest

WORKOUT LEVEL 2

BEGINNER ROUTINE 2

Day One:
C 3 sets 12–15
F 3 sets 8–10
H 3 sets 10–12
I 3 sets 12–15
K 3 sets 12–15
L 3 sets 10–12

Day Two:
Rest

Day Three:
C 3 sets 12–15
F 3 sets 8–10
H 3 sets 10–12
I 3 sets 12–15
K 3 sets 12–15
L 3 sets 10–12

Day Four:
Rest

Day Five:
C 3 sets 12–15
F 3 sets 8–10
H 3 sets 10–12
I 3 sets 12–15
K 3 sets 12–15
L 3 sets 10–12

Day Six:
Cardio 30–45 minutes

Day Seven:
Rest

INTERMEDIATE ROUTINE 2

Day One:
C 3 sets 12–15
F 3 sets 8–10
H 3 sets 10–12
I 3 sets 12–15
K 3 sets 12–15
L 3 sets 10–12
O 3 sets 12–15
P 3 sets 20

Day Two:
Cardio 30–45 minutes

Day Three:
C 3 sets 12–15
F 3 sets 8–10
H 3 sets 10–12
I 3 sets 12–15
K 3 sets 12–15
L 3 sets 10–12
O 3 sets 12–15
P 3 sets 20

Day Four:
Rest

Day Five:
C 3 sets 12–15
F 3 sets 8–10
H 3 sets 10–12
I 3 sets 12–15
K 3 sets 12–15
L 3 sets 10–12
O 3 sets 12–15
P 3 sets 20

Day Six:
Cardio 30–45 minutes

Day Seven:
Rest

ADVANCED ROUTINE 2

Day One:
C 3 sets 12–15
F 3 sets 8–10
H 3 sets 10–12
I 3 sets 12–15
K 3 sets 12–15
L 3 sets 10–12
O 3 sets 12–15
P 3 sets 20
R 3 sets 20
T 3 sets 30–60 seconds

Day Two:
Cardio 30–45 minutes

Day Three:
C 3 sets 12–15
F 3 sets 8–10
H 3 sets 10–12
I 3 sets 12–15
K 3 sets 12–15
L 3 sets 10–12
O 3 sets 12–15
P 3 sets 20
R 3 sets 20
T 3 sets 30–60 seconds

Day Four:
Cardio 30–45 minutes

Day Five:
C 3 sets 12–15
F 3 sets 8–10
H 3 sets 10–12
I 3 sets 12–15
K 3 sets 12–15
L 3 sets 10–12
O 3 sets 12–15
P 3 sets 20
R 3 sets 20
T 3 sets 30–60 seconds

Day Six:
Cardio 30–45 minutes

Day Seven:
Rest

AMERICAN FOOTBALL WORKOUTS

A Barbell Deadlift
page 34
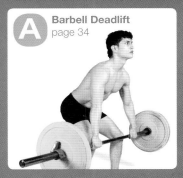

B Barbell Row
page 36
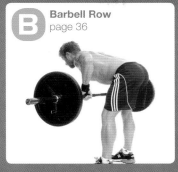

C Flat Bench Hyperextension
page 56
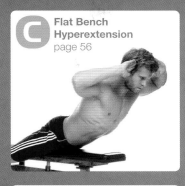

D Barbell Bench Press
page 60
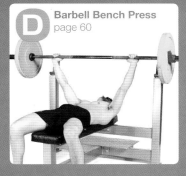

E Dips
page 68
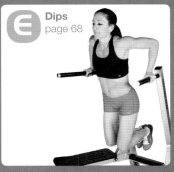

F Overhead Press
page 76
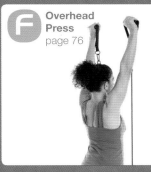

G Barbell Shoulder Shrug
page 94
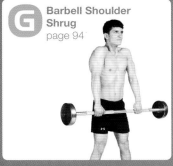

H Rope Pushdown
page 106
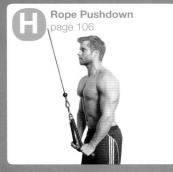

I Wrist Flexion
page 116
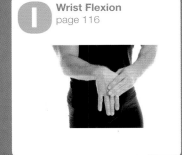

J Swiss Ball Wall Sit
page 134
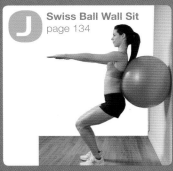

K High Lunge
page 146
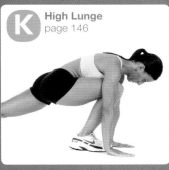

L Goblet Squat
page 150
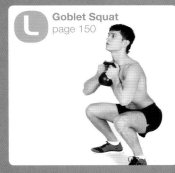

M Swiss Ball Hamstring Curl
page 164
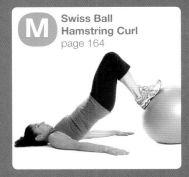

N Dumbbell Calf Raise
page 178
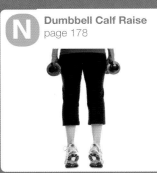

O Turkish Get-Up
page 188
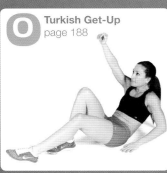

P Bicycle Crunch
page 190
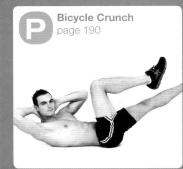

Q Plank Press-Up
page 198
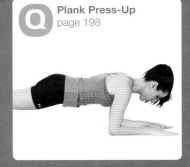

R Seated Russian Twist
page 200
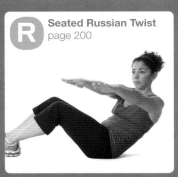

S Medicine Ball Wood Chop
page 130
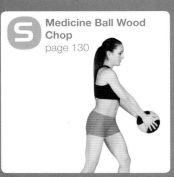

T T-Stabilization
page 124
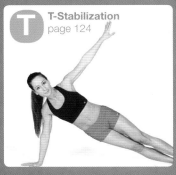

ARCHERY

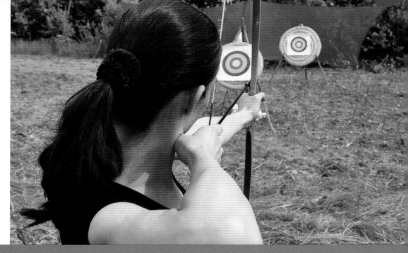

Archery is as much about using muscles as it is about using angles and sight lines. You need a strong back, shoulders and biceps to draw back the bowstring. Strong forearms are required for static gripping as you steadily take aim at the target. A strong core is vital for stability and for balance. Proper extension at the hips and knees is aided by strong glutes, hamstrings and quadriceps. This workout will help to put you right on target to achieve your ambitions in archery.

WORKOUT LEVEL 1

BEGINNER ROUTINE 1

Day One:
A 3 sets 8–10
C 3 sets 8–10
D 3 sets 8–10
E 3 sets 8–10
G 3 sets 12–15
H 3 sets 10–12

Day Two:
Rest

Day Three:
A 3 sets 8–10
C 3 sets 8–10
D 3 sets 8–10
E 3 sets 8–10
G 3 sets 12–15
H 3 sets 10–12

Day Four:
Rest

Day Five:
A 3 sets 8–10
C 3 sets 8–10
D 3 sets 8–10
E 3 sets 8–10
G 3 sets 12–15
H 3 sets 10–12

Day Six:
Cardio 30–45 minutes

Day Seven:
Rest

INTERMEDIATE ROUTINE 1

Day One:
A 3 sets 8–10
C 3 sets 8–10
D 3 sets 8–10
E 3 sets 8–10
G 3 sets 12–15
H 3 sets 10–12
J 3 sets 15–20
K 3 sets 15–20

Day Two:
Cardio 30–45 minutes

Day Three:
A 3 sets 8–10
C 3 sets 8–10
D 3 sets 8–10
E 3 sets 8–10
G 3 sets 12–15
H 3 sets 10–12
J 3 sets 15–20
K 3 sets 15–20

Day Four:
Rest

Day Five:
A 3 sets 8–10
C 3 sets 8–10
D 3 sets 8–10
E 3 sets 8–10
G 3 sets 12–15
H 3 sets 10–12
J 3 sets 15–20
K 3 sets 15–20

Day Six:
Cardio 30–45 minutes

Day Seven:
Rest

ADVANCED ROUTINE 1

Day One:
A 3 sets 8–10
C 3 sets 8–10
D 3 sets 8–10
E 3 sets 8–10
G 3 sets 12–15
H 3 sets 10–12
J 3 sets 15–20
K 3 sets 15–20
Q 30 per side
R 3 sets 8–10

Day Two:
Cardio 30–45 minutes

Day Three:
A 3 sets 8–10
C 3 sets 8–10
D 3 sets 8–10
E 3 sets 8–10
G 3 sets 12–15
H 3 sets 10–12
J 3 sets 15–20
K 3 sets 15–20
Q 30 per side
R 3 sets 8–10

Day Four:
Cardio 30–45 minutes

Day Five:
A 3 sets 8–10
C 3 sets 8–10
D 3 sets 8–10
E 3 sets 8–10
G 3 sets 12–15
H 3 sets 10–12
J 3 sets 15–20
K 3 sets 15–20
Q 30 per side
R 3 sets 8–10

Day Six:
Cardio 30–45 minutes

Day Seven:
Rest

WORKOUT LEVEL 2

BEGINNER ROUTINE 2

Day One:
B 3 sets 8–10
F 3 sets 10–12
I 3 sets 12–15
L 3 sets 12–15
M 3 sets 12–15
N 3 sets 25

Day Two:
Rest

Day Three:
B 3 sets 8–10
F 3 sets 10–12
I 3 sets 12–15
L 3 sets 12–15
M 3 sets 12–15
N 3 sets 25

Day Four:
Rest

Day Five:
B 3 sets 8–10
F 3 sets 10–12
I 3 sets 12–15
L 3 sets 12–15
M 3 sets 12–15
N 3 sets 25

Day Six:
Cardio 30–45 minutes

Day Seven:
Rest

INTERMEDIATE ROUTINE 2

Day One:
B 3 sets 8–10
F 3 sets 10–12
I 3 sets 12–15
L 3 sets 12–15
M 3 sets 12–15
N 3 sets 25
O 3 sets 15
P 3 sets 25

Day Two:
Cardio 30–45 minutes

Day Three:
B 3 sets 8–10
F 3 sets 10–12
I 3 sets 12–15
L 3 sets 12–15
M 3 sets 12–15
N 3 sets 25
O 3 sets 15
P 3 sets 25

Day Four:
Rest

Day Five:
B 3 sets 8–10
F 3 sets 10–12
I 3 sets 12–15
L 3 sets 12–15
M 3 sets 12–15
N 3 sets 25
O 3 sets 15
P 3 sets 25

Day Six:
Cardio 30–45 minutes

Day Seven:
Rest

ADVANCED ROUTINE 2

Day One:
B 3 sets 8–10
F 3 sets 10–12
I 3 sets 12–15
L 3 sets 12–15
M 3 sets 12–15
N 3 sets 25
O 3 sets 15
P 3 sets 25
S 3 sets 20
T 3 sets 20

Day Two:
Cardio 30–45 minutes

Day Three:
B 3 sets 8–10
F 3 sets 10–12
I 3 sets 12–15
L 3 sets 12–15
M 3 sets 12–15
N 3 sets 25
O 3 sets 15
P 3 sets 25
S 3 sets 20
T 3 sets 20

Day Four:
Cardio 30–45 minutes

Day Five:
B 3 sets 8–10
F 3 sets 10–12
I 3 sets 12–15
L 3 sets 12–15
M 3 sets 12–15
N 3 sets 25
O 3 sets 15
P 3 sets 25
S 3 sets 20
T 3 sets 20

Day Six:
Cardio 30–45 minutes

Day Seven:
Rest

ARCHERY WORKOUTS

A Dumbbell Row
page 38

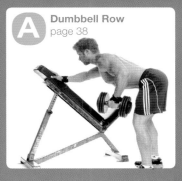

B Lat Pulldown
page 42

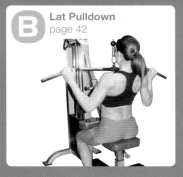

C Reverse Close-Grip Front Chin
page 54

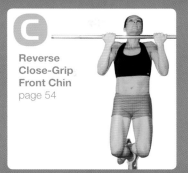

D Dips
page 68

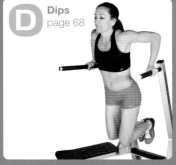

E Dumbbell Shoulder Press
page 74

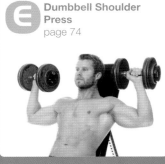

F Alternating Hammer Curl
page 98

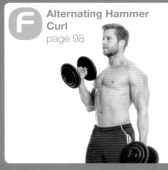

G Wrist Flexion and Wrist Extension
pages 116 and 117

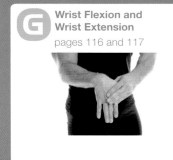

H Swiss Ball Wall Sit
page 134

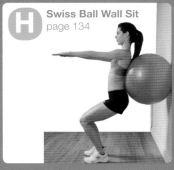

I Crossover Step
page 148

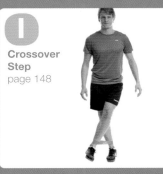

J Adductor Extension
page 162

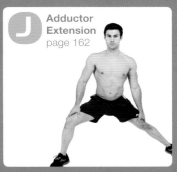

K Hamstring Abductor
page 163

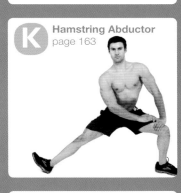

L Stiff-Legged Deadlift
page 174

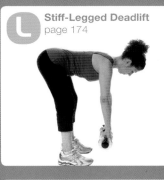

M Hamstring Pull-In
page 170

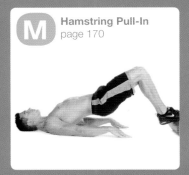

N Crunch
page 118

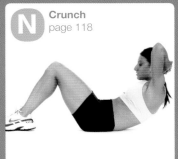

O Plank Press-Up
page 198

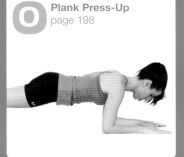

P Swiss Ball Walk-Around
page 126

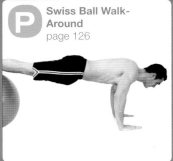

Q Wood Chop with Resistance Band
page 202

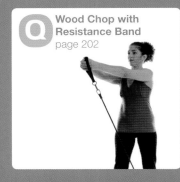

R Triceps Roll-Out
page 110

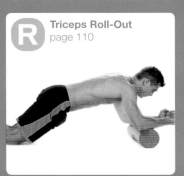

S Swiss Ball Jackknife
page 128

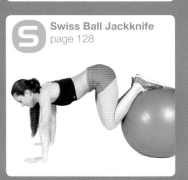

T Swiss Ball Roll-Out
page 206

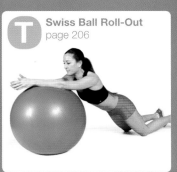

AUSTRALIAN-RULES FOOTBALL

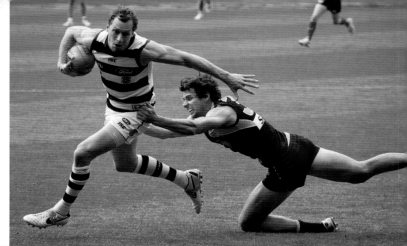

In this fast-paced contact sport, which is something of a hybrid between football and rugby, you can tackle with your hands or use your whole body to obstruct an opponent. You need powerful lower-body muscles as well as a strong core for proper stabilization. Strong legs are especially important as a player can cover long distances over the course of the match.

BEGINNER ROUTINE 1

Day One:
A 3 sets of 8–10
B 3 sets of 12–15
D 3 sets of 10–12
H 3 sets of 12–15
K 3 sets of 10–12
P 3 sets of 15

Day Two:
Rest

Day Three:
A 3 sets of 8–10
B 3 sets of 12–15
D 3 sets of 10–12
H 3 sets of 12–15
K 3 sets of 10–12
P 3 sets of 15

Day Four:
Rest

Day Five:
A 3 sets of 8–10
B 3 sets of 12–15
D 3 sets of 10–12
H 3 sets of 12–15
K 3 sets of 10–12
P 3 sets of 15

Day Six:
Cardio 30–45 minutes

Day Seven:
Rest

INTERMEDIATE ROUTINE 1

Day One:
A 3 sets of 8–10
B 3 sets of 12–15
D 3 sets of 10–12
G 3 sets of 12–15
H 3 sets of 12–15
K 3 sets of 10–12
O 3 sets of 12–15
P 3 sets of 15

Day Two:
Cardio 30–45 minutes

Day Three:
A 3 sets of 8–10
B 3 sets of 12–15
D 3 sets of 10–12
G 3 sets of 12–15
H 3 sets of 12–15
K 3 sets of 10–12
O 3 sets of 12–15
P 3 sets of 15

Day Four:
Rest

Day Five:
A 3 sets of 8–10
B 3 sets of 12–15
D 3 sets of 10–12
G 3 sets of 12–15
H 3 sets of 12–15
K 3 sets of 10–12
O 3 sets of 12–15
P 3 sets of 15

Day Six:
Cardio 30–45 minutes

Day Seven:
Rest

ADVANCED ROUTINE 1

Day One:
A 3 sets of 8–10
B 3 sets of 12–15
D 3 sets of 10–12
G 3 sets of 12–15
H 3 sets of 12–15
K 3 sets of 10–12
L 3 sets of 12–15
O 3 sets of 12–15
P 3 sets of 15
Q 2 minutes

Day Two:
Cardio 30–45 minutes

Day Three:
A 3 sets of 8–10
B 3 sets of 12–15
D 3 sets of 10–12
G 3 sets of 12–15
H 3 sets of 12–15
K 3 sets of 10–12
L 3 sets of 12–15
O 3 sets of 12–15
P 3 sets of 15
Q 2 minutes

Day Four:
Cardio 30–45 minutes

Day Five:
A 3 sets of 8–10
B 3 sets of 12–15
D 3 sets of 10–12
G 3 sets of 12–15
H 3 sets of 12–15
K 3 sets of 10–12
L 3 sets of 12–15
O 3 sets of 12–15
P 3 sets of 15
Q 2 minutes

Day Six:
Cardio 30–45 minutes

Day Seven:
Rest

BEGINNER ROUTINE 2

Day One:
C 3 sets 10–12
E 3 sets 12–15
F 3 sets 12–15
I 3 sets 15–20
J 3 sets 15–20
M 3 sets 12–15

Day Two:
Rest

Day Three:
C 3 sets 10–12
E 3 sets 12–15
F 3 sets 12–15
I 3 sets 15–20
J 3 sets 15–20
M 3 sets 12–15

Day Four:
Rest

Day Five:
C 3 sets 10–12
E 3 sets 12–15
F 3 sets 12–15
I 3 sets 15–20
J 3 sets 15–20
M 3 sets 12–15

Day Six:
Cardio 30–45 minutes

Day Seven:
Rest:

INTERMEDIATE ROUTINE 2

Day One:
C 3 sets 10–12
E 3 sets 12–15
F 3 sets 12–15
I 3 sets 15–20
J 3 sets 15–20
M 3 sets 12–15
N 3 sets 10–12
R 3 sets 30

Day Two:
Cardio 30–45 minutes

Day Three:
C 3 sets 10–12
E 3 sets 12–15
F 3 sets 12–15
I 3 sets 15–20
J 3 sets 15–20
M 3 sets 12–15
N 3 sets 10–12
R 3 sets 30

Day Four:
Rest

Day Five:
C 3 sets 10–12
E 3 sets 12–15
F 3 sets 12–15
I 3 sets 15–20
J 3 sets 15–20
M 3 sets 12–15
N 3 sets 10–12
R 3 sets 30

Day Six:
Cardio 30–45 minutes

Day Seven:
Rest

ADVANCED ROUTINE 2

Day One:
C 3 sets 10–12
E 3 sets 12–15
F 3 sets 12–15
I 3 sets 15–20
J 3 sets 15–20
M 3 sets 12–15
N 3 sets 10–12
R 3 sets 30
S 3 sets 20
T 3 sets 20

Day Two:
Cardio 30–45 minutes

Day Three:
C 3 sets 10–12
E 3 sets 12–15
F 3 sets 12–15
I 3 sets 15–20
J 3 sets 15–20
M 3 sets 12–15
N 3 sets 10–12
R 3 sets 30
S 3 sets 20
T 3 sets 20

Day Four:
Cardio 30–45 minutes

Day Five:
C 3 sets 10–12
E 3 sets 12–15
F 3 sets 12–15
I 3 sets 15–20
J 3 sets 15–20
M 3 sets 12–15
N 3 sets 10–12
R 3 sets 30
S 3 sets 20
T 3 sets 20

Day Six:
Cardio 30–45 minutes

Day Seven:
Rest

AUSTRALIAN-RULES FOOTBALL WORKOUTS

A Dumbbell Pullover
page 40

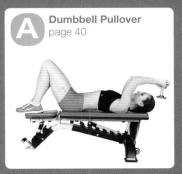

B Flat Bench Hyperextension
page 56

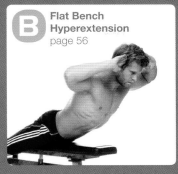

C Barbell Shoulder Shrug
page 94

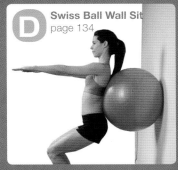

D Swiss Ball Wall Sit
page 134

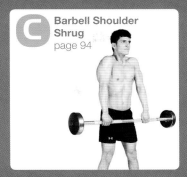

E Dumbbell Lunge
page 138

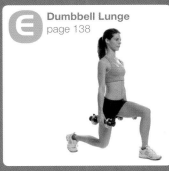

F Reverse Lunge
page 140

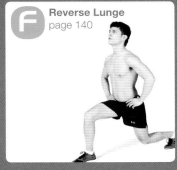

G Dumbbell Walking Lunge
page 144

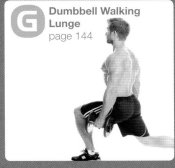

H One-Legged Step-Down
page 152

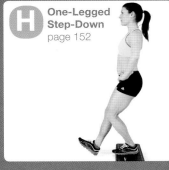

I Adductor Extension
page 162

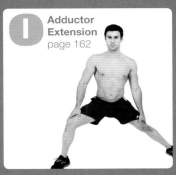

J Hamstring Abductor
page 163

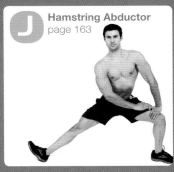

K Swiss Ball Hamstring Curl
page 164

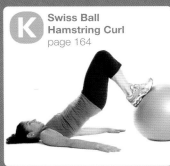

L Hamstring Pull-In
page 170

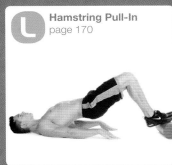

M Sumo Squat
page 172

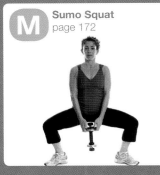

N Stiff-Legged Deadlift
page 174

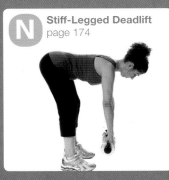

O Single-Leg Calf Press
page 176

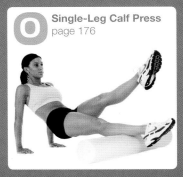

P Star Jump
page 156

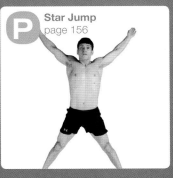

Q Mountain Climber
page 158

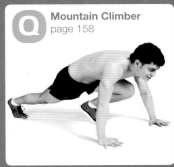

R Wood Chop with Resistance Band
page 202

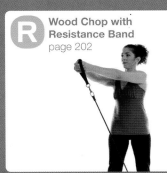

S Swiss Ball Jackknife
page 128

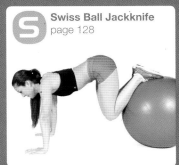

T Swiss Ball Hip Crossover
page 210

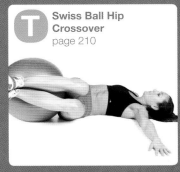

BADMINTON

The basic aim in badminton is to prevent the shuttlecock from landing on your side of the court. It's a sport in which a lot of internal shoulder and core muscles are continuously fired up for fast, deliberate and immediate performance — it requires great reflexes. Your shoulders and core need to be exercised regularly for strength, flexibility and endurance. Your arms need to be strong, too, as points are often won with powerful "smashes" from high above the net.

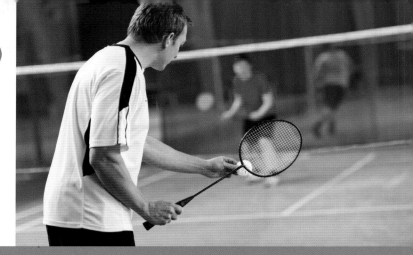

BEGINNER ROUTINE 1

Day One:
B 3 sets of 8–10
E 3 sets of 12–15
F 3 sets of 15
H 3 sets of 25 per side
N 3 sets of 30 per side
P 3 sets of 15

Day Two:
Rest

Day Three:
B 3 sets of 8–10
E 3 sets of 12–15
F 3 sets of 15
H 3 sets of 25 per side
N 3 sets of 30 per side
P 3 sets of 15

Day Four:
Rest

Day Five:
B 3 sets of 8–10
E 3 sets of 12–15
F 3 sets of 15
H 3 sets of 25 per side
N 3 sets of 30 per side
P 3 sets of 15

Day Six:
Cardio 30–45 minutes

Day Seven:
Rest

INTERMEDIATE ROUTINE 1

Day One:
B 3 sets of 8–10
E 3 sets of 12–15
F 3 sets of 15
G 3 sets of 15
H 3 sets of 25 per side
K 3 sets of 15
N 3 sets of 30 per side
P 3 sets of 15

Day Two:
Cardio 30–45 minutes

Day Three:
B 3 sets of 8–10
E 3 sets of 12–15
F 3 sets of 15
G 3 sets of 15
H 3 sets of 25 per side
K 3 sets of 15
N 3 sets of 30 per side
P 3 sets of 15

Day Four:
Rest

Day Five:
B 3 sets of 8–10
E 3 sets of 12–15
F 3 sets of 15
G 3 sets of 15
H 3 sets of 25 per side
K 3 sets of 15
N 3 sets of 30 per side
P 3 sets of 15

Day Six:
Cardio 30–45 minutes

Day Seven:
Rest

ADVANCED ROUTINE 1

Day One:
B 3 sets of 8–10
D 3 sets of 10–12
E 3 sets of 12–15
F 3 sets of 15
G 3 sets of 15
H 3 sets of 25 per side
K 3 sets of 15
N 3 sets of 30 per side
O 30–60 seconds per side
P 3 sets of 15

Day Two:
Cardio 30–45 minutes

Day Three:
B 3 sets of 8–10
D 3 sets of 10–12
E 3 sets of 12–15
F 3 sets of 15
G 3 sets of 15
H 3 sets of 25 per side
K 3 sets of 15
N 3 sets of 30 per side
O 30–60 seconds per side

P 3 sets of 15

Day Four:
Cardio 30–45 minutes

Day Five:
B 3 sets of 8–10
D 3 sets of 10–12
E 3 sets of 12–15
F 3 sets of 15
G 3 sets of 15
H 3 sets of 25 per side
K 3 sets of 15
N 3 sets of 30 per side
O 30–60 seconds per side
P 3 sets of 15

Day Six:
Cardio 30–45 minutes

Day Seven:
Rest

BEGINNER ROUTINE 2

Day One:
A 3 sets 8–10
C 3 sets 10–12
I 3 sets 30
J 3 sets 20
L 30–120 seconds
M 3 sets 20

Day Two:
Rest

Day Three:
A 3 sets 8–10
C 3 sets 10–12
I 3 sets 30
J 3 sets 20
L 30–120 seconds
M 3 sets 20

Day Four:
Rest

Day Five:
A 3 sets 8–10
C 3 sets 10–12
I 3 sets 30
J 3 sets 20
L 30–120 seconds
M 3 sets 20

Day Six:
Cardio 30–45 minutes

Day Seven:
Rest

INTERMEDIATE ROUTINE 2

Day One:
A 3 sets 8–10
C 3 sets 10–12
I 3 sets 30
J 3 sets 20
L 30–120 seconds
M 3 sets 20
Q 3 sets 20
R 3 sets 20

Day Two:
Cardio 30–45 minutes

Day Three:
A 3 sets 8–10
C 3 sets 10–12
I 3 sets 30
J 3 sets 20
L 30–120 seconds
M 3 sets 20
Q 3 sets 20
R 3 sets 20

Day Four:
Rest

Day Five:
A 3 sets 8–10
C 3 sets 10–12
I 3 sets 30
J 3 sets 20
L 30–120 seconds
M 3 sets 20
Q 3 sets 20
R 3 sets 20

Day Six:
Cardio 30–45 minutes

Day Seven:
Rest

ADVANCED ROUTINE 2

Day One:
A 3 sets 8–10
C 3 sets 10–12
I 3 sets 30
J 3 sets 20
L 30–120 seconds
M 3 sets 20
Q 3 sets 20
R 3 sets 20
S 3 sets 25
T 3 sets 20

Day Two:
Cardio 30–45 minutes

Day Three:
A 3 sets 8–10
C 3 sets 10–12
I 3 sets 30
J 3 sets 20
L 30–120 seconds
M 3 sets 20
Q 3 sets 20
R 3 sets 20
S 3 sets 25
T 3 sets 20

Day Four:
Cardio 30–45 minutes

Day Five:
A 3 sets 8–10
C 3 sets 10–12
I 3 sets 30
J 3 sets 20
L 30–120 seconds
M 3 sets 20
Q 3 sets 20
R 3 sets 20
S 3 sets 25
T 3 sets 20

Day Six:
Cardio 30–45 minutes

Day Seven:
Rest

BADMINTON WORKOUTS

A Lat Pulldown
page 42
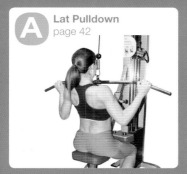

B Dumbbell Shoulder Press
page 74
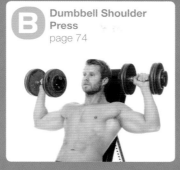

C Rope Pushdown
page 106
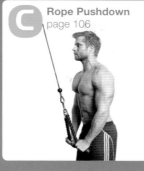

D Lying Triceps Extension
page 108
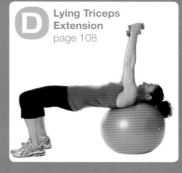

E Scapular Range of Motion
page 44
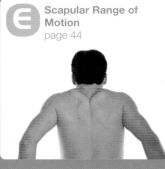

F Rotation Exercises
page 78
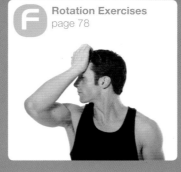

G External Rotation with Band
page 80
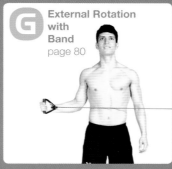

H Abdominal Kick
page 184
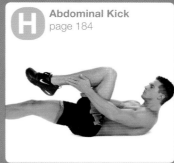

I Turkish Get-Up
page 188
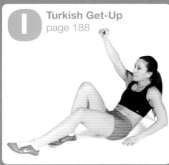

J Bicycle Crunch
page 190
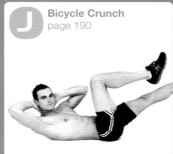

K Plank Press-Up
page 198
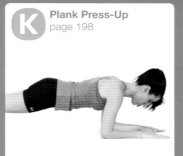

L Plank
page 120
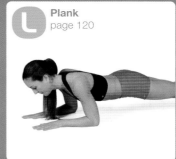

M Seated Russian Twist
page 200
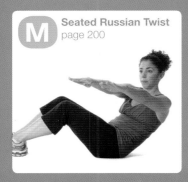

N Wood Chop with Resistance Band
page 202
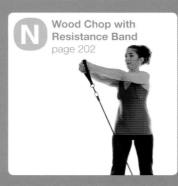

O T-Stabilization
page 124
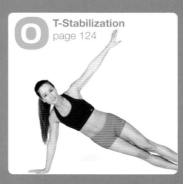

P Hip Abduction and Adduction
page 204
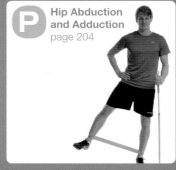

Q Swiss Ball Roll-Out
page 206
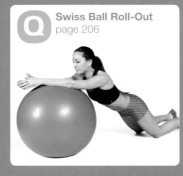

R V-Up
page 212
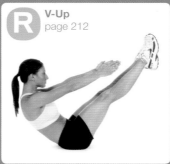

S Medicine Ball Slam
page 214
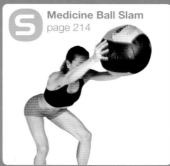

T The Windmill
page 216
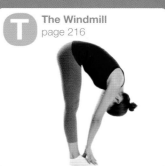

BASEBALL

Whether pitching the ball at tremendous speed or hitting it out of the park, baseball certainly isn't just about having strong arms. The shoulders, back and core also need to be powerful — as do the hips and thighs to help produce all that explosive power. Fielding calls for speed and flexibility, as well as strong arms and shoulders to throw the ball hard and fast. This great workout covers all the bases to keep you on top of your game and help you to hit more home runs.

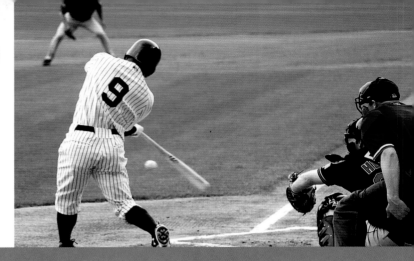

WORKOUT LEVEL 1

BEGINNER ROUTINE 1

Day One:
A 3 sets of 8–10
C 3 sets of 12–15
F 3 sets of 10–12
H 3 sets of 10–12
N 20 rotations
O 20 per side

Day Two:
Rest

Day Three:
A 3 sets of 8–10
C 3 sets of 12–15
F 3 sets of 10–12
H 3 sets of 10–12
N 20 rotations
O 20 per side

Day Four:
Rest

Day Five:
A 3 sets of 8–10
C 3 sets of 12–15
F 3 sets of 10–12
H 3 sets of 10–12
N 20 rotations
O 20 per side

Day Six:
Cardio 30–45 minutes

Day Seven:
Rest

INTERMEDIATE ROUTINE 1

Day One:
A 3 sets of 8–10
C 3 sets of 12–15
F 3 sets of 10–12
H 3 sets of 10–12
J 3 sets of 10–12
N 20 rotations
O 20 per side
T 25 repetitions

Day Two:
Cardio 30–45 minutes

Day Three:
A 3 sets of 8–10
C 3 sets of 12–15
F 3 sets of 10–12
H 3 sets of 10–12
J 3 sets of 10–12
N 20 rotations
O 20 per side
T 25 repetitions

Day Four:
Rest

Day Five:
A 3 sets of 8–10
C 3 sets of 12–15
F 3 sets of 10–12
H 3 sets of 10–12
J 3 sets of 10–12
N 20 rotations
O 20 per side
T 25 repetitions

Day Six:
Cardio 30–45 minutes

Day Seven:
Rest

ADVANCED ROUTINE 1

Day One:
A 3 sets of 8–10
C 3 sets of 12–15
E 3 sets of 10–12
F 3 sets of 10–12
H 3 sets of 10–12
J 3 sets of 10–12
N 20 rotations
O 20 per side
R 20 per side
T 25 repetitions

Day Two:
Cardio 30–45 minutes

Day Three:
A 3 sets of 8–10
C 3 sets of 12–15
E 3 sets of 10–12
F 3 sets of 10–12
H 3 sets of 10–12
J 3 sets of 10–12
N 20 rotations
O 20 per side
R 20 per side
T 25 repetitions

Day Four:
Cardio 30–45 minutes

Day Five:
A 3 sets of 8–10
C 3 sets of 12–15
E 3 sets of 10–12
F 3 sets of 10–12
H 3 sets of 10–12
J 3 sets of 10–12
N 20 rotations
O 20 per side
R 20 per side
T 25 repetitions

Day Six:
Cardio 30–45 minutes

Day Seven:
Rest

WORKOUT LEVEL 2

BEGINNER ROUTINE 2

Day One:
B 3 sets 15
D 3 sets 10–12
G 3 sets 10–12
I 3 sets 12–15
K 3 sets 25
L 3 sets 20

Day Two:
Rest

Day Three:
B 3 sets 15
D 3 sets 10–12
G 3 sets 10–12
I 3 sets 12–15
K 3 sets 25
L 3 sets 20

Day Four:
Rest

Day Five:
B 3 sets 15
D 3 sets 10–12
G 3 sets 10–12
I 3 sets 12–15
K 3 sets 25
L 3 sets 20

Day Six:
Cardio 30–45 minutes

Day Seven:
Rest

INTERMEDIATE ROUTINE 2

Day One:
B 3 sets 15
D 3 sets 10–12
G 3 sets 10–12
I 3 sets 12–15
K 3 sets 25
L 3 sets 20
M 3 sets 20
P 3 sets 12–15

Day Two:
Cardio 30–45 minutes

Day Three:
B 3 sets 15
D 3 sets 10–12
G 3 sets 10–12
I 3 sets 12–15
K 3 sets 25
L 3 sets 20
M 3 sets 20
P 3 sets 12–15

Day Four:
Rest

Day Five:
B 3 sets 15
D 3 sets 10–12
G 3 sets 10–12
I 3 sets 12–15
K 3 sets 25
L 3 sets 20
M 3 sets 20
P 3 sets 12–15

Day Six:
Cardio 30–45 minutes

Day Seven:
Rest

ADVANCED ROUTINE 2

Day One:
B 3 sets 15
D 3 sets 10–12
G 3 sets 10–12
I 3 sets 12–15
K 3 sets 25
L 3 sets 20
M 3 sets 20
P 3 sets 12–15
Q 3 sets 20
S 3 sets 20

Day Two:
Cardio 30–45 minutes

Day Three:
B 3 sets 15
D 3 sets 10–12
G 3 sets 10–12
I 3 sets 12–15
K 3 sets 25
L 3 sets 20
M 3 sets 20
P 3 sets 12–15
Q 3 sets 20
S 3 sets 20

Day Four:
Cardio 30–45 minutes

Day Five:
B 3 sets 15
D 3 sets 10–12
G 3 sets 10–12
I 3 sets 12–15
K 3 sets 25
L 3 sets 20
M 3 sets 20
P 3 sets 12–15
Q 3 sets 20
S 3 sets 20

Day Six:
Cardio 30–45 minutes

Day Seven:
Rest

BASEBALL WORKOUTS

A Dumbbell Shoulder Press
page 74

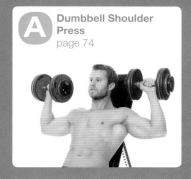

B Incline Bench Row
page 50

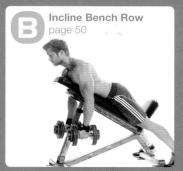

C External Rotation with Band
page 80

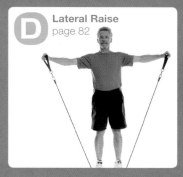

D Lateral Raise
page 82

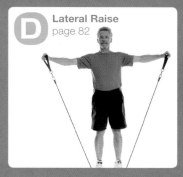

E Swiss Ball Reverse Fly
page 90

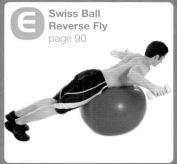

F Rope Pushdown
page 106

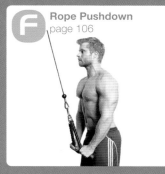

G Lying Triceps Extension
page 108

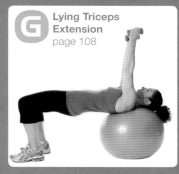

H Swiss Ball Wall Sit
page 134

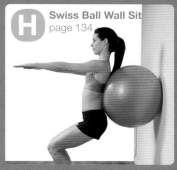

I Dumbbell Lunge
page 138

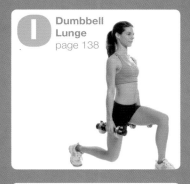

J Goblet Squat
page 150

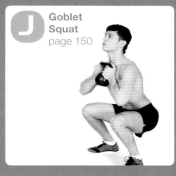

K Abdominal Kick
page 184

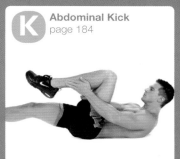

L Bicycle Crunch
page 190

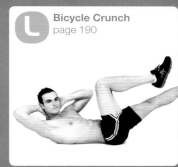

M Side Plank
page 122

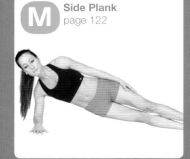

N Seated Russian Twist
page 200

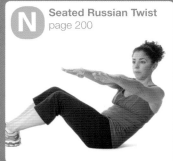

O Medicine Ball Wood Chop
page 130

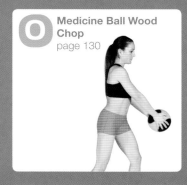

P Single-Arm Concentration Curl
page 102

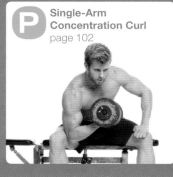

Q Swiss Ball Roll-Out
page 206

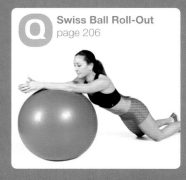

R Thigh Rock-Back
page 208

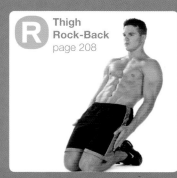

S Swiss Ball Hip Crossover
page 210

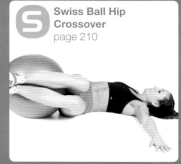

T Medicine Ball Slam
page 214

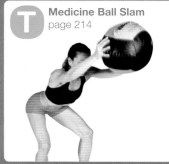

BASKETBALL

Players use a combination of sprinting and jumping, while passing and shooting with great speed and accuracy. Being 7-foot tall is helpful but, whatever your height, basketball prowess is driven predominantly by four powerful muscle groups — the upper arms, shoulders, core and thighs. Use this workout to put a serious spring in your step.

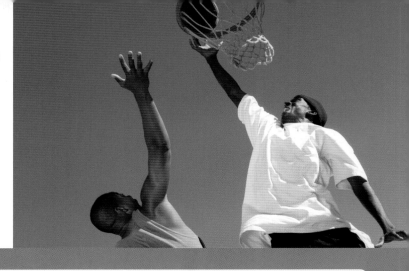

WORKOUT LEVEL 1

BEGINNER ROUTINE I

Day One:
A 3 sets of 8–10
C 3 sets of 8–10
E 3 sets of 10–12
F 3 sets of 12–15
J 3 sets of 12–15
N 15

Day Two:
Rest

Day Three:
A 3 sets of 8–10
C 3 sets of 8–10
E 3 sets of 10–12
F 3 sets of 12–15
J 3 sets of 12–15
N 15

Day Four:
Rest

Day Five:
A 3 sets of 8–10
C 3 sets of 8–10
E 3 sets of 10–12
F 3 sets of 12–15
J 3 sets of 12–15
N 15

Day Six:
Cardio 30–45 minutes

Day Seven:
Rest

INTERMEDIATE ROUTINE I

Day One:
A 3 sets of 8–10
C 3 sets of 8–10
E 3 sets of 10–12
F 3 sets of 12–15
J 3 sets of 12–15
N 15
P 30 per side
S 25

Day Two:
Cardio 30–45 minutes

Day Three:
A 3 sets of 8–10
C 3 sets of 8–10
E 3 sets of 10–12
F 3 sets of 12–15
J 3 sets of 12–15
N 15
P 30 per side
S 25

Day Four:
Rest

Day Five:
A 3 sets of 8–10
C 3 sets of 8–10
E 3 sets of 10–12
F 3 sets of 12–15
J 3 sets of 12–15
N 15
P 30 per side
S 25

Day Six:
Cardio 30–45 minutes

Day Seven:
Rest

ADVANCED ROUTINE I

Day One:
A 3 sets of 8–10
C 3 sets of 8–10
E 3 sets of 10–12
F 3 sets of 12–15
J 3 sets of 12–15
K 3 sets of 10–12
N 15
P 30 per side
R 20
S 25

Day Two:
Cardio 30–45 minutes

Day Three:
A 3 sets of 8–10
C 3 sets of 8–10
E 3 sets of 10–12
F 3 sets of 12–15
J 3 sets of 12–15
K 3 sets of 10–12
N 15
P 30 per side

R 20
S 25

Day Four:
Cardio 30–45 minutes

Day Five:
A 3 sets of 8–10
C 3 sets of 8–10
E 3 sets of 10–12
F 3 sets of 12–15
J 3 sets of 12–15
K 3 sets of 10–12
N 15
P 30 per side
R 20
S 25

Day Six:
Cardio 30–45 minutes

Day Seven:
Rest

WORKOUT LEVEL 2

BEGINNER ROUTINE 2

Day One:
B 3 sets 8–10
D 3 sets 8–10
G 3 sets 12–15
H 3 sets 12–15
I 3 sets 12–15
L 3 sets 12–15

Day Two:
Rest

Day Three:
B 3 sets 8–10
D 3 sets 8–10
G 3 sets 12–15
H 3 sets 12–15
I 3 sets 12–15
L 3 sets 12–15

Day Four:
Rest

Day Five:
B 3 sets 8–10
D 3 sets 8–10
G 3 sets 12–15
H 3 sets 12–15
I 3 sets 12–15
L 3 sets 12–15

Day Six:
Cardio 30–45 minutes

Day Seven:
Rest

INTERMEDIATE ROUTINE 2

Day One:
B 3 sets 8–10
D 3 sets 8–10
G 3 sets 12–15
H 3 sets 12–15
I 3 sets 12–15
L 3 sets 12–15
M 3 sets 20
O 3 sets 30–120 seconds

Day Two:
Cardio 30–45 minutes

Day Three:
B 3 sets 8–10
D 3 sets 8–10
G 3 sets 12–15
H 3 sets 12–15
I 3 sets 12–15
L 3 sets 12–15
M 3 sets 20
O 3 sets 30–120 seconds

Day Four:
Rest

Day Five:
B 3 sets 8–10
D 3 sets 8–10
G 3 sets 12–15
H 3 sets 12–15
I 3 sets 12–15
L 3 sets 12–15
M 3 sets 20
O 3 sets 30–120 seconds

Day Six:
Cardio 30–45 minutes

Day Seven:
Rest

ADVANCED ROUTINE 2

Day One:
B 3 sets 8–10
D 3 sets 8–10
G 3 sets 12–15
H 3 sets 12–15
I 3 sets 12–15
L 3 sets 12–15
M 3 sets 20
O 3 sets 30–120 seconds
Q 3 sets 15
T 3 sets 20

Day Two:
Cardio 30–45 minutes

Day Three:
B 3 sets 8–10
D 3 sets 8–10
G 3 sets 12–15
H 3 sets 12–15
I 3 sets 12–15
L 3 sets 12–15
M 3 sets 20
O 3 sets 30–120 seconds

Q 3 sets 15
T 3 sets 20

Day Four:
Cardio 30–45 minutes

Day Five:
B 3 sets 8–10
D 3 sets 8–10
G 3 sets 12–15
H 3 sets 12–15
I 3 sets 12–15
L 3 sets 12–15
M 3 sets 20
O 3 sets 30–60 seconds
Q 3 sets 15
T 3 sets 20

Day Six:
Cardio 30–45 minutes

Day Seven:
Rest

BASKETBALL WORKOUTS

A Lat Pulldown
page 42
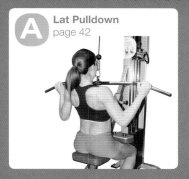

B Dips
page 68
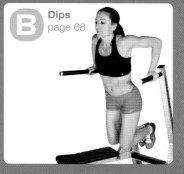

C Overhead Press
page 76
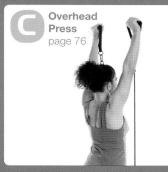

D Barbell Upright Row
page 86
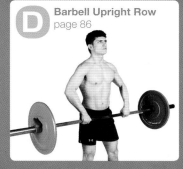

E Rope Overhead Extension
page 114
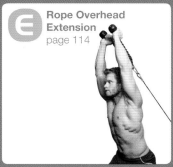

F Reverse Lunge
page 140
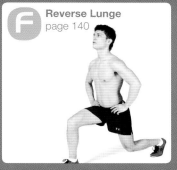

G Lateral Low Lunge
page 142
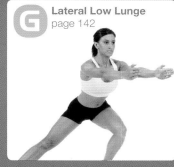

H Dumbbell Walking Lunge
page 144
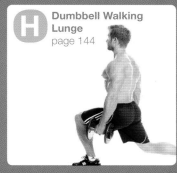

I High Lunge
page 146
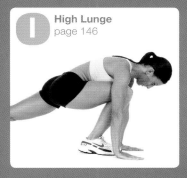

J One-Legged Step-Down
page 152
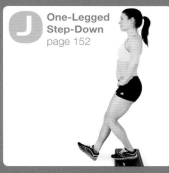

K Swiss Ball Hamstring Curl
page 164
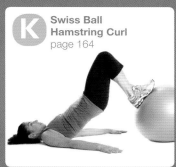

L Dumbbell Calf Raise
page 178
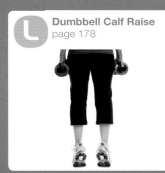

M Abdominal Hip Lift
page 186
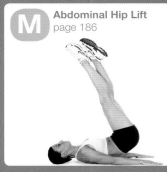

N Star Jump
page 156
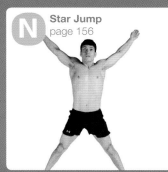

O Mountain Climber
page 158
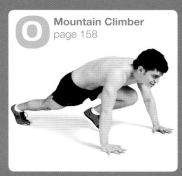

P Wood Chop with Resistance Band
page 202
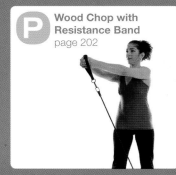

Q Hip Abduction and Adduction
page 204
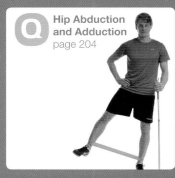

R Swiss Ball Jackknife
page 128
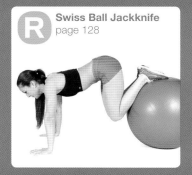

S Medicine Ball Slam
page 214
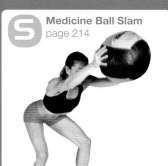

T The Windmill
page 216
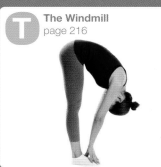

BOXING

A gruelling sport, boxing requires compact muscles that harness explosive power and accuracy. Combinations of punches use all of the major muscles of the body in synergistic movement and the sport requires great stamina as well as strength. Clearly, avoiding punches is even more important than landing them, so core strength and strong legs are needed to successfully "bob and weave" your way around the ring. Enjoy this hard-hitting routine to keep yourself fighting fit.

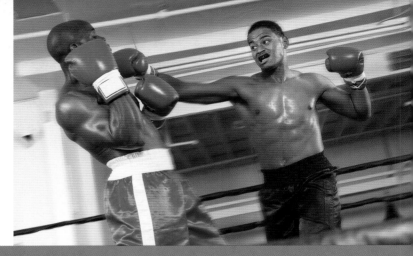

WORKOUT LEVEL 1

BEGINNER ROUTINE 1

Day One:
A 3 sets of 8–10
B 3 sets of 8–10
E 3 sets of 8–10
I 3 sets of 10–12
K 3 sets of 10–12
S 20 per side

Day Two:
Rest

Day Three:
A 3 sets of 8–10
B 3 sets of 8–10
E 3 sets of 8–10
I 3 sets of 10–12
K 3 sets of 10–12
S 20 per side

Day Four:
Rest

Day Five:
A 3 sets of 8–10
B 3 sets of 8–10
E 3 sets of 8–10
I 3 sets of 10–12
K 3 sets of 10–12
S 20 per side

Day Six:
Cardio 30–45 minutes

Day Seven:
Rest

INTERMEDIATE ROUTINE 1

Day One:
A 3 sets of 8–10
B 3 sets of 8–10
E 3 sets of 8–10
F 20
I 3 sets of 10–12
K 3 sets of 10–12
L 3 sets of 12–15
S 20 per side

Day Two:
Cardio 30–45 minutes

Day Three:
A 3 sets of 8–10
B 3 sets of 8–10
E 3 sets of 8–10
F 20
I 3 sets of 10–12
K 3 sets of 10–12
L 3 sets of 12–15
S 20 per side

Day Four:
Rest

Day Five:
A 3 sets of 8–10
B 3 sets of 8–10
E 3 sets of 8–10
F 20
I 3 sets of 10–12
K 3 sets of 10–12
L 3 sets of 12–15
S 20 per side

Day Six:
Cardio 30–45 minutes

Day Seven:
Rest

ADVANCED ROUTINE 1

Day One:
A 3 sets of 8–10
B 3 sets of 8–10
E 3 sets of 8–10
F 20
I 3 sets of 10–12
K 3 sets of 10–12
L 3 sets of 12–15
O 3 sets of 12–15
S 20 per side
T 25

Day Two:
Cardio 30–45 minutes

Day Three:
A 3 sets of 8–10
B 3 sets of 8–10
E 3 sets of 8–10
F 20
I 3 sets of 10–12
K 3 sets of 10–12
L 3 sets of 12–15
O 3 sets of 12–15
S 20 per side
T 25

Day Four:
Cardio 30–45 minutes

Day Five:
A 3 sets of 8–10
B 3 sets of 8–10
E 3 sets of 8–10
F 20
I 3 sets of 10–12
K 3 sets of 10–12
L 3 sets of 12–15
O 3 sets of 12–15
S 20 per side
T 25

Day Six:
Cardio 30–45 minutes

Day Seven:
Rest

WORKOUT LEVEL 2

BEGINNER ROUTINE 2

Day One:
C 3 sets 12–15
D 3 sets 8–10
G 3 sets 15
H 3 sets 12–15
J 3 sets 10–12
M 3 sets 15–20

Day Two:
Rest

Day Three:
C 3 sets 12–15
D 3 sets 8–10
G 3 sets 15
H 3 sets 12–15
J 3 sets 10–12
M 3 sets 15–20

Day Four:
Rest

Day Five:
C 3 sets 12–15
D 3 sets 8–10
G 3 sets 15
H 3 sets 12–15
J 3 sets 10–12
M 3 sets 15–20

Day Six:
Cardio 30–45 minutes

Day Seven:
Rest

INTERMEDIATE ROUTINE 2

Day One:
C 3 sets 12–15
D 3 sets 8–10
G 3 sets 15
H 3 sets 12–15
J 3 sets 10–12
M 3 sets 15–20
N 3 sets 15–20
P 3 sets 12–15

Day Two:
Cardio 30–45 minutes

Day Three:
C 3 sets 12–15
D 3 sets 8–10
G 3 sets 15
H 3 sets 12–15
J 3 sets 10–12
M 3 sets 15–20
N 3 sets 15–20
P 3 sets 12–15

Day Four:
Rest

Day Five:
C 3 sets 12–15
D 3 sets 8–10
G 3 sets 15
H 3 sets 12–15
J 3 sets 10–12
M 3 sets 15–20
N 3 sets 15–20
P 3 sets 12–15

Day Six:
Cardio 30–45 minutes

Day Seven:
Rest

ADVANCED ROUTINE 2

Day One:
C 3 sets 12–15
D 3 sets 8–10
G 3 sets 15
H 3 sets 12–15
J 3 sets 10–12
M 3 sets 15–20
N 3 sets 15–20
P 3 sets 12–15
Q 3 sets 15
R 3 sets 20

Day Two:
Cardio 30–45 minutes

Day Three:
C 3 sets 12–15
D 3 sets 8–10
G 3 sets 15
H 3 sets 12–15
J 3 sets 10–12
M 3 sets 15–20
N 3 sets 15–20
P 3 sets 12–15
Q 3 sets 15
R 3 sets 20

Day Four:
Cardio 30–45 minutes

Day Five:
C 3 sets 12–15
D 3 sets 8–10
G 3 sets 15
H 3 sets 12–15
J 3 sets 10–12
M 3 sets 15–20
N 3 sets 15–20
P 3 sets 12–15
Q 3 sets 15
R 3 sets 20

Day Six:
Cardio 30–45 minutes

Day Seven:
Rest

BOXING WORKOUTS

A Dumbbell Row
page 38

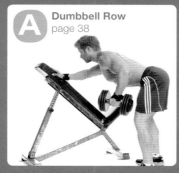

B Rope Pulldown
page 52

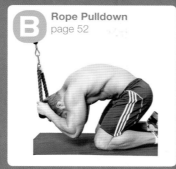

C Rotated Back Extension
page 58

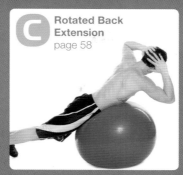

D Roller Push-Up
page 62

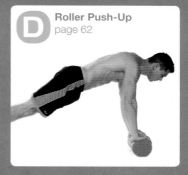

E Dips
page 68

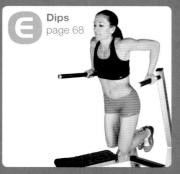

F Push-Up Hand Walk-Over
page 72

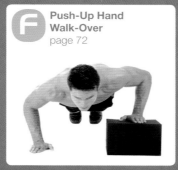

G Rotation Exercises
page 78

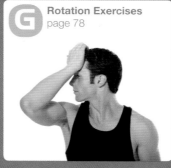

H External Rotation with Band
page 80

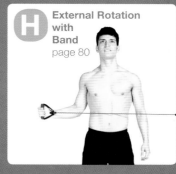

I Front-Plate Raise
page 92

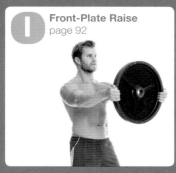

J Alternating Hammer Curl
page 98

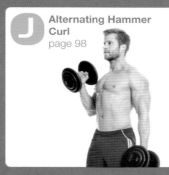

K Swiss Ball Wall Sit
page 134

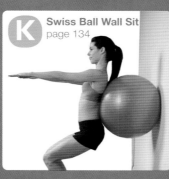

L High Lunge
page 146

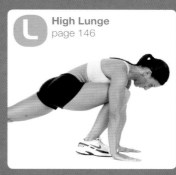

M Adductor Extension
page 162

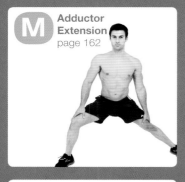

N Hamstring Abductor
page 163

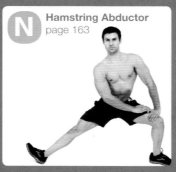

O Hamstring Pull-In
page 170

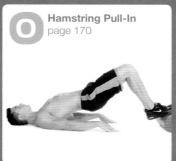

P Dumbbell Shin Raise
page 180

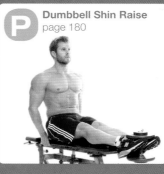

Q Plank Press-Up
page 198

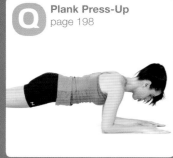

R Burpee
page 160

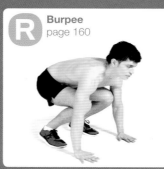

S Medicine Ball Wood Chop
page 130

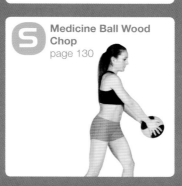

T Medicine Ball Slam
page 214

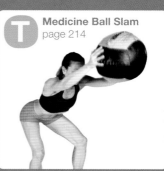

CANOEING

Important muscles to train for canoeing are the obliques, lats, triceps, biceps and forearms, which are all used in the basic paddling action. However, to stabilize your body when counteracting the movement of water you rely heavily on the core muscles. More advanced canoeists use their entire body, especially incorporating the strong muscles of their legs and hips to drive each stroke. This tailored workout will help you to develop serious paddle power.

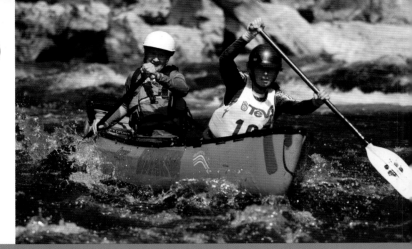

WORKOUT LEVEL 1

BEGINNER ROUTINE 1

Day One:
A 3 sets 8–10
E 3 sets 8–10
F 3 sets of 15
H 3 sets 10–12
I 3 sets 10–12
R 20 per side

Day Two:
Rest

Day Three:
A 3 sets 8–10
E 3 sets 8–10
F 3 sets of 15
H 3 sets 10–12
I 3 sets 10–12
R 20 per side

Day Four:
Rest

Day Five:
A 3 sets 8–10
E 3 sets 8–10
F 3 sets of 15
H 3 sets 10–12
I 3 sets 10–12
R 20 per side

Day Six:
Cardio 30–45 minutes

Day Seven:
Rest

INTERMEDIATE ROUTINE 1

Day One:
A 3 sets 8–10
B 3 sets 8–10
E 3 sets 8–10
F 3 sets of 15
H 3 sets 10–12
I 3 sets 10–12
J 3 sets 12–15
R 20 per side

Day Two:
Cardio 30–45 minutes

Day Three:
A 3 sets 8–10
B 3 sets 8–10
E 3 sets 8–10
F 3 sets of 15
H 3 sets 10–12
I 3 sets 10–12
J 3 sets 12–15
R 20 per side

Day Four:
Rest

Day Five:
A 3 sets 8–10
B 3 sets 8–10
E 3 sets 8–10
F 3 sets of 15
H 3 sets 10–12
I 3 sets 10–12
J 3 sets 12–15
R 20 per side

Day Six:
Cardio 30–45 minutes

Day Seven:
Rest

ADVANCED ROUTINE 1

Day One:
A 3 sets 8–10
B 3 sets 8–10
E 3 sets 8–10
F 3 sets of 15
H 3 sets 10–12
I 3 sets 10–12
J 3 sets 12–15
K 3 sets 12–15
R 20 per side
S 20

Day Two:
Cardio 30–45 minutes

Day Three:
A 3 sets 8–10
B 3 sets 8–10
E 3 sets 8–10
F 3 sets of 15
H 3 sets 10–12
I 3 sets 10–12
J 3 sets 12–15
K 3 sets 12–15
R 20 per side
S 20

Day Four:
Cardio 30–45 minutes

Day Five:
A 3 sets 8–10
B 3 sets 8–10
E 3 sets 8–10
F 3 sets of 15
H 3 sets 10–12
I 3 sets 10–12
J 3 sets 12–15
K 3 sets 12–15
R 20 per side
S 20

Day Six:
Cardio 30–45 minutes

Day Seven:
Rest

WORKOUT LEVEL 2

BEGINNER ROUTINE 2

Day One:
C 3 sets 12–15
D 3 sets 10–12
G 3 sets 8–10
L 3 sets 25
M 3 sets 20
N 3 sets 20

Day Two:
Rest

Day Three:
C 3 sets 12–15
D 3 sets 10–12
G 3 sets 8–10
L 3 sets 25
M 3 sets 20
N 3 sets 20

Day Four:
Rest

Day Five:
C 3 sets 12–15
D 3 sets 10–12
G 3 sets 8–10
L 3 sets 25
M 3 sets 20
N 3 sets 20

Day Six:
Cardio 30–45 minutes

Day Seven:
Rest

INTERMEDIATE ROUTINE 2

Day One:
C 3 sets 12–15
D 3 sets 10–12
G 3 sets 8–10
L 3 sets 25
M 3 sets 20
N 3 sets 20
O 3 sets 30
P 3 sets 30–60 seconds per side

Day Two:
Cardio 30–45 minutes

Day Three:
C 3 sets 12–15
D 3 sets 10–12
G 3 sets 8–10
L 3 sets 25
M 3 sets 20
N 3 sets 20
O 3 sets 30
P 3 sets 30–60 seconds per side

Day Four:
Rest

Day Five:
C 3 sets 12–15
D 3 sets 10–12
G 3 sets 8–10
L 3 sets 25
M 3 sets 20
N 3 sets 20
O 3 sets 30
P 3 sets 30–60 seconds per side

Day Six:
Cardio 30–45 minutes

Day Seven:
Rest

ADVANCED ROUTINE 2

Day One:
C 3 sets 12–15
D 3 sets 10–12
G 3 sets 8–10
L 3 sets 25
M 3 sets 20
N 3 sets 20
O 3 sets 30
P 3 sets 30–60 seconds per side
Q 3 sets 20
T 3 sets 20

Day Two:
Cardio 30–45 minutes

Day Three:
C 3 sets 12–15
D 3 sets 10–12
G 3 sets 8–10
L 3 sets 25
M 3 sets 20
N 3 sets 20
O 3 sets 30
P 3 sets 30–60 seconds per side
Q 3 sets 20
T 3 sets 20

Day Four:
Cardio 30–45 minutes

Day Five:
C 3 sets 12–15
D 3 sets 10–12
G 3 sets 8–10
L 3 sets 25
M 3 sets 20
N 3 sets 20
O 3 sets 30
P 3 sets 30–60 seconds per side
Q 3 sets 20
T 3 sets 20

Day Six:
Cardio 30–45 minutes

Day Seven:
Rest

CANOEING WORKOUTS

A Lat Pulldown
page 42
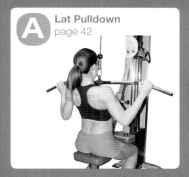

B Alternating Renegade Row
page 48
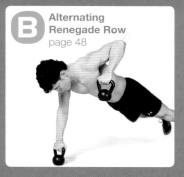

C Flat Bench Hyperextension
page 56
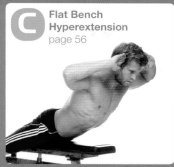

D Dumbbell Fly
page 64
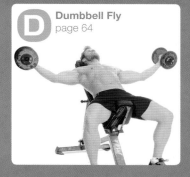

E Dips
page 68
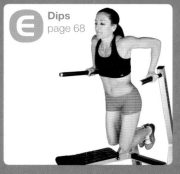

F Rotation Exercises
page 78
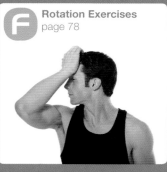

G Shoulder Raise and Pull
page 84
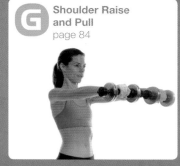

H Alternating Hammer Curl
page 98
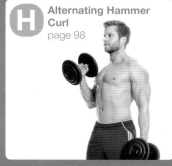

I Lying Triceps Extension
page 108
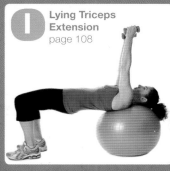

J Wrist Flexion
page 116
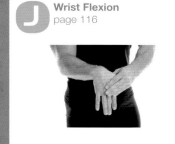

K Wrist Extension
page 117
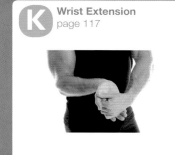

L Crunch
page 118
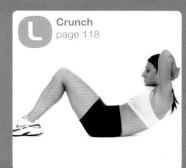

M Reverse Crunch
page 192
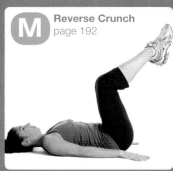

N Seated Russian Twist
page 200
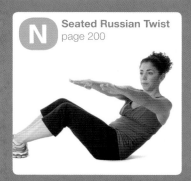

O Wood Chop with Resistance Band
page 202
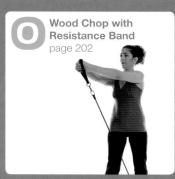

P T-Stabilization
page 124
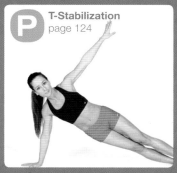

Q Swiss Ball Roll-Out
page 206
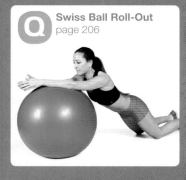

R Thigh Rock-Back
page 208
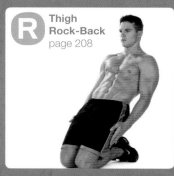

S V-Up
page 212
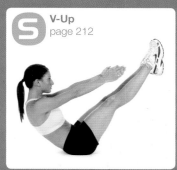

T The Windmill
page 216
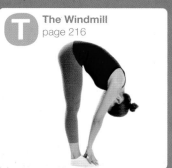

CLIMBING

Climbing involves nearly every major muscle group for proper execution, with particular emphasis on the lower body and core, which help to stabilize and strengthen the body for upward mobility. The quadriceps and calves are critical for climbing, and although climbing does indeed take upper body strength, the true lifting comes from the legs. The calf muscles allow you to rise to tip-toes for a better reach. This exercise routine will build your strength and keep you at peak fitness.

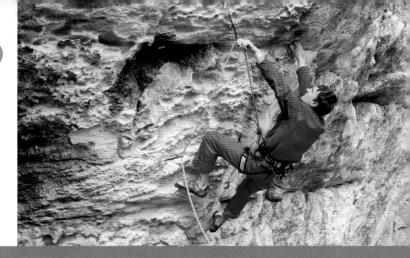

WORKOUT LEVEL 1

BEGINNER ROUTINE I

Day One:
B 3 sets 8–10
C 3 sets 10–12
G 3 sets 12–15
I 3 sets 10–12
N 3 sets 12–15
R 15

Day Two:
Rest

Day Three:
B 3 sets 8–10
C 3 sets 10–12
G 3 sets 12–15
I 3 sets 10–12
N 3 sets 12–15
R 15

Day Four:
Rest

Day Five:
B 3 sets 8–10
C 3 sets 10–12
G 3 sets 12–15
I 3 sets 10–12
N 3 sets 12–15
R 15

Day Six:
Cardio 30–45 minutes

Day Seven:
Rest

INTERMEDIATE ROUTINE I

Day One:
B 3 sets 8–10
C 3 sets 10–12
F 3 sets 10–12
G 3 sets 12–15
I 3 sets 10–12
L 3 sets 12–15
N 3 sets 12–15
R 15

Day Two:
Cardio 30–45 minutes

Day Three:
B 3 sets 8–10
C 3 sets 10–12
F 3 sets 10–12
G 3 sets 12–15
I 3 sets 10–12
L 3 sets 12–15
N 3 sets 12–15
R 15

Day Four:
Rest

Day Five:
B 3 sets 8–10
C 3 sets 10–12
F 3 sets 10–12
G 3 sets 12–15
I 3 sets 10–12
L 3 sets 12–15
N 3 sets 12–15
R 15

Day Six:
Cardio 30–45 minutes

Day Seven:
Rest

ADVANCED ROUTINE I

Day One:
B 3 sets 8–10
C 3 sets 10–12
F 3 sets 10–12
G 3 sets 12–15
I 3 sets 10–12
L 3 sets 12–15
N 3 sets 12–15
O 3 sets 12–15
R 15
S 30–120 seconds

Day Two:
Cardio 30–45 minutes

Day Three:
B 3 sets 8–10
C 3 sets 10–12
F 3 sets 10–12
G 3 sets 12–15
I 3 sets 10–12
L 3 sets 12–15
N 3 sets 12–15
O 3 sets 12–15
R 15
S 30–120 seconds

Day Four:
Cardio 30–45 minutes

Day Five:
B 3 sets 8–10
C 3 sets 10–12
F 3 sets 10–12
G 3 sets 12–15
I 3 sets 10–12
L 3 sets 12–15
N 3 sets 12–15
O 3 sets 12–15
R 15
S 30–120 seconds

Day Six:
Cardio 30–45 minutes

Day Seven:
Rest

WORKOUT LEVEL 2

BEGINNER ROUTINE 2

Day One:
A 3 sets 8–10
D 3 sets 10–12
E 3 sets 10–12
H 3 sets 12–15
J 3 sets 12–15
K 3 sets 12–15

Day Two:
Rest

Day Three:
A 3 sets 8–10
D 3 sets 10–12
E 3 sets 10–12
H 3 sets 12–15
J 3 sets 12–15
K 3 sets 12–15

Day Four:
Rest

Day Five:
A 3 sets 8–10
D 3 sets 10–12
E 3 sets 10–12
H 3 sets 12–15
J 3 sets 12–15
K 3 sets 12–15

Day Six:
Cardio 30–45 minutes

Day Seven:
Rest

INTERMEDIATE ROUTINE 2

Day One:
A 3 sets 8–10
D 3 sets 10–12
E 3 sets 10–12
H 3 sets 12–15
J 3 sets 12–15
K 3 sets 12–15

Day Two:
Cardio 30–45 minutes

Day Three:
A 3 sets 8–10
D 3 sets 10–12
E 3 sets 10–12
H 3 sets 12–15
J 3 sets 12–15
K 3 sets 12–15

Day Four:
Rest

Day Five:
A 3 sets 8–10
D 3 sets 10–12
E 3 sets 10–12
H 3 sets 12–15
J 3 sets 12–15
K 3 sets 12–15

Day Six:
Cardio 30–45 minutes

Day Seven:
Rest

ADVANCED ROUTINE 2

Day One:
A 3 sets 8–10
D 3 sets 10–12
E 3 sets 10–12
H 3 sets 12–15
J 3 sets 12–15
K 3 sets 12–15
M 3 sets 12–15
P 3 sets 20
Q 3 sets 15
T 3 sets 3–5 per side

Day Two:
Cardio 30–45 minutes

Day Three:
A 3 sets 8–10
D 3 sets 10–12
E 3 sets 10–12
H 3 sets 12–15
J 3 sets 12–15
K 3 sets 12–15
M 3 sets 12–15
P 3 sets 20
Q 3 sets 15
T 3 sets 3–5 per side

Day Four:
Cardio 30–45 minutes

Day Five:
A 3 sets 8–10
D 3 sets 10–12
E 3 sets 10–12
H 3 sets 12–15
J 3 sets 12–15
K 3 sets 12–15
M 3 sets 12–15
P 3 sets 20
Q 3 sets 15
T 3 sets 3–5 per side

Day Six:
Cardio 30–45 minutes

Day Seven:
Rest

CLIMBING WORKOUTS

A Lat Pulldown
page 42

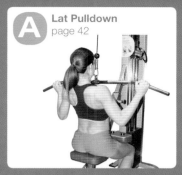

B Reverse Close-Grip Front Chin
page 54

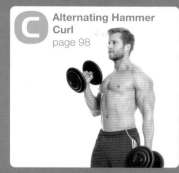

C Alternating Hammer Curl
page 98

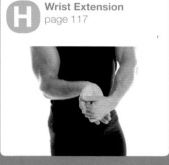

D Rope Hammer Curl
page 104

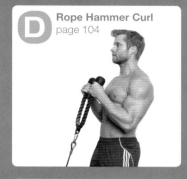

E Rope Pushdown
page 106

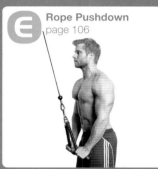

F Lying Triceps Extension
page 108

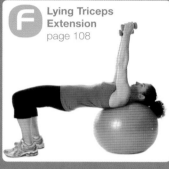

G Wrist Flexion
page 116

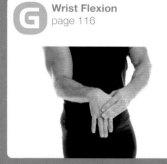

H Wrist Extension
page 117

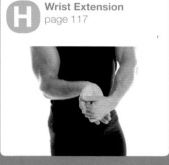

I Barbell Squat
page 136

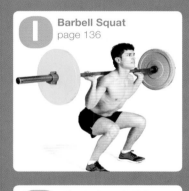

J Lateral Low Lunge
page 142

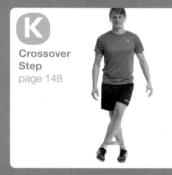

K Crossover Step
page 148

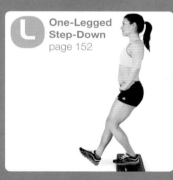

L One-Legged Step-Down
page 152

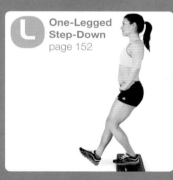

M Single-Leg Calf Press
page 176

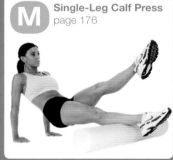

N Dumbbell Calf Raise
page 178

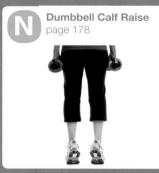

O Dumbbell Shin Raise
page 180

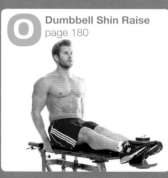

P Abdominal Hip Lift
page 186

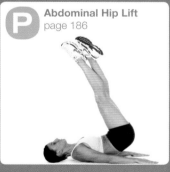

Q Swiss Ball Pelvic Tilt
page 196

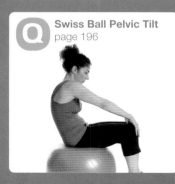

R Plank Press-Up
page 198

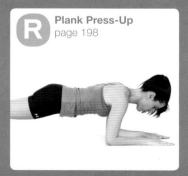

S Mountain Climber
page 158

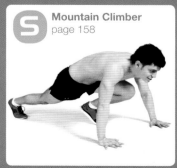

T Swiss Ball Walk-Around
page 126

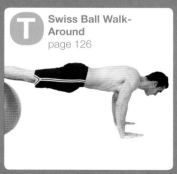

CRICKET

Whether batting, bowling or fielding, the highly tactical game of cricket requires good cardiovascular fitness as well as strength and power. The legs play a key role in providing manoeuvrability and power, with help from the major muscles of the upper body. There is a wide range of defensive and offensive batting strokes that involve an even wider range of muscles. Successful Cricket training focuses on speed, flexibility, strength and explosiveness, rather than sheer bulk.

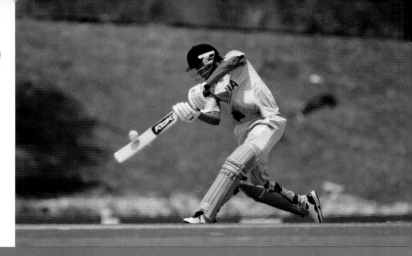

BEGINNER ROUTINE 1

Day One:
A 3 sets of 8–10
C 3 sets of 12–15
F 3 sets of 10–12
H 3 sets of 10–12
N 20 rotations
O 20 per side

Day Two:
Rest

Day Three:
A 3 sets of 8–10
C 3 sets of 12–15
F 3 sets of 10–12
H 3 sets of 10–12
N 20 rotations
O 20 per side

Day Four:
Rest

Day Five:
A 3 sets of 8–10
C 3 sets of 12–15
F 3 sets of 10–12
H 3 sets of 10–12
N 20 rotations
O 20 per side

Day Six:
Cardio 30–45 minutes

Day Seven:
Rest

INTERMEDIATE ROUTINE 1

Day One:
A 3 sets of 8–10
C 3 sets of 12–15
F 3 sets of 10–12
H 3 sets of 10–12
J 3 sets of 10–12
N 20 rotations
O 20 per side
T 25 repetitions

Day Two:
Cardio 30–45 minutes

Day Three:
A 3 sets of 8–10
C 3 sets of 12–15
F 3 sets of 10–12
H 3 sets of 10–12
J 3 sets of 10–12
N 20 rotations
O 20 per side
T 25 repetitions

Day Four:
Rest

Day Five:
A 3 sets of 8–10
C 3 sets of 12–15
F 3 sets of 10–12
H 3 sets of 10–12
J 3 sets of 10–12
N 20 rotations
O 20 per side
T 25 repetitions

Day Six:
Cardio 30–45 minutes

Day Seven:
Rest

ADVANCED ROUTINE 1

Day One:
A 3 sets of 8–10
C 3 sets of 12–15
F 3 sets of 10–12
H 3 sets of 10–12
I 3 sets of 10–12
J 3 sets of 10–12
N 20 rotations
O 20 per side
R 20 per side
T 25 repetitions

Day Two:
Cardio 30–45 minutes

Day Three:
A 3 sets of 8–10
C 3 sets of 12–15
F 3 sets of 10–12
H 3 sets of 10–12
I 3 sets of 10–12
J 3 sets of 10–12
N 20 rotations
O 20 per side
R 20 per side
T 25 repetitions

Day Four:
Cardio 30–45 minutes

Day Five:
A 3 sets of 8–10
C 3 sets of 12–15
F 3 sets of 10–12
H 3 sets of 10–12
I 3 sets of 10–12
J 3 sets of 10–12
N 20 rotations
O 20 per side
R 20 per side
T 25 repetitions

Day Six:
Cardio 30–45 minutes

Day Seven:
Rest

BEGINNER ROUTINE 2

Day One:
B 3 sets 15
D 3 sets 10–12
E 3 sets 10–12
G 3 sets 10–12
K 3 sets 25
L 3 sets 20

Day Two:
Rest

Day Three:
B 3 sets 15
D 3 sets 10–12
E 3 sets 10–12
G 3 sets 10–12
K 3 sets 25
L 3 sets 20

Day Four:
Rest

Day Five:
B 3 sets 15
D 3 sets 10–12
E 3 sets 10–12
G 3 sets 10–12
K 3 sets 25
L 3 sets 20

Day Six:
Cardio 30–45 minutes

Day Seven:
Rest

INTERMEDIATE ROUTINE 2

Day One:
B 3 sets 15
D 3 sets 10–12
E 3 sets 10–12
G 3 sets 10–12
K 3 sets 25
L 3 sets 20
M 3 sets 30–60 seconds
P 3 sets 30–60 seconds

Day Two:
Cardio 30–45 minutes

Day Three:
B 3 sets 15
D 3 sets 10–12
E 3 sets 10–12
G 3 sets 10–12
K 3 sets 25
L 3 sets 20
M 3 sets 30–60 seconds
P 3 sets 30–60 seconds

Day Four:
Rest

Day Five:
B 3 sets 15
D 3 sets 10–12
E 3 sets 10–12
G 3 sets 10–12
K 3 sets 25
L 3 sets 20
M 3 sets 30–60 seconds
P 3 sets 30–60 seconds

Day Six:
Cardio 30–45 minutes

Day Seven:
Rest

ADVANCED ROUTINE 2

Day One:
B 3 sets 15
D 3 sets 10–12
E 3 sets 10–12
G 3 sets 10–12
K 3 sets 25
L 3 sets 20
M 3 sets 30–60 seconds
P 3 sets 30–60 seconds
Q 3 sets 20
S 3 sets 20

Day Two:
Cardio 30–45 minutes

Day Three:
B 3 sets 15
D 3 sets 10–12
E 3 sets 10–12
G 3 sets 10–12
K 3 sets 25
L 3 sets 20
M 3 sets 30–60 seconds
P 3 sets 30–60 seconds
Q 3 sets 20
S 3 sets 20

Day Four:
Cardio 30–45 minutes

Day Five:
B 3 sets 15
D 3 sets 10–12
E 3 sets 10–12
G 3 sets 10–12
K 3 sets 25
L 3 sets 20
M 3 sets 30–60 seconds
P 3 sets 30–60 seconds
Q 3 sets 20
S 3 sets 20

Day Six:
Cardio 30–45 minutes

Day Seven:
Rest

CRICKET WORKOUTS

A Dumbbell Shoulder Press
page 74

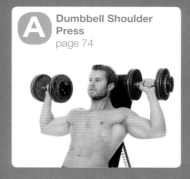

B Rotation Exercises
page 78

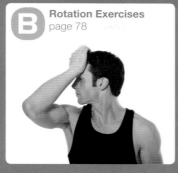

C External Rotation with Band
page 80

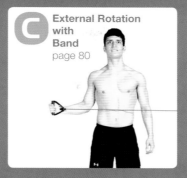

D Lateral Raise
page 82

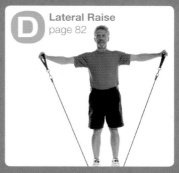

E Swiss Ball Reverse Fly
page 90

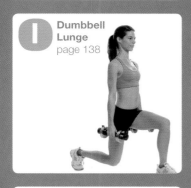

F Rope Pushdown
page 106

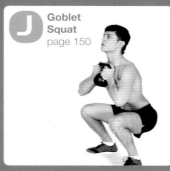

G Lying Triceps Extension
page 108

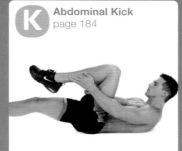

H Swiss Ball Wall Sit
page 134

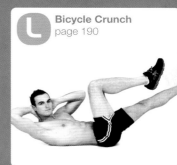

I Dumbbell Lunge
page 138

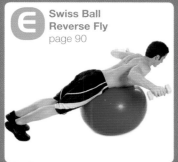

J Goblet Squat
page 150

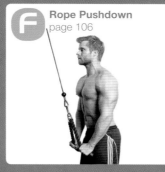

K Abdominal Kick
page 184

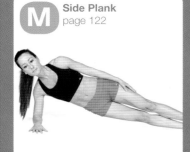

L Bicycle Crunch
page 190

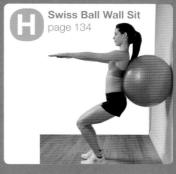

M Side Plank
page 122

N Seated Russian Twist
page 200

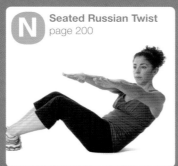

O Medicine Ball Wood Chop
page 130

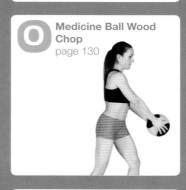

P T-Stabilization
page 124

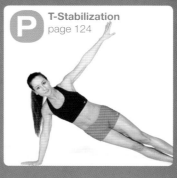

Q Swiss Ball Roll-Out
page 206

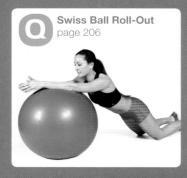

R Thigh Rock-Back
page 208

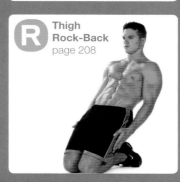

S Swiss Ball Hip Crossover
page 210

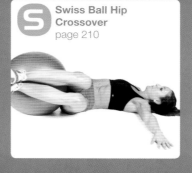

T Medicine Ball Slam
page 214

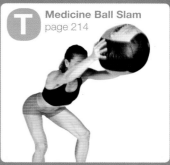

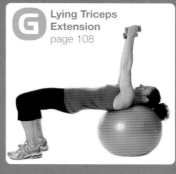

CROSS-COUNTRY SKIING

A long-distance sport usually performed on subtly rolling trails, cross-country skiing draws strength from the lower body and also uses the muscles of the upper body and core for power and performance. Since considerable energy is used while cross-country skiing, this activity makes for an excellent overall calorie burner as well as cardiovascular exercise.

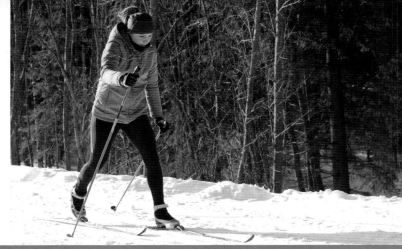

WORKOUT LEVEL 1

BEGINNER ROUTINE 1

Day One:
B 3 sets 10–12
E 3 sets 10–12
F 3 sets 10–12
G 3 sets 10–12
I 3 sets 12–15
P 30–120 seconds

Day Two:
Rest

Day Three:
B 3 sets 10–12
E 3 sets 10–12
F 3 sets 10–12
G 3 sets 10–12
I 3 sets 12–15
P 30–120 seconds

Day Four:
Rest

Day Five:
B 3 sets 10–12
E 3 sets 10–12
F 3 sets 10–12
G 3 sets 10–12
I 3 sets 12–15
P 30–120 seconds

Day Six:
Cardio 30–45 minutes

Day Seven:
Rest

INTERMEDIATE ROUTINE 1

Day One:
A 3 sets 12–15
B 3 sets 10–12
E 3 sets 10–12
F 3 sets 10–12
G 3 sets 10–12
I 3 sets 12–15
M 3 sets 10–12
P 30–120 seconds

Day Two:
Cardio 30–45 minutes

Day Three:
A 3 sets 12–15
B 3 sets 10–12
E 3 sets 10–12
F 3 sets 10–12
G 3 sets 10–12
I 3 sets 12–15
M 3 sets 10–12
P 30–120 seconds

Day Four:
Rest

Day Five:
A 3 sets 12–15
B 3 sets 10–12
E 3 sets 10–12
F 3 sets 10–12
G 3 sets 10–12
I 3 sets 12–15
M 3 sets 10–12
P 30–120 seconds

Day Six:
Cardio 30–45 minutes

Day Seven:
Rest

ADVANCED ROUTINE 1

Day One:
A 3 sets 12–15
B 3 sets 10–12
E 3 sets 10–12
F 3 sets 10–12
G 3 sets 10–12
I 3 sets 12–15
M 3 sets 10–12
O 3 sets 12–15
P 30–120 seconds
T 20

Day Two:
Cardio 30–45 minutes

Day Three:
A 3 sets 12–15
B 3 sets 10–12
E 3 sets 10–12
F 3 sets 10–12
G 3 sets 10–12
I 3 sets 12–15
M 3 sets 10–12
O 3 sets 12–15
P 30–120 seconds
T 20

Day Four:
Cardio 30–45 minutes

Day Five:
A 3 sets 12–15
B 3 sets 10–12
E 3 sets 10–12
F 3 sets 10–12
G 3 sets 10–12
I 3 sets 12–15
M 3 sets 10–12
O 3 sets 12–15
P 30–120 seconds
T 20

Day Six:
Cardio 30–45 minutes

Day Seven:
Rest

WORKOUT LEVEL 2

BEGINNER ROUTINE 2

Day One:
C 3 sets 20
D 3 sets 8–10
H 3 sets 12–15
J 3 sets 12–15
K 3 sets 15–20
L 3 sets 15–20

Day Two:
Rest

Day Three:
C 3 sets 20
D 3 sets 8–10
H 3 sets 12–15
J 3 sets 12–15
K 3 sets 15–20
L 3 sets 15–20

Day Four:
Rest

Day Five:
C 3 sets 20
D 3 sets 8–10
H 3 sets 12–15
J 3 sets 12–15
K 3 sets 15–20
L 3 sets 15–20

Day Six:
Cardio 30–45 minutes

Day Seven:
Rest

INTERMEDIATE ROUTINE 2

Day One:
C 3 sets 20
D 3 sets 8–10
H 3 sets 12–15
J 3 sets 12–15
K 3 sets 15–20
L 3 sets 15–20
N 3 sets 12–15
Q 3 sets 15

Day Two:
Cardio 30–45 minutes

Day Three:
C 3 sets 20
D 3 sets 8–10
H 3 sets 12–15
J 3 sets 12–15
K 3 sets 15–20
L 3 sets 15–20
N 3 sets 12–15
Q 3 sets 15

Day Four:
Rest

Day Five:
C 3 sets 20
D 3 sets 8–10
H 3 sets 12–15
J 3 sets 12–15
K 3 sets 15–20
L 3 sets 15–20
N 3 sets 12–15
Q 3 sets 15

Day Six:
Cardio 30–45 minutes

Day Seven:
Rest

ADVANCED ROUTINE 2

Day One:
C 3 sets 20
D 3 sets 8–10
H 3 sets 12–15
J 3 sets 12–15
K 3 sets 15–20
L 3 sets 15–20
N 3 sets 12–15
Q 3 sets 15
R 3 sets 20
S 3 sets 20

Day Two:
Cardio 30–45 minutes

Day Three:
C 3 sets 20
D 3 sets 8–10
H 3 sets 12–15
J 3 sets 12–15
K 3 sets 15–20
L 3 sets 15–20
N 3 sets 12–15
Q 3 sets 15
R 3 sets 20
S 3 sets 20

Day Four:
Cardio 30–45 minutes

Day Five:
C 3 sets 20
D 3 sets 8–10
H 3 sets 12–15
J 3 sets 12–15
K 3 sets 15–20
L 3 sets 15–20
N 3 sets 12–15
Q 3 sets 15
R 3 sets 20
S 3 sets 20

Day Six:
Cardio 30–45 minutes

Day Seven:
Rest

CROSS-COUNTRY SKIING WORKOUTS

A Scapular Range of Motion
page 44
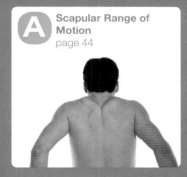

B Dumbbell Fly
page 64
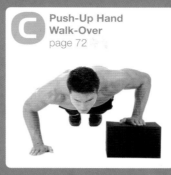

C Push-Up Hand Walk-Over
page 72
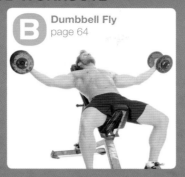

D Shoulder Raise and Pull
page 84
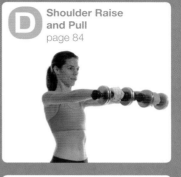

E Reverse Fly
page 88
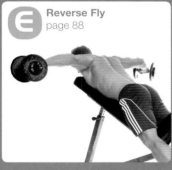

F Rope Hammer Curl
page 104
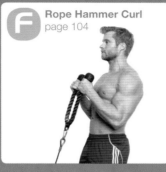

G Lying Triceps Extension
page 108
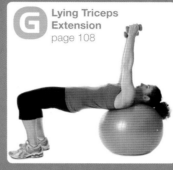

H Wrist Flexion
page 116
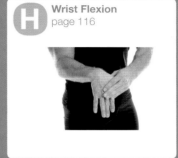

I Dumbbell Lunge
page 138
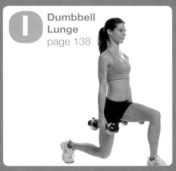

J One-Legged Step-Down
page 152
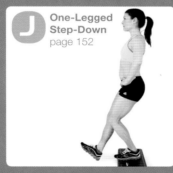

K Adductor Extension
page 162
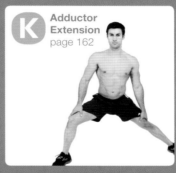

L Hamstring Abductor
page 163
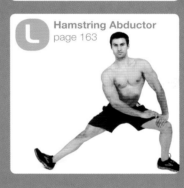

M Swiss Ball Hamstring Curl
page 164
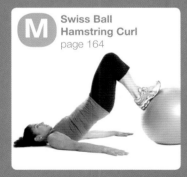

N Inverted Hamstring
page 166
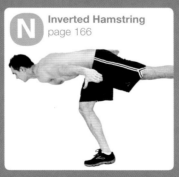

O Dumbbell Calf Raise
page 178
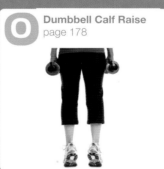

P Mountain Climber
page 158
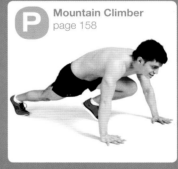

Q Hip Abduction and Adduction
page 204
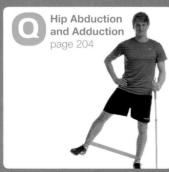

R Swiss Ball Jackknife
page 128
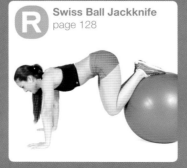

S Swiss Ball Hip Crossover
page 210
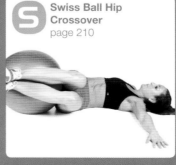

T V-Up
page 212
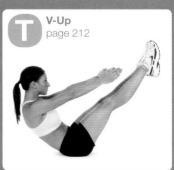

CYCLING

The sport of cycling is part power and part endurance, and varying terrain makes use of different groups of leg muscles. Ascending calls on the quadriceps, while standing brings the gluteal muscles more into play. Riding for speed or against the wind is a test of the synergistic combination of all leg muscles. The biceps and triceps are used when holding onto handlebars and supporting your bodyweight. The back and abdominals are ancillary muscles used for stabilization.

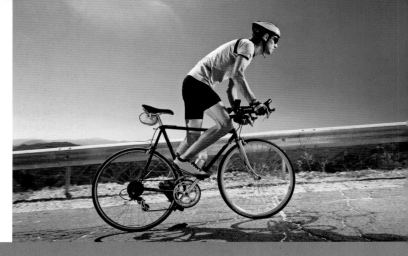

WORKOUT LEVEL 1

BEGINNER ROUTINE 1

Day One:
B 3 sets 8–10
C 3 sets 8–10
D 3 sets 8–10
F 3 sets 12–15
I 3 sets 12–15
L 3 sets 12–15

Day Two:
Rest

Day Three:
B 3 sets 8–10
C 3 sets 8–10
D 3 sets 8–10
F 3 sets 12–15
I 3 sets 12–15
L 3 sets 12–15

Day Four:
Rest

Day Five:
B 3 sets 8–10
C 3 sets 8–10
D 3 sets 8–10
F 3 sets 12–15
I 3 sets 12–15
L 3 sets 12–15

Day Six:
Cardio 30–45 minutes

Day Seven:
Rest

INTERMEDIATE ROUTINE 1

Day One:
B 3 sets 8–10
C 3 sets 8–10
D 3 sets 8–10
E 3 sets 10–12
F 3 sets 12–15
I 3 sets 12–15
L 3 sets 12–15
Q 30–60 seconds per side

Day Two:
Cardio 30–45 minutes

Day Three:
B 3 sets 8–10
C 3 sets 8–10
D 3 sets 8–10
E 3 sets 10–12
F 3 sets 12–15
I 3 sets 12–15
L 3 sets 12–15
Q 30–60 seconds per side

Day Four:
Rest

Day Five:
B 3 sets 8–10
C 3 sets 8–10
D 3 sets 8–10
E 3 sets 10–12
F 3 sets 12–15
I 3 sets 12–15
L 3 sets 12–15
Q 30–60 seconds per side

Day Six:
Cardio 30–45 minutes

Day Seven:
Rest

ADVANCED ROUTINE 1

Day One:
B 3 sets 8–10
C 3 sets 8–10
D 3 sets 8–10
E 3 sets 10–12
F 3 sets 12–15
I 3 sets 12–15
L 3 sets 12–15
K 3 sets 12–15
Q 30–60 seconds per side
S 20

Day Two:
Cardio 30–45 minutes

Day Three:
B 3 sets 8–10
C 3 sets 8–10
D 3 sets 8–10
E 3 sets 10–12
F 3 sets 12–15
I 3 sets 12–15
L 3 sets 12–15
K 3 sets 12–15
Q 30–60 seconds per side
S 20

Day Four:
Cardio 30–45 minutes

Day Five:
B 3 sets 8–10
C 3 sets 8–10
D 3 sets 8–10
E 3 sets 10–12
F 3 sets 12–15
I 3 sets 12–15
L 3 sets 12–15
K 3 sets 12–15
Q 30–60 seconds per side
S 20

Day Six:
Cardio 30–45 minutes

Day Seven:
Rest

WORKOUT LEVEL 2

BEGINNER ROUTINE 2

Day One:
A 3 sets 8–10
G 3 sets 12–15
H 3 sets 12–15
J 3 sets 12–15
K 3 sets 12–15
M 3 sets 25

Day Two:
Rest

Day Three:
A 3 sets 8–10
G 3 sets 12–15
H 3 sets 12–15
J 3 sets 12–15
K 3 sets 12–15
M 3 sets 25

Day Four:
Rest

Day Five:
A 3 sets 8–10
G 3 sets 12–15
H 3 sets 12–15
J 3 sets 12–15
K 3 sets 12–15
M 3 sets 25

Day Six:
Cardio 30–45 minutes

Day Seven:
Rest

INTERMEDIATE ROUTINE 2

Day One:
A 3 sets 8–10
G 3 sets 12–15
H 3 sets 12–15
J 3 sets 12–15
K 3 sets 12–15
M 3 sets 25
N 3 sets 30
O 3 sets 15

Day Two:
Cardio 30–45 minutes

Day Three:
A 3 sets 8–10
G 3 sets 12–15
H 3 sets 12–15
J 3 sets 12–15
K 3 sets 12–15
M 3 sets 25
N 3 sets 30
O 3 sets 15

Day Four:
Rest

Day Five:
A 3 sets 8–10
G 3 sets 12–15
H 3 sets 12–15
J 3 sets 12–15
K 3 sets 12–15
M 3 sets 25
N 3 sets 30
O 3 sets 15

Day Six:
Cardio 30–45 minutes

Day Seven:
Rest

ADVANCED ROUTINE 2

Day One:
A 3 sets 8–10
G 3 sets 12–15
H 3 sets 12–15
J 3 sets 12–15
M 3 sets 25
N 3 sets 30
O 3 sets 15
P 3 sets 30–60 seconds
R 3 sets 15
T 3 sets 20

Day Two:
Cardio 30–45 minutes

Day Three:
A 3 sets 8–10
G 3 sets 12–15
H 3 sets 12–15
J 3 sets 12–15
M 3 sets 25
N 3 sets 30
O 3 sets 15
P 3 sets 30–60 seconds
R 3 sets 15
T 3 sets 20

Day Four:
Cardio 30–45 minutes

Day Five:
A 3 sets 8–10
G 3 sets 12–15
H 3 sets 12–15
J 3 sets 12–15
M 3 sets 25
N 3 sets 30
O 3 sets 15
P 3 sets 30–60 seconds
R 3 sets 15
T 3 sets 20

Day Six:
Cardio 30–45 minutes

Day Seven:
Rest

CYCLING WORKOUTS

A Barbell Row
page 36
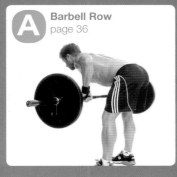

B Lat Pulldown
page 42
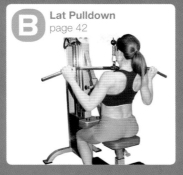

C Dips
page 68
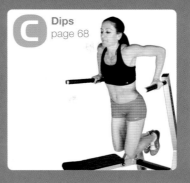

D Bicep Curl
page 96
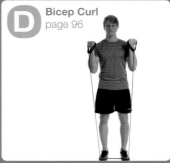

E Swiss Ball Wall Sit
page 134
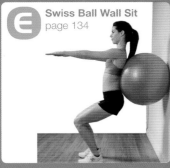

F Reverse Lunge
page 140
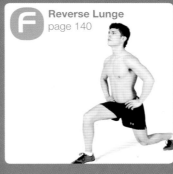

G Dumbbell Walking Lunge
page 144
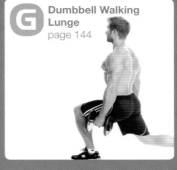

H One-Legged Step-Down
page 152
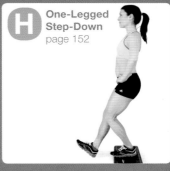

I Inverted Hamstring
page 166
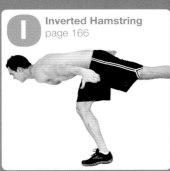

J Stiff-Legged Deadlift
page 174
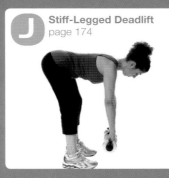

K Single-Leg Calf Press
page 176
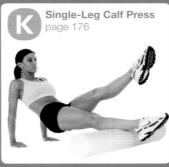

L Dumbbell Shin Raise
page 180
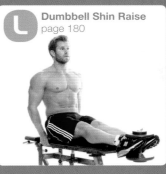

M Abdominal Kick
page 184
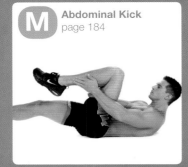

N Turkish Get-Up
page 188
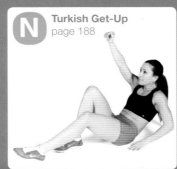

O Swiss Ball Pelvic Tilt
page 196
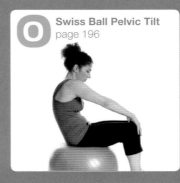

P Side Plank
page 122
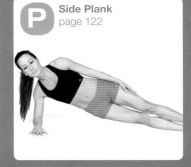

Q T-Stabilization
page 124
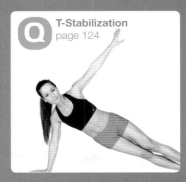

R Hip Abduction and Adduction
page 204
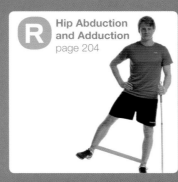

S Swiss Ball Jackknife
page 128
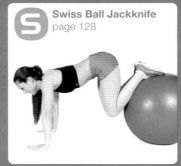

T Swiss Ball Hip Crossover
page 210
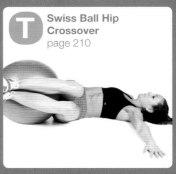

DIVING

Most of the major muscles in the human body are needed just to propel the diver from the springboard or diving platform, while strength, flexibility and acute awareness are needed to control the shape of the body through the air. Diving is a sport of precision and grace and the muscles used vary according to the type of dive being performed. "Dryland" training is carried out with a trampoline and a specialist "spotting rig," but a regular fitness routine biased toward core strength is a must.

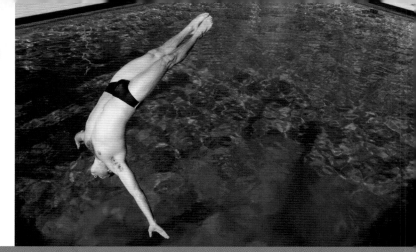

BEGINNER ROUTINE 1

Day One:
A 3 sets 8–10
C 3 sets 10–12
F 3 sets 15
I 3 sets 10–12
L 3 sets 10–12
R 30–120 seconds

Day Two:
Rest

Day Three:
A 3 sets 8–10
C 3 sets 10–12
F 3 sets 15
I 3 sets 10–12
L 3 sets 10–12
R 30–120 seconds

Day Four:
Rest

Day Five:
A 3 sets 8–10
C 3 sets 10–12
F 3 sets 15
I 3 sets 10–12
L 3 sets 10–12
R 30–120 seconds

Day Six:
Cardio 30–45 minutes

Day Seven:
Rest

INTERMEDIATE ROUTINE 1

Day One:
A 3 sets 8–10
C 3 sets 10–12
D 3 sets 12–15
E 3 sets 8–10
F 3 sets 15
I 3 sets 10–12
L 3 sets 10–12
R 30–120 seconds

Day Two:
Cardio 30–45 minutes

Day Three:
A 3 sets 8–10
C 3 sets 10–12
D 3 sets 12–15
E 3 sets 8–10
F 3 sets 15
I 3 sets 10–12
L 3 sets 10–12
R 30–120 seconds

Day Four:
Rest

Day Five:
A 3 sets 8–10
C 3 sets 10–12
D 3 sets 12–15
E 3 sets 8–10
F 3 sets 15
I 3 sets 10–12
L 3 sets 10–12
R 30–120 seconds

Day Six:
Cardio 30–45 minutes

Day Seven:
Rest

ADVANCED ROUTINE 1

Day One:
A 3 sets 8–10
C 3 sets 10–12
D 3 sets 12–15
E 3 sets 8–10
F 3 sets 15
I 3 sets 10–12
L 3 sets 10–12
M 3 sets 12–15
R 30–120 seconds
T 20

Day Two:
Cardio 30–45 minutes

Day Three:
A 3 sets 8–10
C 3 sets 10–12
D 3 sets 12–15
E 3 sets 8–10
F 3 sets 15
I 3 sets 10–12
L 3 sets 10–12
M 3 sets 12–15
R 30–120 seconds
T 20

Day Four:
Cardio 30–45 minutes

Day Five:
A 3 sets 8–10
C 3 sets 10–12
D 3 sets 12–15
E 3 sets 8–10
F 3 sets 15
I 3 sets 10–12
L 3 sets 10–12
M 3 sets 12–15
R 30–120 seconds
T 20

Day Six:
Cardio 30–45 minutes

Day Seven:
Rest

BEGINNER ROUTINE 2

Day One:
B 3 sets 12–15
G 3 sets 12–15
H 3 sets 8–10
J 3 sets 12–15
K 3 sets 10–12
N 3 sets 12–15

Day Two:
Rest

Day Three:
B 3 sets 12–15
G 3 sets 12–15
H 3 sets 8–10
J 3 sets 12–15
K 3 sets 10–12
N 3 sets 12–15

Day Four:
Rest

Day Five:
B 3 sets 12–15
G 3 sets 12–15
H 3 sets 8–10
J 3 sets 12–15
K 3 sets 10–12
N 3 sets 12–15

Day Six:
Cardio 30–45 minutes

Day Seven:
Rest

INTERMEDIATE ROUTINE 2

Day One:
B 3 sets 12–15
G 3 sets 12–15
H 3 sets 8–10
J 3 sets 12–15
K 3 sets 10–12
N 3 sets 12–15
O 3 sets 12–15
P 3 sets 12–15

Day Two:
Cardio 30–45 minutes

Day Three:
B 3 sets 8–10
F 3 sets 8–10
I 3 sets 8–10
L 3 sets 8–10
M 3 sets 12–15
N 3 sets 10–12
O 3 sets 15–20
P 3 sets 15–20

Day Four:
Rest

Day Five:
B 3 sets 8–10
F 3 sets 8–10
I 3 sets 8–10
L 3 sets 8–10
M 3 sets 12–15
N 3 sets 10–12
O 3 sets 15–20
P 3 sets 15–20

Day Six:
Cardio 30–45 minutes

Day Seven:
Rest

ADVANCED ROUTINE 2

Day One:
B 3 sets 12–15
G 3 sets 12–15
H 3 sets 8–10
J 3 sets 12–15
K 3 sets 10–12
N 3 sets 12–15
O 3 sets 12–15
P 3 sets 12–15
Q 3 sets 15
S 3 sets 30–60 seconds

Day Two:
Cardio 30–45 minutes

Day Three:
B 3 sets 12–15
G 3 sets 12–15
H 3 sets 8–10
J 3 sets 12–15
K 3 sets 10–12
N 3 sets 12–15
O 3 sets 12–15
P 3 sets 12–15
Q 3 sets 15

S 3 sets 30–60 seconds

Day Four:
Cardio 30–45 minutes

Day Five:
B 3 sets 12–15
G 3 sets 12–15
H 3 sets 8–10
J 3 sets 12–15
K 3 sets 10–12
N 3 sets 12–15
O 3 sets 12–15
P 3 sets 12–15
Q 3 sets 15
S 3 sets 30–60 seconds

Day Six:
Cardio 30–45 minutes

Day Seven:
Rest

DIVING WORKOUTS

A Lat Pulldown
page 42
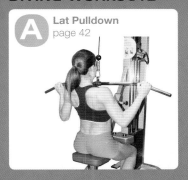

B Scapular Range of Motion
page 44
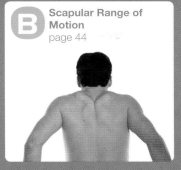

C Dumbbell Fly
page 64
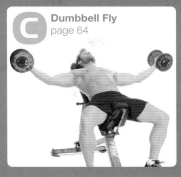

D Cable Fly
page 66
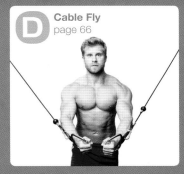

E Dumbbell Shoulder Press
page 74
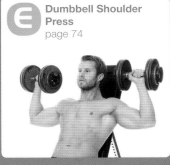

F Rotation Exercises
page 78
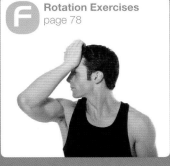

G External Rotation with Band
page 80
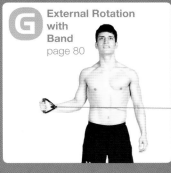

H Shoulder Raise and Pull
page 84
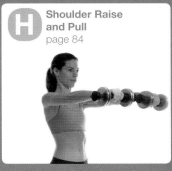

I Swiss Ball Wall Sit
page 134
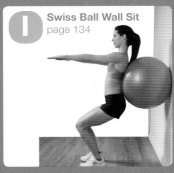

J Reverse Lunge
page 140
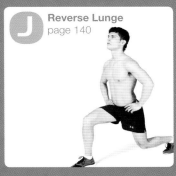

K Goblet Squat
page 150
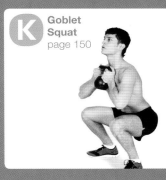

L Swiss Ball Hamstring Curl
page 164
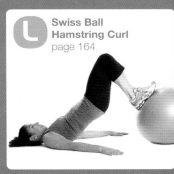

M Inverted Hamstring
page 166
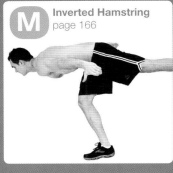

N Stiff-Legged Barbell Deadlift
page 168
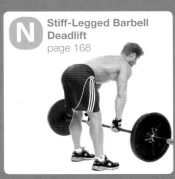

O Hamstring Pull-In
page 170
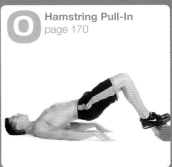

P Sumo Squat
page 172
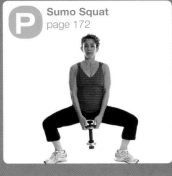

Q Cobra Stretch
page 194
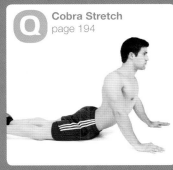

R Plank
page 120
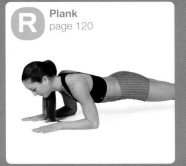

S Side Plank
page 122
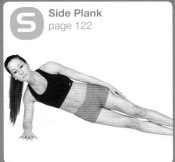

T Swiss Ball Jackknife
page 128
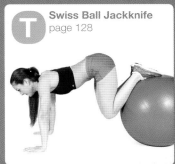

EQUESTRIANISM

Because so much effort is invested in keeping relatively still in equestrian sports, it is often difficult for the untrained observer to appreciate that the rider's entire body is involved in subtly shifting at all times to maintain control and balance. Your abdominals and spinal erectors help stabilization and your thighs in particular are called upon to maintain a correct "seat" and to cue the horse to change direction or pace. Training should be geared toward strength, balance and endurance.

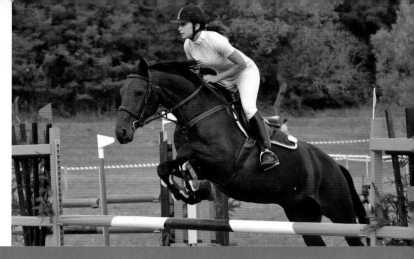

BEGINNER ROUTINE I

Day One:
A 3 sets 8–10
C 3 sets 12–15
D 3 sets 10–12
F 3 sets 10–12
K 3 sets 12–15
O 30–120 seconds

Day Two:
Rest

Day Three:
A 3 sets 8–10
C 3 sets 12–15
D 3 sets 10–12
F 3 sets 10–12
K 3 sets 12–15
O 30–120 seconds

Day Four:
Rest

Day Five:
A 3 sets 8–10
C 3 sets 12–15
D 3 sets 10–12
F 3 sets 10–12
K 3 sets 12–15
O 30–120 seconds

Day Six:
Cardio 30–45 minutes

Day Seven:
Rest

INTERMEDIATE ROUTINE I

Day One:
A 3 sets 8–10
C 3 sets 12–15
D 3 sets 10–12
F 3 sets 10–12
H 3 sets 15–20
I 3 sets 15–20
K 3 sets 12–15
O 30–120 seconds

Day Two:
Cardio 30–45 minutes

Day Three:
A 3 sets 8–10
C 3 sets 12–15
D 3 sets 10–12
F 3 sets 10–12
H 3 sets 15–20
I 3 sets 15–20
K 3 sets 12–15
O 30–120 seconds

Day Four:
Rest

Day Five:
A 3 sets 8–10
C 3 sets 12–15
D 3 sets 10–12
F 3 sets 10–12
H 3 sets 15–20
I 3 sets 15–20
K 3 sets 12–15
O 30–120 seconds

Day Six:
Cardio 30–45 minutes

Day Seven:
Rest

ADVANCED ROUTINE I

Day One:
A 3 sets 8–10
C 3 sets 12–15
D 3 sets 10–12
F 3 sets 10–12
H 3 sets 15–20
I 3 sets 15–20
K 3 sets 12–15
O 30–120 seconds
Q 30–60 seconds per side
R 15

Day Two:
Cardio 30–45 minutes

Day Three:
A 3 sets 8–10
C 3 sets 12–15
D 3 sets 10–12
F 3 sets 10–12
H 3 sets 15–20
I 3 sets 15–20
K 3 sets 12–15
O 30–120 seconds
Q 30–60 seconds per side
R 15

Day Four:
Cardio 30–45 minutes

Day Five:
A 3 sets 8–10
C 3 sets 12–15
D 3 sets 10–12
F 3 sets 10–12
H 3 sets 15–20
I 3 sets 15–20
K 3 sets 12–15
O 30–120 seconds
Q 30–60 seconds per side
R 15

Day Six:
Cardio 30–45 minutes

Day Seven:
Rest

BEGINNER ROUTINE 2

Day One:
B 3 sets 8–10
E 3 sets 12–15
G 3 sets 12–15
J 3 sets 12–15
L 3 sets 12–15
M 3 sets 15

Day Two:
Rest

Day Three:
B 3 sets 8–10
E 3 sets 12–15
G 3 sets 12–15
J 3 sets 12–15
L 3 sets 12–15
M 3 sets 15

Day Four:
Rest

Day Five:
B 3 sets 8–10
E 3 sets 12–15
G 3 sets 12–15
J 3 sets 12–15
L 3 sets 12–15
M 3 sets 15

Day Six:
Cardio 30–45 minutes

Day Seven:
Rest

INTERMEDIATE ROUTINE 2

Day One:
B 3 sets 8–10
E 3 sets 12–15
G 3 sets 12–15
J 3 sets 12–15
L 3 sets 12–15
M 3 sets 15
N 3 sets 15
P 3 sets 30–60 seconds

Day Two:
Cardio 30–45 minutes

Day Three:
B 3 sets 8–10
E 3 sets 12–15
G 3 sets 12–15
J 3 sets 12–15
L 3 sets 12–15
M 3 sets 15
N 3 sets 15
P 3 sets 30–60 seconds

Day Four:
Rest

Day Five:
B 3 sets 8–10
E 3 sets 12–15
G 3 sets 12–15
J 3 sets 12–15
L 3 sets 12–15
M 3 sets 15
N 3 sets 15
P 3 sets 30–60 seconds

Day Six:
Cardio 30–45 minutes

Day Seven:
Rest

ADVANCED ROUTINE 2

Day One:
B 3 sets 8–10
E 3 sets 12–15
G 3 sets 12–15
J 3 sets 12–15
L 3 sets 12–15
M 3 sets 15
N 3 sets 15
P 3 sets 30–60 seconds
S 3 sets 20
T 3 sets 20

Day Two:
Cardio 30–45 minutes

Day Three:
B 3 sets 8–10
E 3 sets 12–15
G 3 sets 12–15
J 3 sets 12–15
L 3 sets 12–15
M 3 sets 15
N 3 sets 15
P 3 sets 30–60 seconds
S 3 sets 20
T 3 sets 20

Day Four:
Cardio 30–45 minutes

Day Five:
B 3 sets 8–10
E 3 sets 12–15
G 3 sets 12–15
J 3 sets 12–15
L 3 sets 12–15
M 3 sets 15
N 3 sets 15
P 3 sets 30–60 seconds
S 3 sets 20
T 3 sets 20

Day Six:
Cardio 30–45 minutes

Day Seven:
Rest

EQUESTRIANISM WORKOUTS

A Rope Pulldown
page 52

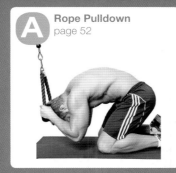

B Roller Push-Up
page 62

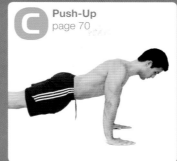

C Push-Up
page 70

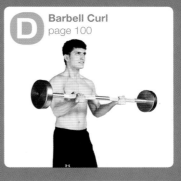

D Barbell Curl
page 100

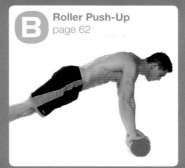

E Wrist Flexion
page 116

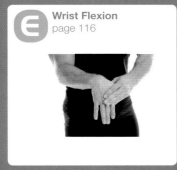

F Swiss Ball Wall Sit
page 134

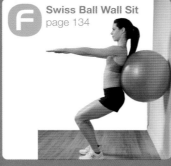

G Knee Extension with Rotation
page 154

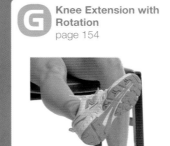

H Adductor Extension
page 162

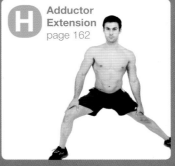

I Hamstring Abductor
page 163

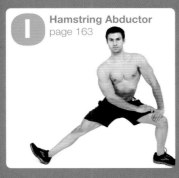

J Inverted Hamstring
page 166

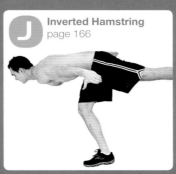

K Single-Leg Calf Press
page 176

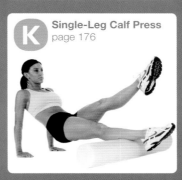

L Dumbbell Shin Raise
page 180

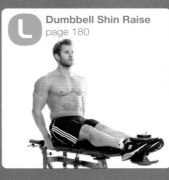

M Cobra Stretch
page 194

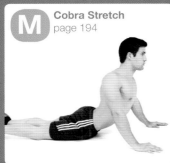

N Plank Press-Up
page 198

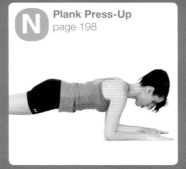

O Plank
page 120

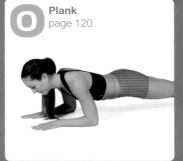

P Side Plank
page 122

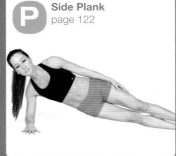

Q T-Stabilization
page 124

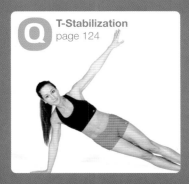

R Hip Abduction and Adduction
page 204

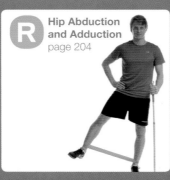

S Swiss Ball Hip Crossover
page 210

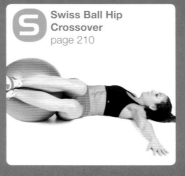

T V-Up
page 212

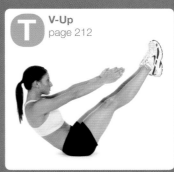

FENCING

Balance, posture and stability are the mainstays of fencing and originate from a toned and developed core as well as a strong lower back for flexibility during combat, where lightning-fast changes of direction are needed. The quads are largely responsible for the dramatic lunges and your shoulders must be powerful to either dart forward to attack or to pull backward to avoid being hit. All-round explosive power can be developed by following the program set out below.

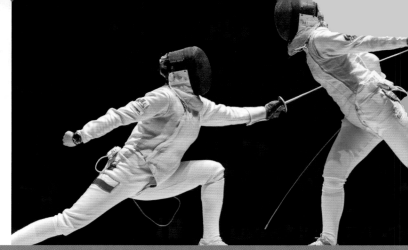

WORKOUT LEVEL 1

BEGINNER ROUTINE I

Day One:
C 3 sets 8–10
D 3 sets of 15
I 3 sets of 12–15
K 3 sets of 12–15
O 3 sets of 15
S 20 per side

Day Two:
Rest

Day Three:
C 3 sets 8–10
D 3 sets of 15
I 3 sets of 12–15
K 3 sets of 12–15
O 3 sets of 15
S 20 per side

Day Four:
Rest

Day Five:
C 3 sets 8–10
D 3 sets of 15
I 3 sets of 12–15
K 3 sets of 12–15
O 3 sets of 15
S 20 per side

Day Six:
Cardio 30–45 minutes

Day Seven:
Rest

INTERMEDIATE ROUTINE I

Day One:
A 3 sets 12–15
C 3 sets 8–10
D 3 sets of 15
E 3 sets 12–15
I 3 sets of 12–15
K 3 sets of 12–15
O 3 sets of 15
S 20 per side

Day Two:
Cardio 30–45 minutes

Day Three:
A 3 sets 12–15
C 3 sets 8–10
D 3 sets of 15
E 3 sets 12–15
I 3 sets of 12–15
K 3 sets of 12–15
O 3 sets of 15
S 20 per side

Day Four:
Rest

Day Five:
A 3 sets 12–15
C 3 sets 8–10
D 3 sets of 15
E 3 sets 12–15
I 3 sets of 12–15
K 3 sets of 12–15
O 3 sets of 15
S 20 per side

Day Six:
Cardio 30–45 minutes

Day Seven:
Rest

ADVANCED ROUTINE I

Day One:
A 3 sets 12–15
B 3 sets 12–15
C 3 sets 8–10
D 3 sets of 15
E 3 sets 12–15
I 3 sets of 12–15
K 3 sets of 12–15
L 3 sets 12–15
O 3 sets of 15
S 20 per side

Day Two:
Cardio 30–45 minutes

Day Three:
A 3 sets 12–15
B 3 sets 12–15
C 3 sets 8–10
D 3 sets of 15
E 3 sets 12–15
I 3 sets of 12–15
K 3 sets of 12–15
L 3 sets 12–15

O 3 sets of 15
S 20 per side

Day Four:
Cardio 30–45 minutes

Day Five:
A 3 sets 12–15
B 3 sets 12–15
C 3 sets 8–10
D 3 sets of 15
E 3 sets 12–15
I 3 sets of 12–15
K 3 sets of 12–15
L 3 sets 12–15
O 3 sets of 15
S 20 per side

Day Six:
Cardio 30–45 minutes

Day Seven:
Rest

WORKOUT LEVEL 2

BEGINNER ROUTINE 2

Day One:
F 3 sets 8–10
G 3 sets 10–12
H 3 sets 10–12
J 3 sets 12–15
M 3 sets 12–15
N 3 sets 12–15

Day Two:
Rest

Day Three:
F 3 sets 8–10
G 3 sets 10–12
H 3 sets 10–12
J 3 sets 12–15
M 3 sets 12–15
N 3 sets 12–15

Day Four:
Rest

Day Five:
F 3 sets 8–10
G 3 sets 10–12
H 3 sets 10–12
J 3 sets 12–15
M 3 sets 12–15
N 3 sets 12–15

Day Six:
Cardio 30–45 minutes

Day Seven:
Rest

INTERMEDIATE ROUTINE 2

Day One:
F 3 sets 8–10
G 3 sets 10–12
H 3 sets 10–12
J 3 sets 12–15
M 3 sets 12–15
N 3 sets 12–15
P 3 sets 30–60 seconds
Q 3 sets 30–60 seconds

Day Two:
Cardio 30–45 minutes

Day Three:
F 3 sets 8–10
G 3 sets 10–12
H 3 sets 10–12
J 3 sets 12–15
M 3 sets 12–15
N 3 sets 12–15
P 3 sets 30–60 seconds
Q 3 sets 30–60 seconds

Day Four:
Rest

Day Five:
F 3 sets 8–10
G 3 sets 10–12
H 3 sets 10–12
J 3 sets 12–15
M 3 sets 12–15
N 3 sets 12–15
P 3 sets 30–60 seconds
Q 3 sets 30–60 seconds

Day Six:
Cardio 30–45 minutes

Day Seven:
Rest

ADVANCED ROUTINE 2

Day One:
F 3 sets 8–10
G 3 sets 10–12
H 3 sets 10–12
J 3 sets 12–15
M 3 sets 12–15
N 3 sets 12–15
P 3 sets 30–60 seconds
Q 3 sets 30–60 seconds
R 3 sets 20
T 3 sets 25

Day Two:
Cardio 30–45 minutes

Day Three:
F 3 sets 8–10
G 3 sets 10–12
H 3 sets 10–12
J 3 sets 12–15
M 3 sets 12–15
N 3 sets 12–15
P 3 sets 30–60 seconds

Q 3 sets 30–60 seconds
R 3 sets 20
T 3 sets 25

Day Four:
Cardio 30–45 minutes

Day Five:
F 3 sets 8–10
G 3 sets 10–12
H 3 sets 10–12
J 3 sets 12–15
M 3 sets 12–15
N 3 sets 12–15
P 3 sets 30–60 seconds
Q 3 sets 30–60 seconds
R 3 sets 20
T 3 sets 25

Day Six:
Cardio 30–45 minutes

Day Seven:
Rest

FENCING WORKOUTS

A Scapular Range of Motion
page 44
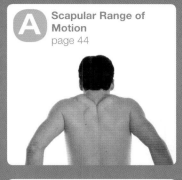

B Flat Bench Hyperextension
page 56
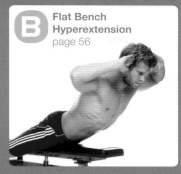

C Dumbbell Shoulder Press
page 74
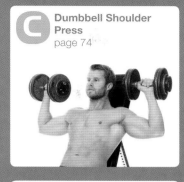

D Rotation Exercises
page 78
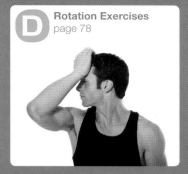

E External Rotation with Band
page 80
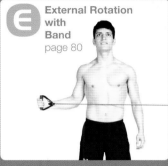

F Shoulder Raise and Pull
page 84
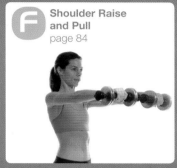

G Reverse Fly
page 88
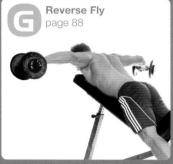

H Barbell Squat
page 136
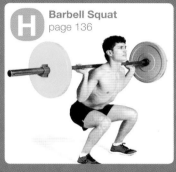

I Reverse Lunge
page 140
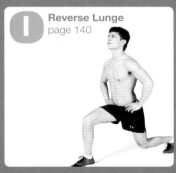

J Lateral Low Lunge
page 142
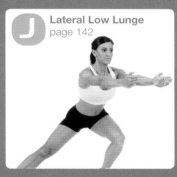

K Dumbbell Walking Lunge
page 144
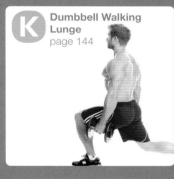

L High Lunge
page 146
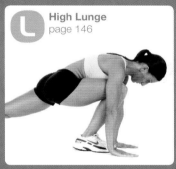

M Crossover Step
page 148
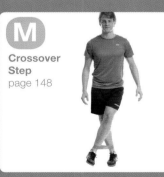

N One-Legged Step-Down
page 152
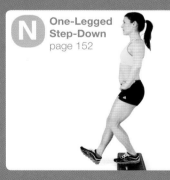

O Cobra Stretch
page 194
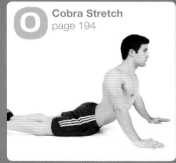

P Plank
page 120
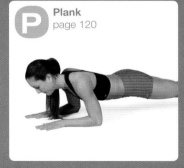

Q T-Stabilization
page 124
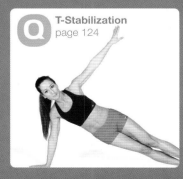

R Swiss Ball Jackknife
page 128
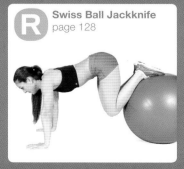

S Thigh Rock-Back
page 208
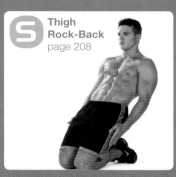

T Medicine Ball Slam
page 214
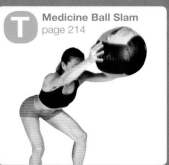

FIELD HOCKEY

Field hockey is very cardiovascular in nature, and involves the legs for running; the arms for dribbling, hitting and flicking; the chest and back for power and the abdomen for stabilizing and turning. A few more "explosive" exercises — using medicine balls — have been added to the program to increase your power while giving you a good cardio workout. You can make most of the other exercises similarly explosive simply by performing them as quickly as possible.

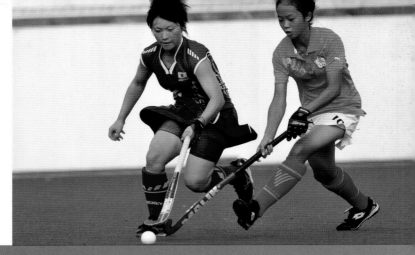

BEGINNER ROUTINE 1

Day One:
A 3 sets 8–10
C 3 sets 8–10
E 3 sets 15
H 3 sets 10–12
I 3 sets 10–12
N 20 per side

Day Two:
Rest

Day Three:
A 3 sets 8–10
C 3 sets 8–10
E 3 sets 15
H 3 sets 10–12
I 3 sets 10–12
N 20 per side

Day Four:
Rest

Day Five:
A 3 sets 8–10
C 3 sets 8–10
E 3 sets 15
H 3 sets 10–12
I 3 sets 10–12
N 20 per side

Day Six:
Cardio 30–45 minutes

Day Seven:
Rest

INTERMEDIATE ROUTINE 1

Day One:
A 3 sets 8–10
C 3 sets 8–10
D 3 sets 8–10
E 3 sets 15
H 3 sets 10–12
I 3 sets 10–12
K 3 sets 12–15
N 20 per side

Day Two:
Cardio 30–45 minutes

Day Three:
A 3 sets 8–10
C 3 sets 8–10
D 3 sets 8–10
E 3 sets 15
H 3 sets 10–12
I 3 sets 10–12
K 3 sets 12–15
N 20 per side

Day Four:
Rest

Day Five:
A 3 sets 8–10
C 3 sets 8–10
D 3 sets 8–10
E 3 sets 15
H 3 sets 10–12
I 3 sets 10–12
K 3 sets 12–15
N 20 per side

Day Six:
Cardio 30–45 minutes

Day Seven:
Rest

ADVANCED ROUTINE 1

Day One:
A 3 sets 8–10
C 3 sets 8–10
D 3 sets 8–10
E 3 sets 15
F 3 sets 10–12
H 3 sets 10–12
I 3 sets 10–12
K 3 sets 12–15
L 3 sets 10–12
N 20 per side

Day Two:
Cardio 30–45 minutes

Day Three:
A 3 sets 8–10
C 3 sets 8–10
D 3 sets 8–10
E 3 sets 15
F 3 sets 10–12
H 3 sets 10–12
I 3 sets 10–12
K 3 sets 12–15
L 3 sets 10–12
N 20 per side

Day Four:
Cardio 30–45 minutes

Day Five:
A 3 sets 8–10
C 3 sets 8–10
D 3 sets 8–10
E 3 sets 15
F 3 sets 10–12
H 3 sets 10–12
I 3 sets 10–12
K 3 sets 12–15
L 3 sets 10–12
N 20 per side

Day Six:
Cardio 30–45 minutes

Day Seven:
Rest

BEGINNER ROUTINE 2

Day One:
B 3 sets 8–10
G 3 sets 10–12
J 3 sets 12–15
M 3 sets 20
O 3 sets 30–60 seconds
P 3 sets 20

Day Two:
Rest

Day Three:
B 3 sets 8–10
G 3 sets 10–12
J 3 sets 12–15
M 3 sets 20
O 3 sets 30–60 seconds
P 3 sets 20

Day Four:
Rest

Day Five:
B 3 sets 8–10
G 3 sets 10–12
J 3 sets 12–15
M 3 sets 20
O 3 sets 30–60 seconds
P 3 sets 20

Day Six:
Cardio 30–45 minutes

Day Seven:
Rest

INTERMEDIATE ROUTINE 2

Day One:
B 3 sets 8–10
G 3 sets 10–12
J 3 sets 12–15
M 3 sets 20
O 3 sets 30–60 seconds
P 3 sets 20
Q 3 sets 20
R 3 sets 20

Day Two:
Cardio 30–45 minutes

Day Three:
B 3 sets 8–10
G 3 sets 10–12
J 3 sets 12–15
M 3 sets 20
O 3 sets 30–60 seconds
P 3 sets 20
Q 3 sets 20
R 3 sets 20

Day Four:
Rest

Day Five:
B 3 sets 8–10
G 3 sets 10–12
J 3 sets 12–15
M 3 sets 20
O 3 sets 30–60 seconds
P 3 sets 20
Q 3 sets 20
R 3 sets 20

Day Six:
Cardio 30–45 minutes

Day Seven:
Rest

ADVANCED ROUTINE 2

Day One:
B 3 sets 8–10
G 3 sets 10–12
J 3 sets 12–15
M 3 sets 20
O 3 sets 30–60 seconds
P 3 sets 20
Q 3 sets 20
R 3 sets 20
S 3 sets 20
T 3 sets 25

Day Two:
Cardio 30–45 minutes

Day Three:
B 3 sets 8–10
G 3 sets 10–12
J 3 sets 12–15
M 3 sets 20
O 3 sets 30–60 seconds
P 3 sets 20
Q 3 sets 20
R 3 sets 20
S 3 sets 20
T 3 sets 25

Day Four:
Cardio 30–45 minutes

Day Five:
B 3 sets 8–10
G 3 sets 10–12
J 3 sets 12–15
M 3 sets 20
O 3 sets 30–60 seconds
P 3 sets 20
Q 3 sets 20
R 3 sets 20
S 3 sets 20
T 3 sets 25

Day Six:
Cardio 30–45 minutes

Day Seven:
Rest

FIELD HOCKEY WORKOUTS

A Dumbbell Row
page 38
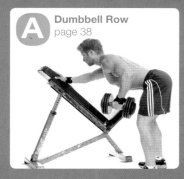

B Incline Bench Row
page 50
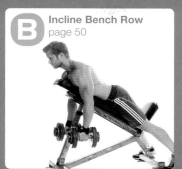

C Barbell Bench Press
page 60
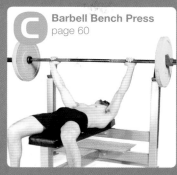

D Dips
page 68
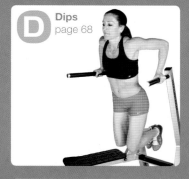

E Rotation Exercises
page 78
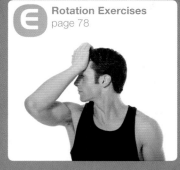

F Front-Plate Raise
page 92
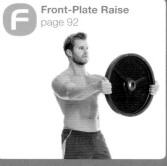

G Barbell Shoulder Shrug
page 94
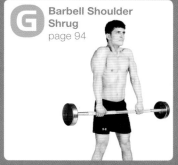

H Alternating Hammer Curl
page 98
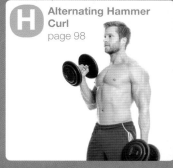

I Swiss Ball Wall Sit
page 134
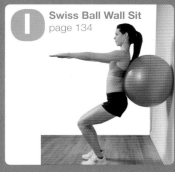

J Lateral Low Lunge
page 142
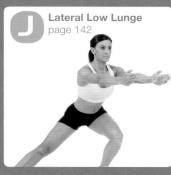

K Dumbbell Walking Lunge
page 144
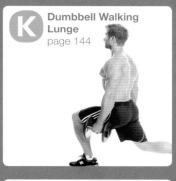

L Swiss Ball Hamstring Curl
page 164
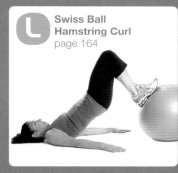

M Seated Russian Twist
page 200
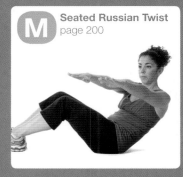

N Medicine Ball Wood Chop
page 130
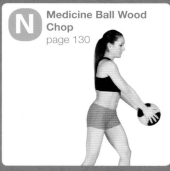

O T-Stabilization
page 124
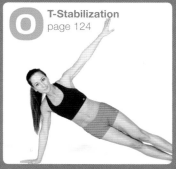

P Swiss Ball Jackknife
page 128
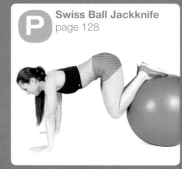

Q Swiss Ball Roll-Out
page 206
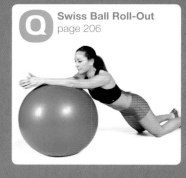

R Thigh Rock-Back
page 208
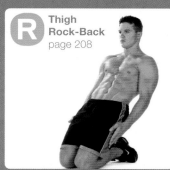

S V-Up
page 212
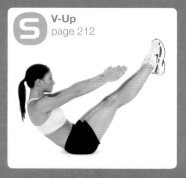

T Medicine Ball Slam
page 214
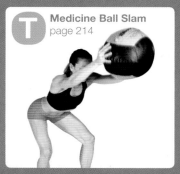

FIGURE SKATING

Heavily reliant on the leg and hip musculature for performance, the figure skater is a study in balance, grace, athleticism, patience and skill, and training is geared toward strength, balance and endurance. The powerful glute muscles are used when skating backward, the quads when skating forward or laterally, with secondary assistance from the abductors, hamstrings and calves. The male partner needs great upper-body strength to perform the ever-popular lifts.

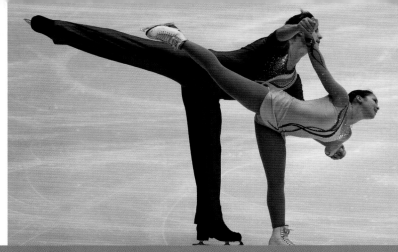

WORKOUT LEVEL 1

BEGINNER ROUTINE I

Day One:
A 3 sets 10–12
B 3 sets 12–15
H 3 sets 15–20
J 3 sets 12–15
K 3 sets 12–15
O 15

Day Two:
Rest

Day Three:
A 3 sets 10–12
B 3 sets 12–15
H 3 sets 15–20
J 3 sets 12–15
K 3 sets 12–15
O 15

Day Four:
Rest

Day Five:
A 3 sets 10–12
B 3 sets 12–15
H 3 sets 15–20
J 3 sets 12–15
K 3 sets 12–15
O 15

Day Six:
Cardio 30–45 minutes

Day Seven:
Rest

INTERMEDIATE ROUTINE I

Day One:
A 3 sets 10–12
B 3 sets 12–15
D 3 sets 12–15
G 3 sets 15–20
H 3 sets 15–20
J 3 sets 12–15
K 3 sets 12–15
O 15

Day Two:
Cardio 30–45 minutes

Day Three:
A 3 sets 10–12
B 3 sets 12–15
D 3 sets 12–15
G 3 sets 15–20
H 3 sets 15–20
J 3 sets 12–15
K 3 sets 12–15
O 15

Day Four:
Rest

Day Five:
A 3 sets 10–12
B 3 sets 12–15
D 3 sets 12–15
G 3 sets 15–20
H 3 sets 15–20
J 3 sets 12–15
K 3 sets 12–15
O 15

Day Six:
Cardio 30–45 minutes

Day Seven:
Rest

ADVANCED ROUTINE I

Day One:
A 3 sets 10–12
B 3 sets 12–15
D 3 sets 12–15
G 3 sets 15–20
H 3 sets 15–20
J 3 sets 12–15
K 3 sets 12–15
O 15
R 30–60 seconds per side
S 15

Day Two:
Cardio 30–45 minutes

Day Three:
A 3 sets 10–12
B 3 sets 12–15
D 3 sets 12–15
G 3 sets 15–20
H 3 sets 15–20
J 3 sets 12–15
K 3 sets 12–15
O 15
R 30

Day Four:
Cardio 30–45 minutes

Day Five:
A 3 sets 10–12
B 3 sets 12–15
D 3 sets 12–15
G 3 sets 15–20
H 3 sets 15–20
J 3 sets 12–15
K 3 sets 12–15
O 15
R 30–60 seconds per side
S 15

Day Six:
Cardio 30–45 minutes

Day Seven:
Rest

WORKOUT LEVEL 2

BEGINNER ROUTINE 2

Day One:
C 3 sets 12–15
E 3 sets 12–15
F 3 sets 12–15
I 3 sets 10–12
L 3 sets 12–15
M 3 sets 20

Day Two:
Rest

Day Three:
C 3 sets 12–15
E 3 sets 12–15
F 3 sets 12–15
I 3 sets 10–12
L 3 sets 12–15
M 3 sets 20

Day Four:
Rest

Day Five:
C 3 sets 12–15
E 3 sets 12–15
F 3 sets 12–15
I 3 sets 10–12
L 3 sets 12–15
M 3 sets 20

Day Six:
Cardio 30–45 minutes

Day Seven:
Rest

INTERMEDIATE ROUTINE 2

Day One:
C 3 sets 12–15
E 3 sets 12–15
F 3 sets 12–15
I 3 sets 10–12
L 3 sets 12–15
M 3 sets 20
N 3 sets 15
P 3 sets 30–120 seconds

Day Two:
Cardio 30–45 minutes

Day Three:
C 3 sets 12–15
E 3 sets 12–15
F 3 sets 12–15
I 3 sets 10–12
L 3 sets 12–15
M 3 sets 20
N 3 sets 15
P 3 sets 30–120 seconds

Day Four:
Rest

Day Five:
C 3 sets 12–15
E 3 sets 12–15
F 3 sets 12–15
I 3 sets 10–12
L 3 sets 12–15
M 3 sets 20
N 3 sets 15
P 3 sets 30–120 seconds

Day Six:
Cardio 30–45 minutes

Day Seven:
Rest

ADVANCED ROUTINE 2

Day One:
C 3 sets 12–15
E 3 sets 12–15
F 3 sets 12–15
I 3 sets 10–12
L 3 sets 12–15
M 3 sets 20
N 3 sets 15
P 3 sets 30–120 seconds
Q 3 sets 20
T 3 sets 20

Day Two:
Cardio 30–45 minutes

Day Three:
C 3 sets 12–15
E 3 sets 12–15
F 3 sets 12–15
I 3 sets 10–12
L 3 sets 12–15
M 3 sets 20
N 3 sets 15
P 3 sets 30–120 seconds
Q 3 sets 20
T 3 sets 20

Day Four:
Cardio 30–45 minutes

Day Five:
C 3 sets 12–15
E 3 sets 12–15
F 3 sets 12–15
I 3 sets 10–12
L 3 sets 12–15
M 3 sets 20
N 3 sets 15
P 3 sets 30–120 seconds
Q 3 sets 20
T 3 sets 20

Day Six:
Cardio 30–45 minutes

Day Seven:
Rest

FIGURE SKATING WORKOUTS

A Swiss Ball Wall Sit
page 134
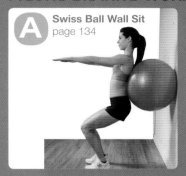

B Reverse Lunge
page 140
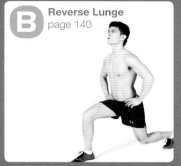

C Lateral Low Lunge
page 142
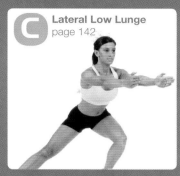

D Dumbbell Walking Lunge
page 144
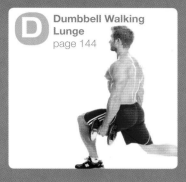

E High Lunge
page 146
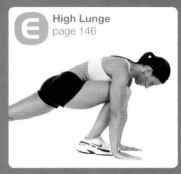

F Crossover Step
page 148
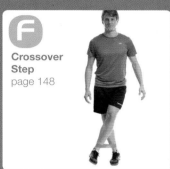

G Adductor Extension
page 162
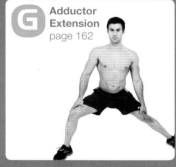

H Hamstring Abductor
page 163
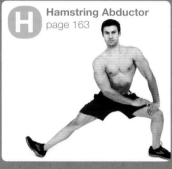

I Swiss Ball Hamstring Curl
page 164
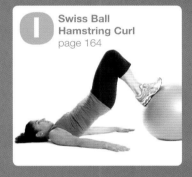

J Stiff-Legged Barbell Deadlift
page 168
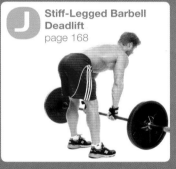

K Dumbbell Calf Raise
page 178
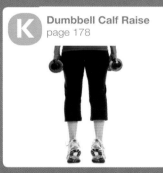

L Dumbbell Shin Raise
page 180
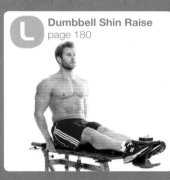

M Bicycle Crunch
page 190
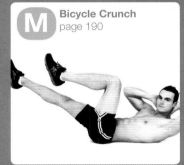

N Swiss Ball Pelvic Tilt
page 196
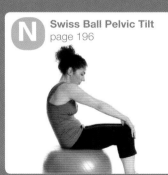

O Star Jump
page 156
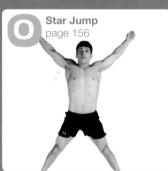

P Mountain Climber
page 158
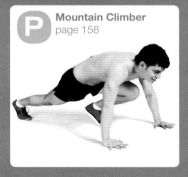

Q Burpee
page 160
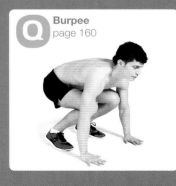

R T-Stabilization
page 124
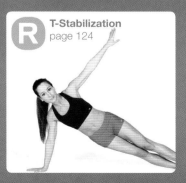

S Hip Abduction and Adduction
page 204
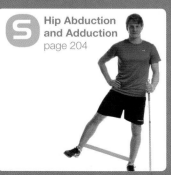

T Swiss Ball Roll-Out
page 206
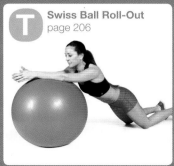

FLY FISHING

This sport makes much use of the "casting" muscles in the back, shoulders, arms and forearms, and requires a strong core for stability. The repetitive nature of the casting action means that good technique is doubly important. A common mistake is to throw the arm too far forward, which tires the wrist and forearm. It's vital to keep fit during the closed season. Practice "lawn casting" once a week and make time for this great routine to get the most out of the open season.

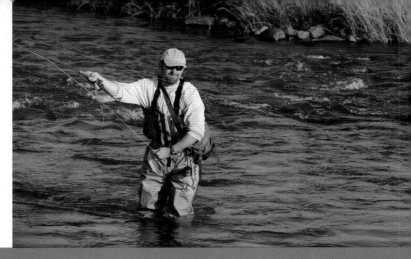

BEGINNER ROUTINE I

Day One:
C 3 sets of 10–12
G 3 sets of 12–15
K 3 sets of 10–12
L 3 sets of 12–15
Q 20 per side
T 3 sets of 20

Day Two:
Rest

Day Three:
C 3 sets of 10–12
G 3 sets of 12–15
K 3 sets of 10–12
L 3 sets of 12–15
Q 20 per side
T 3 sets of 20

Day Four:
Rest

Day Five:
C 3 sets of 10–12
G 3 sets of 12–15
K 3 sets of 10–12
L 3 sets of 12–15
Q 20 per side
T 3 sets of 20

Day Six:
Cardio 30–45 minutes

Day Seven:
Rest

INTERMEDIATE ROUTINE I

Day One:
A 3 sets of 12–15
C 3 sets of 10–12
E 3 sets of 8–10
G 3 sets of 12–15
K 3 sets of 10–12
L 3 sets of 12–15
Q 20 per side
T 3 sets of 20

Day Two:
Cardio 30–45 minutes

Day Three:
A 3 sets of 12–15
C 3 sets of 10–12
E 3 sets of 8–10
G 3 sets of 12–15
K 3 sets of 10–12
L 3 sets of 12–15
Q 20 per side
T 3 sets of 20

Day Four:
Rest

Day Five:
A 3 sets of 12–15
C 3 sets of 10–12
E 3 sets of 8–10
G 3 sets of 12–15
K 3 sets of 10–12
L 3 sets of 12–15
Q 20 per side
T 3 sets of 20

Day Six:
Cardio 30–45 minutes

Day Seven:
Rest

ADVANCED ROUTINE I

Day One:
A 3 sets of 12–15
C 3 sets of 10–12
E 3 sets of 8–10
G 3 sets of 12–15
K 3 sets of 10–12
L 3 sets of 12–15
N 15
R 3 sets 8–10
Q 20 per side
T 3 sets of 20

Day Two:
Cardio 30–45 minutes

Day Three:
A 3 sets of 12–15
C 3 sets of 10–12
E 3 sets of 8–10
G 3 sets of 12–15
K 3 sets of 10–12
L 3 sets of 12–15
N 15
R 3 sets 8–10
Q 20 per side
T 3 sets of 20

Day Four:
Cardio 30–45 minutes

Day Five:
A 3 sets of 12–15
C 3 sets of 10–12
E 3 sets of 8–10
G 3 sets of 12–15
K 3 sets of 10–12
L 3 sets of 12–15
N 15
R 3 sets 8–10
Q 20 per side
T 3 sets of 20

Day Six:
Cardio 30–45 minutes

Day Seven:
Rest

BEGINNER ROUTINE 2

Day One:
B 3 sets 12–15
D 3 sets 8–10
F 3 sets 15
H 3 sets 8–10
I 3 sets 8–10
J 3 sets 10–12

Day Two:
Rest

Day Three:
B 3 sets 12–15
D 3 sets 8–10
F 3 sets 15
H 3 sets 8–10
I 3 sets 8–10
J 3 sets 10–12

Day Four:
Rest

Day Five:
B 3 sets 12–15
D 3 sets 8–10
F 3 sets 15
H 3 sets 8–10
I 3 sets 8–10
J 3 sets 10–12

Day Six:
Cardio 30–45 minutes

Day Seven:
Rest

INTERMEDIATE ROUTINE 2

Day One:
B 3 sets 12–15
D 3 sets 8–10
F 3 sets 15
H 3 sets 8–10
I 3 sets 8–10
J 3 sets 10–12
M 3 sets 12–15
O 3 sets 30–60 seconds

Day Two:
Cardio 30–45 minutes

Day Three:
B 3 sets 12–15
D 3 sets 8–10
F 3 sets 15
H 3 sets 8–10
I 3 sets 8–10
J 3 sets 10–12
M 3 sets 12–15
O 3 sets 30–60 seconds

Day Four:
Rest

Day Five:
B 3 sets 12–15
D 3 sets 8–10
F 3 sets 15
H 3 sets 8–10
I 3 sets 8–10
J 3 sets 10–12
M 3 sets 12–15
O 3 sets 30–60 seconds

Day Six:
Cardio 30–45 minutes

Day Seven:
Rest

ADVANCED ROUTINE 2

Day One:
B 3 sets 12–15
D 3 sets 8–10
F 3 sets 15
H 3 sets 8–10
I 3 sets 8–10
J 3 sets 10–12
M 3 sets 12–15
O 3 sets 30–60 seconds
P 3 sets 30
S 3 sets 20

Day Two:
Cardio 30–45 minutes

Day Three:
B 3 sets 12–15
D 3 sets 8–10
F 3 sets 15
H 3 sets 8–10
I 3 sets 8–10
J 3 sets 10–12
M 3 sets 12–15
O 3 sets 30–60 seconds
P 3 sets 30
S 3 sets 20

Day Four:
Cardio 30–45 minutes

Day Five:
B 3 sets 12–15
D 3 sets 8–10
F 3 sets 15
H 3 sets 8–10
I 3 sets 8–10
J 3 sets 10–12
M 3 sets 12–15
O 3 sets 30–60 seconds
P 3 sets 30
S 3 sets 20

Day Six:
Cardio 30–45 minutes

Day Seven:
Rest

FLY FISHING WORKOUTS

A Scapular Range of Motion
page 44
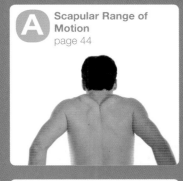

B Flat Bench Hyperextension
page 56
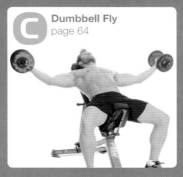

C Dumbbell Fly
page 64
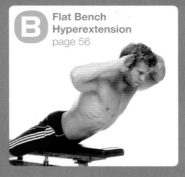

D Dumbbell Shoulder Press
page 74
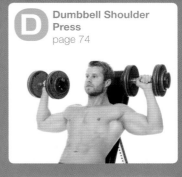

E Overhead Press
page 76
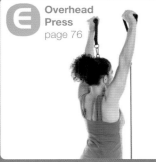

F Rotation Exercises
page 78
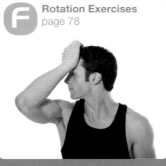

G External Rotation with Band
page 80
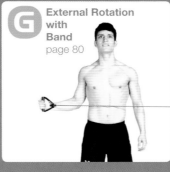

H Shoulder Raise and Pull
page 84
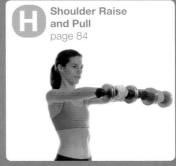

I Barbell Upright Row
page 86
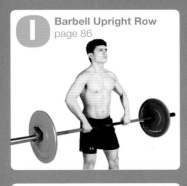

J Alternating Hammer Curl
page 98
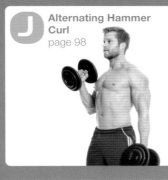

K Rope Hammer Curl
page 104
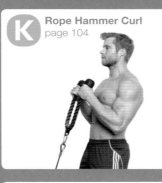

L Wrist Flexion
page 116
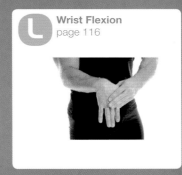

M Wrist Extension
page 117
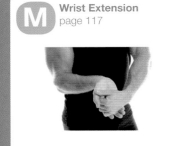

N Plank Press-Up
page 198
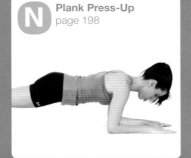

O Side Plank
page 122
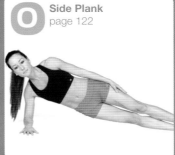

P Wood Chop with Resistance Band
page 202
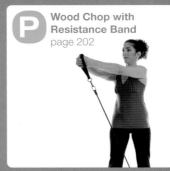

Q Medicine Ball Wood Chop
page 130
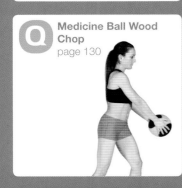

R Triceps Roll-Out
page 110
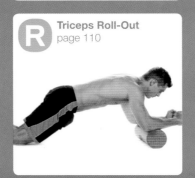

S Swiss Ball Jackknife
page 128
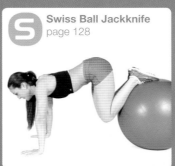

T Swiss Ball Roll-Out
page 206
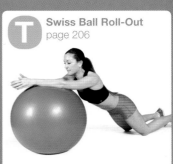

GAELIC FOOTBALL

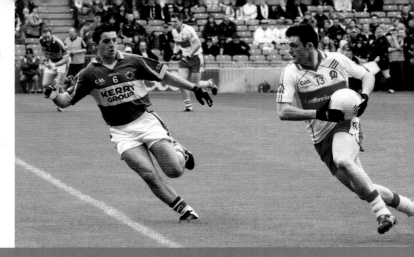

Gaelic football is in many ways a hybrid of soccer and American football and, as such, employs most of the major muscles of the body. The legs need to be strong for running and kicking, and the upper body must be powerful for passing and "shoulder-charging." The ball can be carried, as long as it is bounced every few steps, so the arms need to be strong — particularly the forearms and wrists. As for all such relentlessly active sports, rapid repetitions can help to increase your stamina.

WORKOUT LEVEL 1

BEGINNER ROUTINE 1

Day One:
A 3 sets 6–8
D 3 sets 8–10
G 3 sets 10–12
J 3 sets 10–12
M 3 sets 10–12
Q 15

Day Two:
Rest

Day Three:
A 3 sets 6–8
D 3 sets 8–10
G 3 sets 10–12
J 3 sets 10–12
M 3 sets 10–12
Q 15

Day Four:
Rest

Day Five:
A 3 sets 6–8
D 3 sets 8–10
G 3 sets 10–12
J 3 sets 10–12
M 3 sets 10–12
Q 15

Day Six:
Cardio 30–45 minutes

Day Seven:
Rest

INTERMEDIATE ROUTINE 1

Day One:
A 3 sets 6–8
B 3 sets of 8–10
D 3 sets 8–10
E 3 sets of 8–10
G 3 sets 10–12
J 3 sets 10–12
M 3 sets 10–12
Q 15

Day Two:
Cardio 30–45 minutes

Day Three:
A 3 sets 6–8
B 3 sets of 8–10
D 3 sets 8–10
E 3 sets of 8–10
G 3 sets 10–12
J 3 sets 10–12
M 3 sets 10–12
Q 15

Day Four:
Rest

Day Five:
A 3 sets 6–8
B 3 sets of 8–10
D 3 sets 8–10
E 3 sets of 8–10
G 3 sets 10–12
J 3 sets 10–12
M 3 sets 10–12
Q 15

Day Six:
Cardio 30–45 minutes

Day Seven:
Rest

ADVANCED ROUTINE 1

Day One:
A 3 sets 6–8
B 3 sets of 8–10
D 3 sets 8–10
E 3 sets of 8–10
G 3 sets 10–12
J 3 sets 10–12
M 3 sets 10–12
N 3 sets 12–15
Q 15
S 20 per side

Day Two:
Cardio 30–45 minutes

Day Three:
A 3 sets 6–8
B 3 sets of 8–10
D 3 sets 8–10
E 3 sets of 8–10
G 3 sets 10–12
J 3 sets 10–12
M 3 sets 10–12
N 3 sets 12–15
Q 15
S 20 per side

Day Four:
Cardio 30–45 minutes

Day Five:
A 3 sets 6–8
B 3 sets of 8–10
D 3 sets 8–10
E 3 sets of 8–10
G 3 sets 10–12
J 3 sets 10–12
M 3 sets 10–12
N 3 sets 12–15
Q 15
S 20 per side

Day Six:
Cardio 30–45 minutes

Day Seven:
Rest

WORKOUT LEVEL 2

BEGINNER ROUTINE 2

Day One:
C 3 sets 8–10
F 3 sets 8–10
H 3 sets 10–12
I 3 sets 12–15
K 3 sets 12–15
L 3 sets 10–12

Day Two:
Rest

Day Three:
C 3 sets 8–10
F 3 sets 8–10
H 3 sets 10–12
I 3 sets 12–15
K 3 sets 12–15
L 3 sets 10–12

Day Four:
Rest

Day Five:
C 3 sets 8–10
F 3 sets 8–10
H 3 sets 10–12
I 3 sets 12–15
K 3 sets 12–15
L 3 sets 10–12

Day Six:
Cardio 30–45 minutes

Day Seven:
Rest

INTERMEDIATE ROUTINE 2

Day One:
C 3 sets 8–10
F 3 sets 8–10
H 3 sets 10–12
I 3 sets 12–15
K 3 sets 12–15
L 3 sets 10–12
O 3 sets 30
P 3 sets 20

Day Two:
Cardio 30–45 minutes

Day Three:
C 3 sets 8–10
F 3 sets 8–10
H 3 sets 10–12
I 3 sets 12–15
K 3 sets 12–15
L 3 sets 10–12
O 3 sets 30
P 3 sets 20

Day Four:
Rest

Day Five:
C 3 sets 8–10
F 3 sets 8–10
H 3 sets 10–12
I 3 sets 12–15
K 3 sets 12–15
L 3 sets 10–12
O 3 sets 30
P 3 sets 20

Day Six:
Cardio 30–45 minutes

Day Seven:
Rest

ADVANCED ROUTINE 2

Day One:
C 3 sets 8–10
F 3 sets 8–10
H 3 sets 10–12
I 3 sets 12–15
K 3 sets 12–15
L 3 sets 10–12
O 3 sets 30
P 3 sets 20
R 3 sets 20
T 3 sets 30–60 seconds

Day Two:
Cardio 30–45 minutes

Day Three:
C 3 sets 8–10
F 3 sets 8–10
H 3 sets 10–12
I 3 sets 12–15
K 3 sets 12–15
L 3 sets 10–12
O 3 sets 30
P 3 sets 20
R 3 sets 20

Day Four:
T 3 sets 30–60 seconds

Day Four:
Cardio 30–45 minutes

Day Five:
C 3 sets 8–10
F 3 sets 8–10
H 3 sets 10–12
I 3 sets 12–15
K 3 sets 12–15
L 3 sets 10–12
O 3 sets 30
P 3 sets 20
R 3 sets 20
T 3 sets 30–60 seconds

Day Six:
Cardio 30–45 minutes

Day Seven:
Rest

GAELIC FOOTBALL WORKOUTS

A Barbell Deadlift
page 34
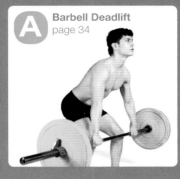

B Barbell Row
page 36
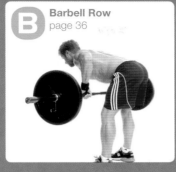

C Flat Bench Hyperextension
page 56
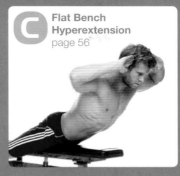

D Barbell Bench Press
page 60
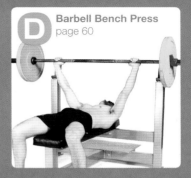

E Dips
page 68
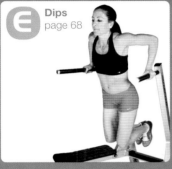

F Overhead Press
page 76
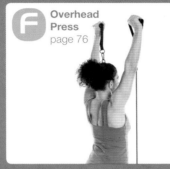

G Barbell Shoulder Shrug
page 94
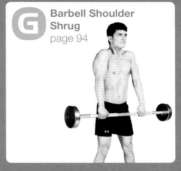

H Rope Pushdown
page 106
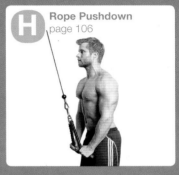

I Wrist Flexion
page 116
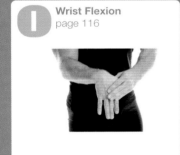

J Swiss Ball Wall Sit
page 134
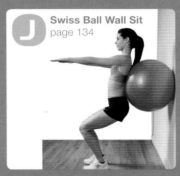

K High Lunge
page 146
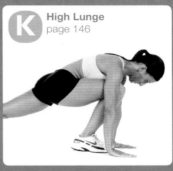

L Goblet Squat
page 150
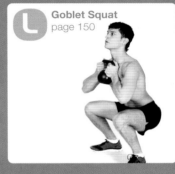

M Swiss Ball Hamstring Curl
page 164
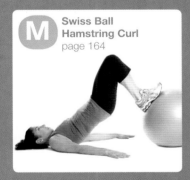

N Dumbbell Calf Raise
page 178
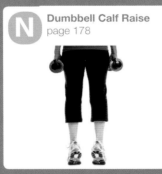

O Turkish Get-Up
page 188
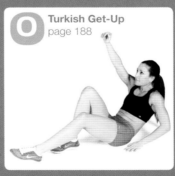

P Bicycle Crunch
page 190
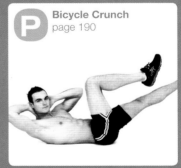

Q Plank Press-Up
page 198
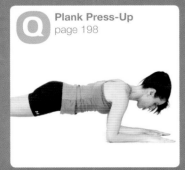

R Seated Russian Twist
page 200
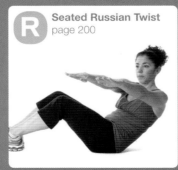

S Medicine Ball Wood Chop
page 130
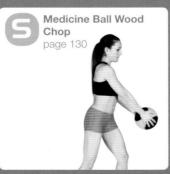

T T-Stabilization
page 124
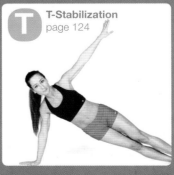

GOLF

Golf is more of a workout than most of us think. A good swing works muscles throughout the body. Since the back and core are the driving forces behind your swing, these areas need to be strong and developed. The pectorals, whose function is to draw the arms across, help to extend the arm and flex the shoulder, as do the lats. The gluteus maximus provides lower-body support and allows you to drive through the hips and, lastly, the forearms allow for proper gripping in mid swing.

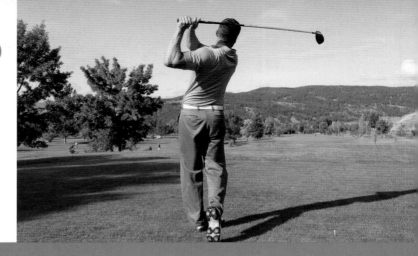

BEGINNER ROUTINE 1

Day One:
A 3 sets 8–10
B 3 sets 8–10
D 3 sets 10–12
H 3 sets 12–15
J 3 sets 10–12
P 20 per side

Day Two:
Rest

Day Three:
A 3 sets 8–10
B 3 sets 8–10
D 3 sets 10–12
H 3 sets 12–15
J 3 sets 10–12
P 20 per side

Day Four:
Rest

Day Five:
A 3 sets 8–10
B 3 sets 8–10
D 3 sets 10–12
H 3 sets 12–15
J 3 sets 10–12
P 20 per side

Day Six:
Cardio 30–45 minutes

Day Seven:
Rest

INTERMEDIATE ROUTINE 1

Day One:
A 3 sets 8–10
B 3 sets 8–10
D 3 sets 10–12
G 3 sets 10–12
H 3 sets 12–15
J 3 sets 10–12
K 3 sets 12–15
P 20 per side

Day Two:
Cardio 30–45 minutes

Day Three:
A 3 sets 8–10
B 3 sets 8–10
D 3 sets 10–12
G 3 sets 10–12
H 3 sets 12–15
J 3 sets 10–12
K 3 sets 12–15
P 20 per side

Day Four:
Rest

Day Five:
A 3 sets 8–10
B 3 sets 8–10
D 3 sets 10–12
G 3 sets 10–12
H 3 sets 12–15
J 3 sets 10–12
K 3 sets 12–15
P 20 per side

Day Six:
Cardio 30–45 minutes

Day Seven:
Rest

ADVANCED ROUTINE 1

Day One:
A 3 sets 8–10
B 3 sets 8–10
D 3 sets 10–12
G 3 sets 10–12
H 3 sets 12–15
J 3 sets 10–12
K 3 sets 12–15
O 30 per side
P 20 per side
R 15

Day Two:
Cardio 30–45 minutes

Day Three:
A 3 sets 8–10
B 3 sets 8–10
D 3 sets 10–12
G 3 sets 10–12
H 3 sets 12–15
J 3 sets 10–12
K 3 sets 12–15
O 30 per side

P 20 per side
R 15

Day Four:
Cardio 30–45 minutes

Day Five:
A 3 sets 8–10
B 3 sets 8–10
D 3 sets 10–12
G 3 sets 10–12
H 3 sets 12–15
J 3 sets 10–12
K 3 sets 12–15
O 30 per side
P 20 per side
R 15

Day Six:
Cardio 30–45 minutes

Day Seven:
Rest

BEGINNER ROUTINE 2

Day One:
C 3 sets 10–12
E 3 sets 12–15
F 3 sets 8–10
I 3 sets 12–15
L 3 sets 25
M 3 sets 20

Day Two:
Rest

Day Three:
C 3 sets 10–12
E 3 sets 12–15
F 3 sets 8–10
I 3 sets 12–15
L 3 sets 25
M 3 sets 20

Day Four:
Rest

Day Five:
C 3 sets 10–12
E 3 sets 12–15
F 3 sets 8–10
I 3 sets 12–15
L 3 sets 25
M 3 sets 20

Day Six:
Cardio 30–45 minutes

Day Seven:
Rest

INTERMEDIATE ROUTINE 2

Day One:
C 3 sets 10–12
E 3 sets 12–15
F 3 sets 8–10
I 3 sets 12–15
L 3 sets 25
M 3 sets 20
N 3 sets 20
Q 3 sets 8–10

Day Two:
Cardio 30–45 minutes

Day Three:
C 3 sets 10–12
E 3 sets 12–15
F 3 sets 8–10
I 3 sets 12–15
L 3 sets 25
M 3 sets 20
N 3 sets 20
Q 3 sets 8–10

Day Four:
Rest

Day Five:
C 3 sets 10–12
E 3 sets 12–15
F 3 sets 8–10
I 3 sets 12–15
L 3 sets 25
M 3 sets 20
N 3 sets 20
Q 3 sets 8–10

Day Six:
Cardio 30–45 minutes

Day Seven:
Rest

ADVANCED ROUTINE 2

Day One:
C 3 sets 10–12
E 3 sets 12–15
F 3 sets 8–10
I 3 sets 12–15
L 3 sets 25
M 3 sets 20
N 3 sets 20
Q 3 sets 8–10
S 3 sets 25
T 3 sets 20

Day Two:
Cardio 30–45 minutes

Day Three:
C 3 sets 10–12
E 3 sets 12–15
F 3 sets 8–10
I 3 sets 12–15
L 3 sets 25
M 3 sets 20
N 3 sets 20
Q 3 sets 8–10
S 3 sets 25
T 3 sets 20

Day Four:
Cardio 30–45 minutes

Day Five:
C 3 sets 10–12
E 3 sets 12–15
F 3 sets 8–10
I 3 sets 12–15
L 3 sets 25
M 3 sets 20
N 3 sets 20
Q 3 sets 8–10
S 3 sets 25
T 3 sets 20

Day Six:
Cardio 30–45 minutes

Day Seven:
Rest

GOLF WORKOUTS

A Lat Pulldown
page 42
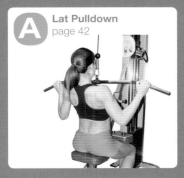

B Alternating Kettlebell Row
page 46
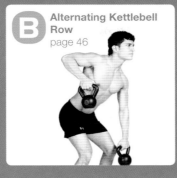

C Flat Bench Hyperextension
page 56
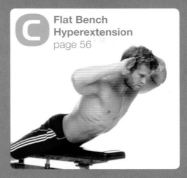

D Dumbbell Fly
page 64
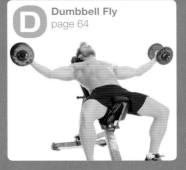

E External Rotation with Band
page 80
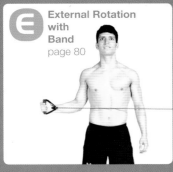

F Shoulder Raise and Pull
page 84
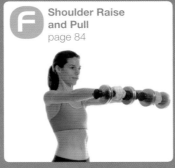

G Rope Pushdown
page 106
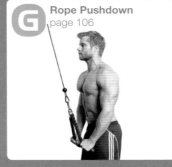

H Wrist Flexion
page 116
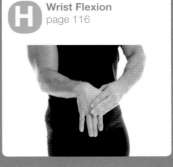

I Wrist Extension
page 117
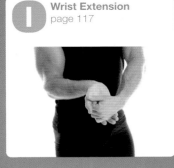

J Swiss Ball Wall Sit
page 134
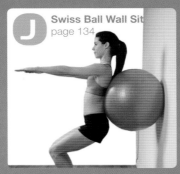

K Crossover Step
page 148
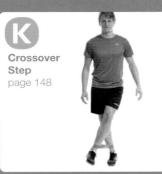

L Abdominal Kick
page 184
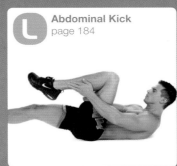

M Bicycle Crunch
page 190
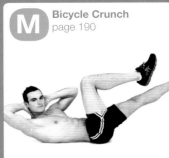

N Seated Russian Twist
page 200
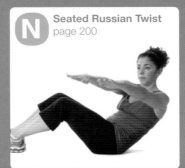

O Wood Chop with Resistance Band
page 202
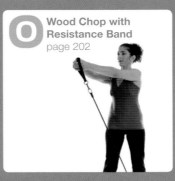

P Medicine Ball Wood Chop
page 130
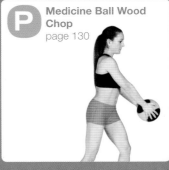

Q Alternating Renegade Row
page 48
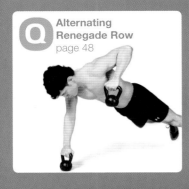

R Hip Abduction and Adduction
page 204
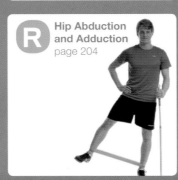

S Medicine Ball Slam
page 214
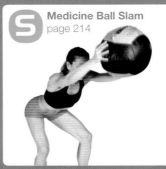

T The Windmill
page 216
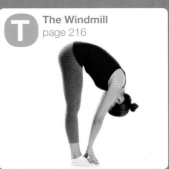

GYMNASTICS

Gymnastics involves the synergistic use of most of the major muscles in the human body to perform graceful and often spectacular feats of agility, strength, balance, flexibility and, not least, courage on a variety of apparatus. In gymnastic training, the goal is to achieve an exceptional level of strength without building excessive mass so that you can lift your own body weight as comfortably as possible. This routine is largely comprised of such "calisthenic" exercises.

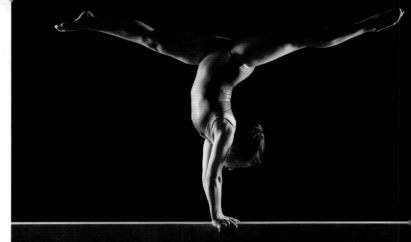

WORKOUT LEVEL 1

BEGINNER ROUTINE 1

Day One:
A 3 sets 8–10
E 3 sets 8–10
G 20
K 3 sets 10–12
Q 15
S 30–60 seconds per side

Day Two:
Rest

Day Three:
A 3 sets 8–10
E 3 sets 8–10
G 20
K 3 sets 10–12
Q 15
S 30–60 seconds per side

Day Four:
Rest

Day Five:
A 3 sets 8–10
E 3 sets 8–10
G 20
K 3 sets 10–12
Q 15
S 30–60 seconds per side

Day Six:
Cardio 30–45 minutes

Day Seven:
Rest

INTERMEDIATE ROUTINE 1

Day One:
A 3 sets 8–10
C 3 sets 12–15
E 3 sets 8–10
G 20
I 3 sets 12–15
K 3 sets 10–12
Q 15
S 30–60 seconds per side

Day Two:
Cardio 30–45 minutes

Day Three:
A 3 sets 8–10
C 3 sets 12–15
E 3 sets 8–10
G 20
I 3 sets 12–15
K 3 sets 10–12
Q 15
S 30–60 seconds per side

Day Four:
Rest

Day Five:
A 3 sets 8–10
C 3 sets 12–15
E 3 sets 8–10
G 20
I 3 sets 12–15
K 3 sets 10–12
Q 15
S 30–60 seconds per side

Day Six:
Cardio 30–45 minutes

Day Seven:
Rest

ADVANCED ROUTINE 1

Day One:
A 3 sets 8–10
C 3 sets 12–15
E 3 sets 8–10
G 20
I 3 sets 12–15
K 3 sets 10–12
Q 15
R 30–120 seconds
S 30–60 seconds per side
T 20 per side

Day Two:
Cardio 30–45 minutes

Day Three:
A 3 sets 8–10
C 3 sets 12–15
E 3 sets 8–10
G 20
I 3 sets 12–15
K 3 sets 10–12
Q 15
R 30–120 seconds

S 30–60 seconds per side
T 20 per side

Day Four:
Cardio 30–45 minutes

Day Five:
A 3 sets 8–10
C 3 sets 12–15
E 3 sets 8–10
G 20
I 3 sets 12–15
K 3 sets 10–12
Q 15
R 30–120 seconds
S 30–60 seconds per side
T 20 per side

Day Six:
Cardio 30–45 minutes

Day Seven:
Rest

WORKOUT LEVEL 2

BEGINNER ROUTINE 2

Day One:
B 3 sets 8–10
D 3 sets 12–15
F 3 sets 12–15
H 3 sets 15
J 3 sets 12–15
L 3 sets 15–20

Day Two:
Rest

Day Three:
B 3 sets 8–10
D 3 sets 12–15
F 3 sets 12–15
H 3 sets 15
J 3 sets 12–15
L 3 sets 15–20

Day Four:
Rest

Day Five:
B 3 sets 8–10
D 3 sets 12–15
F 3 sets 12–15
H 3 sets 15
J 3 sets 12–15
L 3 sets 15–20

Day Six:
Cardio 30–45 minutes

Day Seven:
Rest

INTERMEDIATE ROUTINE 2

Day One:
B 3 sets 8–10
D 3 sets 12–15
F 3 sets 12–15
H 3 sets 15
J 3 sets 12–15
L 3 sets 15–20
M 3 sets 15–20
N 3 sets 12–15

Day Two:
Cardio 30–45 minutes

Day Three:
B 3 sets 8–10
D 3 sets 12–15
F 3 sets 12–15
H 3 sets 15
J 3 sets 12–15
L 3 sets 15–20
M 3 sets 15–20
N 3 sets 12–15

Day Four:
Rest

Day Five:
B 3 sets 8–10
D 3 sets 12–15
F 3 sets 12–15
H 3 sets 15
J 3 sets 12–15
L 3 sets 15–20
M 3 sets 15–20
N 3 sets 12–15

Day Six:
Cardio 30–45 minutes

Day Seven:
Rest

ADVANCED ROUTINE 2

Day One:
B 3 sets 8–10
D 3 sets 12–15
F 3 sets 12–15
H 3 sets 15
J 3 sets 12–15
L 3 sets 15–20
M 3 sets 15–20
N 3 sets 12–15
O 3 sets 12–15
P 3 sets 20

Day Two:
Cardio 30–45 minutes

Day Three:
B 3 sets 8–10
D 3 sets 12–15
F 3 sets 12–15
H 3 sets 15
J 3 sets 12–15
L 3 sets 15–20
M 3 sets 15–20
N 3 sets 12–15
O 3 sets 12–15
P 3 sets 20

Day Four:
Cardio 30–45 minutes

Day Five:
B 3 sets 8–10
D 3 sets 12–15
F 3 sets 12–15
H 3 sets 15
J 3 sets 12–15
L 3 sets 15–20
M 3 sets 15–20
N 3 sets 12–15
O 3 sets 12–15
P 3 sets 20

Day Six:
Cardio 30–45 minutes

Day Seven:
Rest

GYMNASTICS WORKOUTS

A Rope Pulldown
page 52

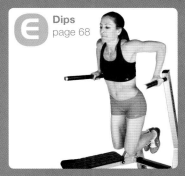

B Reverse Close-Grip Front Chin
page 54

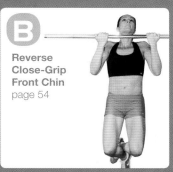

C Flat Bench Hyperextension
page 56

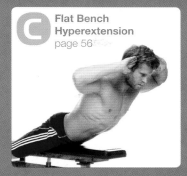

D Rotated Back Extension
page 58

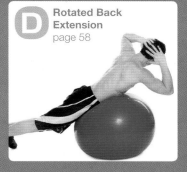

E Dips
page 68

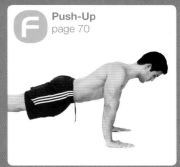

F Push-Up
page 70

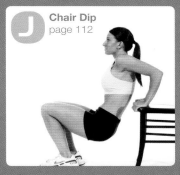

G Push-Up Hand Walk-Over
page 72

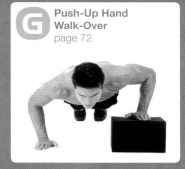

H Rotation Exercises
page 78

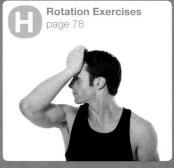

I External Rotation with Band
page 80

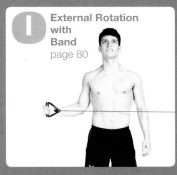

J Chair Dip
page 112

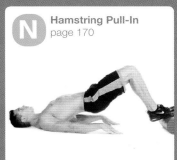

K Swiss Ball Wall Sit
page 134

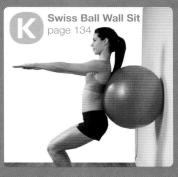

L Adductor Extension
page 162

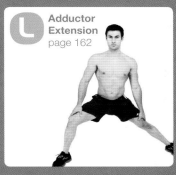

M Hamstring Abductor
page 163

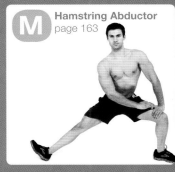

N Hamstring Pull-In
page 170

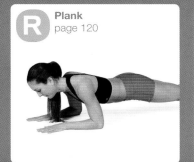

O Sumo Squat
page 172

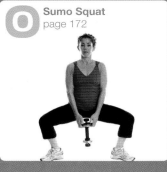

P Abdominal Hip Lift
page 186

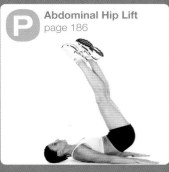

Q Plank Press-Up
page 198

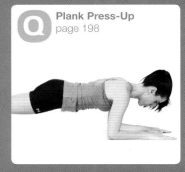

R Plank
page 120

S T-Stabilization
page 124

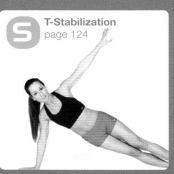

T Swiss Ball Hip Crossover
page 210

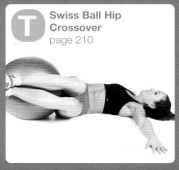

HANDBALL

An intense and fast-paced game, in handball it is the shoulders that are the primary muscles used for firing the ball toward a teammate or in an attempt on goal. The triceps support throwing power, and the core helps use motion from the lower body to augment upper-body power. Handball players also need powerful legs for continuous running, usually at speed. Attackers often leap spectacularly before attempting a shot on goal, which also demands great leg strength.

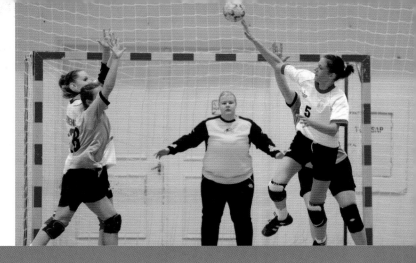

BEGINNER ROUTINE 1

Day One:
A 3 sets 6–8
B 3 sets 8–10
C 3 sets 15
G 3 sets 10–12
L 3 sets 10–12
P 30

Day Two:
Rest

Day Three:
A 3 sets 6–8
B 3 sets 8–10
C 3 sets 15
G 3 sets 10–12
L 3 sets 10–12
P 30

Day Four:
Rest

Day Five:
A 3 sets 6–8
B 3 sets 8–10
C 3 sets 15
G 3 sets 10–12
L 3 sets 10–12
P 30

Day Six:
Cardio 30–45 minutes

Day Seven:
Rest

INTERMEDIATE ROUTINE 1

Day One:
A 3 sets 6–8
B 3 sets 8–10
C 3 sets 15
F 3 sets 10–12
G 3 sets 10–12
L 3 sets 10–12
P 30
R 30–120 seconds

Day Two:
Cardio 30–45 minutes

Day Three:
A 3 sets 6–8
B 3 sets 8–10
C 3 sets 15
F 3 sets 10–12
G 3 sets 10–12
L 3 sets 10–12
P 30
R 30–120 seconds

Day Four:
Rest

Day Five:
A 3 sets 6–8
B 3 sets 8–10
C 3 sets 15
F 3 sets 10–12
G 3 sets 10–12
L 3 sets 10–12
P 30
R 30–120 seconds

Day Six:
Cardio 30–45 minutes

Day Seven:
Rest

ADVANCED ROUTINE 1

Day One:
A 3 sets 6–8
B 3 sets 8–10
C 3 sets 15
F 3 sets 10–12
G 3 sets 10–12
J 3 sets 10–12
L 3 sets 10–12
P 30
R 30–120 seconds
S 20 per side

Day Two:
Cardio 30–45 minutes

Day Three:
A 3 sets 6–8
B 3 sets 8–10
C 3 sets 15
F 3 sets 10–12
G 3 sets 10–12
J 3 sets 10–12
L 3 sets 10–12
P 30
R 30–120 seconds
S 20 per side

Day Four:
Cardio 30–45 minutes

Day Five:
A 3 sets 6–8
B 3 sets 8–10
C 3 sets 15
F 3 sets 10–12
G 3 sets 10–12
J 3 sets 10–12
L 3 sets 10–12
P 30
R 30–120 seconds
S 20 per side

Day Six:
Cardio 30–45 minutes

Day Seven:
Rest

BEGINNER ROUTINE 2

Day One:
D 3 sets 10–12
E 3 sets 10–12
H 3 sets 10–12
I 3 sets 10–12
K 3 sets 12–15
M 3 sets 12–15

Day Two:
Rest

Day Three:
D 3 sets 10–12
E 3 sets 10–12
H 3 sets 10–12
I 3 sets 10–12
K 3 sets 12–15
M 3 sets 12–15

Day Four:
Rest

Day Five:
D 3 sets 10–12
E 3 sets 10–12
H 3 sets 10–12
I 3 sets 10–12
K 3 sets 12–15
M 3 sets 12–15

Day Six:
Cardio 30–45 minutes

Day Seven:
Rest

INTERMEDIATE ROUTINE 2

Day One:
D 3 sets 10–12
E 3 sets 10–12
H 3 sets 10–12
I 3 sets 10–12
K 3 sets 12–15
M 3 sets 12–15
N 3 sets 25
O 3 sets 20

Day Two:
Cardio 30–45 minutes

Day Three:
D 3 sets 10–12
E 3 sets 10–12
H 3 sets 10–12
I 3 sets 10–12
K 3 sets 12–15
M 3 sets 12–15
N 3 sets 25
O 3 sets 20

Day Four:
Rest

Day Five:
D 3 sets 10–12
E 3 sets 10–12
H 3 sets 10–12
I 3 sets 10–12
K 3 sets 12–15
M 3 sets 12–15
N 3 sets 25
O 3 sets 20

Day Six:
Cardio 30–45 minutes

Day Seven:
Rest

ADVANCED ROUTINE 2

Day One:
D 3 sets 10–12
E 3 sets 10–12
H 3 sets 10–12
I 3 sets 10–12
K 3 sets 12–15
M 3 sets 12–15
N 3 sets 25
O 3 sets 20
Q 3 sets 20
T 3 sets 25

Day Two:
Cardio 30–45 minutes

Day Three:
D 3 sets 10–12
E 3 sets 10–12
H 3 sets 10–12
I 3 sets 10–12
K 3 sets 12–15
M 3 sets 12–15
N 3 sets 25
O 3 sets 20
Q 3 sets 20
T 3 sets 25

Day Four:
Cardio 30–45 minutes

Day Five:
D 3 sets 10–12
E 3 sets 10–12
H 3 sets 10–12
I 3 sets 10–12
K 3 sets 12–15
M 3 sets 12–15
N 3 sets 25
O 3 sets 20
Q 3 sets 20
T 3 sets 25

Day Six:
Cardio 30–45 minutes

Day Seven:
Rest

HANDBALL WORKOUTS

A Barbell Deadlift
page 34
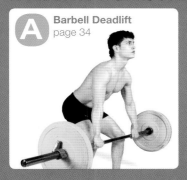

B Overhead Press
page 76
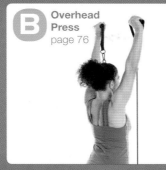

C Rotation Exercises
page 78
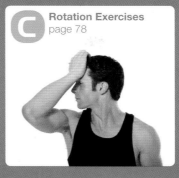

D Lateral Raise
page 82
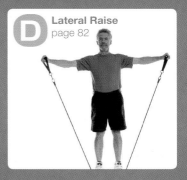

E Reverse Fly
page 88
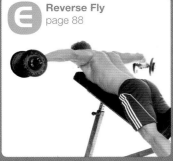

F Front-Plate Raise
page 92
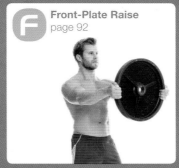

G Rope Pushdown
page 106
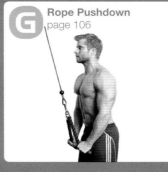

H Lying Triceps Extension
page 108
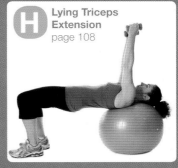

I Swiss Ball Wall Sit
page 134
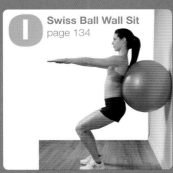

J Goblet Squat
page 150
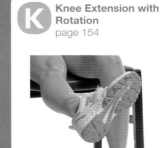

K Knee Extension with Rotation
page 154
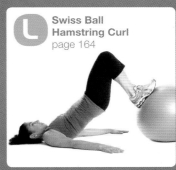

L Swiss Ball Hamstring Curl
page 164
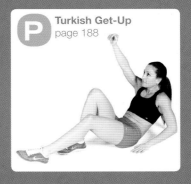

M Stiff-Legged Barbell Deadlift
page 168
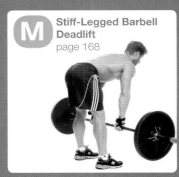

N Abdominal Kick
page 184
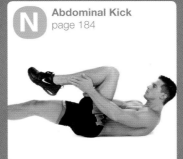

O Abdominal Hip Lift
page 286
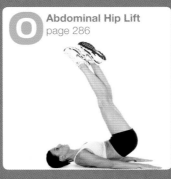

P Turkish Get-Up
page 188
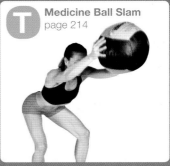

Q Reverse Crunch
page 192
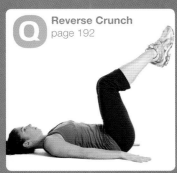

R Mountain Climber
page 158
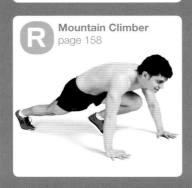

S Medicine Ball Wood Chop
page 130
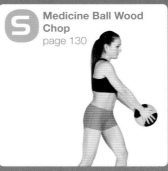

T Medicine Ball Slam
page 214

301

HURLING

Hurling is one of the fastest field-ball sports in the world. Training should center around three major lifts: deadlifts, squats and bench presses. In addition, good wrist strength is needed for hurling, as well as a strong core capable of powerful rotation. For variety and increased stamina, you should occasionally practice each of the weight-lifting exercises with relatively small weights and additional repetitions at a quicker pace. However, maintain good form at all times.

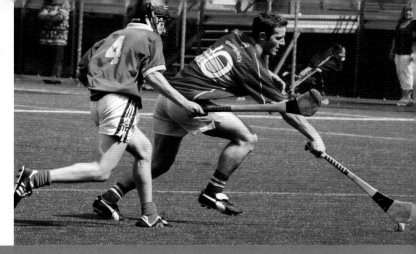

BEGINNER ROUTINE 1

Day One:
A 3 sets 6–8
C 3 sets 8–10
D 3 sets 8–10
H 3 sets 10–12
K 20 per side
Q 20 per side

Day Two:
Rest

Day Three:
A 3 sets 6–8
C 3 sets 8–10
D 3 sets 8–10
H 3 sets 10–12
K 20 per side
Q 20 per side

Day Four:
Rest

Day Five:
A 3 sets 6–8
C 3 sets 8–10
D 3 sets 8–10
H 3 sets 10–12
K 20 per side
Q 20 per side

Day Six:
Cardio 30–45 minutes

Day Seven:
Rest

INTERMEDIATE ROUTINE 1

Day One:
A 3 sets 6–8
C 3 sets 8–10
D 3 sets 8–10
E 3 sets 15
G 3 sets 12–15
H 3 sets 10–12
K 20 per side
Q 20 per side

Day Two:
Cardio 30–45 minutes

Day Three:
A 3 sets 6–8
C 3 sets 8–10
D 3 sets 8–10
E 3 sets 15
G 3 sets 12–15
H 3 sets 10–12
K 20 per side
Q 20 per side

Day Four:
Rest

Day Five:
A 3 sets 6–8
C 3 sets 8–10
D 3 sets 8–10
E 3 sets 15
G 3 sets 12–15
H 3 sets 10–12
K 20 per side
Q 20 per side

Day Six:
Cardio 30–45 minutes

Day Seven:
Rest

ADVANCED ROUTINE 1

Day One:
A 3 sets 6–8
C 3 sets 8–10
D 3 sets 8–10
E 3 sets 15
G 3 sets 12–15
H 3 sets 10–12
J 3 sets 10–12
K 20 per side
Q 20 per side
S 25

Day Two:
Cardio 30–45 minutes

Day Three:
A 3 sets 6–8
C 3 sets 8–10
D 3 sets 8–10
E 3 sets 15
G 3 sets 12–15
H 3 sets 10–12
J 3 sets 10–12
K 20 per side

Q 20 per side
S 25

Day Four:
Cardio 30–45 minutes

Day Five:
A 3 sets 6–8
C 3 sets 8–10
D 3 sets 8–10
E 3 sets 15
G 3 sets 12–15
H 3 sets 10–12
J 3 sets 10–12
K 20 per side
Q 20 per side
S 25

Day Six:
Cardio 30–45 minutes

Day Seven:
Rest

BEGINNER ROUTINE 2

Day One:
B 3 sets 8–10
F 3 sets 12–15
I 3 sets 10–12
L 3 sets 15
M 3 sets 30–60 seconds
N 3 sets 20

Day Two:
Rest

Day Three:
B 3 sets 8–10
F 3 sets 12–15
I 3 sets 10–12
L 3 sets 15
M 3 sets 30–60 seconds
N 3 sets 20

Day Four:
Rest

Day Five:
B 3 sets 8–10
F 3 sets 12–15
I 3 sets 10–12
L 3 sets 15
M 3 sets 30–60 seconds
N 3 sets 20

Day Six:
Cardio 30–45 minutes

Day Seven:
Rest

INTERMEDIATE ROUTINE 2

Day One:
B 3 sets 8–10
F 3 sets 12–15
I 3 sets 10–12
L 3 sets 15
M 3 sets 30–60 seconds
N 3 sets 20
O 3 sets 30–60 seconds
P 3 sets 20

Day Two:
Cardio 30–45 minutes

Day Three:
B 3 sets 8–10
F 3 sets 12–15
I 3 sets 10–12
L 3 sets 15
M 3 sets 30–60 seconds
N 3 sets 20
O 3 sets 30–60 seconds
P 3 sets 20

Day Four:
Rest

Day Five:
B 3 sets 8–10
F 3 sets 12–15
I 3 sets 10–12
L 3 sets 15
M 3 sets 30–60 seconds
N 3 sets 20
O 3 sets 30–60 seconds
P 3 sets 20

Day Six:
Cardio 30–45 minutes

Day Seven:
Rest

ADVANCED ROUTINE 2

Day One:
B 3 sets 8–10
F 3 sets 12–15
I 3 sets 10–12
L 3 sets 15
M 3 sets 30–60 seconds
N 3 sets 20
O 3 sets 30–60 seconds
P 3 sets 20
R 3 sets 20
T 3 sets 20

Day Two:
Cardio 30–45 minutes

Day Three:
B 3 sets 8–10
F 3 sets 12–15
I 3 sets 10–12
L 3 sets 15
M 3 sets 30–60 seconds
N 3 sets 20
O 3 sets 30–60 seconds

P 3 sets 20
R 3 sets 20
T 3 sets 20

Day Four:
Cardio 30–45 minutes

Day Five:
B 3 sets 8–10
F 3 sets 12–15
I 3 sets 10–12
L 3 sets 15
M 3 sets 30–60 seconds
N 3 sets 20
O 3 sets 30–60 seconds
P 3 sets 20
R 3 sets 20
T 3 sets 20

Day Six:
Cardio 30–45 minutes

Day Seven:
Rest

HURLING WORKOUTS

A Barbell Deadlift
page 34

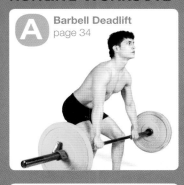

B Barbell Row
page 36

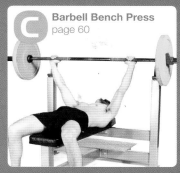

C Barbell Bench Press
page 60

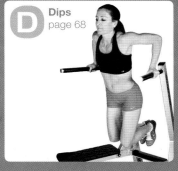

D Dips
page 68

E Rotation Exercises
page 78

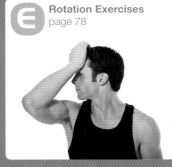

F Wrist Flexion
page 116

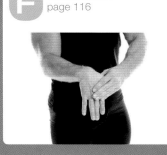

G Wrist Extension
page 117

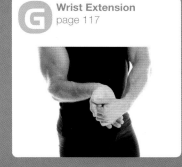

H Swiss Ball Wall Sit
page 134

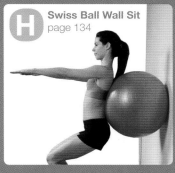

I Goblet Squat
page 150

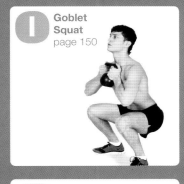

J Swiss Ball Hamstring Curl
page 164

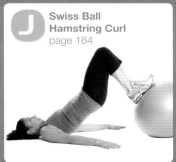

K Bicycle Crunch
page 190

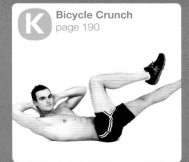

L Swiss Ball Pelvic Tilt
page 196

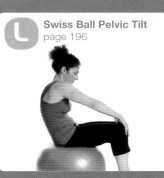

M Side Plank
page 122

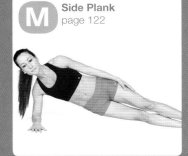

N Medicine Ball Wood Chop
page 130

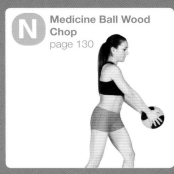

O T-Stabilization
page 124

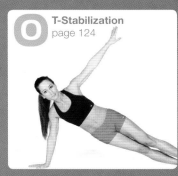

P Swiss Ball Jackknife
page 128

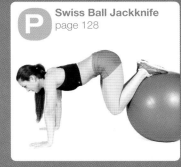

Q Thigh Rock-Back
page 208

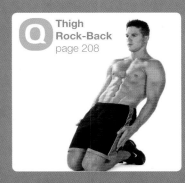

R V-Up
page 212

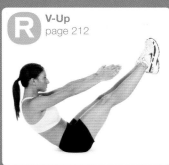

S Medicine Ball Slam
page 214

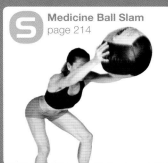

T The Windmill
page 216

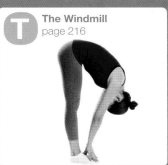

ICE HOCKEY

Ice hockey is a fast-paced and often aggressive contact sport notorious for its brutal body checks and even fighting. Consequently, training needs to be focused on strength and stamina. It is very cardiovascular in nature, involving mostly the core and leg muscles to propel the players across the ice. However, the shoulders and arms also need to be powerful to strike the puck, while the forearms need to be particularly strong to manipulate the hockey stick.

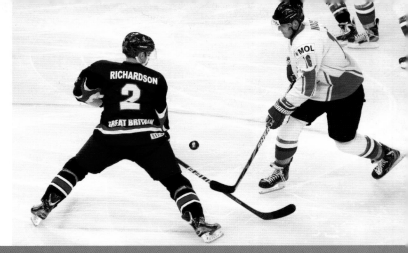

WORKOUT LEVEL 1

BEGINNER ROUTINE 1

Day One:
A 3 sets 6–8
B 3 sets 12–15
C 3 sets 10–12
F 3 sets 15–20
I 3 sets 12–15
T 20 per side

Day Two:
Rest

Day Three:
A 3 sets 6–8
B 3 sets 12–15
C 3 sets 10–12
F 3 sets 15–20
I 3 sets 12–15
T 20 per side

Day Four:
Rest

Day Five:
A 3 sets 6–8
B 3 sets 12–15
C 3 sets 10–12
F 3 sets 15–20
I 3 sets 12–15
T 20 per side

Day Six:
Cardio 30–45 minutes

Day Seven:
Rest

INTERMEDIATE ROUTINE 1

Day One:
A 3 sets 6–8
B 3 sets 12–15
C 3 sets 10–12
E 3 sets 12–15
F 3 sets 15–20
H 3 sets 10–12
I 3 sets 12–15
T 20 per side

Day Two:
Cardio 30–45 minutes

Day Three:
A 3 sets 6–8
B 3 sets 12–15
C 3 sets 10–12
E 3 sets 12–15
F 3 sets 15–20
H 3 sets 10–12
I 3 sets 12–15
T 20 per side

Day Four:
Rest

Day Five:
A 3 sets 6–8
B 3 sets 12–15
C 3 sets 10–12
E 3 sets 12–15
F 3 sets 15–20
H 3 sets 10–12
I 3 sets 12–15
T 20 per side

Day Six:
Cardio 30–45 minutes

Day Seven:
Rest

ADVANCED ROUTINE 1

Day One:
A 3 sets 6–8
B 3 sets 12–15
C 3 sets 10–12
E 3 sets 12–15
F 3 sets 15–20
H 3 sets 10–12
I 3 sets 12–15
L 20 per side
Q 20 per side
T 20 per side

Day Two:
Cardio 30–45 minutes

Day Three:
A 3 sets 6–8
B 3 sets 12–15
C 3 sets 10–12
E 3 sets 12–15
F 3 sets 15–20
H 3 sets 10–12
I 3 sets 12–15
L 20 per side
Q 20 per side
T 20 per side

Day Four:
Cardio 30–45 minutes

Day Five:
A 3 sets 6–8
B 3 sets 12–15
C 3 sets 10–12
E 3 sets 12–15
F 3 sets 15–20
H 3 sets 10–12
I 3 sets 12–15
L 20 per side
Q 20 per side
T 20 per side

Day Six:
Cardio 30–45 minutes

Day Seven:
Rest

WORKOUT LEVEL 2

BEGINNER ROUTINE 2

Day One:
D 3 sets 12–15
G 3 sets 15–20
J 3 sets 20
K 3 sets 30
M 3 sets 30–60 seconds
N 3 sets 15

Day Two:
Rest

Day Three:
D 3 sets 12–15
G 3 sets 15–20
J 3 sets 20
K 3 sets 30
M 3 sets 30–60 seconds
N 3 sets 15

Day Four:
Rest

Day Five:
D 3 sets 12–15
G 3 sets 15–20
J 3 sets 20
K 3 sets 30
M 3 sets 30–60 seconds
N 3 sets 15

Day Six:
Cardio 30–45 minutes

Day Seven:
Rest

INTERMEDIATE ROUTINE 2

Day One:
D 3 sets 12–15
G 3 sets 15–20
J 3 sets 20
K 3 sets 30
M 3 sets 30–60 seconds
N 3 sets 15
O 3 sets 20
P 3 sets 20

Day Two:
Cardio 30–45 minutes

Day Three:
D 3 sets 12–15
G 3 sets 15–20
J 3 sets 20
K 3 sets 30
M 3 sets 30–60 seconds
N 3 sets 15
O 3 sets 20
P 3 sets 20

Day Four:
Rest

Day Five:
D 3 sets 12–15
G 3 sets 15–20
J 3 sets 20
K 3 sets 30
M 3 sets 30–60 seconds
N 3 sets 15
O 3 sets 20
P 3 sets 20

Day Six:
Cardio 30–45 minutes

Day Seven:
Rest

ADVANCED ROUTINE 2

Day One:
D 3 sets 12–15
G 3 sets 15–20
J 3 sets 20
K 3 sets 30
M 3 sets 30–60 seconds
N 3 sets 15
O 3 sets 20
P 3 sets 20
R 3 sets 20
S 3 sets 25

Day Two:
Cardio 30–45 minutes

Day Three:
D 3 sets 12–15
G 3 sets 15–20
J 3 sets 20
K 3 sets 30
M 3 sets 30–60 seconds
N 3 sets 15
O 3 sets 20
P 3 sets 20

R 3 sets 20
S 3 sets 25

Day Four:
Cardio 30–45 minutes

Day Five:
D 3 sets 12–15
G 3 sets 15–20
J 3 sets 20
K 3 sets 30
M 3 sets 30–60 seconds
N 3 sets 15
O 3 sets 20
P 3 sets 20
R 3 sets 20
S 3 sets 25

Day Six:
Cardio 30–45 minutes

Day Seven:
Rest

ICE HOCKEY WORKOUTS

A Barbell Deadlift
page 34
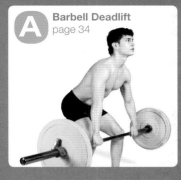

B Flat Bench Hyperextension
page 56
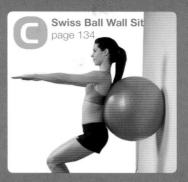

C Swiss Ball Wall Sit
page 134
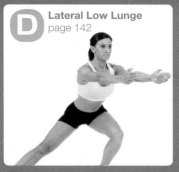

D Lateral Low Lunge
page 142
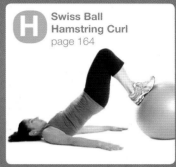

E Dumbbell Walking Lunge
page 144
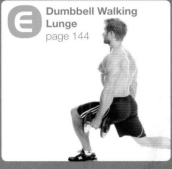

F Adductor Extension
page 162
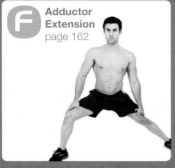

G Hamstring Abductor
page 163
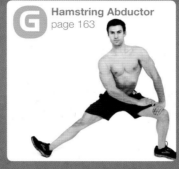

H Swiss Ball Hamstring Curl
page 164
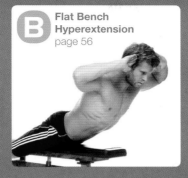

I Stiff-Legged Barbell Deadlift
page 168
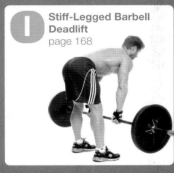

J Seated Russian Twist
page 200
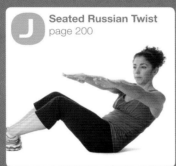

K Wood Chop with Resistance Band
page 202
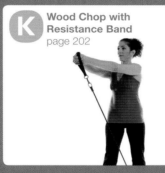

L Medicine Ball Wood Chop
page 130
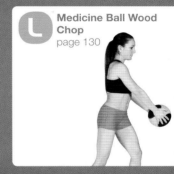

M T-Stabilization
page 124
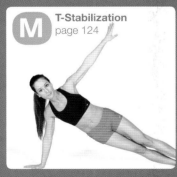

N Hip Abduction and Adduction
page 204
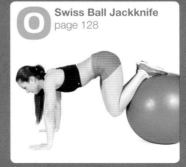

O Swiss Ball Jackknife
page 128
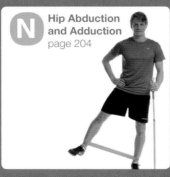

P Swiss Ball Roll-Out
page 206
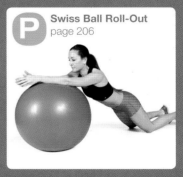

Q Thigh Rock-Back
page 208
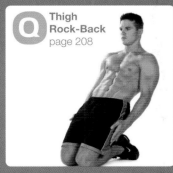

R V-Up
page 212
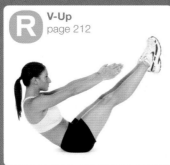

S Medicine Ball Slam
page 214
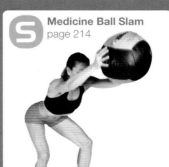

T The Windmill
page 216
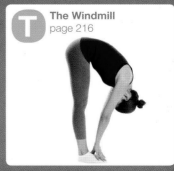

JUDO

Judo is a combative sport where, for beginners at least, strength can be a disadvantage because you may rely on your strength to the detriment of proper technique. A small woman, who is expert at judo, should have no problem defeating a much larger man with little or no training in the sport. However, when faced with an equally experienced opponent, size and strength do matter. For competitive judo at a higher level, add more strength-training exercises (see page 372) to your routine.

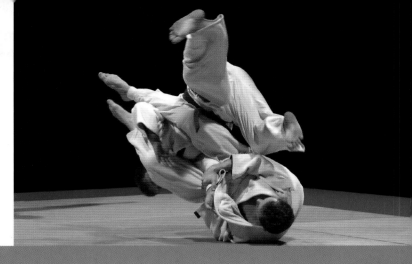

BEGINNER ROUTINE I

Day One:
A 3 sets 6–8
B 3 sets 8–10
D 3 sets 8–10
E 3 sets 10–12
M 20 rotations
P 20

Day Two:
Rest

Day Three:
A 3 sets 6–8
B 3 sets 8–10
D 3 sets 8–10
E 3 sets 10–12
M 20 rotations
P 20

Day Four:
Rest

Day Five:
A 3 sets 6–8
B 3 sets 8–10
D 3 sets 8–10
E 3 sets 10–12
M 20 rotations
P 20

Day Six:
Cardio 30–45 minutes

Day Seven:
Rest

INTERMEDIATE ROUTINE I

Day One:
A 3 sets 6–8
B 3 sets 8–10
C 3 sets 12–15
D 3 sets 8–10
E 3 sets 10–12
G 3 sets 10–12
M 20 rotations
P 20

Day Two:
Cardio 30–45 minutes

Day Three:
A 3 sets 6–8
B 3 sets 8–10
C 3 sets 12–15
D 3 sets 8–10
E 3 sets 10–12
G 3 sets 10–12
M 20 rotations
P 20

Day Four:
Rest

Day Five:
A 3 sets 6–8
B 3 sets 8–10
C 3 sets 12–15
D 3 sets 8–10
E 3 sets 10–12
G 3 sets 10–12
M 20 rotations
P 20

Day Six:
Cardio 30–45 minutes

Day Seven:
Rest

ADVANCED ROUTINE I

Day One:
A 3 sets 6–8
B 3 sets 8–10
C 3 sets 12–15
D 3 sets 8–10
E 3 sets 10–12
F 3 sets 10–12
G 3 sets 10–12
M 20 rotations
P 20
Q 20

Day Two:
Cardio 30–45 minutes

Day Three:
A 3 sets 6–8
B 3 sets 8–10
C 3 sets 12–15
D 3 sets 8–10
E 3 sets 10–12
F 3 sets 10–12
G 3 sets 10–12
M 20 rotations
P 20
Q 20

Day Four:
Cardio 30–45 minutes

Day Five:
A 3 sets 6–8
B 3 sets 8–10
C 3 sets 12–15
D 3 sets 8–10
E 3 sets 10–12
F 3 sets 10–12
G 3 sets 10–12
M 20 rotations
P 20
Q 20

Day Six:
Cardio 30–45 minutes

Day Seven:
Rest

BEGINNER ROUTINE 2

Day One:
H 3 sets 25
I 3 sets 25
J 3 sets 20
K 3 sets 15
L 3 sets 30–60 seconds
N 3 sets 30

Day Two:
Rest

Day Three:
H 3 sets 25
I 3 sets 25
J 3 sets 20
K 3 sets 15
L 3 sets 30–60 seconds
N 3 sets 30

Day Four:
Rest

Day Five:
H 3 sets 25
I 3 sets 25
J 3 sets 20
K 3 sets 15
L 3 sets 30–60 seconds
N 3 sets 30

Day Six:
Cardio 30–45 minutes

Day Seven:
Rest

INTERMEDIATE ROUTINE 2

Day One:
H 3 sets 25
I 3 sets 25
J 3 sets 20
K 3 sets 15
L 3 sets 30–60 seconds
N 3 sets 30
O 3 sets 3–5 per side
R 3 sets 20

Day Two:
Cardio 30–45 minutes

Day Three:
H 3 sets 25
I 3 sets 25
J 3 sets 20
K 3 sets 15
L 3 sets 30–60 seconds
N 3 sets 30
O 3 sets 3–5 per side
R 3 sets 20

Day Four:
Rest

Day Five:
H 3 sets 25
I 3 sets 25
J 3 sets 20
K 3 sets 15
L 3 sets 30–60 seconds
N 3 sets 30
O 3 sets 3–5 per side
R 3 sets 20

Day Six:
Cardio 30–45 minutes

Day Seven:
Rest

ADVANCED ROUTINE 2

Day One:
H 3 sets 25
I 3 sets 25
J 3 sets 20
K 3 sets 15
L 3 sets 30–60 seconds
N 3 sets 30
O 3 sets 3–5 per side
R 3 sets 20
S 3 sets 25
T 3 sets 20

Day Two:
Cardio 30–45 minutes

Day Three:
H 3 sets 25
I 3 sets 25
J 3 sets 20
K 3 sets 15
L 3 sets 30–60 seconds
N 3 sets 30
O 3 sets 3–5 per side
R 3 sets 20

S 3 sets 25
T 3 sets 20

Day Four:
Cardio 30–45 minutes

Day Five:
H 3 sets 25
I 3 sets 25
J 3 sets 20
K 3 sets 15
L 3 sets 30–60 seconds
N 3 sets 30
O 3 sets 3–5 per side
R 3 sets 20
S 3 sets 25
T 3 sets 20

Day Six:
Cardio 30–45 minutes

Day Seven:
Rest

JUDO WORKOUTS

A Alternating Kettlebell Row
page 46
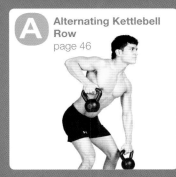

B Rope Pulldown
page 52
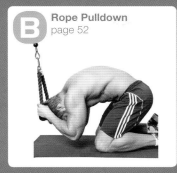

C Rotated Back Extension
page 58
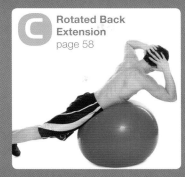

D Roller Push-Up
page 62
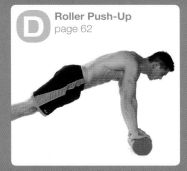

E Barbell Squat
page 136
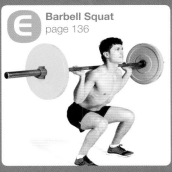

F Swiss Ball Hamstring Curl
page 164
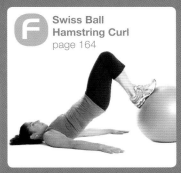

G Stiff-Legged Deadlift
page 174
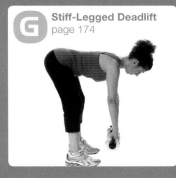

H Crunch
page 118
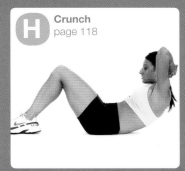

I Abdominal Kick
page 184
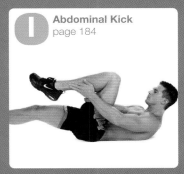

J Abdominal Hip Lift
page 186
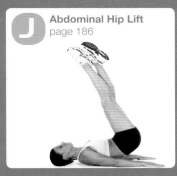

K Plank Press-Up
page 198
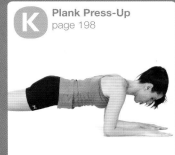

L Side Plank
page 122
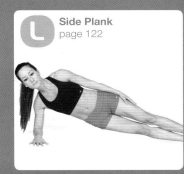

M Seated Russian Twist
page 200
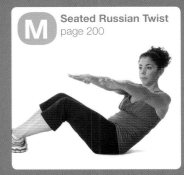

N Wood Chop with Resistance Band
page 202
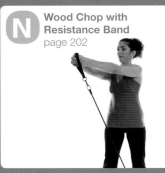

O Swiss Ball Walk-Around
page 126
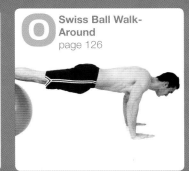

P Push-Up
page 70
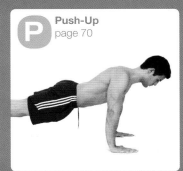

Q Swiss Ball Roll-Out
page 206
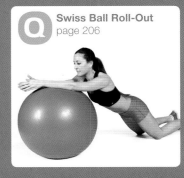

R Swiss Ball Hip Crossover
page 210
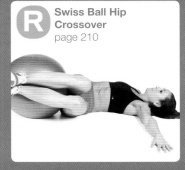

S Medicine Ball Slam
page 214
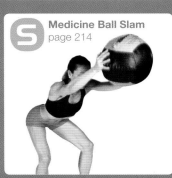

T The Windmill
page 216
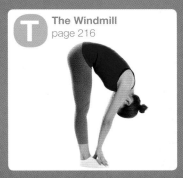

KARATE

For excellence in karate, you need explosive power, flexibility and stamina. Leg and core work — in addition to extensive stretching and some basic upper-body strengthening — is the key to mastering this martial art. Many of the exercises included in this routine are calisthenic because the aim in karate is to increase power without increasing bulk. In competitive karate, maximum points are awarded for kicks to the head, so leg stretches are particularly important in this sport.

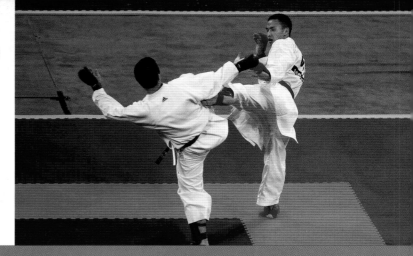

WORKOUT LEVEL 1

BEGINNER ROUTINE 1

Day One:
B 3 sets 8–10
C 3 sets 20
F 3 sets 10–12
I 3 sets 12–15
Q 30 per side
S 3 sets 15

Day Two:
Rest

Day Three:
B 3 sets 8–10
C 3 sets 20
F 3 sets 10–12
I 3 sets 12–15
Q 30 per side
S 3 sets 15

Day Four:
Rest

Day Five:
B 3 sets 8–10
C 3 sets 20
F 3 sets 10–12
I 3 sets 12–15
Q 30 per side
S 3 sets 15

Day Six:
Cardio 30–45 minutes

Day Seven:
Rest

INTERMEDIATE ROUTINE 1

Day One:
B 3 sets 8–10
C 3 sets 20
D 3 sets 15
F 3 sets 10–12
I 3 sets 12–15
Q 30 per side
R 30–60 seconds per side
S 3 sets 15

Day Two:
Cardio 30–45 minutes

Day Three:
B 3 sets 8–10
C 3 sets 20
D 3 sets 15
F 3 sets 10–12
I 3 sets 12–15
Q 30 per side
R 30–60 seconds per side
S 3 sets 15

Day Four:
Rest

Day Five:
B 3 sets 8–10
C 3 sets 20
D 3 sets 15
F 3 sets 10–12
I 3 sets 12–15
Q 30 per side
R 30–60 seconds per side
S 3 sets 15

Day Six:
Cardio 30–45 minutes

Day Seven:
Rest

ADVANCED ROUTINE 1

Day One:
B 3 sets 8–10
C 3 sets 20
D 3 sets 15
F 3 sets 10–12
I 3 sets 12–15
Q 30 per side
P 20 rotations
R 30–60 seconds per side
S 3 sets 15
T 20

Day Two:
Cardio 30–45 minutes

Day Three:
B 3 sets 8–10
C 3 sets 20
D 3 sets 15
F 3 sets 10–12
I 3 sets 12–15
Q 30 per side
P 20 rotations
R 30–60 seconds per side

S 3 sets 15
T 20

Day Four:
Cardio 30–45 minutes

Day Five:
B 3 sets 8–10
C 3 sets 20
D 3 sets 15
F 3 sets 10–12
I 3 sets 12–15
Q 30 per side
P 20 rotations
R 30–60 seconds per side
S 3 sets 15
T 20

Day Six:
Cardio 30–45 minutes

Day Seven:
Rest

WORKOUT LEVEL 2

BEGINNER ROUTINE 2

Day One:
A 3 sets 8–10
E 3 sets 12–15
G 3 sets 12–15
H 3 sets 12–15
J 3 sets 15–20
K 3 sets 15–20

Day Two:
Rest

Day Three:
A 3 sets 8–10
E 3 sets 12–15
G 3 sets 12–15
H 3 sets 12–15
J 3 sets 15–20
K 3 sets 15–20

Day Four:
Rest

Day Five:
A 3 sets 8–10
E 3 sets 12–15
G 3 sets 12–15
H 3 sets 12–15
J 3 sets 15–20
K 3 sets 15–20

Day Six:
Cardio 30–45 minutes

Day Seven:
Rest

INTERMEDIATE ROUTINE 2

Day One:
A 3 sets 8–10
E 3 sets 12–15
G 3 sets 12–15
H 3 sets 12–15
J 3 sets 15–20
K 3 sets 15–20
L 3 sets 12–15
M 3 sets 12–15

Day Two:
Cardio 30–45 minutes

Day Three:
A 3 sets 8–10
E 3 sets 12–15
G 3 sets 12–15
H 3 sets 12–15
J 3 sets 15–20
K 3 sets 15–20
L 3 sets 12–15
M 3 sets 12–15

Day Four:
Rest

Day Five:
A 3 sets 8–10
E 3 sets 12–15
G 3 sets 12–15
H 3 sets 12–15
J 3 sets 15–20
K 3 sets 15–20
L 3 sets 12–15
M 3 sets 12–15

Day Six:
Cardio 30–45 minutes

Day Seven:
Rest

ADVANCED ROUTINE 2

Day One:
A 3 sets 8–10
E 3 sets 12–15
G 3 sets 12–15
H 3 sets 12–15
J 3 sets 15–20
K 3 sets 15–20
L 3 sets 12–15
M 3 sets 12–15
N 3 sets 20
O 3 sets 30–60 seconds

Day Two:
Cardio 30–45 minutes

Day Three:
A 3 sets 8–10
E 3 sets 12–15
G 3 sets 12–15
H 3 sets 12–15
J 3 sets 15–20
K 3 sets 15–20
L 3 sets 12–15
M 3 sets 12–15

N 3 sets 20
O 3 sets 30–60 seconds

Day Four:
Cardio 30–45 minutes

Day Five:
A 3 sets 8–10
E 3 sets 12–15
G 3 sets 12–15
H 3 sets 12–15
J 3 sets 15–20
K 3 sets 15–20
L 3 sets 12–15
M 3 sets 12–15
N 3 sets 20
O 3 sets 30–60 seconds

Day Six:
Cardio 30–45 minutes

Day Seven:
Rest

KARATE WORKOUTS

A Rope Pulldown
page 52
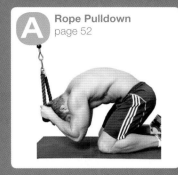

B Dips
page 68
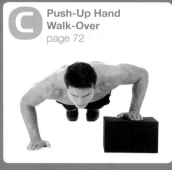

C Push-Up Hand Walk-Over
page 72
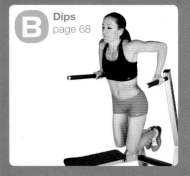

D Rotation Exercises
page 78
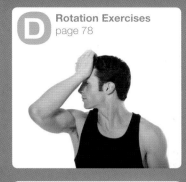

E Wrist Flexion
page 116
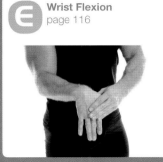

F Swiss Ball Wall Sit
page 134
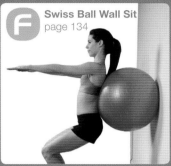

G Dumbbell Walking Lunge
page 144
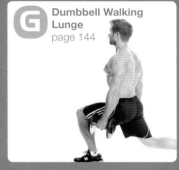

H High Lunge
page 146
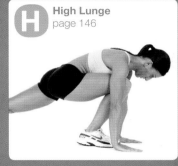

I One-Legged Step-Down
page 152
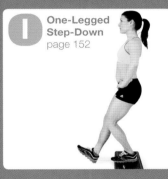

J Adductor Extension
page 162
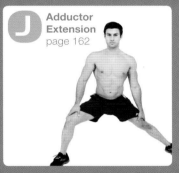

K Hamstring Abductor
page 163
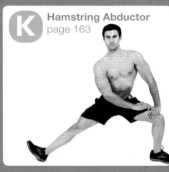

L Stiff-Legged Barbell Deadlift
page 168
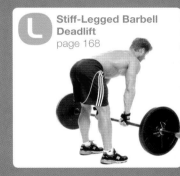

M Hamstring Pull-In
page 170
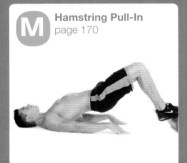

N Abdominal Hip Lift
page 186
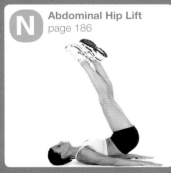

O Side Plank
page 122
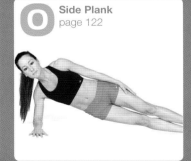

P Seated Russian Twist
page 200
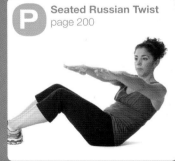

Q Wood Chop with Resistance Band
page 202
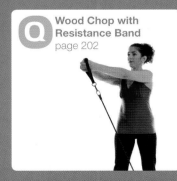

R T-Stabilization
page 124
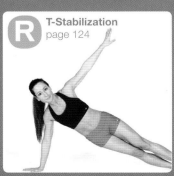

S Hip Abduction and Adduction
page 204
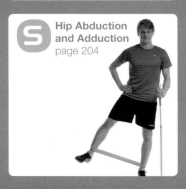

T Swiss Ball Jackknife
page 128
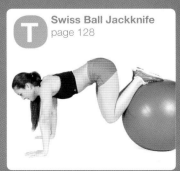

KAYAKING

Kayaking provides a great cardiovascular as well as strength workout depending on the current of the waters. The double-bladed paddle demands a characteristic technique that builds strong shoulders and lats as well as powerful triceps, forearms and wrists. When proper form is used, however, your core muscles are the primary parts of the body that stabilize the body and propel the kayak. And don't neglect the legs. In conjunction with the hips, they help to turn, stabilize, brace and roll the kayak.

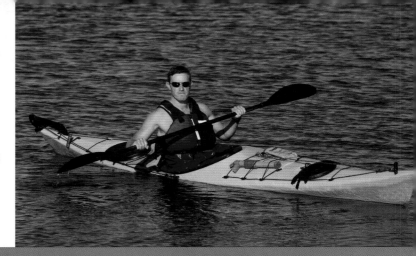

WORKOUT LEVEL 1

BEGINNER ROUTINE 1

Day One:
A 3 sets 8–10
B 3 sets 8–10
D 3 sets 12–15
F 3 sets 10–12
K 3 sets 15–20
S 20 per side

Day Two:
Rest

Day Three:
A 3 sets 8–10
B 3 sets 8–10
D 3 sets 12–15
F 3 sets 10–12
K 3 sets 15–20
S 20 per side

Day Four:
Rest

Day Five:
A 3 sets 8–10
B 3 sets 8–10
D 3 sets 12–15
F 3 sets 10–12
K 3 sets 15–20
S 20 per side

Day Six:
Cardio 30–45 minutes

Day Seven:
Rest

INTERMEDIATE ROUTINE 1

Day One:
A 3 sets 8–10
B 3 sets 8–10
C 3 sets 12–15
D 3 sets 12–15
F 3 sets 10–12
K 3 sets 15–20
L 3 sets 15–20
S 20 per side

Day Two:
Cardio 30–45 minutes

Day Three:
A 3 sets 8–10
B 3 sets 8–10
C 3 sets 12–15
D 3 sets 12–15
F 3 sets 10–12
K 3 sets 15–20
L 3 sets 15–20
S 20 per side

Day Four:
Rest

Day Five:
A 3 sets 8–10
B 3 sets 8–10
C 3 sets 12–15
D 3 sets 12–15
F 3 sets 10–12
K 3 sets 15–20
L 3 sets 15–20
S 20 per side

Day Six:
Cardio 30–45 minutes

Day Seven:
Rest

ADVANCED ROUTINE 1

Day One:
A 3 sets 8–10
B 3 sets 8–10
C 3 sets 12–15
D 3 sets 12–15
F 3 sets 10–12
J 3 sets 12–15
K 3 sets 15–20
L 3 sets 15–20
Q 3 sets 8–10
S 20 per side

Day Two:
Cardio 30–45 minutes

Day Three:
A 3 sets 8–10
B 3 sets 8–10
C 3 sets 12–15
D 3 sets 12–15
F 3 sets 10–12
J 3 sets 12–15
K 3 sets 15–20
L 3 sets 15–20
Q 3 sets 8–10
S 20 per side

Day Four:
Cardio 30–45 minutes

Day Five:
A 3 sets 8–10
B 3 sets 8–10
C 3 sets 12–15
D 3 sets 12–15
F 3 sets 10–12
J 3 sets 12–15
K 3 sets 15–20
L 3 sets 15–20
Q 3 sets 8–10
S 20 per side

Day Six:
Cardio 30–45 minutes

Day Seven:
Rest

WORKOUT LEVEL 2

BEGINNER ROUTINE 2

Day One:
E 3 sets 15
G 3 sets 10–12
H 3 sets 10–12
I 3 sets 10–12
M 3 sets 25
N 3 sets 20

Day Two:
Rest

Day Three:
E 3 sets 15
G 3 sets 10–12
H 3 sets 10–12
I 3 sets 10–12
M 3 sets 25
N 3 sets 20

Day Four:
Rest

Day Five:
E 3 sets 15
G 3 sets 10–12
H 3 sets 10–12
I 3 sets 10–12
M 3 sets 25
N 3 sets 20

Day Six:
Cardio 30–45 minutes

Day Seven:
Rest

INTERMEDIATE ROUTINE 2

Day One:
E 3 sets 15
G 3 sets 10–12
H 3 sets 10–12
I 3 sets 10–12
M 3 sets 25
N 3 sets 20
O 3 sets 20
P 3 sets 30

Day Two:
Cardio 30–45 minutes

Day Three:
E 3 sets 15
G 3 sets 10–12
H 3 sets 10–12
I 3 sets 10–12
M 3 sets 25
N 3 sets 20
O 3 sets 20
P 3 sets 30

Day Four:
Rest

Day Five:
E 3 sets 15
G 3 sets 10–12
H 3 sets 10–12
I 3 sets 10–12
M 3 sets 25
N 3 sets 20
O 3 sets 20
P 3 sets 30

Day Six:
Cardio 30–45 minutes

Day Seven:
Rest

ADVANCED ROUTINE 2

Day One:
E 3 sets 15
G 3 sets 10–12
H 3 sets 10–12
I 3 sets 10–12
M 3 sets 25
N 3 sets 20
O 3 sets 20
P 3 sets 30
R 3 sets 20
T 3 sets 20

Day Two:
Cardio 30–45 minutes

Day Three:
E 3 sets 15
G 3 sets 10–12
H 3 sets 10–12
I 3 sets 10–12
M 3 sets 25
N 3 sets 20
O 3 sets 20
P 3 sets 30
R 3 sets 20
T 3 sets 20

Day Four:
Cardio 30–45 minutes

Day Five:
E 3 sets 15
G 3 sets 10–12
H 3 sets 10–12
I 3 sets 10–12
M 3 sets 25
N 3 sets 20
O 3 sets 20
P 3 sets 30
R 3 sets 20
T 3 sets 20

Day Six:
Cardio 30–45 minutes

Day Seven:
Rest

KAYAKING WORKOUTS

A Dumbbell Pullover
page 40
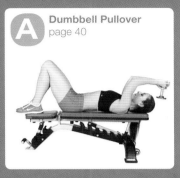

B Lat Pulldown
page 42
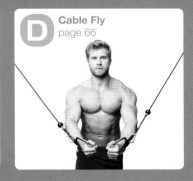

C Flat Bench Hyperextension
page 56
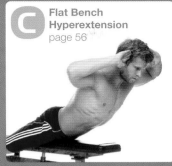

D Cable Fly
page 66
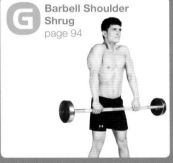

E Rotation Exercises
page 78
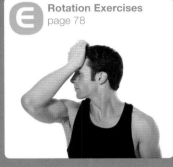

F Reverse Fly
page 88
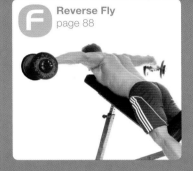

G Barbell Shoulder Shrug
page 94
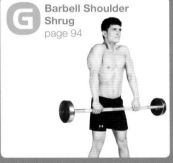

H Alternating Hammer Curl
page 98
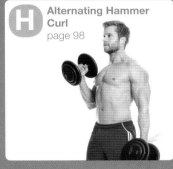

I Lying Triceps Extension
page 108
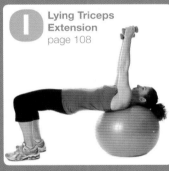

J Wrist Flexion
page 116
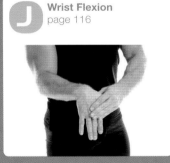

K Adductor Extension
page 162
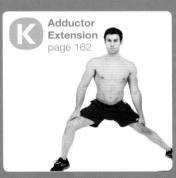

L Hamstring Abductor
page 163
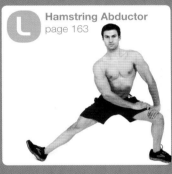

M Crunch
page 118
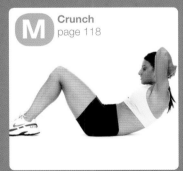

N Reverse Crunch
page 192
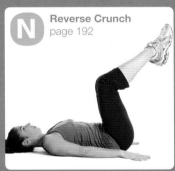

O Seated Russian Twist
page 200
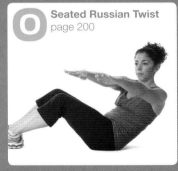

P Wood Chop with Resistance Band
page 202
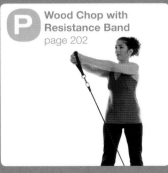

Q Alternating Renegade Row
page 48
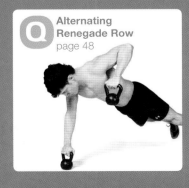

R Swiss Ball Roll-Out
page 206
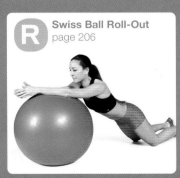

S Thigh Rock-Back
page 208
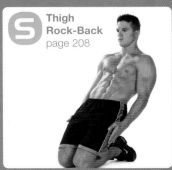

T The Windmill
page 216
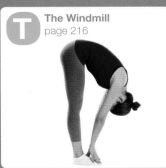

LACROSSE

The major muscles used in the fast-paced sport of lacrosse are the shoulder, trapezius, arm and leg muscles, with secondary assistance from the abdominals, pectorals and lats. Lacrosse is an "explosive" sport. You need endurance in the lower part of your body, while in the upper body you tend to need explosive strength more than endurance. It is a contact sport and defenders need good upper-body strength to block an opponent's advance.

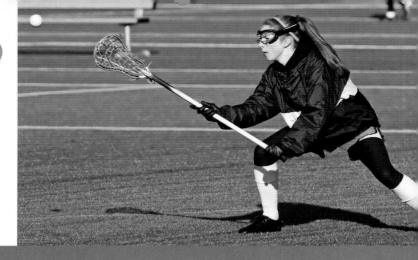

BEGINNER ROUTINE I

Day One:
A 3 sets 8–10
C 3 sets 8–10
F 3 sets 10–12
G 3 sets 10–12
I 3 sets 12–15
L 3 sets 12–15

Day Two:
Rest

Day Three:
A 3 sets 8–10
C 3 sets 8–10
F 3 sets 10–12
G 3 sets 10–12
I 3 sets 12–15
L 3 sets 12–15

Day Four:
Rest

Day Five:
A 3 sets 8–10
C 3 sets 8–10
F 3 sets 10–12
G 3 sets 10–12
I 3 sets 12–15
L 3 sets 12–15

Day Six:
Cardio 30–45 minutes

Day Seven:
Rest

INTERMEDIATE ROUTINE I

Day One:
A 3 sets 8–10
C 3 sets 8–10
F 3 sets 10–12
G 3 sets 10–12
I 3 sets 12–15
L 3 sets 12–15
O 20 per side
Q 15

Day Two:
Cardio 30–45 minutes

Day Three:
A 3 sets 8–10
C 3 sets 8–10
F 3 sets 10–12
G 3 sets 10–12
I 3 sets 12–15
L 3 sets 12–15
O 20 per side
Q 15

Day Four:
Rest

Day Five:
A 3 sets 8–10
C 3 sets 8–10
F 3 sets 10–12
G 3 sets 10–12
I 3 sets 12–15
L 3 sets 12–15
O 20 per side
Q 15

Day Six:
Cardio 30–45 minutes

Day Seven:
Rest

ADVANCED ROUTINE I

Day One:
A 3 sets 8–10
C 3 sets 8–10
F 3 sets 10–12
G 3 sets 10–12
I 3 sets 12–15
K 3 sets 10–12
L 3 sets 12–15
O 20 per side
Q 15
R 20 per side

Day Two:
Cardio 30–45 minutes

Day Three:
A 3 sets 8–10
C 3 sets 8–10
F 3 sets 10–12
G 3 sets 10–12
I 3 sets 12–15
K 3 sets 10–12
L 3 sets 12–15
O 20 per side
Q 15
R 20 per side

Day Four:
Cardio 30–45 minutes

Day Five:
A 3 sets 8–10
C 3 sets 8–10
F 3 sets 10–12
G 3 sets 10–12
I 3 sets 12–15
K 3 sets 10–12
L 3 sets 12–15
O 20 per side
Q 15
R 20 per side

Day Six:
Cardio 30–45 minutes

Day Seven:
Rest

BEGINNER ROUTINE 2

Day One:
B 3 sets 10–12
D 3 sets 15
E 3 sets 10–12
H 3 sets 12–15
J 3 sets 10–12
M 3 sets 25

Day Two:
Rest

Day Three:
B 3 sets 10–12
D 3 sets 15
E 3 sets 10–12
H 3 sets 12–15
J 3 sets 10–12
M 3 sets 25

Day Four:
Rest

Day Five:
B 3 sets 10–12
D 3 sets 15
E 3 sets 10–12
H 3 sets 12–15
J 3 sets 10–12
M 3 sets 25

Day Six:
Cardio 30–45 minutes

Day Seven:
Rest

INTERMEDIATE ROUTINE 2

Day One:
B 3 sets 10–12
D 3 sets 15
E 3 sets 10–12
H 3 sets 12–15
J 3 sets 10–12
M 3 sets 25
N 3 sets 20
P 3 sets 12–15

Day Two:
Cardio 30–45 minutes

Day Three:
B 3 sets 10–12
D 3 sets 15
E 3 sets 10–12
H 3 sets 12–15
J 3 sets 10–12
M 3 sets 25
N 3 sets 20
P 3 sets 12–15

Day Four:
Rest

Day Five:
B 3 sets 10–12
D 3 sets 15
E 3 sets 10–12
H 3 sets 12–15
J 3 sets 10–12
M 3 sets 25
N 3 sets 20
P 3 sets 12–15

Day Six:
Cardio 30–45 minutes

Day Seven:
Rest

ADVANCED ROUTINE 2

Day One:
B 3 sets 10–12
D 3 sets 15
E 3 sets 10–12
H 3 sets 12–15
J 3 sets 10–12
M 3 sets 25
N 3 sets 20
P 3 sets 12–15
S 3 sets 20
T 3 sets 20

Day Two:
Cardio 30–45 minutes

Day Three:
B 3 sets 10–12
D 3 sets 15
E 3 sets 10–12
H 3 sets 12–15
J 3 sets 10–12
M 3 sets 25
N 3 sets 20
P 3 sets 12–15
S 3 sets 20
T 3 sets 20

Day Four:
Cardio 30–45 minutes

Day Five:
B 3 sets 10–12
D 3 sets 15
E 3 sets 10–12
H 3 sets 12–15
J 3 sets 10–12
M 3 sets 25
N 3 sets 20
P 3 sets 12–15
S 3 sets 20
T 3 sets 20

Day Six:
Cardio 30–45 minutes

Day Seven:
Rest

LACROSSE WORKOUTS

A Lat Pulldown
page 42
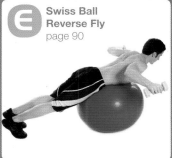

B Reverse Fly
page 88
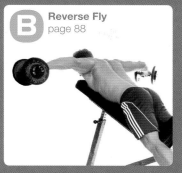

C Dumbbell Shoulder Press
page 74
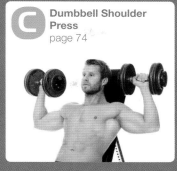

D Rotation Exercises
page 78
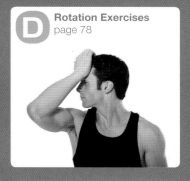

E Swiss Ball Reverse Fly
page 90
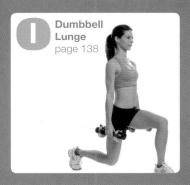

F Barbell Shoulder Shrug
page 94
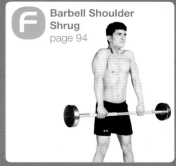

G Alternating Hammer Curl
page 98
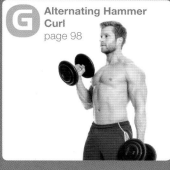

H Chair Dip
page 112
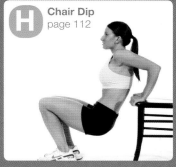

I Dumbbell Lunge
page 138
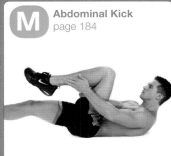

J Goblet Squat
page 150
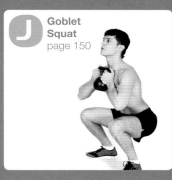

K Swiss Ball Hamstring Curl
page 164
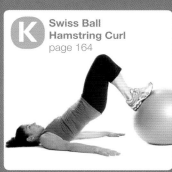

L Dumbbell Calf Raise
page 178
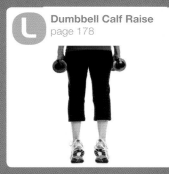

M Abdominal Kick
page 184
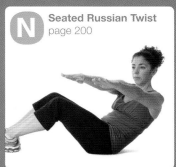

N Seated Russian Twist
page 200
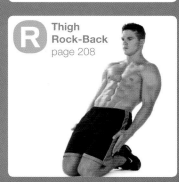

O Medicine Ball Wood Chop
page 130
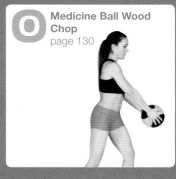

P Single-Arm Concentration Curl
page 102
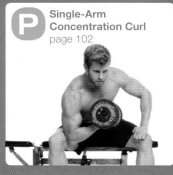

Q Hip Abduction and Adduction
page 204
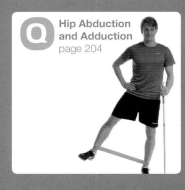

R Thigh Rock-Back
page 208
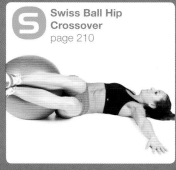

S Swiss Ball Hip Crossover
page 210
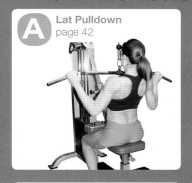

T The Windmill
page 216
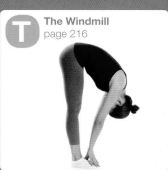

MOUNTAIN BIKING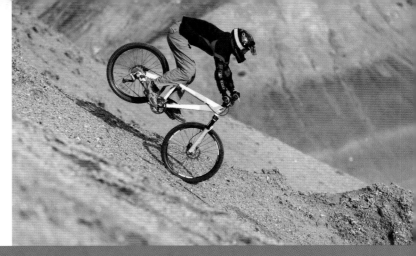

Core strength, conditioning and balance are some of the ingredients needed for successful runs on a mountain bike. Although the leg muscles are clearly paramount, many challenges such as steep-hill descents and ascents require strong upper-body musculature for successful completion. For example, the biceps, forearms and abdominal muscles are important for steering and stabilizing during an uphill climb. The core muscles are engaged almost constantly.

WORKOUT LEVEL 1

BEGINNER ROUTINE 1

Day One:
A 3 sets 8–10
C 3 sets 8–10
G 3 sets 8–10
H 3 sets 10–12
K 3 sets 10–12
M 3 sets 15–20

Day Two:
Rest

Day Three:
A 3 sets 8–10
C 3 sets 8–10
G 3 sets 8–10
H 3 sets 10–12
K 3 sets 10–12
M 3 sets 15–20

Day Four:
Rest

Day Five:
A 3 sets 8–10
C 3 sets 8–10
G 3 sets 8–10
H 3 sets 10–12
K 3 sets 10–12
M 3 sets 15–20

Day Six:
Cardio 30–45 minutes

Day Seven:
Rest

INTERMEDIATE ROUTINE 1

Day One:
A 3 sets 8–10
C 3 sets 8–10
G 3 sets 8–10
H 3 sets 10–12
K 3 sets 10–12
M 3 sets 15–20
N 3 sets 15–20
O 3 sets 12–15

Day Two:
Cardio 30–45 minutes

Day Three:
A 3 sets 8–10
C 3 sets 8–10
G 3 sets 8–10
H 3 sets 10–12
K 3 sets 10–12
M 3 sets 15–20
N 3 sets 15–20
O 3 sets 12–15

Day Four:
Rest

Day Five:
A 3 sets 8–10
C 3 sets 8–10
G 3 sets 8–10
H 3 sets 10–12
K 3 sets 10–12
M 3 sets 15–20
N 3 sets 15–20
O 3 sets 12–15

Day Six:
Cardio 30–45 minutes

Day Seven:
Rest

ADVANCED ROUTINE 1

Day One:
A 3 sets 8–10
C 3 sets 8–10
G 3 sets 8–10
H 3 sets 10–12
K 3 sets 10–12
M 3 sets 15–20
N 3 sets 15–20
O 3 sets 12–15
P 3 sets 12–15
Q 25 per side

Day Two:
Cardio 30–45 minutes

Day Three:
A 3 sets 8–10
C 3 sets 8–10
G 3 sets 8–10
H 3 sets 10–12
K 3 sets 10–12
M 3 sets 15–20
N 3 sets 15–20
O 3 sets 12–15
P 3 sets 12–15
Q 25 per side

Day Four:
Cardio 30–45 minutes

Day Five:
A 3 sets 8–10
C 3 sets 8–10
G 3 sets 8–10
H 3 sets 10–12
K 3 sets 10–12
M 3 sets 15–20
N 3 sets 15–20
O 3 sets 12–15
P 3 sets 12–15
Q 25 per side

Day Six:
Cardio 30–45 minutes

Day Seven:
Rest

WORKOUT LEVEL 2

BEGINNER ROUTINE 2

Day One:
B 3 sets 8–10
D 3 sets 12–15
E 3 sets 15
F 3 sets 12–15
I 3 sets 12–15
J 3 sets 12–15

Day Two:
Rest

Day Three:
B 3 sets 8–10
D 3 sets 12–15
E 3 sets 15
F 3 sets 12–15
I 3 sets 12–15
J 3 sets 12–15

Day Four:
Rest

Day Five:
B 3 sets 8–10
D 3 sets 12–15
E 3 sets 15
F 3 sets 12–15
I 3 sets 12–15
J 3 sets 12–15

Day Six:
Cardio 30–45 minutes

Day Seven:
Rest

INTERMEDIATE ROUTINE 2

Day One:
B 3 sets 8–10
D 3 sets 12–15
E 3 sets 15
F 3 sets 12–15
I 3 sets 12–15
J 3 sets 12–15
L 3 sets 12–15
R 3 sets 20

Day Two:
Cardio 30–45 minutes

Day Three:
B 3 sets 8–10
D 3 sets 12–15
E 3 sets 15
F 3 sets 12–15
I 3 sets 12–15
J 3 sets 12–15
L 3 sets 12–15
R 3 sets 20

Day Four:
Rest

Day Five:
B 3 sets 8–10
D 3 sets 12–15
E 3 sets 15
F 3 sets 12–15
I 3 sets 12–15
J 3 sets 12–15
L 3 sets 12–15
R 3 sets 20

Day Six:
Cardio 30–45 minutes

Day Seven:
Rest

ADVANCED ROUTINE 2

Day One:
B 3 sets 8–10
D 3 sets 12–15
E 3 sets 15
F 3 sets 12–15
I 3 sets 12–15
J 3 sets 12–15
L 3 sets 12–15
R 3 sets 20
S 3 sets 15
T 3 sets 15

Day Two:
Cardio 30–45 minutes

Day Three:
B 3 sets 8–10
D 3 sets 12–15
E 3 sets 15
F 3 sets 12–15
I 3 sets 12–15
J 3 sets 12–15
L 3 sets 12–15
R 3 sets 20
S 3 sets 15
T 3 sets 15

Day Four:
Cardio 30–45 minutes

Day Five:
B 3 sets 8–10
D 3 sets 12–15
E 3 sets 15
F 3 sets 12–15
I 3 sets 12–15
J 3 sets 12–15
L 3 sets 12–15
R 3 sets 20
S 3 sets 15
T 3 sets 15

Day Six:
Cardio 30–45 minutes

Day Seven:
Rest

MOUNTAIN BIKING WORKOUTS

A Dumbbell Pullover
page 40

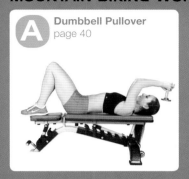

B Alternating Renegade Row
page 48

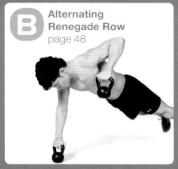

C Reverse Close-Grip Front Chin
page 54

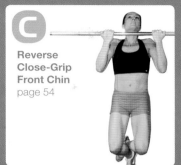

D Flat Bench Hyperextension
page 56

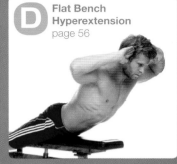

E Incline Bench Row
page 50

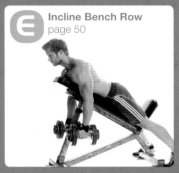

F External Rotation with Band
page 80

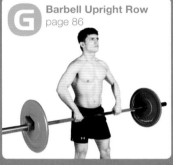

G Barbell Upright Row
page 86

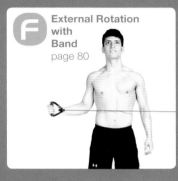

H Barbell Curl
page 100

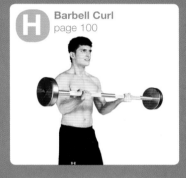

I Wrist Flexion
page 116

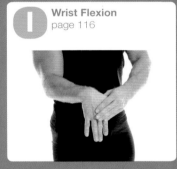

J Wrist Extension
page 117

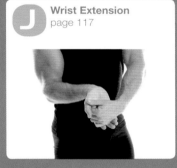

K Swiss Ball Wall Sit
page 134

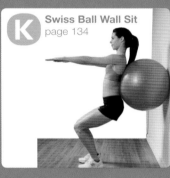

L Reverse Lunge
page 140

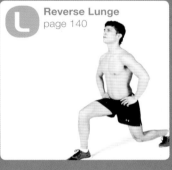

M Adductor Extension
page 162

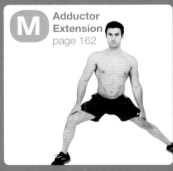

N Hamstring Abductor
page 163

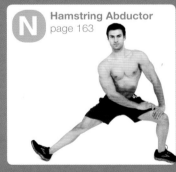

O Stiff-Legged Barbell Deadlift
page 168

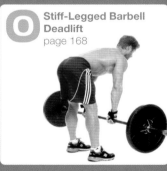

P Single-Leg Calf Press
page 176

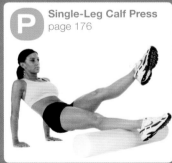

Q Abdominal Kick
page 184

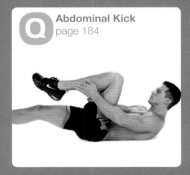

R Abdominal Hip Lift
page 186

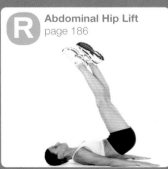

S Plank Press-Up
page 198

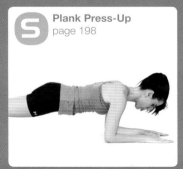

T Hip Abduction and Adduction
page 204

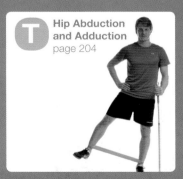

PADDLE BOARD

Paddle boarding, specifically, stand up paddle boarding (SUP), offers a great full-body workout. Here, the core is of paramount importance in stabilizing the athlete and offering ancillary assistance to other muscle groups. The paddling technique itself engages the deltoid, triceps and upper back, even on flat water. Changes in the water surface and the strength of the current affect the muscles being used but, generally speaking, the legs become more involved as the current increases.

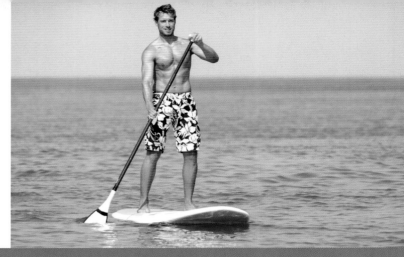

BEGINNER ROUTINE I

Day One:
B 3 sets 8–10
D 3 sets 10–12
E 3 sets 15
G 3 sets 10–12
J 3 sets 12–15
P 30–60 seconds per side

Day Two:
Rest

Day Three:
B 3 sets 8–10
D 3 sets 10–12
E 3 sets 15
G 3 sets 10–12
J 3 sets 12–15
P 30–60 seconds per side

Day Four:
Rest

Day Five:
B 3 sets 8–10
D 3 sets 10–12
E 3 sets 15
G 3 sets 10–12
J 3 sets 12–15
P 30–60 seconds per side

Day Six:
Cardio 30–45 minutes

Day Seven:
Rest

INTERMEDIATE ROUTINE I

Day One:
B 3 sets 8–10
D 3 sets 10–12
E 3 sets 15
G 3 sets 10–12
J 3 sets 12–15
K 3 sets 15–20
L 3 sets 15–20
P 30–60 seconds per side

Day Two:
Cardio 30–45 minutes

Day Three:
B 3 sets 8–10
D 3 sets 10–12
E 3 sets 15
G 3 sets 10–12
J 3 sets 12–15
K 3 sets 15–20
L 3 sets 15–20
P 30–60 seconds per side

Day Four:
Rest

Day Five:
B 3 sets 8–10
D 3 sets 10–12
E 3 sets 15
G 3 sets 10–12
J 3 sets 12–15
K 3 sets 15–20
L 3 sets 15–20
P 30–60 seconds per side

Day Six:
Cardio 30–45 minutes

Day Seven:
Rest

ADVANCED ROUTINE I

Day One:
B 3 sets 8–10
D 3 sets 10–12
E 3 sets 15
G 3 sets 10–12
J 3 sets 12–15
K 3 sets 15–20
L 3 sets 15–20
N 30 per side
P 30–60 seconds per side
T 25

Day Two:
Cardio 30–45 minutes

Day Three:
B 3 sets 8–10
D 3 sets 10–12
E 3 sets 15
G 3 sets 10–12
J 3 sets 12–15
K 3 sets 15–20
L 3 sets 15–20
N 30 per side

P 30–60 seconds per side
T 25

Day Four:
Cardio 30–45 minutes

Day Five:
B 3 sets 8–10
D 3 sets 10–12
E 3 sets 15
G 3 sets 10–12
J 3 sets 12–15
K 3 sets 15–20
L 3 sets 15–20
N 30 per side
P 30–60 seconds per side
T 25

Day Six:
Cardio 30–45 minutes

Day Seven:
Rest

BEGINNER ROUTINE 2

Day One:
A 3 sets 8–10
C 3 sets 10–12
F 3 sets 12–15
H 3 sets 12–15
I 3 sets 12–15
M 3 sets 25

Day Two:
Rest

Day Three:
A 3 sets 8–10
C 3 sets 10–12
F 3 sets 12–15
H 3 sets 12–15
I 3 sets 12–15
M 3 sets 25

Day Four:
Rest

Day Five:
A 3 sets 8–10
C 3 sets 10–12
F 3 sets 12–15
H 3 sets 12–15
I 3 sets 12–15
M 3 sets 25

Day Six:
Cardio 30–45 minutes

Day Seven:
Rest

INTERMEDIATE ROUTINE 2

Day One:
A 3 sets 8–10
C 3 sets 10–12
F 3 sets 12–15
H 3 sets 12–15
I 3 sets 12–15
M 3 sets 25
O 3 sets 20
Q 3 sets 15

Day Two:
Cardio 30–45 minutes

Day Three:
A 3 sets 8–10
C 3 sets 10–12
F 3 sets 12–15
H 3 sets 12–15
I 3 sets 12–15
M 3 sets 25
O 3 sets 20
Q 3 sets 15

Day Four:
Rest

Day Five:
A 3 sets 8–10
C 3 sets 10–12
F 3 sets 12–15
H 3 sets 12–15
I 3 sets 12–15
M 3 sets 25
O 3 sets 20
Q 3 sets 15

Day Six:
Cardio 30–45 minutes

Day Seven:
Rest

ADVANCED ROUTINE 2

Day One:
A 3 sets 8–10
C 3 sets 10–12
F 3 sets 12–15
H 3 sets 12–15
I 3 sets 12–15
M 3 sets 25
O 3 sets 20
Q 3 sets 15
R 3 sets 20
S 3 sets 20

Day Two:
Cardio 30–45 minutes

Day Three:
A 3 sets 8–10
C 3 sets 10–12
F 3 sets 12–15
H 3 sets 12–15
I 3 sets 12–15
M 3 sets 25
O 3 sets 20
Q 3 sets 15
R 3 sets 20
S 3 sets 20

Day Four:
Cardio 30–45 minutes

Day Five:
A 3 sets 8–10
C 3 sets 10–12
F 3 sets 12–15
H 3 sets 12–15
I 3 sets 12–15
M 3 sets 25
O 3 sets 20
Q 3 sets 15
R 3 sets 20
S 3 sets 20

Day Six:
Cardio 30–45 minutes

Day Seven:
Rest

PADDLE BOARD WORKOUTS

A Dumbbell Pullover
page 40
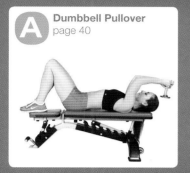

B Lat Pulldown
page 42
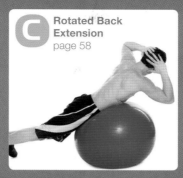

C Rotated Back Extension
page 58
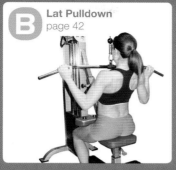

D Dumbbell Fly
page 64
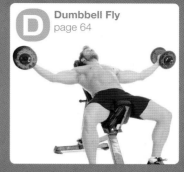

E Incline Bench Row
page 50
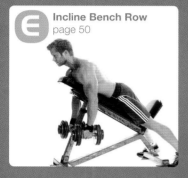

F External Rotation with Band
page 80
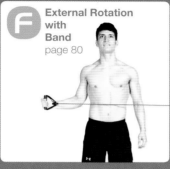

G Alternating Hammer Curl
page 98
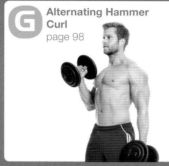

H Chair Dip
page 112
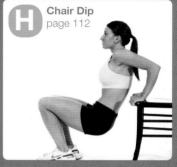

I Wrist Extension
page 117
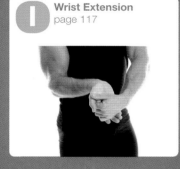

J Crossover Step
page 148
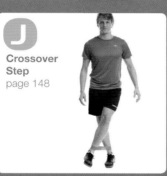

K Adductor Extension
page 162
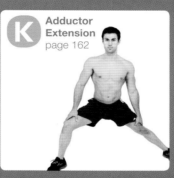

L Hamstring Abductor
page 163
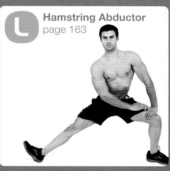

M Abdominal Kick
page 184
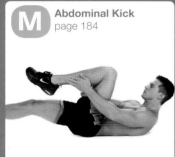

N Wood Chop with Resistance Band
page 202
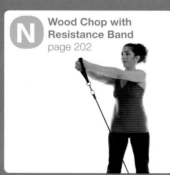

O Medicine Ball Wood Chop
page 130
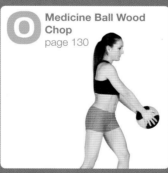

P T-Stabilization
page 124
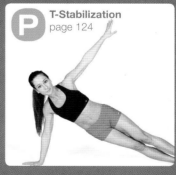

Q Hip Abduction and Adduction
page 204
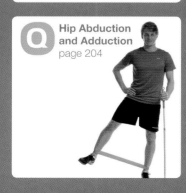

R Thigh Rock-Back
page 208
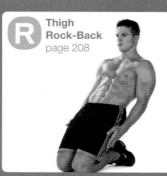

S Swiss Ball Hip Crossover
page 210
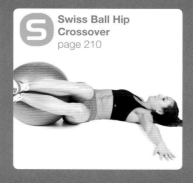

T Medicine Ball Slam
page 214
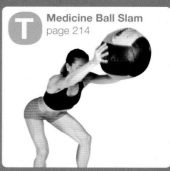

RACQUETBALL

Racquetball is a fast-paced sport that demands quick reflexes and great flexibility to rapidly change direction. It works just about every muscle group in the body, especially the lower body and the core. In addition to strength and speed, playing racquetball improves coordination, agility, balance and suppleness. The back, shoulders and triceps are the primary muscles used to direct a shot. The legs need strength to lunge for low shots and reach — or even leap — for overhead shots.

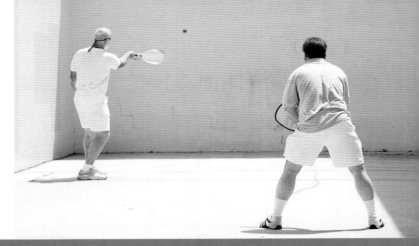

BEGINNER ROUTINE 1

Day One:
A 3 sets 6–8
B 3 sets 8–10
C 3 sets 15
G 3 sets 10–12
L 3 sets 10–12
P 30

Day Two:
Rest

Day Three:
A 3 sets 6–8
B 3 sets 8–10
C 3 sets 15
G 3 sets 10–12
L 3 sets 10–12
P 30

Day Four:
Rest

Day Five:
A 3 sets 6–8
B 3 sets 8–10
C 3 sets 15
G 3 sets 10–12
L 3 sets 10–12
P 30

Day Six:
Cardio 30–45 minutes

Day Seven:
Rest

INTERMEDIATE ROUTINE 1

Day One:
A 3 sets 6–8
B 3 sets 8–10
C 3 sets 15
F 3 sets 10–12
G 3 sets 10–12
L 3 sets 10–12
P 30
R 30–120 seconds

Day Two:
Cardio 30–45 minutes

Day Three:
A 3 sets 6–8
B 3 sets 8–10
C 3 sets 15
F 3 sets 10–12
G 3 sets 10–12
L 3 sets 10–12
P 30
R 30–120 seconds

Day Four:
Rest

Day Five:
A 3 sets 6–8
B 3 sets 8–10
C 3 sets 15
F 3 sets 10–12
G 3 sets 10–12
L 3 sets 10–12
P 30
R 30–120 seconds

Day Six:
Cardio 30–45 minutes

Day Seven:
Rest

ADVANCED ROUTINE 1

Day One:
A 3 sets 6–8
B 3 sets 8–10
C 3 sets 15
F 3 sets 10–12
G 3 sets 10–12
J 3 sets 10–12
L 3 sets 10–12
P 30
R 30–120 seconds
S 20 per side

Day Two:
Cardio 30–45 minutes

Day Three:
A 3 sets 6–8
B 3 sets 8–10
C 3 sets 15
F 3 sets 10–12
G 3 sets 10–12
J 3 sets 10–12
L 3 sets 10–12
P 30
R 30–120 seconds
S 20 per side

Day Four:
Cardio 30–45 minutes

Day Five:
A 3 sets 6–8
B 3 sets 8–10
C 3 sets 15
F 3 sets 10–12
G 3 sets 10–12
J 3 sets 10–12
L 3 sets 10–12
P 30
R 30–120 seconds
S 20 per side

Day Six:
Cardio 30–45 minutes

Day Seven:
Rest

BEGINNER ROUTINE 2

Day One:
D 3 sets 10–12
E 3 sets 10–12
H 3 sets 10–12
I 3 sets 10–12
K 3 sets 12–15
M 3 sets 12–15

Day Two:
Rest

Day Three:
D 3 sets 10–12
E 3 sets 10–12
H 3 sets 10–12
I 3 sets 10–12
K 3 sets 12–15
M 3 sets 12–15

Day Four:
Rest

Day Five:
D 3 sets 10–12
E 3 sets 10–12
H 3 sets 10–12
I 3 sets 10–12
K 3 sets 12–15
M 3 sets 12–15

Day Six:
Cardio 30–45 minutes

Day Seven:
Rest

INTERMEDIATE ROUTINE 2

Day One:
D 3 sets 10–12
E 3 sets 10–12
H 3 sets 10–12
I 3 sets 10–12
K 3 sets 12–15
M 3 sets 12–15
N 3 sets 25
O 3 sets 20

Day Two:
Cardio 30–45 minutes

Day Three:
D 3 sets 10–12
E 3 sets 10–12
H 3 sets 10–12
I 3 sets 10–12
K 3 sets 12–15
M 3 sets 12–15
N 3 sets 25
O 3 sets 20

Day Four:
Rest

Day Five:
D 3 sets 10–12
E 3 sets 10–12
H 3 sets 10–12
I 3 sets 10–12
K 3 sets 12–15
M 3 sets 12–15
N 3 sets 25
O 3 sets 20

Day Six:
Cardio 30–45 minutes

Day Seven:
Rest

ADVANCED ROUTINE 2

Day One:
D 3 sets 10–12
E 3 sets 10–12
H 3 sets 10–12
I 3 sets 10–12
K 3 sets 12–15
M 3 sets 12–15
N 3 sets 25
O 3 sets 20
Q 3 sets 20
T 3 sets 25

Day Two:
Cardio 30–45 minutes

Day Three:
D 3 sets 10–12
E 3 sets 10–12
H 3 sets 10–12
I 3 sets 10–12
K 3 sets 12–15
M 3 sets 12–15
N 3 sets 25
O 3 sets 20
Q 3 sets 20
T 3 sets 25

Day Four:
Cardio 30–45 minutes

Day Five:
D 3 sets 10–12
E 3 sets 10–12
H 3 sets 10–12
I 3 sets 10–12
K 3 sets 12–15
M 3 sets 12–15
N 3 sets 25
O 3 sets 20
Q 3 sets 20
T 3 sets 25

Day Six:
Cardio 30–45 minutes

Day Seven:
Rest

RACQUETBALL WORKOUTS

A Barbell Deadlift
page 34

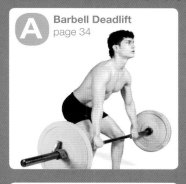

B Overhead Press
page 76

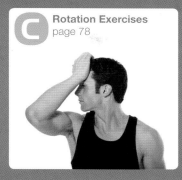

C Rotation Exercises
page 78

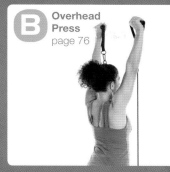

D Lateral Raise
page 82

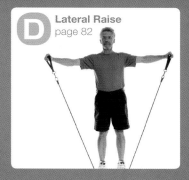

E Reverse Fly
page 88

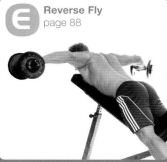

F Front-Plate Raise
page 92

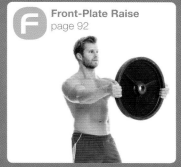

G Rope Pushdown
page 106

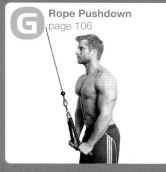

H Lying Triceps Extension
page 108

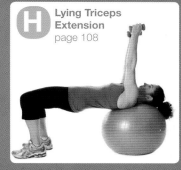

I Swiss Ball Wall Sit
page 134

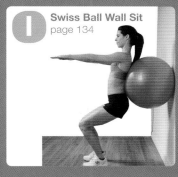

J Goblet Squat
page 150

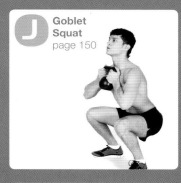

K Knee Extension with Rotation
page 154

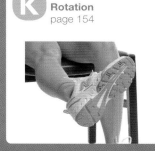

L Swiss Ball Hamstring Curl
page 164

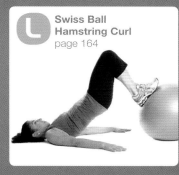

M Stiff-Legged Barbell Deadlift
page 168

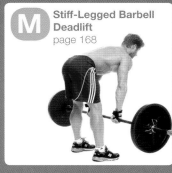

N Abdominal Kick
page 184

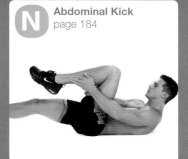

O Abdominal Hip Lift
page 186

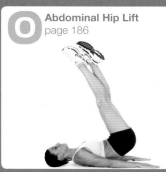

P Turkish Get-Up
page 188

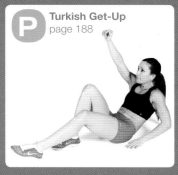

Q Reverse Crunch
page 192

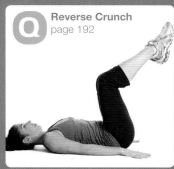

R Mountain Climber
page 158

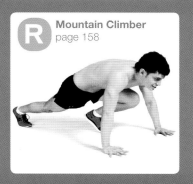

S Medicine Ball Wood Chop
page 130

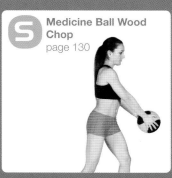

T Medicine Ball Slam
page 214

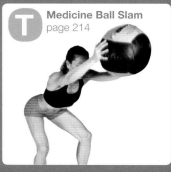

ROWING

Rowing is an excellent full-body and cardiovascular workout. The true power of the stroke is in your legs. The seat slides on rollers so that your legs can be extended to direct energy through the core and back. The shoulders and arms complete the stroke before the oars are raised from the water and your forearms and wrists come into play to rotate the oar so the blade is parallel to the water. You then engage the chest muscles to push the oars away and begin the next stroke.

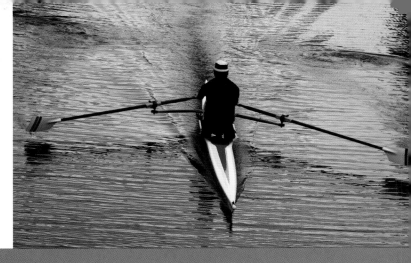

WORKOUT LEVEL 1

BEGINNER ROUTINE 1

Day One:
A 3 sets 8–10
C 3 sets 8–10
E 3 sets 8–10
F 3 sets 15
J 3 sets 10–12
N 3 sets 20

Day Two:
Rest

Day Three:
A 3 sets 8–10
C 3 sets 8–10
E 3 sets 8–10
F 3 sets 15
J 3 sets 10–12
N 3 sets 20

Day Four:
Rest

Day Five:
A 3 sets 8–10
C 3 sets 8–10
E 3 sets 8–10
F 3 sets 15
J 3 sets 10–12
N 3 sets 20

Day Six:
Cardio 30–45 minutes

Day Seven:
Rest

INTERMEDIATE ROUTINE 1

Day One:
A 3 sets 8–10
C 3 sets 8–10
E 3 sets 8–10
F 3 sets 15
H 3 sets 10–12
I 3 sets 10–12
J 3 sets 10–12
N 3 sets 20

Day Two:
Cardio 30–45 minutes

Day Three:
A 3 sets 8–10
C 3 sets 8–10
E 3 sets 8–10
F 3 sets 15
H 3 sets 10–12
I 3 sets 10–12
J 3 sets 10–12
N 3 sets 20

Day Four:
Rest

Day Five:
A 3 sets 8–10
C 3 sets 8–10
E 3 sets 8–10
F 3 sets 15
H 3 sets 10–12
I 3 sets 10–12
J 3 sets 10–12
N 3 sets 20

Day Six:
Cardio 30–45 minutes

Day Seven:
Rest

ADVANCED ROUTINE 1

Day One:
A 3 sets 8–10
C 3 sets 8–10
E 3 sets 8–10
F 3 sets 15
H 3 sets 10–12
I 3 sets 10–12
J 3 sets 10–12
N 3 sets 20
P 20
T 25

Day Two:
Cardio 30–45 minutes

Day Three:
A 3 sets 8–10
C 3 sets 8–10
E 3 sets 8–10
F 3 sets 15
H 3 sets 10–12
I 3 sets 10–12
J 3 sets 10–12
N 3 sets 20
P 20
T 25

Day Four:
Cardio 30–45 minutes

Day Five:
A 3 sets 8–10
C 3 sets 8–10
E 3 sets 8–10
F 3 sets 15
H 3 sets 10–12
I 3 sets 10–12
J 3 sets 10–12
N 3 sets 20
P 20
T 25

Day Six:
Cardio 30–45 minutes

Day Seven:
Rest

WORKOUT LEVEL 2

BEGINNER ROUTINE 2

Day One:
B 3 sets 8–10
D 3 sets 8–10
G 3 sets 10–12
K 3 sets 12–15
L 3 sets 12–15
M 3 sets 25

Day Two:
Rest

Day Three:
B 3 sets 8–10
D 3 sets 8–10
G 3 sets 10–12
K 3 sets 12–15
L 3 sets 12–15
M 3 sets 25

Day Four:
Rest

Day Five:
B 3 sets 8–10
D 3 sets 8–10
G 3 sets 10–12
K 3 sets 12–15
L 3 sets 12–15
M 3 sets 25

Day Six:
Cardio 30–45 minutes

Day Seven:
Rest

INTERMEDIATE ROUTINE 2

Day One:
B 3 sets 8–10
D 3 sets 8–10
G 3 sets 10–12
K 3 sets 12–15
L 3 sets 12–15
M 3 sets 25
O 3 sets 15
Q 3 sets 20

Day Two:
Cardio 30–45 minutes

Day Three:
B 3 sets 8–10
D 3 sets 8–10
G 3 sets 10–12
K 3 sets 12–15
L 3 sets 12–15
M 3 sets 25
O 3 sets 15
Q 3 sets 20

Day Four:
Rest

Day Five:
B 3 sets 8–10
D 3 sets 8–10
G 3 sets 10–12
K 3 sets 12–15
L 3 sets 12–15
M 3 sets 25
O 3 sets 15
Q 3 sets 20

Day Six:
Cardio 30–45 minutes

Day Seven:
Rest

ADVANCED ROUTINE 2

Day One:
B 3 sets 8–10
D 3 sets 8–10
G 3 sets 10–12
K 3 sets 12–15
L 3 sets 12–15
M 3 sets 25
O 3 sets 15
Q 3 sets 20
R 3 sets 20
S 3 sets 20

Day Two:
Cardio 30–45 minutes

Day Three:
B 3 sets 8–10
D 3 sets 8–10
G 3 sets 10–12
K 3 sets 12–15
L 3 sets 12–15
M 3 sets 25
O 3 sets 15
Q 3 sets 20

R 3 sets 20
S 3 sets 20

Day Four:
Cardio 30–45 minutes

Day Five:
B 3 sets 8–10
D 3 sets 8–10
G 3 sets 10–12
K 3 sets 12–15
L 3 sets 12–15
M 3 sets 25
O 3 sets 15
Q 3 sets 20
R 3 sets 20
S 3 sets 20

Day Six:
Cardio 30–45 minutes

Day Seven:
Rest

ROWING WORKOUTS

A Dumbbell Row
page 38

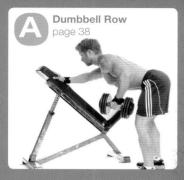

B Dumbbell Pullover
page 40

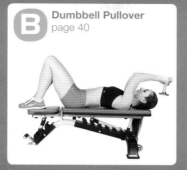

C Lat Pulldown
page 42

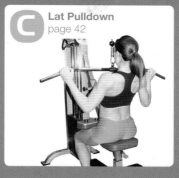

D Incline Bench Row
page 50

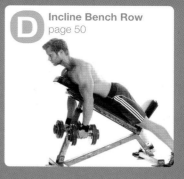

E Roller Push-Up
page 62

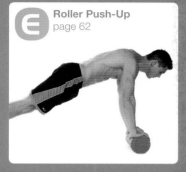

F Rotation Exercises
page 78

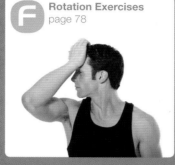

G Swiss Ball Reverse Fly
page 90

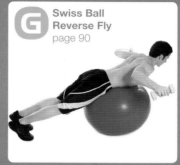

H Bicep Curl
page 96

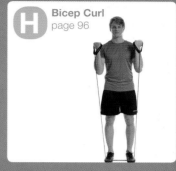

I Rope Pushdown
page 106

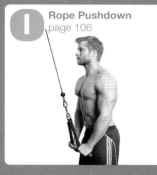

J Goblet Squat
page 150

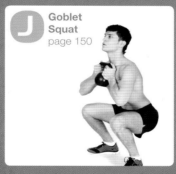

K Knee Extension with Rotation
page 154

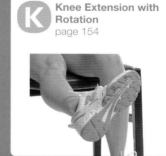

L Inverted Hamstring
page 166

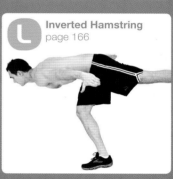

M Crunch
page 118

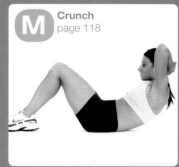

N Reverse Crunch
page 192

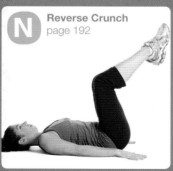

O Plank
page 120

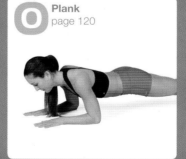

P Push-Up
page 70

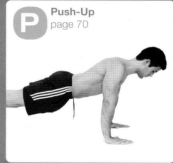

Q Swiss Ball Roll-Out
page 206

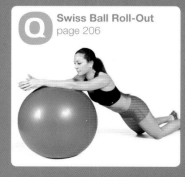

R Swiss Ball Hip Crossover
page 210

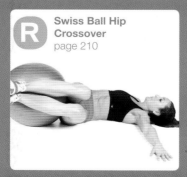

S V-Up
page 212

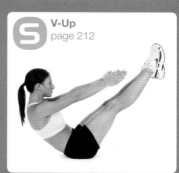

T Medicine Ball Slam
page 214

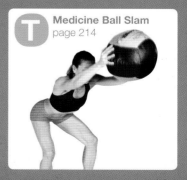

RUGBY

Not for the faint hearted, rugby is, nevertheless, a highly tactical sport that demands enormous strength whatever your position in the team. The forward, perhaps surprisingly, actually tend to be the biggest and strongest players — they're the ones who battle for the ball in set plays such as scrums and line outs. The backs tend to be smaller (relatively) and usually have greater individual skills in running, passing, catching, kicking and tackling, which require speed and flexibility.

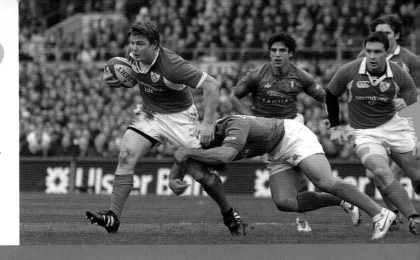

WORKOUT LEVEL 1

BEGINNER ROUTINE 1

Day One:
A 3 sets 6–8
D 3 sets 8–10
G 3 sets 10–12
J 3 sets 10–12
M 3 sets 10–12
Q 15

Day Two:
Rest

Day Three:
A 3 sets 6–8
D 3 sets 8–10
G 3 sets 10–12
J 3 sets 10–12
M 3 sets 10–12
Q 15

Day Four:
Rest

Day Five:
A 3 sets 6–8
D 3 sets 8–10
G 3 sets 10–12
J 3 sets 10–12
M 3 sets 10–12
Q 15

Day Six:
Cardio 30–45 minutes

Day Seven:
Rest

INTERMEDIATE ROUTINE 1

Day One:
A 3 sets 6–8
B 3 sets of 8–10
D 3 sets 8–10
E 3 sets of 8–10
G 3 sets 10–12
J 3 sets 10–12
M 3 sets 10–12
Q 15

Day Two:
Cardio 30–45 minutes

Day Three:
A 3 sets 6–8
B 3 sets of 8–10
D 3 sets 8–10
E 3 sets of 8–10
G 3 sets 10–12
J 3 sets 10–12
M 3 sets 10–12
Q 15

Day Four:
Rest

Day Five:
A 3 sets 6–8
B 3 sets of 8–10
D 3 sets 8–10
E 3 sets of 8–10
G 3 sets 10–12
J 3 sets 10–12
M 3 sets 10–12
Q 15

Day Six:
Cardio 30–45 minutes

Day Seven:
Rest

ADVANCED ROUTINE 1

Day One:
A 3 sets 6–8
B 3 sets of 8–10
D 3 sets 8–10
E 3 sets of 8–10
G 3 sets 10–12
J 3 sets 10–12
M 3 sets 10–12
N 3 sets 12–15
Q 15
S 20 per side

Day Two:
Cardio 30–45 minutes

Day Three:
A 3 sets 6–8
B 3 sets of 8–10
D 3 sets 8–10
E 3 sets of 8–10
G 3 sets 10–12
J 3 sets 10–12
M 3 sets 10–12
N 3 sets 12–15
Q 15
S 20 per side

Day Four:
Cardio 30–45 minutes

Day Five:
A 3 sets 6–8
B 3 sets of 8–10
D 3 sets 8–10
E 3 sets of 8–10
G 3 sets 10–12
J 3 sets 10–12
M 3 sets 10–12
N 3 sets 12–15
Q 15
S 20 per side

Day Six:
Cardio 30–45 minutes

Day Seven:
Rest

WORKOUT LEVEL 2

BEGINNER ROUTINE 2

Day One:
C 3 sets 12–15
F 3 sets 8–10
H 3 sets 10–12
I 3 sets 12–15
K 3 sets 12–15
L 3 sets 10–12

Day Two:
Rest

Day Three:
C 3 sets 12–15
F 3 sets 8–10
H 3 sets 10–12
I 3 sets 12–15
K 3 sets 12–15
L 3 sets 10–12

Day Four:
Rest

Day Five:
C 3 sets 12–15
F 3 sets 8–10
H 3 sets 10–12
I 3 sets 12–15
K 3 sets 12–15
L 3 sets 10–12

Day Six:
Cardio 30–45 minutes

Day Seven:
Rest

INTERMEDIATE ROUTINE 2

Day One:
C 3 sets 12–15
F 3 sets 8–10
H 3 sets 10–12
I 3 sets 12–15
K 3 sets 12–15
L 3 sets 10–12
O 3 sets 30
P 3 sets 20

Day Two:
Cardio 30–45 minutes

Day Three:
C 3 sets 12–15
F 3 sets 8–10
H 3 sets 10–12
I 3 sets 12–15
K 3 sets 12–15
L 3 sets 10–12
O 3 sets 30
P 3 sets 20

Day Four:
Rest

Day Five:
C 3 sets 12–15
F 3 sets 8–10
H 3 sets 10–12
I 3 sets 12–15
K 3 sets 12–15
L 3 sets 10–12
O 3 sets 30
P 3 sets 20

Day Six:
Cardio 30–45 minutes

Day Seven:
Rest

ADVANCED ROUTINE 2

Day One:
C 3 sets 12–15
F 3 sets 8–10
H 3 sets 10–12
I 3 sets 12–15
K 3 sets 12–15
L 3 sets 10–12
O 3 sets 30
P 3 sets 20
R 3 sets 20
T 3 sets 30–60 seconds

Day Two:
Cardio 30–45 minutes

Day Three:
C 3 sets 12–15
F 3 sets 8–10
H 3 sets 10–12
I 3 sets 12–15
K 3 sets 12–15
L 3 sets 10–12
O 3 sets 30
P 3 sets 20
R 3 sets 20

T 3 sets 30–60 seconds

Day Four:
Cardio 30–45 minutes

Day Five:
C 3 sets 12–15
F 3 sets 8–10
H 3 sets 10–12
I 3 sets 12–15
K 3 sets 12–15
L 3 sets 10–12
O 3 sets 30
P 3 sets 20
R 3 sets 20
T 3 sets 30–60 seconds

Day Six:
Cardio 30–45 minutes

Day Seven:
Rest

RUGBY WORKOUTS

A Barbell Deadlift
page 34
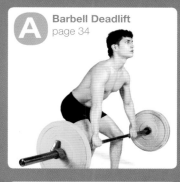

B Barbell Row
page 36
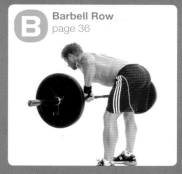

C Flat Bench Hyperextension
page 56
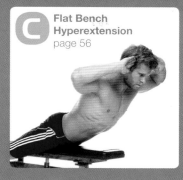

D Barbell Bench Press
page 60
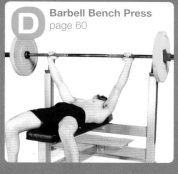

E Rope Overhead Extension
page 114
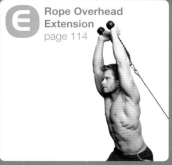

F Overhead Press
page 76
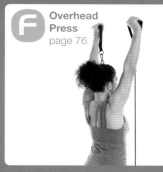

G Barbell Shoulder Shrug
page 94
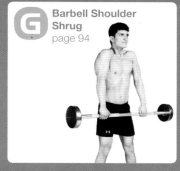

H Rope Pushdown
page 106
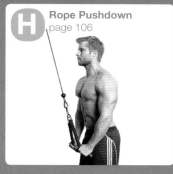

I Wrist Flexion
page 116
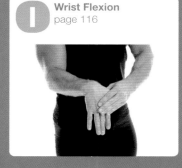

J Swiss Ball Wall Sit
page 134
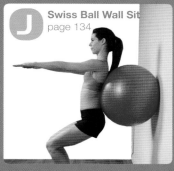

K High Lunge
page 146
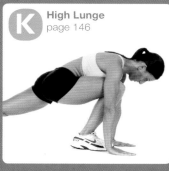

L Goblet Squat
page 150
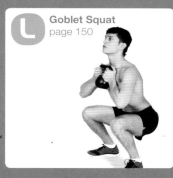

M Swiss Ball Hamstring Curl
page 164
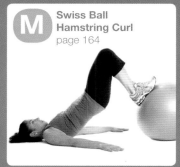

N Dumbbell Calf Raise
page 178
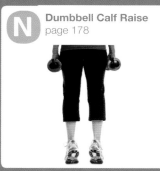

O Turkish Get-Up
page 188
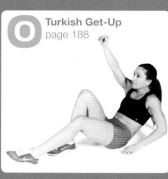

P Bicycle Crunch
page 190
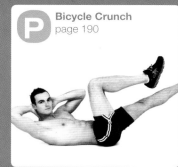

Q Plank Press-Up
page 198
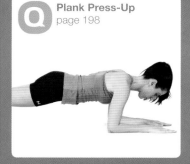

R Seated Russian Twist
page 200
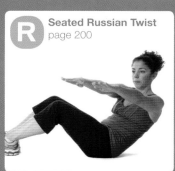

S Medicine Ball Wood Chop
page 130
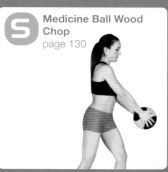

T T-Stabilization
page 124
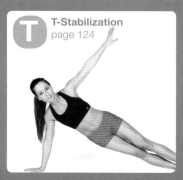

RUNNING

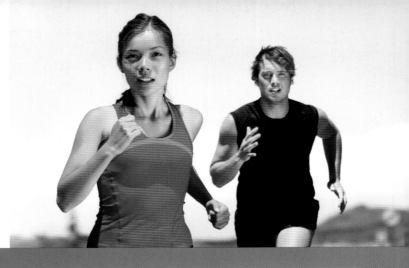

Required for survival in prehistoric times, running has been developed into a sport that is globally popular and highly competitive, providing an excellent cardiovascular workout. The muscles of the legs, hips, feet and abdomen are all critical to success, but they cannot function without a strong core for stabilization and balance. Long-distance runners particularly need to avoid building bulk during training. This workout is designed to get you on the fast track to running fitness.

WORKOUT LEVEL I

BEGINNER ROUTINE I

Day One:
A 3 sets 10–12
C 3 sets 12–15
E 3 sets 15–20
F 3 sets 15–20
H 3 sets 12–15
I 3 sets 12–15

Day Two:
Rest

Day Three:
A 3 sets 10–12
C 3 sets 12–15
E 3 sets 15–20
F 3 sets 15–20
H 3 sets 12–15
I 3 sets 12–15

Day Four:
Rest

Day Five:
A 3 sets 10–12
C 3 sets 12–15
E 3 sets 15–20
F 3 sets 15–20
H 3 sets 12–15
I 3 sets 12–15

Day Six:
Cardio 30–45 minutes

Day Seven:
Rest

INTERMEDIATE ROUTINE I

Day One:
A 3 sets 10–12
C 3 sets 12–15
D 3 sets 12–15
E 3 sets 15–20
F 3 sets 15–20
G 3 sets 12–15
H 3 sets 12–15
I 3 sets 12–15

Day Two:
Cardio 30–45 minutes

Day Three:
A 3 sets 10–12
C 3 sets 12–15
D 3 sets 12–15
E 3 sets 15–20
F 3 sets 15–20
G 3 sets 12–15
H 3 sets 12–15
I 3 sets 12–15

Day Four:
Rest

Day Five:
A 3 sets 10–12
C 3 sets 12–15
D 3 sets 12–15
E 3 sets 15–20
F 3 sets 15–20
G 3 sets 12–15
H 3 sets 12–15
I 3 sets 12–15

Day Six:
Cardio 30–45 minutes

Day Seven:
Rest

ADVANCED ROUTINE I

Day One:
A 3 sets 10–12
C 3 sets 12–15
D 3 sets 12–15
E 3 sets 15–20
F 3 sets 15–20
G 3 sets 12–15
H 3 sets 12–15
I 3 sets 12–15
Q 30–60 seconds per side
S 20

Day Two:
Cardio 30–45 minutes

Day Three:
A 3 sets 10–12
C 3 sets 12–15
D 3 sets 12–15
E 3 sets 15–20
F 3 sets 15–20
G 3 sets 12–15
H 3 sets 12–15
I 3 sets 12–15

Q 30–60 seconds per side
S 20

Day Four:
Cardio 30–45 minutes

Day Five:
A 3 sets 10–12
C 3 sets 12–15
D 3 sets 12–15
E 3 sets 15–20
F 3 sets 15–20
G 3 sets 12–15
H 3 sets 12–15
I 3 sets 12–15
Q 30–60 seconds per side
S 20

Day Six:
Cardio 30–45 minutes

Day Seven:
Rest

WORKOUT LEVEL 2

BEGINNER ROUTINE 2

Day One:
B 3 sets 12–15
J 3 sets 12–15
K 3 sets 25
L 3 sets 25
M 3 sets 30
N 3 sets 20

Day Two:
Rest

Day Three:
B 3 sets 12–15
J 3 sets 12–15
K 3 sets 25
L 3 sets 25
M 3 sets 30
N 3 sets 20

Day Four:
Rest

Day Five:
B 3 sets 12–15
J 3 sets 12–15
K 3 sets 25
L 3 sets 25
M 3 sets 30
N 3 sets 20

Day Six:
Cardio 30–45 minutes

Day Seven:
Rest

INTERMEDIATE ROUTINE 2

Day One:
B 3 sets 12–15
J 3 sets 12–15
K 3 sets 25
L 3 sets 25
M 3 sets 30
N 3 sets 20
O 3 sets 15
P 3 sets 30–60 seconds

Day Two:
Cardio 30–45 minutes

Day Three:
B 3 sets 12–15
J 3 sets 12–15
K 3 sets 25
L 3 sets 25
M 3 sets 30
N 3 sets 20
O 3 sets 15
P 3 sets 30–60 seconds

Day Four:
Rest

Day Five:
B 3 sets 12–15
J 3 sets 12–15
K 3 sets 25
L 3 sets 25
M 3 sets 30
N 3 sets 20
O 3 sets 15
P 3 sets 30–60 seconds

Day Six:
Cardio 30–45 minutes

Day Seven:
Rest

ADVANCED ROUTINE 2

Day One:
B 3 sets 12–15
J 3 sets 12–15
K 3 sets 25
L 3 sets 25
M 3 sets 30
N 3 sets 20
O 3 sets 15
P 3 sets 30–60 seconds
R 3 sets 15
T 3 sets 20

Day Two:
Cardio 30–45 minutes

Day Three:
B 3 sets 12–15
J 3 sets 12–15
K 3 sets 25
L 3 sets 25
M 3 sets 30
N 3 sets 20
O 3 sets 15
P 3 sets 30–60 seconds

R 3 sets 15
T 3 sets 20

Day Four:
Cardio 30–45 minutes

Day Five:
B 3 sets 12–15
J 3 sets 12–15
K 3 sets 25
L 3 sets 25
M 3 sets 30
N 3 sets 20
O 3 sets 15
P 3 sets 30–60 seconds
R 3 sets 15
T 3 sets 20

Day Six:
Cardio 30–45 minutes

Day Seven:
Rest

RUNNING WORKOUTS

A Swiss Ball Wall Sit
page 134
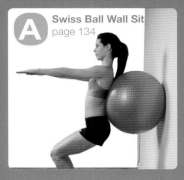

B Reverse Lunge
page 140
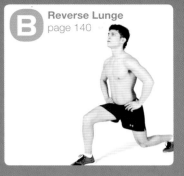

C Dumbbell Walking Lunge
page 144
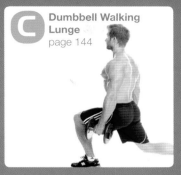

D Knee Extension with Rotation
page 154
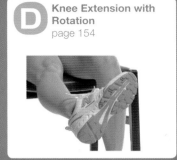

E Adductor Extension
page 162
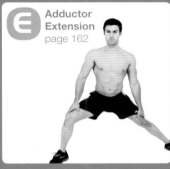

F Hamstring Abductor
page 163
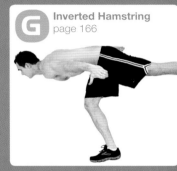

G Inverted Hamstring
page 166
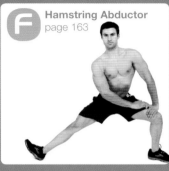

H Stiff-Legged Deadlift
page 174
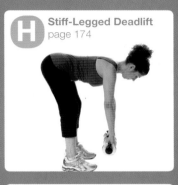

I Single-Leg Calf Press
page 176
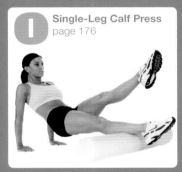

J Dumbbell Shin Raise
page 180
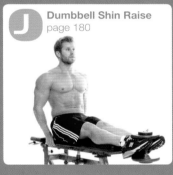

K Crunch
page 118
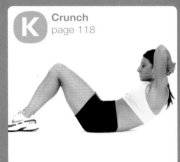

L Abdominal Kick
page 184
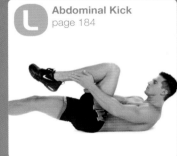

M Turkish Get-Up
page 188
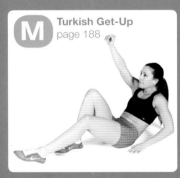

N Reverse Crunch
page 192
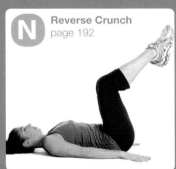

O Swiss Ball Pelvic Tilt
page 196
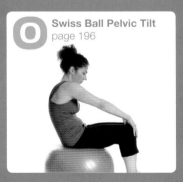

P Side Plank
page 122
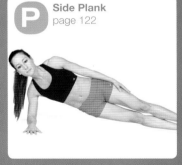

Q T-Stabilization
page 124
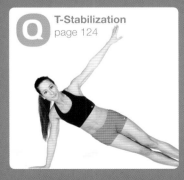

R Hip Abduction and Adduction
page 204
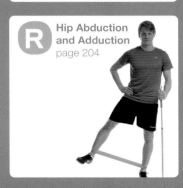

S Swiss Ball Jackknife
page 128
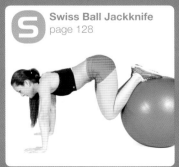

T Swiss Ball Hip Crossover
page 210
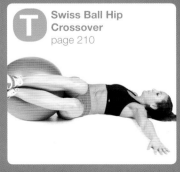

SAILING

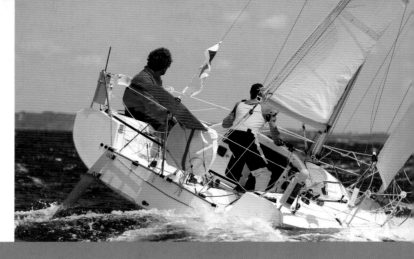

Racing a sailing dinghy or keelboat on a breezy day can be extremely demanding physically. "Hiking out" by leaning backward over the side to balance the boat needs strength in the quads, abs, lower back, knees, ankles, neck and shoulders. Meanwhile, you need arm and hand strength to hold the "sheet" (the rope that adjusts – trims – the sail) and prevent it sliding through the ratchet block. A small boat is very responsive to adjustments in your position and core strength is a must.

BEGINNER ROUTINE 1

Day One:
A 3 sets 8–10
B 3 sets 12–15
D 3 sets 8–10
G 3 sets 8–10
K 3 sets 12–15
N 3 sets 12–15

Day Two:
Rest

Day Three:
A 3 sets 8–10
B 3 sets 12–15
D 3 sets 8–10
G 3 sets 8–10
K 3 sets 12–15
N 3 sets 12–15

Day Four:
Rest

Day Five:
A 3 sets 8–10
B 3 sets 12–15
D 3 sets 8–10
G 3 sets 8–10
K 3 sets 12–15
N 3 sets 12–15

Day Six:
Cardio 30–45 minutes

Day Seven:
Rest

INTERMEDIATE ROUTINE 1

Day One:
A 3 sets 8–10
B 3 sets 12–15
D 3 sets 8–10
E 3 sets 12–15
F 20
G 3 sets 8–10
K 3 sets 12–15
N 3 sets 12–15

Day Two:
Cardio 30–45 minutes

Day Three:
A 3 sets 8–10
B 3 sets 12–15
D 3 sets 8–10
E 3 sets 12–15
F 20
G 3 sets 8–10
K 3 sets 12–15
N 3 sets 12–15

Day Four:
Rest

Day Five:
A 3 sets 8–10
B 3 sets 12–15
D 3 sets 8–10
E 3 sets 12–15
F 20
G 3 sets 8–10
K 3 sets 12–15
N 3 sets 12–15

Day Six:
Cardio 30–45 minutes

Day Seven:
Rest

ADVANCED ROUTINE 1

Day One:
A 3 sets 8–10
B 3 sets 12–15
D 3 sets 8–10
E 3 sets 12–15
F 20
G 3 sets 8–10
J 3 sets 10–12
K 3 sets 12–15
N 3 sets 12–15
R 3 sets 3–5 per side

Day Two:
Cardio 30–45 minutes

Day Three:
A 3 sets 8–10
B 3 sets 12–15
D 3 sets 8–10
E 3 sets 12–15
F 20
G 3 sets 8–10
J 3 sets 10–12
K 3 sets 12–15
N 3 sets 12–15
R 3 sets 3–5 per side

Day Four:
Cardio 30–45 minutes

Day Five:
A 3 sets 8–10
B 3 sets 12–15
D 3 sets 8–10
E 3 sets 12–15
F 20
G 3 sets 8–10
J 3 sets 10–12
K 3 sets 12–15
N 3 sets 12–15
R 3 sets 3–5 per side

Day Six:
Cardio 30–45 minutes

Day Seven:
Rest

BEGINNER ROUTINE 2

Day One:
C 3 sets 8–10
H 3 sets 8–10
I 3 sets 10–12
L 3 sets 12–15
M 3 sets 12–15
O 3 sets 15

Day Two:
Rest

Day Three:
C 3 sets 8–10
H 3 sets 8–10
I 3 sets 10–12
L 3 sets 12–15
M 3 sets 12–15
O 3 sets 15

Day Four:
Rest

Day Five:
C 3 sets 8–10
H 3 sets 8–10
I 3 sets 10–12
L 3 sets 12–15
M 3 sets 12–15
O 3 sets 15

Day Six:
Cardio 30–45 minutes

Day Seven:
Rest

INTERMEDIATE ROUTINE 2

Day One:
C 3 sets 8–10
H 3 sets 8–10
I 3 sets 10–12
L 3 sets 12–15
M 3 sets 12–15
O 3 sets 15
P 3 sets 30–120 seconds
Q 3 sets 30–60 seconds

Day Two:
Cardio 30–45 minutes

Day Three:
C 3 sets 8–10
H 3 sets 8–10
I 3 sets 10–12
L 3 sets 12–15
M 3 sets 12–15
O 3 sets 15
P 3 sets 30–120 seconds
Q 3 sets 30–60 seconds

Day Four:
Rest

Day Five:
C 3 sets 8–10
H 3 sets 8–10
I 3 sets 10–12
L 3 sets 12–15
M 3 sets 12–15
O 3 sets 15
P 3 sets 30–120 seconds
Q 3 sets 30–60 seconds

Day Six:
Cardio 30–45 minutes

Day Seven:
Rest

ADVANCED ROUTINE 2

Day One:
C 3 sets 8–10
H 3 sets 8–10
I 3 sets 10–12
L 3 sets 12–15
M 3 sets 12–15
O 3 sets 15
P 3 sets 30–120 seconds
Q 3 sets 30–60 seconds
S 20
T 3 sets 20

Day Two:
Cardio 30–45 minutes

Day Three:
C 3 sets 8–10
H 3 sets 8–10
I 3 sets 10–12
L 3 sets 12–15
M 3 sets 12–15
O 3 sets 15
P 3 sets 30–120 seconds
Q 3 sets 30–60 seconds
S 20
T 3 sets 20

Day Four:
Cardio 30–45 minutes

Day Five:
C 3 sets 8–10
H 3 sets 8–10
I 3 sets 10–12
L 3 sets 12–15
M 3 sets 12–15
O 3 sets 15
P 3 sets 30–120 seconds
Q 3 sets 30–60 seconds
S 20
T 3 sets 20

Day Six:
Cardio 30–45 minutes

Day Seven:
Rest

SAILING WORKOUTS

A Dumbbell Row
page 38

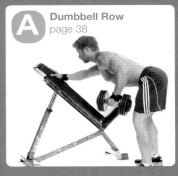

B Scapular Range of Motion
page 44

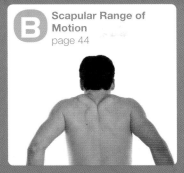

C Rope Pulldown
page 52

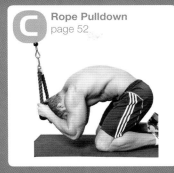

D Reverse Close-Grip Front Chin
page 54

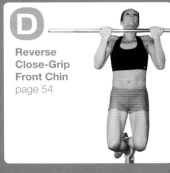

E Flat Bench Hyperextension
page 56

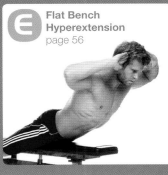

F Push-Up Hand Walk-Over
page 72

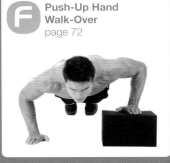

G Shoulder Raise and Pull
page 84

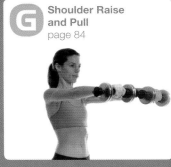

H Barbell Upright Row
page 86

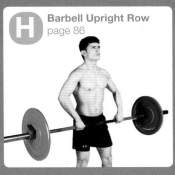

I Barbell Curl
page 100

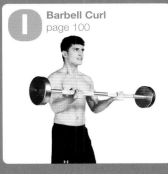

J Swiss Ball Wall Sit
page 134

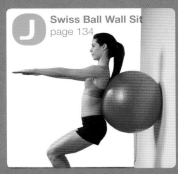

K Dumbbell Lunge
page 138

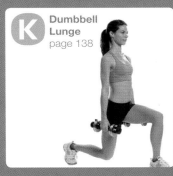

L Inverted Hamstring
page 166

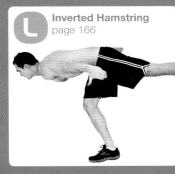

M Hamstring Pull-In
page 170

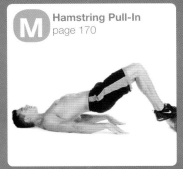

N Sumo Squat
page 172

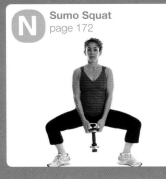

O Plank Press-Up
page 198

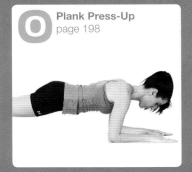

P Plank
page 120

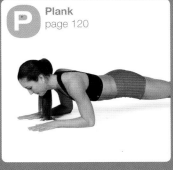

Q Side Plank
page 122

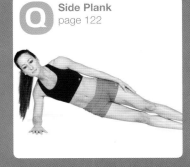

R Swiss Ball Walk-Around
page 126

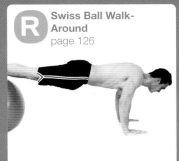

S Push-Up
page 70

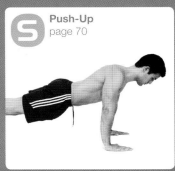

T The Windmill
page 216

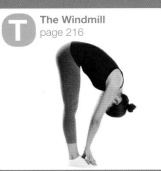

SHOOTING

It takes a lot of practice and conditioning to be able to hold a rifle steady, looking through the sight lines to correctly assess the location of the target and take an accurate shot. Upper-body muscles are at work for stabilization and strength, supported by the glutes, hamstrings and quads for proper extension at the hips and knees. However, if your core is not strong, you will experience difficulty holding a rifle with any degree of steadiness so core strength is paramount.

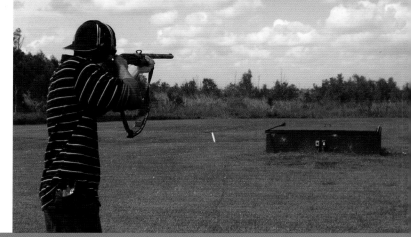

WORKOUT LEVEL 1

BEGINNER ROUTINE 1

Day One:
A 3 sets 8–10
C 3 sets 8–10
D 3 sets 8–10
E 3 sets 8–10
G 3 sets 12–15
H 3 sets 10–12

Day Two:
Rest

Day Three:
A 3 sets 8–10
C 3 sets 8–10
D 3 sets 8–10
E 3 sets 8–10
G 3 sets 12–15
H 3 sets 10–12

Day Four:
Rest

Day Five:
A 3 sets 8–10
C 3 sets 8–10
D 3 sets 8–10
E 3 sets 8–10
G 3 sets 12–15
H 3 sets 10–12

Day Six:
Cardio 30–45 minutes

Day Seven:
Rest

INTERMEDIATE ROUTINE 1

Day One:
A 3 sets 8–10
C 3 sets 8–10
D 3 sets 8–10
E 3 sets 8–10
G 3 sets 12–15
H 3 sets 10–12
J 3 sets 15–20
K 3 sets 15–20

Day Two:
Cardio 30–45 minutes

Day Three:
A 3 sets 8–10
C 3 sets 8–10
D 3 sets 8–10
E 3 sets 8–10
G 3 sets 12–15
H 3 sets 10–12
J 3 sets 15–20
K 3 sets 15–20

Day Four:
Rest

Day Five:
A 3 sets 8–10
C 3 sets 8–10
D 3 sets 8–10
E 3 sets 8–10
G 3 sets 12–15
H 3 sets 10–12
J 3 sets 15–20
K 3 sets 15–20

Day Six:
Cardio 30–45 minutes

Day Seven:
Rest

ADVANCED ROUTINE 1

Day One:
A 3 sets 8–10
C 3 sets 8–10
D 3 sets 8–10
E 3 sets 8–10
G 3 sets 12–15
H 3 sets 10–12
J 3 sets 15–20
K 3 sets 15–20
Q 30 per side
R 3 sets 8–10

Day Two:
Cardio 30–45 minutes

Day Three:
A 3 sets 8–10
C 3 sets 8–10
D 3 sets 8–10
E 3 sets 8–10
G 3 sets 12–15
H 3 sets 10–12
J 3 sets 15–20
K 3 sets 15–20
Q 30 per side
R 3 sets 8–10

Day Four:
Cardio 30–45 minutes

Day Five:
A 3 sets 8–10
C 3 sets 8–10
D 3 sets 8–10
E 3 sets 8–10
G 3 sets 12–15
H 3 sets 10–12
J 3 sets 15–20
K 3 sets 15–20
Q 30 per side
R 3 sets 8–10

Day Six:
Cardio 30–45 minutes

Day Seven:
Rest

WORKOUT LEVEL 2

BEGINNER ROUTINE 2

Day One:
B 3 sets 8–10
F 3 sets 10–12
I 3 sets 12–15
L 3 sets 12–15
M 3 sets 12–15
N 3 sets 25

Day Two:
Rest

Day Three:
B 3 sets 8–10
F 3 sets 10–12
I 3 sets 12–15
L 3 sets 12–15
M 3 sets 12–15
N 3 sets 25

Day Four:
Rest

Day Five:
B 3 sets 8–10
F 3 sets 10–12
I 3 sets 12–15
L 3 sets 12–15
M 3 sets 12–15
N 3 sets 25

Day Six:
Cardio 30–45 minutes

Day Seven:
Rest

INTERMEDIATE ROUTINE 2

Day One:
B 3 sets 8–10
F 3 sets 10–12
I 3 sets 12–15
L 3 sets 12–15
M 3 sets 12–15
N 3 sets 25
O 3 sets 15
P 3 sets 25

Day Two:
Cardio 30–45 minutes

Day Three:
B 3 sets 8–10
F 3 sets 10–12
I 3 sets 12–15
L 3 sets 12–15
M 3 sets 12–15
N 3 sets 25
O 3 sets 15
P 3 sets 25

Day Four:
Rest

Day Five:
B 3 sets 8–10
F 3 sets 10–12
I 3 sets 12–15
L 3 sets 12–15
M 3 sets 12–15
N 3 sets 25
O 3 sets 15
P 3 sets 25

Day Six:
Cardio 30–45 minutes

Day Seven:
Rest

ADVANCED ROUTINE 2

Day One:
B 3 sets 8–10
F 3 sets 10–12
I 3 sets 12–15
L 3 sets 12–15
M 3 sets 12–15
N 3 sets 25
O 3 sets 15
P 3 sets 25
S 3 sets 20
T 3 sets 20

Day Two:
Cardio 30–45 minutes

Day Three:
B 3 sets 8–10
F 3 sets 10–12
I 3 sets 12–15
L 3 sets 12–15
M 3 sets 12–15
N 3 sets 25
O 3 sets 15
P 3 sets 25
S 3 sets 20
T 3 sets 20

Day Four:
Cardio 30–45 minutes

Day Five:
B 3 sets 8–10
F 3 sets 10–12
I 3 sets 12–15
L 3 sets 12–15
M 3 sets 12–15
N 3 sets 25
O 3 sets 15
P 3 sets 25
S 3 sets 20
T 3 sets 20

Day Six:
Cardio 30–45 minutes

Day Seven:
Rest

SHOOTING WORKOUTS

A Dumbbell Row
page 38
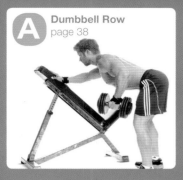

B Lat Pulldown
page 42
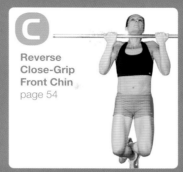

C Reverse Close-Grip Front Chin
page 54
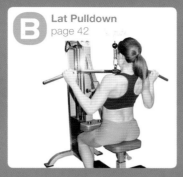

D Dips
page 68
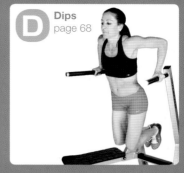

E Dumbbell Shoulder Press
page 74
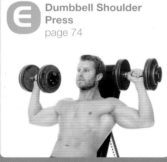

F Alternating Hammer Curl
page 98
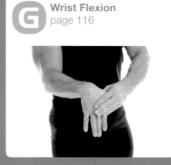

G Wrist Flexion
page 116
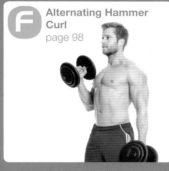

H Swiss Ball Wall-Sit
page 134
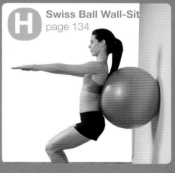

I Crossover Step
page 148
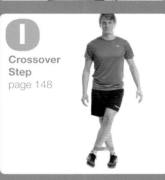

J Adductor Extension
page 162
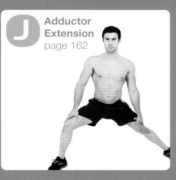

K Hamstring Abductor
page 163
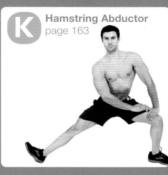

L Stiff-Legged Deadlift
page 174
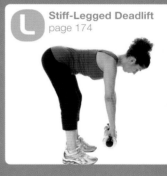

M Hamstring Pull-In
page 170
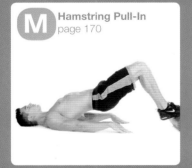

N Crunch
page 118
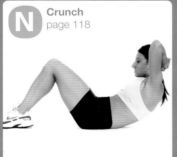

O Plank Press-Up
page 198
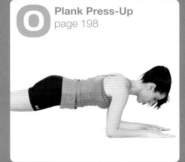

P Swiss Ball Walk-Around
page 126
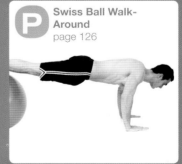

Q Wood Chop with Resistance Band
page 202
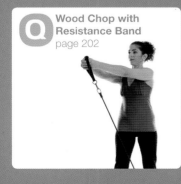

R Triceps Roll-Out
page 110
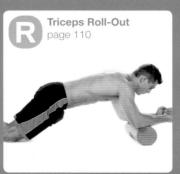

S Swiss Ball Jackknife
page 128
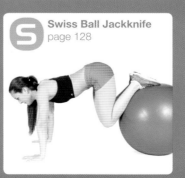

T Swiss Ball Roll-Out
page 206
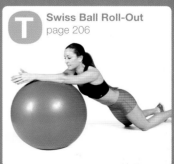

SKATEBOARDING

Once again, a good strong core is the basis for keeping the torso stabilized and strong when constantly adjusting your body position to stay balanced on your skateboard. Since the legs are doing most of the work in skateboarding, leg muscles need to be well conditioned and powerful, especially the biceps femoris and other hamstring muscles that are responsible for bending the legs. The trapezius muscle is used for shifting the shoulders during turning maneuvers.

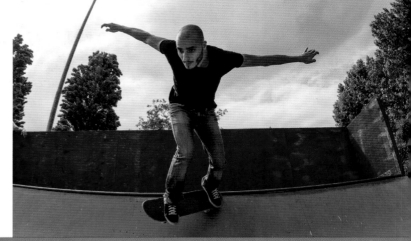

BEGINNER ROUTINE 1

Day One:
A 3 sets 12–15
D 3 sets 10–12
E 3 sets 10–12
G 3 sets 10–12
I 3 sets 12–15
M 30–120 seconds

Day Two:
Rest

Day Three:
A 3 sets 12–15
D 3 sets 10–12
E 3 sets 10–12
G 3 sets 10–12
I 3 sets 12–15
M 30–120 seconds

Day Four:
Rest

Day Five:
A 3 sets 12–15
D 3 sets 10–12
E 3 sets 10–12
G 3 sets 10–12
I 3 sets 12–15
M 30–120 seconds

Day Six:
Cardio 30–45 minutes

Day Seven:
Rest

INTERMEDIATE ROUTINE 1

Day One:
A 3 sets 12–15
D 3 sets 10–12
E 3 sets 10–12
G 3 sets 10–12
I 3 sets 12–15
M 30–120 seconds
N 30–60 seconds
O 3 sets 3–5 per side

Day Two:
Cardio 30–45 minutes

Day Three:
A 3 sets 12–15
D 3 sets 10–12
E 3 sets 10–12
G 3 sets 10–12
I 3 sets 12–15
M 30–120 seconds
N 30–60 seconds
O 3 sets 3–5 per side

Day Four:
Rest

Day Five:
A 3 sets 12–15
D 3 sets 10–12
E 3 sets 10–12
G 3 sets 10–12
I 3 sets 12–15
M 30–120 seconds
N 30–60 seconds
O 3 sets 3–5 per side

Day Six:
Cardio 30–45 minutes

Day Seven:
Rest

ADVANCED ROUTINE 1

Day One:
A 3 sets 12–15
D 3 sets 10–12
E 3 sets 10–12
G 3 sets 10–12
I 3 sets 12–15
M 30–120 seconds
N 30–60 seconds
O 3 sets 3–5 per side
P 3 sets 15
S 3 sets 25

Day Two:
Cardio 30–45 minutes

Day Three:
A 3 sets 12–15
D 3 sets 10–12
E 3 sets 10–12
G 3 sets 10–12
I 3 sets 12–15
M 30–120 seconds
N 30–60 seconds
O 3 sets 3–5 per side

P 3 sets 15
S 3 sets 25

Day Four:
Cardio 30–45 minutes

Day Five:
A 3 sets 12–15
D 3 sets 10–12
E 3 sets 10–12
G 3 sets 10–12
I 3 sets 12–15
M 30–120 seconds
N 30–60 seconds
O 3 sets 3–5 per side
P 3 sets 15
S 3 sets 25

Day Six:
Cardio 30–45 minutes

Day Seven:
Rest

BEGINNER ROUTINE 2

Day One:
B 3 sets 12–15
C 3 sets 8–10
F 3 sets 10–12
H 3 sets 12–15
J 3 sets 15
K 3 sets 15

Day Two:
Rest

Day Three:
B 3 sets 12–15
C 3 sets 8–10
F 3 sets 10–12
H 3 sets 12–15
J 3 sets 15
K 3 sets 15

Day Four:
Rest

Day Five:
B 3 sets 12–15
C 3 sets 8–10
F 3 sets 10–12
H 3 sets 12–15
J 3 sets 15
K 3 sets 15

Day Six:
Cardio 30–45 minutes

Day Seven:
Rest

INTERMEDIATE ROUTINE 2

Day One:
B 3 sets 12–15
C 3 sets 8–10
F 3 sets 10–12
H 3 sets 12–15
J 3 sets 15
K 3 sets 15
L 3 sets 15
Q 3 sets 20

Day Two:
Cardio 30–45 minutes

Day Three:
B 3 sets 12–15
C 3 sets 8–10
F 3 sets 10–12
H 3 sets 12–15
J 3 sets 15
K 3 sets 15
L 3 sets 15
Q 3 sets 20

Day Four:
Rest

Day Five:
B 3 sets 12–15
C 3 sets 8–10
F 3 sets 10–12
H 3 sets 12–15
J 3 sets 15
K 3 sets 15
L 3 sets 15
Q 3 sets 20

Day Six:
Cardio 30–45 minutes

Day Seven:
Rest

ADVANCED ROUTINE 2

Day One:
B 3 sets 12–15
C 3 sets 8–10
F 3 sets 10–12
H 3 sets 12–15
J 3 sets 15
K 3 sets 15
L 3 sets 15
Q 3 sets 20
R 3 sets 20
T 3 sets 20

Day Two:
Cardio 30–45 minutes

Day Three:
B 3 sets 12–15
C 3 sets 8–10
F 3 sets 10–12
H 3 sets 12–15
J 3 sets 15
K 3 sets 15
L 3 sets 15
Q 3 sets 20
R 3 sets 20
T 3 sets 20

Day Four:
Cardio 30–45 minutes

Day Five:
B 3 sets 12–15
C 3 sets 8–10
F 3 sets 10–12
H 3 sets 12–15
J 3 sets 15
K 3 sets 15
L 3 sets 15
Q 3 sets 20
R 3 sets 20
T 3 sets 20

Day Six:
Cardio 30–45 minutes

Day Seven:
Rest

SKATEBOARDING WORKOUTS

A Flat Bench Hyperextension
page 56
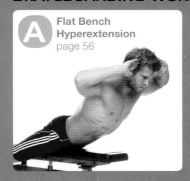

B Rotated Back Extension
page 58
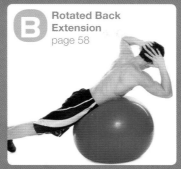

C Barbell Upright Row
page 86
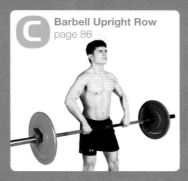

D Barbell Shoulder Shrug
page 94
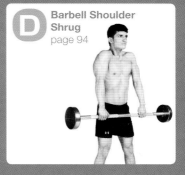

E Swiss Ball Wall Sit
page 134
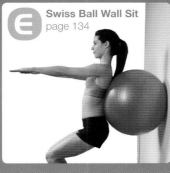

F Goblet Squat
page 150
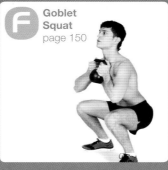

G Swiss Ball Hamstring Curl
page 164
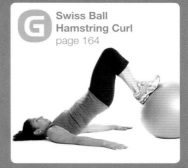

H Inverted Hamstring
page 166
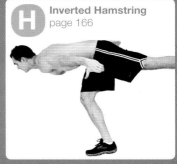

I Dumbbell Calf Raise
page 178
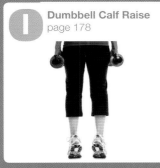

J Cobra Stretch
page 194
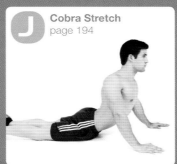

K Swiss Ball Pelvic Tilt
page 196
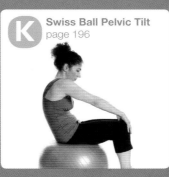

L Plank Press-Up
page 198
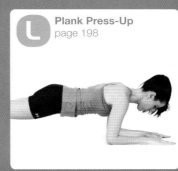

M Plank
page 120
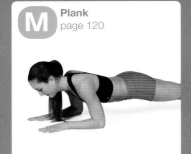

N Side Plank
page 122
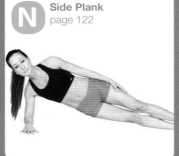

O Swiss Ball Walk-Around
page 126
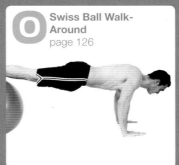

P Hip Abduction and Adduction
page 204
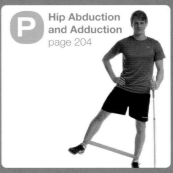

Q Swiss Ball Jackknife
page 128
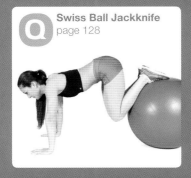

R Swiss Ball Roll-Out
page 206
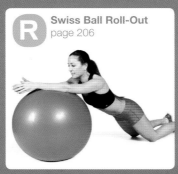

S Medicine Ball Slam
page 214
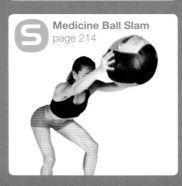

T The Windmill
page 216
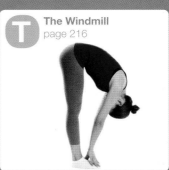

SKIING

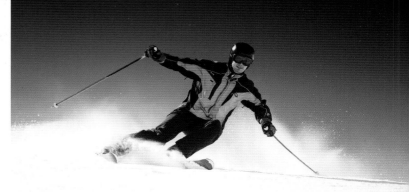

Skiing demands a series of complex interactions between your upper- and lower-body muscles. The core muscles orchestrate this interaction and help you maintain balance, which is the most essential skiing skill. Strong hamstrings perform the vital role of bending your knees and protecting your cruciate ligament — a highly sensitive knee ligament that is all-too-commonly damaged when skiing. The glutes assist in external leg rotation, which helps you to steer your skis.

WORKOUT LEVEL 1

BEGINNER ROUTINE I

Day One:
B 3 sets 10–12
E 3 sets 10–12
F 3 sets 10–12
G 3 sets 10–12
I 3 sets 12–15
P 30–120 seconds

Day Two:
Rest

Day Three:
B 3 sets 10–12
E 3 sets 10–12
F 3 sets 10–12
G 3 sets 10–12
I 3 sets 12–15
P 30 seconds - 2 minutes

Day Four:
Rest

Day Five:
B 3 sets 10–12
E 3 sets 10–12
F 3 sets 10–12
G 3 sets 10–12
I 3 sets 12–15
P 30 seconds - 2 minutes

Day Six:
Cardio 30–45 minutes

Day Seven:
Rest

INTERMEDIATE ROUTINE I

Day One:
A 3 sets 12–15
B 3 sets 10–12
E 3 sets 10–12
F 3 sets 10–12
G 3 sets 10–12
I 3 sets 12–15
M 3 sets 10–12
P 30–120 seconds

Day Two:
Cardio 30–45 minutes

Day Three:
A 3 sets 12–15
B 3 sets 10–12
E 3 sets 10–12
F 3 sets 10–12
G 3 sets 10–12
I 3 sets 12–15
M 3 sets 10–12
P 30–120 seconds

Day Four:
Rest

Day Five:
A 3 sets 12–15
B 3 sets 10–12
E 3 sets 10–12
F 3 sets 10–12
G 3 sets 10–12
I 3 sets 12–15
M 3 sets 10–12
P 30–120 seconds

Day Six:
Cardio 30–45 minutes

Day Seven:
Rest

ADVANCED ROUTINE I

Day One:
A 3 sets 12–15
B 3 sets 10–12
E 3 sets 10–12
F 3 sets 10–12
G 3 sets 10–12
I 3 sets 12–15
M 3 sets 10–12
O 3 sets 12–15
P 30–120 seconds
T 20

Day Two:
Cardio 30–45 minutes

Day Three:
A 3 sets 12–15
B 3 sets 10–12
E 3 sets 10–12
F 3 sets 10–12
G 3 sets 10–12
I 3 sets 12–15
M 3 sets 10–12
O 3 sets 12–15
P 30–120 seconds
T 20

Day Four:
Cardio 30–45 minutes

Day Five:
A 3 sets 12–15
B 3 sets 10–12
E 3 sets 10–12
F 3 sets 10–12
G 3 sets 10–12
I 3 sets 12–15
M 3 sets 10–12
O 3 sets 12–15
P 30–120 seconds
T 20

Day Six:
Cardio 30–45 minutes

Day Seven:
Rest

WORKOUT LEVEL 2

BEGINNER ROUTINE 2

Day One:
C 3 sets 20
D 3 sets 8–10
H 3 sets 12–15
J 3 sets 12–15
K 3 sets 15–20
L 3 sets 15–20

Day Two:
Rest

Day Three:
C 3 sets 20
D 3 sets 8–10
H 3 sets 12–15
J 3 sets 12–15
K 3 sets 15–20
L 3 sets 15–20

Day Four:
Rest

Day Five:
C 3 sets 20
D 3 sets 8–10
H 3 sets 12–15
J 3 sets 12–15
K 3 sets 15–20
L 3 sets 15–20

Day Six:
Cardio 30–45 minutes

Day Seven:
Rest

INTERMEDIATE ROUTINE 2

Day One:
C 3 sets 20
D 3 sets 8–10
H 3 sets 12–15
J 3 sets 12–15
K 3 sets 15–20
L 3 sets 15–20
N 3 sets 12–15
Q 3 sets 15

Day Two:
Cardio 30–45 minutes

Day Three:
C 3 sets 20
D 3 sets 8–10
H 3 sets 12–15
J 3 sets 12–15
K 3 sets 15–20
L 3 sets 15–20
N 3 sets 12–15
Q 3 sets 15

Day Four:
Rest

Day Five:
C 3 sets 20
D 3 sets 8–10
H 3 sets 12–15
J 3 sets 12–15
K 3 sets 15–20
L 3 sets 15–20
N 3 sets 12–15
Q 3 sets 15

Day Six:
Cardio 30–45 minutes

Day Seven:
Rest

ADVANCED ROUTINE 2

Day One:
C 3 sets 20
D 3 sets 8–10
H 3 sets 12–15
J 3 sets 12–15
K 3 sets 15–20
L 3 sets 15–20
N 3 sets 12–15
Q 3 sets 15
R 3 sets 20
S 3 sets 20

Day Two:
Cardio 30–45 minutes

Day Three:
C 3 sets 20
D 3 sets 8–10
H 3 sets 12–15
J 3 sets 12–15
K 3 sets 15–20
L 3 sets 15–20
N 3 sets 12–15
Q 3 sets 15
R 3 sets 20
S 3 sets 20

Day Four:
Cardio 30–45 minutes

Day Five:
C 3 sets 20
D 3 sets 8–10
H 3 sets 12–15
J 3 sets 12–15
K 3 sets 15–20
L 3 sets 15–20
N 3 sets 12–15
Q 3 sets 15
R 3 sets 20
S 3 sets 20

Day Six:
Cardio 30–45 minutes

Day Seven:
Rest

SKIING WORKOUTS

A Scapular Range of Motion
page 44
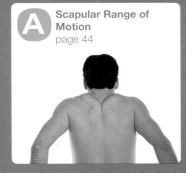

B Dumbbell Fly
page 64
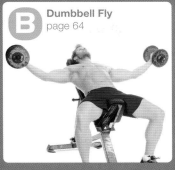

C Push-Up Hand Walk-Over
page 72
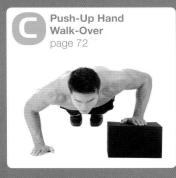

D Shoulder Raise and Pull
page 84
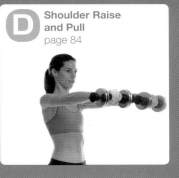

E Reverse Fly
page 88
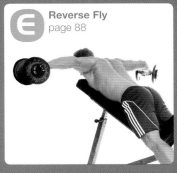

F Rope Hammer Curl
page 104
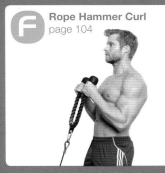

G Lying Triceps Extension
page 108
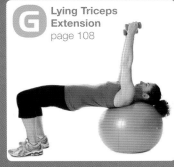

H Wrist Flexion
page 116
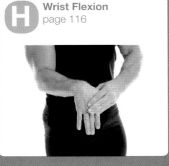

I Dumbbell Lunge
page 138
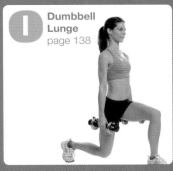

J One-Legged Step-Down
page 152
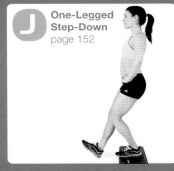

K Adductor Extension
page 162
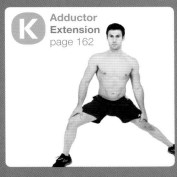

L Hamstring Abductor
page 163
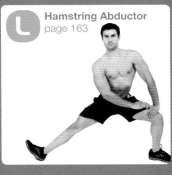

M Swiss-Ball Hamstring Curl
page 164
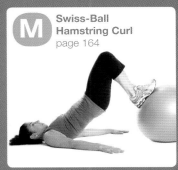

N Inverted Hamstring
page 166
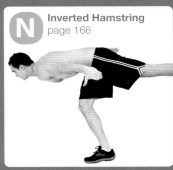

O Dumbbell Calf Raise
page 178
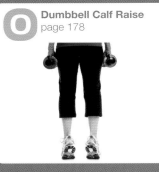

P Mountain Climber
page 158
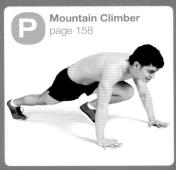

Q Hip Abduction and Adduction
page 204
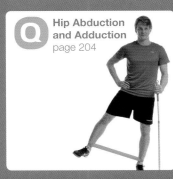

R Swiss Ball Jackknife
page 128
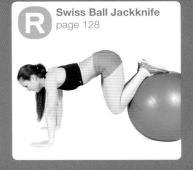

S Swiss Ball Hip Crossover
page 210
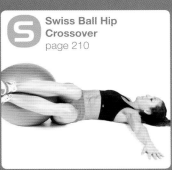

T V-Up
page 212
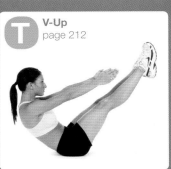

SNOWBOARDING

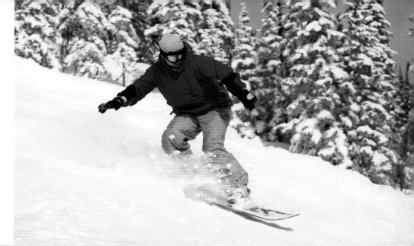

When snowboarding, the core needs to be strong to provide balance and stability. The quadriceps and hamstrings are used when boarding downhill as you continually adjust your center of gravity by flexing and extending the knees. The glute and hip muscles help with steering, and the muscles of the ankles and feet are key to turning. The shin and calf muscles need to be strong to support the flexion and extension of your feet while snow boarding over rapidly undulating surfaces.

WORKOUT LEVEL 1

BEGINNER ROUTINE I

Day One:
B 3 sets 8–10
C 3 sets 12–15
D 3 sets 10–12
J 3 sets 12–15
K 3 sets 12–15
Q 30–60 seconds per side

Day Two:
Rest

Day Three:
B 3 sets 8–10
C 3 sets 12–15
D 3 sets 10–12
J 3 sets 12–15
K 3 sets 12–15
Q 30–60 seconds per side

Day Four:
Rest

Day Five:
B 3 sets 8–10
C 3 sets 12–15
D 3 sets 10–12
J 3 sets 12–15
K 3 sets 12–15
Q 30–60 seconds per side

Day Six:
Cardio 30–45 minutes

Day Seven:
Rest

INTERMEDIATE ROUTINE I

Day One:
B 3 sets 8–10
C 3 sets 12–15
D 3 sets 10–12
G 3 sets 15–20
H 3 sets 15–20
J 3 sets 12–15
K 3 sets 12–15
Q 30–60 seconds per side

Day Two:
Cardio 30–45 minutes

Day Three:
B 3 sets 8–10
C 3 sets 12–15
D 3 sets 10–12
G 3 sets 15–20
H 3 sets 15–20
J 3 sets 12–15
K 3 sets 12–15
Q 30–60 seconds per side

Day Four:
Rest

Day Five:
B 3 sets 8–10
C 3 sets 12–15
D 3 sets 10–12
G 3 sets 15–20
H 3 sets 15–20
J 3 sets 12–15
K 3 sets 12–15
Q 30–60 seconds per side

Day Six:
Cardio 30–45 minutes

Day Seven:
Rest

ADVANCED ROUTINE I

Day One:
B 3 sets 8–10
C 3 sets 12–15
D 3 sets 10–12
G 3 sets 15–20
H 3 sets 15–20
J 3 sets 12–15
K 3 sets 12–15
O 30–120 seconds
Q 30–60 seconds per side
T 3 sets 20

Day Two:
Cardio 30–45 minutes

Day Three:
B 3 sets 8–10
C 3 sets 12–15
D 3 sets 10–12
G 3 sets 15–20
H 3 sets 15–20
J 3 sets 12–15
K 3 sets 12–15
O 30–120 seconds
Q 30–60 seconds per side
T 3 sets 20

Day Four:
Cardio 30–45 minutes

Day Five:
B 3 sets 8–10
C 3 sets 12–15
D 3 sets 10–12
G 3 sets 15–20
H 3 sets 15–20
J 3 sets 12–15
K 3 sets 12–15
O 30–120 seconds
Q 30–60 seconds per side
T 3 sets 20

Day Six:
Cardio 30–45 minutes

Day Seven:
Rest

WORKOUT LEVEL 2

BEGINNER ROUTINE 2

Day One:
A 3 sets 8–10
E 3 sets 12–15
F 3 sets 12–15
I 3 sets 10–12
L 3 sets 20
M 3 sets 30

Day Two:
Rest

Day Three:
A 3 sets 8–10
E 3 sets 12–15
F 3 sets 12–15
I 3 sets 10–12
L 3 sets 20
M 3 sets 30

Day Four:
Rest

Day Five:
A 3 sets 8–10
E 3 sets 12–15
F 3 sets 12–15
I 3 sets 10–12
L 3 sets 20
M 3 sets 30

Day Six:
Cardio 30–45 minutes

Day Seven:
Rest

INTERMEDIATE ROUTINE 2

Day One:
A 3 sets 8–10
E 3 sets 12–15
F 3 sets 12–15
I 3 sets 10–12
L 3 sets 20
M 3 sets 30
N 3 sets 15
P 3 sets 30

Day Two:
Cardio 30–45 minutes

Day Three:
A 3 sets 8–10
E 3 sets 12–15
F 3 sets 12–15
I 3 sets 10–12
L 3 sets 20
M 3 sets 30
N 3 sets 15
P 3 sets 30

Day Four:
Rest

Day Five:
A 3 sets 8–10
E 3 sets 12–15
F 3 sets 12–15
I 3 sets 10–12
L 3 sets 20
M 3 sets 30
N 3 sets 15
P 3 sets 30

Day Six:
Cardio 30–45 minutes

Day Seven:
Rest

ADVANCED ROUTINE 2

Day One:
A 3 sets 8–10
E 3 sets 12–15
F 3 sets 12–15
I 3 sets 10–12
L 3 sets 20
M 3 sets 30
N 3 sets 15
P 3 sets 30
R 3 sets 15
S 3 sets 20

Day Two:
Cardio 30–45 minutes

Day Three:
A 3 sets 8–10
E 3 sets 12–15
F 3 sets 12–15
I 3 sets 10–12
L 3 sets 20
M 3 sets 30
N 3 sets 15
P 3 sets 30
R 3 sets 15
S 3 sets 20

Day Four:
Cardio 30–45 minutes

Day Five:
A 3 sets 8–10
E 3 sets 12–15
F 3 sets 12–15
I 3 sets 10–12
L 3 sets 20
M 3 sets 30
N 3 sets 15
P 3 sets 30
R 3 sets 15
S 3 sets 20

Day Six:
Cardio 30–45 minutes

Day Seven:
Rest

SNOWBOARDING WORKOUTS

A Alternating Kettlebell Row
page 46
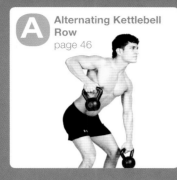

B Alternating Renegade Row
page 48
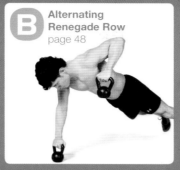

C Flat Bench Hyperextension
page 56
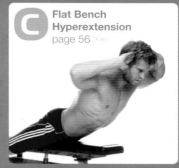

D Swiss Ball Wall Sit
page 134
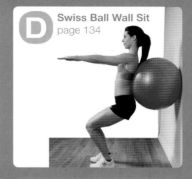

E Dumbbell Walking Lunge
page 144
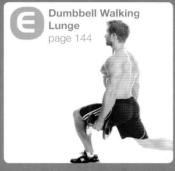

F Crossover Step
page 148
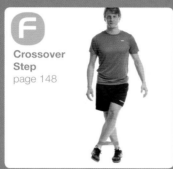

G Adductor Extension
page 162
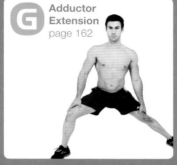

H Hamstring Abductor
page 163
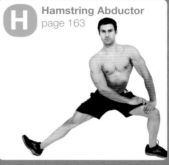

I Swiss Ball Hamstring Curl
page 164
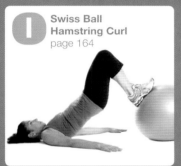

J Stiff-Legged Barbell Deadlift
page 168
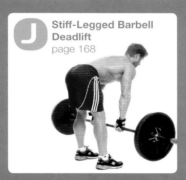

K Dumbbell Calf Raise
page 178
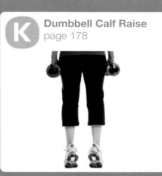

L Abdominal Hip Lift
page 186
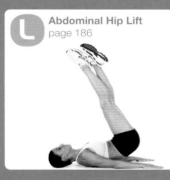

M Turkish Get-Up
page 188
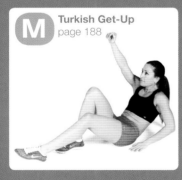

N Cobra Stretch
page 194
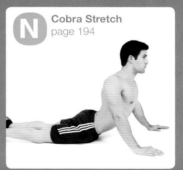

O Mountain Climber
page 158
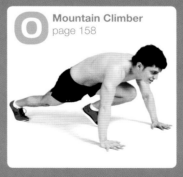

P Wood Chop with Resistance Band
page 202
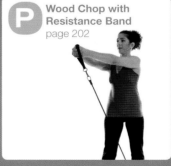

Q T-Stabilization
page 124
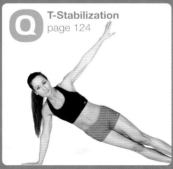

R Hip Abduction and Adduction
page 204
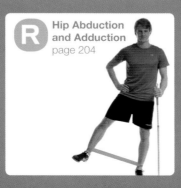

S Swiss Ball Hip Crossover
page 210
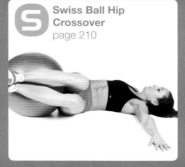

T V-Up
page 212
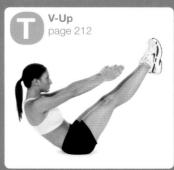

SOCCER

Soccer requires strong cardiovascular reserves and powerful legs as players cover many miles during the course of a game. Development of the leg muscles is also, of course, key to passing and shooting. Strong quads and hamstrings provide kicking power, while the ankles and calves aid balance and are particularly important when dribbling the ball. The core helps with stabilization and stamina, while upper-body strength is important when jostling for the ball during set pieces, such as corners.

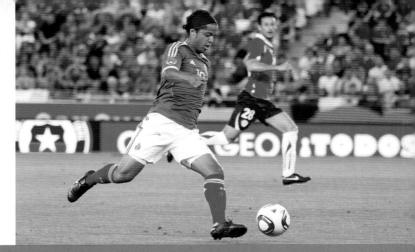

BEGINNER ROUTINE 1

Day One:
A 3 sets 8–10
D 3 sets 10–12
E 3 sets 12–15
F 3 sets 10–12
I 3 sets 12–15
J 3 sets 12–15

Day Two:
Rest

Day Three:
A 3 sets 8–10
D 3 sets 10–12
E 3 sets 12–15
F 3 sets 10–12
I 3 sets 12–15
J 3 sets 12–15

Day Four:
Rest

Day Five:
A 3 sets 8–10
D 3 sets 10–12
E 3 sets 12–15
F 3 sets 10–12
I 3 sets 12–15
J 3 sets 12–15

Day Six:
Cardio 30–45 minutes

Day Seven:
Rest

INTERMEDIATE ROUTINE 1

Day One:
A 3 sets 8–10
D 3 sets 10–12
E 3 sets 12–15
F 3 sets 10–12
G 3 sets 12–15
I 3 sets 12–15
J 3 sets 12–15
K 3 sets 12–15

Day Two:
Cardio 30–45 minutes

Day Three:
A 3 sets 8–10
D 3 sets 10–12
E 3 sets 12–15
F 3 sets 10–12
G 3 sets 12–15
I 3 sets 12–15
J 3 sets 12–15
K 3 sets 12–15

Day Four:
Rest

Day Five:
A 3 sets 8–10
D 3 sets 10–12
E 3 sets 12–15
F 3 sets 10–12
G 3 sets 12–15
I 3 sets 12–15
J 3 sets 12–15
K 3 sets 12–15

Day Six:
Cardio 30–45 minutes

Day Seven:
Rest

ADVANCED ROUTINE 1

Day One:
A 3 sets 8–10
D 3 sets 10–12
E 3 sets 12–15
F 3 sets 10–12
G 3 sets 12–15
I 3 sets 12–15
J 3 sets 12–15
K 3 sets 12–15
P 3 sets 20
S 3 sets 20

Day Two:
Cardio 30–45 minutes

Day Three:
A 3 sets 8–10
D 3 sets 10–12
E 3 sets 12–15
F 3 sets 10–12
G 3 sets 12–15
I 3 sets 12–15
J 3 sets 12–15
K 3 sets 12–15

P 3 sets 20
S 3 sets 20

Day Four:
Cardio 30–45 minutes

Day Five:
A 3 sets 8–10
D 3 sets 10–12
E 3 sets 12–15
F 3 sets 10–12
G 3 sets 12–15
I 3 sets 12–15
J 3 sets 12–15
K 3 sets 12–15
P 3 sets 20
S 3 sets 20

Day Six:
Cardio 30–45 minutes

Day Seven:
Rest

BEGINNER ROUTINE 2

Day One:
B 3 sets 12–15
C 3 sets 10–12
H 3 sets 12–15
L 3 sets 20
M 3 sets 30
N 3 sets 15

Day Two:
Rest

Day Three:
B 3 sets 12–15
C 3 sets 10–12
H 3 sets 12–15
L 3 sets 20
M 3 sets 30
N 3 sets 15

Day Four:
Rest

Day Five:
B 3 sets 12–15
C 3 sets 10–12
H 3 sets 12–15
L 3 sets 20
M 3 sets 30
N 3 sets 15

Day Six:
Cardio 30–45 minutes

Day Seven:
Rest

INTERMEDIATE ROUTINE 2

Day One:
B 3 sets 12–15
C 3 sets 10–12
H 3 sets 12–15
L 3 sets 20
M 3 sets 30
N 3 sets 15
O 3 sets 30–120 seconds
Q 3 sets 30

Day Two:
Cardio 30–45 minutes

Day Three:
B 3 sets 12–15
C 3 sets 10–12
H 3 sets 12–15
L 3 sets 20
M 3 sets 30
N 3 sets 15
O 3 sets 30–120 seconds
Q 3 sets 30

Day Four:
Rest

Day Five:
B 3 sets 12–15
C 3 sets 10–12
H 3 sets 12–15
L 3 sets 20
M 3 sets 30
N 3 sets 15
O 3 sets 30–120 seconds
Q 3 sets 30

Day Six:
Cardio 30–45 minutes

Day Seven:
Rest

ADVANCED ROUTINE 2

Day One:
B 3 sets 12–15
C 3 sets 10–12
H 3 sets 12–15
L 3 sets 20
M 3 sets 30
N 3 sets 15
O 3 sets 30–120 seconds
Q 3 sets 30
R 3 sets 15
T 3 sets 20

Day Two:
Cardio 30–45 minutes

Day Three:
B 3 sets 12–15
C 3 sets 10–12
H 3 sets 12–15
L 3 sets 20
M 3 sets 30
N 3 sets 15
O 3 sets 30–120 seconds
Q 3 sets 30

R 3 sets 15
T 3 sets 20

Day Four:
Cardio 30–45 minutes

Day Five:
B 3 sets 12–15
C 3 sets 10–12
H 3 sets 12–15
L 3 sets 20
M 3 sets 30
N 3 sets 15
O 3 sets 30–120 seconds
Q 3 sets 30
R 3 sets 15
T 3 sets 20

Day Six:
Cardio 30–45 minutes

Day Seven:
Rest

SOCCER WORKOUTS

A Overhead Press
page 76
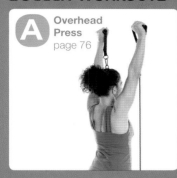

B External Rotation with Band
page 80
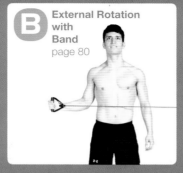

C Reverse Fly
page 88
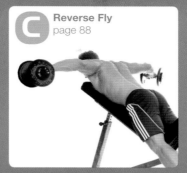

D Barbell Curl
page 100
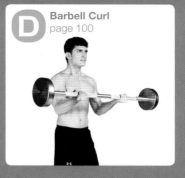

E Chair Dip
page 112
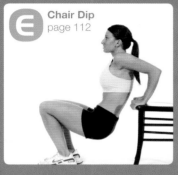

F Barbell Squat
page 136
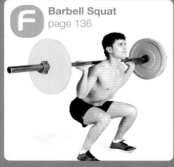

G Dumbbell Lunge
page 138
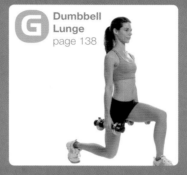

H One-Legged Step-Down
page 152
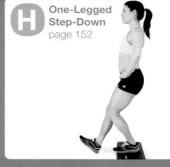

I Stiff-Legged Barbell Deadlift
page 168
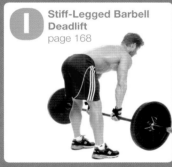

J Dumbbell Calf Raise
page 178
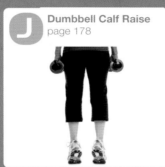

K Dumbbell Shin Raise
page 180
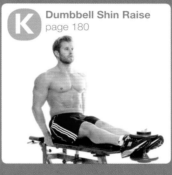

L Abdominal Hip Lift
page 186
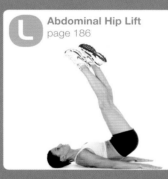

M Turkish Get-Up
page 188
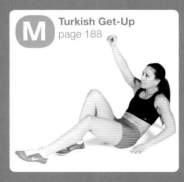

N Star Jump
page 156
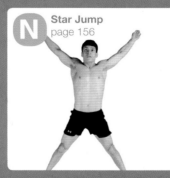

O Mountain Climber
page 158
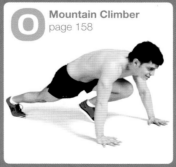

P Burpee
page 160
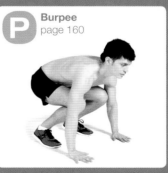

Q Wood Chop with Resistance Band
page 202
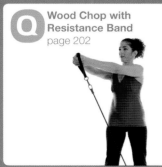

R Hip Abduction and Adduction
page 204
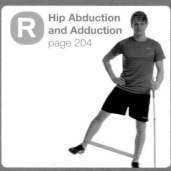

S Swiss Ball Roll-Out
page 206
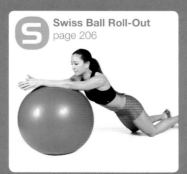

T The Windmill
page 216
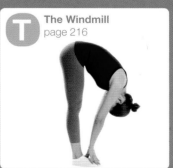

SQUASH

Squash is a high-speed racquet game that requires all-round strength and stamina to move rapidly around the court, and great reflexes and flexibility to quickly change direction. The shoulders are the primary muscles used for firing the ball, while strong triceps increase power. The forearms and wrists need to be strong to perform more subtle shots such as spins and drop shots. The core aids stabilization, while the leg muscles need to be strong for extension, flexion and running.

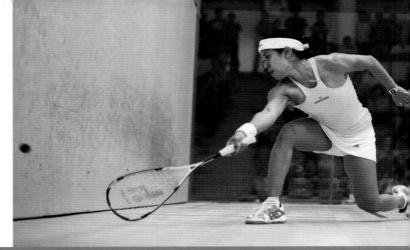

BEGINNER ROUTINE 1

Day One:
A 3 sets 6–8
B 3 sets 8–10
C 3 sets 15
G 3 sets 10–12
L 3 sets 10–12
P 30

Day Two:
Rest

Day Three:
A 3 sets 6–8
B 3 sets 8–10
C 3 sets 15
G 3 sets 10–12
L 3 sets 10–12
P 30

Day Four:
Rest

Day Five:
A 3 sets 6–8
B 3 sets 8–10
C 3 sets 15
G 3 sets 10–12
L 3 sets 10–12
P 30

Day Six:
Cardio 30–45 minutes

Day Seven:
Rest

INTERMEDIATE ROUTINE 1

Day One:
A 3 sets 6–8
B 3 sets 8–10
C 3 sets 15
F 3 sets 10–12
G 3 sets 10–12
L 3 sets 10–12
P 30
R 30–120 seconds

Day Two:
Cardio 30–45 minutes

Day Three:
A 3 sets 6–8
B 3 sets 8–10
C 3 sets 15
F 3 sets 10–12
G 3 sets 10–12
L 3 sets 10–12
P 30
R 30–120 seconds

Day Four:
Rest

Day Five:
A 3 sets 6–8
B 3 sets 8–10
C 3 sets 15
F 3 sets 10–12
G 3 sets 10–12
L 3 sets 10–12
P 30
R 30–120 seconds

Day Six:
Cardio 30–45 minutes

Day Seven:
Rest

ADVANCED ROUTINE 1

Day One:
A 3 sets 6–8
B 3 sets 8–10
C 3 sets 15
F 3 sets 10–12
G 3 sets 10–12
J 3 sets 10–12
L 3 sets 10–12
P 30
R 30–120 seconds
S 20 per side

Day Two:
Cardio 30–45 minutes

Day Three:
A 3 sets 6–8
B 3 sets 8–10
C 3 sets 15
F 3 sets 10–12
G 3 sets 10–12
J 3 sets 10–12
L 3 sets 10–12
P 30
R 30–120 seconds
S 20 per side

Day Four:
Cardio 30–45 minutes

Day Five:
A 3 sets 6–8
B 3 sets 8–10
C 3 sets 15
F 3 sets 10–12
G 3 sets 10–12
J 3 sets 10–12
L 3 sets 10–12
P 30
R 30–120 seconds
S 20 per side

Day Six:
Cardio 30–45 minutes

Day Seven:
Rest

BEGINNER ROUTINE 2

Day One
D 3 sets 10–12
E 3 sets 10–12
H 3 sets 10–12
I 3 sets 10–12
K 3 sets 12–15
M 3 sets 12–15

Day Two:
Rest

Day Three:
D 3 sets 10–12
E 3 sets 10–12
H 3 sets 10–12
I 3 sets 10–12
K 3 sets 12–15
M 3 sets 12–15

Day Four:
Rest

Day Five:
D 3 sets 10–12
E 3 sets 10–12
H 3 sets 10–12
I 3 sets 10–12
K 3 sets 12–15
M 3 sets 12–15

Day Six:
Cardio 30–45 minutes

Day Seven
Rest

INTERMEDIATE ROUTINE 2

Day One
D 3 sets 10–12
E 3 sets 10–12
H 3 sets 10–12
I 3 sets 10–12
K 3 sets 12–15
M 3 sets 12–15
N 3 sets 25
O 3 sets 20

Day Two:
Cardio 30–45 minutes

Day Three:
D 3 sets 10–12
E 3 sets 10–12
H 3 sets 10–12
I 3 sets 10–12
K 3 sets 12–15
M 3 sets 12–15
N 3 sets 25
O 3 sets 20

Day Four:
Rest

Day Five:
D 3 sets 10–12
E 3 sets 10–12
H 3 sets 10–12
I 3 sets 10–12
K 3 sets 12–15
M 3 sets 12–15
N 3 sets 25
O 3 sets 20

Day Six:
Cardio 30–45 minutes

Day Seven
Rest

ADVANCED ROUTINE 2

Day One
D 3 sets 10–12
E 3 sets 10–12
H 3 sets 10–12
I 3 sets 10–12
K 3 sets 12–15
M 3 sets 12–15
N 3 sets 25
O 3 sets 20
Q 3 sets 20
T 3 sets 25

Day Two:
Cardio 30–45 minutes

Day Three:
D 3 sets 10–12
E 3 sets 10–12
H 3 sets 10–12
I 3 sets 10–12
K 3 sets 12–15
M 3 sets 12–15
N 3 sets 25
O 3 sets 20
Q 3 sets 20
T 3 sets 25

Day Four:
Cardio 30–45 minutes

Day Five:
D 3 sets 10–12
E 3 sets 10–12
H 3 sets 10–12
I 3 sets 10–12
K 3 sets 12–15
M 3 sets 12–15
N 3 sets 25
O 3 sets 20
Q 3 sets 20
T 3 sets 25

Day Six:
Cardio 30–45 minutes

Day Seven
Rest

SQUASH WORKOUTS

A Barbell Deadlift
page 34

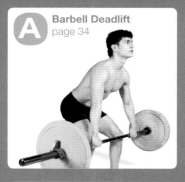

B Overhead Press
page 76

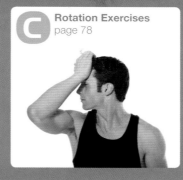

C Rotation Exercises
page 78

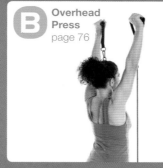

D Lateral Raise
page 82

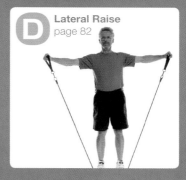

E Reverse Fly
page 88

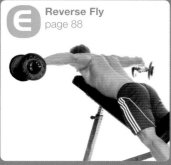

F Front-Plate Raise
page 92

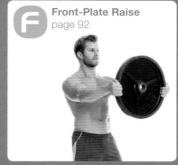

G Rope Pushdown
page 106

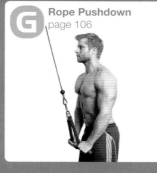

H Lying Triceps Extension
page 108

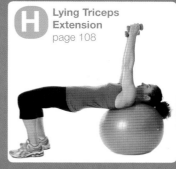

I Swiss Ball Wall Sit
page 134

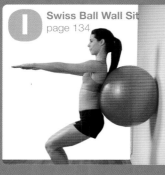

J Goblet Squat
page 150

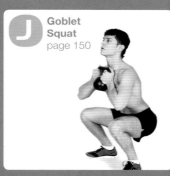

K Knee Extension with Rotation
page 154

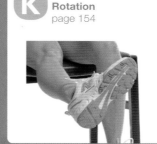

L Swiss Ball Hamstring Curl
page 164

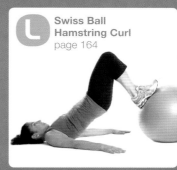

M Stiff-Legged Barbell Deadlift
page 168

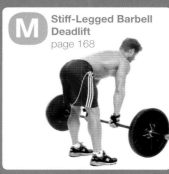

N Abdominal Kick
page 184

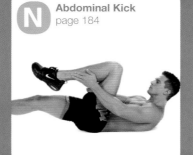

O Abdominal Hip Lift
page 186

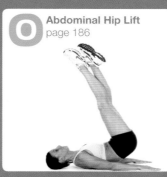

P Turkish Get-Up
page 188

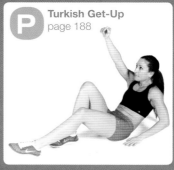

Q Reverse Crunch
page 192

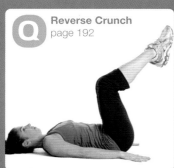

R Mountain Climber
page 158

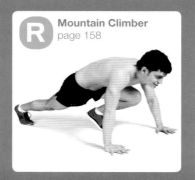

S Medicine Ball Wood Chop
page 130

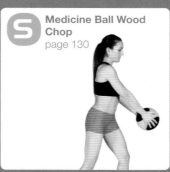

T Medicine Ball Slam
page 214

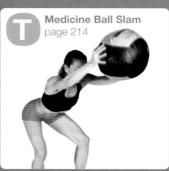

SURFING

The shoulders and arms are used when paddling out to catch a wave. The core is mainly responsible for stability while standing on the surfboard as the surfer constantly adjusts the position of the torso to maintain balance. The legs, too, are clearly hugely important when riding a wave. The hamstrings particularly need to be powerful to lower your center of gravity by bending the knees while travelling at speed. The calves, ankles and feet also need to be strong to help maintain balance.

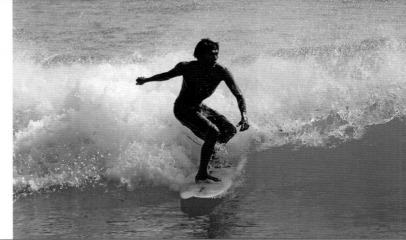

WORKOUT LEVEL 1

BEGINNER ROUTINE 1

Day One:
B 3 sets 8–10
E 3 sets 10–12
F 3 sets 10–12
G 3 sets 10–12
H 3 sets 10–12
T 3 sets 20

Day Two:
Rest

Day Three:
B 3 sets 8–10
E 3 sets 10–12
F 3 sets 10–12
G 3 sets 10–12
H 3 sets 10–12
T 3 sets 20

Day Four:
Rest

Day Five:
B 3 sets 8–10
E 3 sets 10–12
F 3 sets 10–12
G 3 sets 10–12
H 3 sets 10–12
T 3 sets 20

Day Six:
Cardio 30–45 minutes

Day Seven:
Rest

INTERMEDIATE ROUTINE 1

Day One:
B 3 sets 8–10
E 3 sets 10–12
F 3 sets 10–12
G 3 sets 10–12
H 3 sets 10–12
I 3 sets 12–15
O 3 sets 15
T 3 sets 20

Day Two:
Cardio 30–45 minutes

Day Three:
B 3 sets 8–10
E 3 sets 10–12
F 3 sets 10–12
G 3 sets 10–12
H 3 sets 10–12
I 3 sets 12–15
O 3 sets 15
T 3 sets 20

Day Four:
Rest

Day Five:
B 3 sets 8–10
E 3 sets 10–12
F 3 sets 10–12
G 3 sets 10–12
H 3 sets 10–12
I 3 sets 12–15
O 3 sets 15
T 3 sets 20

Day Six:
Cardio 30–45 minutes

Day Seven:
Rest

ADVANCED ROUTINE 1

Day One:
B 3 sets 8–10
E 3 sets 10–12
F 3 sets 10–12
G 3 sets 10–12
H 3 sets 10–12
I 3 sets 12–15
O 3 sets 15
P 30–120 seconds
Q 3 sets 20
T 3 sets 20

Day Two:
Cardio 30–45 minutes

Day Three:
B 3 sets 8–10
E 3 sets 10–12
F 3 sets 10–12
G 3 sets 10–12
H 3 sets 10–12
I 3 sets 12–15
O 3 sets 15
P 30–120 seconds
Q 3 sets 20
T 3 sets 20

Day Four:
Cardio 30–45 minutes

Day Five:
B 3 sets 8–10
E 3 sets 10–12
F 3 sets 10–12
G 3 sets 10–12
H 3 sets 10–12
I 3 sets 12–15
O 3 sets 15
P 30–120 seconds
Q 3 sets 20
T 3 sets 20

Day Six:
Cardio 30–45 minutes

Day Seven:
Rest

WORKOUT LEVEL 2

BEGINNER ROUTINE 2

Day One:
A 3 sets 8–10
C 3 sets 12–15
D 3 sets 10–12
J 3 sets 25
K 3 sets 30
L 3 sets 20

Day Two:
Rest

Day Three:
A 3 sets 8–10
C 3 sets 12–15
D 3 sets 10–12
J 3 sets 25
K 3 sets 30
L 3 sets 20

Day Four:
Rest

Day Five:
A 3 sets 8–10
C 3 sets 12–15
D 3 sets 10–12
J 3 sets 25
K 3 sets 30
L 3 sets 20

Day Six:
Cardio 30–45 minutes

Day Seven:
Rest

INTERMEDIATE ROUTINE 2

Day One:
A 3 sets 8–10
C 3 sets 12–15
D 3 sets 10–12
J 3 sets 25
K 3 sets 30
L 3 sets 20
M 3 sets 15
N 3 sets 15

Day Two:
Cardio 30–45 minutes

Day Three:
A 3 sets 8–10
C 3 sets 12–15
D 3 sets 10–12
J 3 sets 25
K 3 sets 30
L 3 sets 20
M 3 sets 15
N 3 sets 15

Day Four:
Rest

Day Five:
A 3 sets 8–10
C 3 sets 12–15
D 3 sets 10–12
J 3 sets 25
K 3 sets 30
L 3 sets 20
M 3 sets 15
N 3 sets 15

Day Six:
Cardio 30–45 minutes

Day Seven:
Rest

ADVANCED ROUTINE 2

Day One:
A 3 sets 8–10
C 3 sets 12–15
D 3 sets 10–12
J 3 sets 25
K 3 sets 30
L 3 sets 20
M 3 sets 15
N 3 sets 15
R 3 sets 20
S 3 sets 20

Day Two:
Cardio 30–45 minutes

Day Three:
A 3 sets 8–10
C 3 sets 12–15
D 3 sets 10–12
J 3 sets 25
K 3 sets 30
L 3 sets 20
M 3 sets 15
N 3 sets 15

R 3 sets 20
S 3 sets 20

Day Four:
Cardio 30–45 minutes

Day Five:
A 3 sets 8–10
C 3 sets 12–15
D 3 sets 10–12
J 3 sets 25
K 3 sets 30
L 3 sets 20
M 3 sets 15
N 3 sets 15
R 3 sets 20
S 3 sets 20

Day Six:
Cardio 30–45 minutes

Day Seven:
Rest

SURFING WORKOUTS

A Dips
page 68
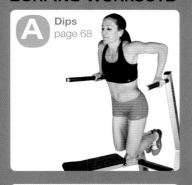

B Overhead Press
page 76
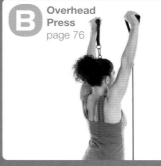

C External Rotation with Band
page 80
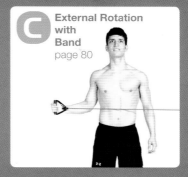

D Swiss Ball Reverse Fly
page 90
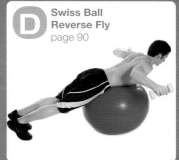

E Barbell Shoulder Shrug
page 94
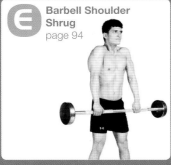

F Barbell Curl
page 100
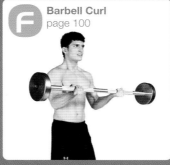

G Rope Pushdown
page 106
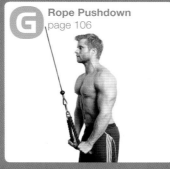

H Swiss Ball Wall Sit
page 134
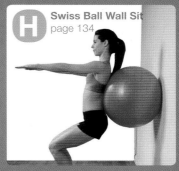

I Stiff-Legged Barbell Deadlift
page 168
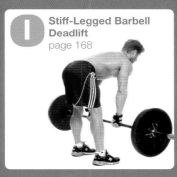

J Abdominal Kick
page 184
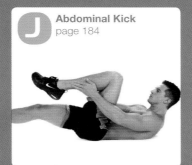

K Turkish Get-Up
page 188
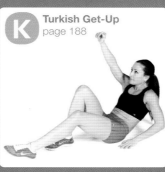

L Bicycle Crunch
page 190
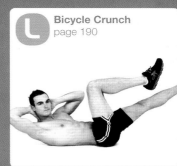

M Cobra Stretch
page 194
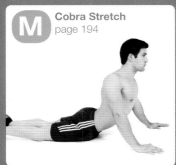

N Plank Press-Up
page 198
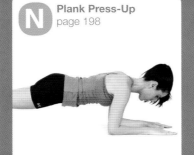

O Star Jump
page 156
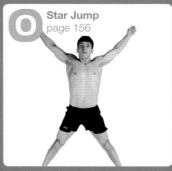

P Mountain Climber
page 158
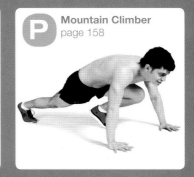

Q Burpee
page 160
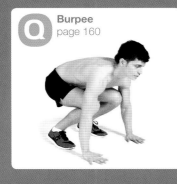

R Seated Russian Twist
page 200
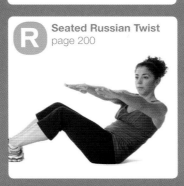

S Medicine Ball Wood Chop
page 130
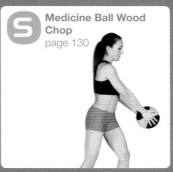

T Swiss Ball Jackknife
page 128
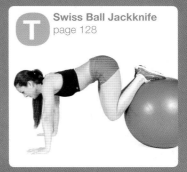

SWIMMING

The four recognised strokes in competitive swimming are freestyle, backstroke, butterfly and breaststroke. In order to maintain a hydrodynamic form in the water and faster propulsion, the entire upper body is used. The glute and hamstring muscles are particularly important for an efficient kick and stabilization. Whichever stroke you employ, the shoulders and back need to be especially powerful. A strong trapezius and neck is important for lifting or turning the head to breathe.

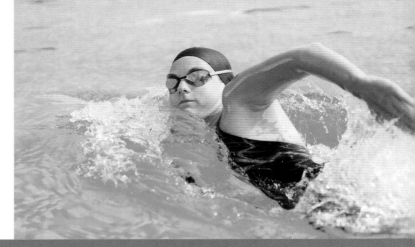

WORKOUT LEVEL 1

BEGINNER ROUTINE 1

Day One:
A 3 sets 8–10
D 3 sets 12–15
E 3 sets 12–15
G 3 sets 15
K 3 sets 10–12
Q 3 sets 8–10

Day Two:
Rest

Day Three:
A 3 sets 8–10
D 3 sets 12–15
E 3 sets 12–15
G 3 sets 15
K 3 sets 10–12

Day Four:
Rest

Day Five:
A 3 sets 8–10
D 3 sets 12–15
E 3 sets 12–15
G 3 sets 15
K 3 sets 10–12
Q 3 sets 8–10

Day Six:
Cardio 30–45 minutes

Day Seven:
Rest

INTERMEDIATE ROUTINE 1

Day One:
A 3 sets 8–10
D 3 sets 12–15
E 3 sets 12–15
G 3 sets 15
I 3 sets 10–12
J 3 sets 8–10
K 3 sets 10–12
Q 3 sets 8–10

Day Two:
Cardio 30–45 minutes

Day Three:
A 3 sets 8–10
D 3 sets 12–15
E 3 sets 12–15
G 3 sets 15
I 3 sets 10–12
J 3 sets 8–10
K 3 sets 10–12

Day Four:
Rest

Day Five:
A 3 sets 8–10
D 3 sets 12–15
E 3 sets 12–15
G 3 sets 15
I 3 sets 10–12
J 3 sets 8–10
K 3 sets 10–12
Q 3 sets 8–10

Day Six:
Cardio 30–45 minutes

Day Seven:
Rest

ADVANCED ROUTINE 1

Day One:
A 3 sets 8–10
D 3 sets 12–15
E 3 sets 12–15
G 3 sets 15
I 3 sets 10–12
J 3 sets 8–10
K 3 sets 10–12
Q 3 sets 8–10
R 3 sets 15
T 3 sets 25

Day Two:
Cardio 30–45 minutes

Day Three:
A 3 sets 8–10
D 3 sets 12–15
E 3 sets 12–15
G 3 sets 15
I 3 sets 10–12
J 3 sets 8–10
K 3 sets 10–12
Q 3 sets 8–10
R 3 sets 15
T 3 sets 25

Day Four:
Cardio 30–45 minutes

Day Five:
A 3 sets 8–10
D 3 sets 12–15
E 3 sets 12–15
G 3 sets 15
I 3 sets 10–12
J 3 sets 8–10
K 3 sets 10–12
Q 3 sets 8–10
R 3 sets 15
T 3 sets 25

Day Six:
Cardio 30–45 minutes

Day Seven:
Rest

WORKOUT LEVEL 2

BEGINNER ROUTINE 2

Day One:
B 3 sets 8–10
C 3 sets 8–10
F 3 sets 8–10
H 3 sets 10–12
L 3 sets 12–15
M 3 sets 12–15

Day Two:
Rest

Day Three:
B 3 sets 8–10
C 3 sets 8–10
F 3 sets 8–10
H 3 sets 10–12
L 3 sets 12–15
M 3 sets 12–15

Day Four:
Rest

Day Five:
B 3 sets 8–10
C 3 sets 8–10
F 3 sets 8–10
H 3 sets 10–12
L 3 sets 12–15
M 3 sets 12–15

Day Six:
Cardio 30–45 minutes

Day Seven:
Rest

INTERMEDIATE ROUTINE 2

Day One:
B 3 sets 8–10
C 3 sets 8–10
F 3 sets 8–10
H 3 sets 10–12
L 3 sets 12–15
M 3 sets 12–15
N 3 sets 25
O 3 sets 25

Day Two:
Cardio 30–45 minutes

Day Three:
B 3 sets 8–10
C 3 sets 8–10
F 3 sets 8–10
H 3 sets 10–12
L 3 sets 12–15
M 3 sets 12–15
N 3 sets 25
O 3 sets 25

Day Four:
Rest

Day Five:
B 3 sets 8–10
C 3 sets 8–10
F 3 sets 8–10
H 3 sets 10–12
L 3 sets 12–15
M 3 sets 12–15
N 3 sets 25
O 3 sets 25

Day Six:
Cardio 30–45 minutes

Day Seven:
Rest

ADVANCED ROUTINE 2

Day One:
B 3 sets 8–10
C 3 sets 8–10
F 3 sets 8–10
H 3 sets 10–12
L 3 sets 12–15
M 3 sets 12–15
N 3 sets 25
O 3 sets 25
P 3 sets 30
S 3 sets 20

Day Two:
Cardio 30–45 minutes

Day Three:
B 3 sets 8–10
C 3 sets 8–10
F 3 sets 8–10
H 3 sets 10–12
L 3 sets 12–15
M 3 sets 12–15
N 3 sets 25
O 3 sets 25
P 3 sets 30
S 3 sets 20

Day Four:
Cardio 30–45 minutes

Day Five:
B 3 sets 8–10
C 3 sets 8–10
F 3 sets 8–10
H 3 sets 10–12
L 3 sets 12–15
M 3 sets 12–15
N 3 sets 25
O 3 sets 25
P 3 sets 30
S 3 sets 20

Day Six:
Cardio 30–45 minutes

Day Seven:
Rest

SWIMMING WORKOUTS

A Dumbbell Row
page 38
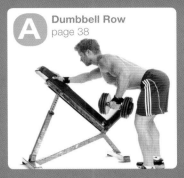

B Dumbbell Pullover
page 40
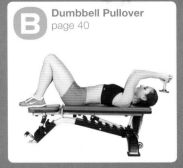

C Lat Pulldown
page 42
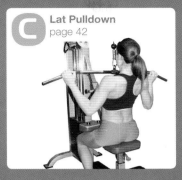

D Alternating Kettlebell Row
page 46
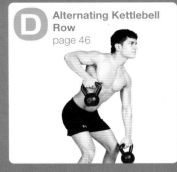

E Cable Fly
page 66
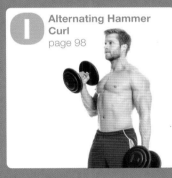

F Dumbbell Shoulder Press
page 74
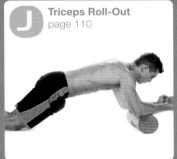

G Incline Bench Row
page 50
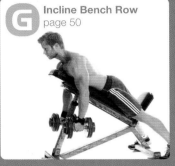

H Reverse Fly
page 88
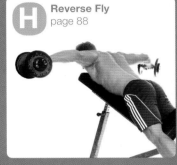

I Alternating Hammer Curl
page 98
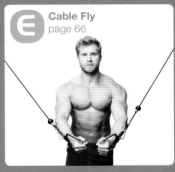

J Triceps Roll-Out
page 110
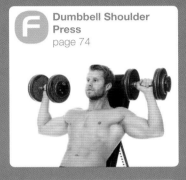

K Swiss Ball Hamstring Curl
page 164
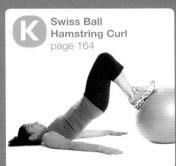

L Stiff-Legged Barbell Deadlift
page 168
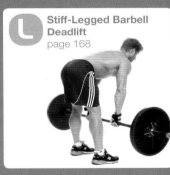

M Hamstring Pull-In
page 170
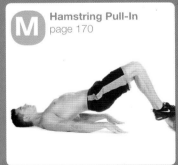

N Crunch
page 118
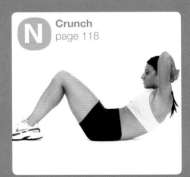

O Swiss Ball Walk-Around
page 126
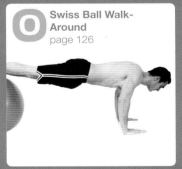

P Wood Chop with Resistance Band
page 202
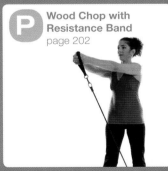

Q Alternating Renegade Row
page 48
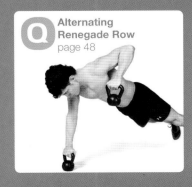

R Hip Abduction and Adduction
page 204
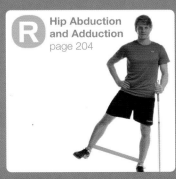

S Swiss Ball Jackknife
page 128
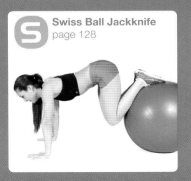

T Medicine Ball Slam
page 214
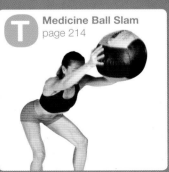

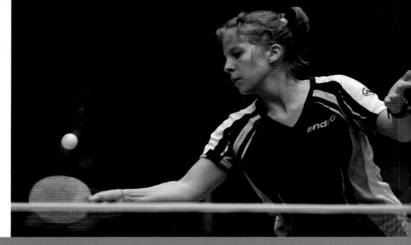

TABLE TENNIS

Table tennis is very fast-paced and necessitates quick reactions and good timing. It is a fun calorie burner while at the same time improving coordination. Numerous muscles are employed in playing this game, including those of the shoulders, arms, forearms, core and chest, with secondary assistance from muscles in the upper back and calves, the quads and the hip abductors. The wrists and forearms help perform spin shots effectively.

SPORT-SPECIFIC WORKOUTS

WORKOUT LEVEL 1

BEGINNER ROUTINE 1

Day One:
A 3 sets 8–10
C 3 sets 10–12
E 3 sets 12–15
G 3 sets 10–12
H 3 sets 12–15
I 3 sets 12–15

Day Two:
Rest

Day Three:
A 3 sets 8–10
C 3 sets 10–12
E 3 sets 12–15
G 3 sets 10–12
H 3 sets 12–15
I 3 sets 12–15

Day Four:
Rest

Day Five:
A 3 sets 8–10
C 3 sets 10–12
E 3 sets 12–15
G 3 sets 10–12
H 3 sets 12–15
I 3 sets 12–15

Day Six:
Cardio 30–45 minutes

Day Seven:
Rest

INTERMEDIATE ROUTINE 1

Day One:
A 3 sets 8–10
C 3 sets 10–12
E 3 sets 12–15
G 3 sets 10–12
H 3 sets 12–15
I 3 sets 12–15
L 3 sets 10–12
N 3 sets 15–20

Day Two:
Cardio 30–45 minutes

Day Three:
A 3 sets 8–10
C 3 sets 10–12
E 3 sets 12–15
G 3 sets 10–12
H 3 sets 12–15
I 3 sets 12–15
L 3 sets 10–12
N 3 sets 15–20

Day Four:
Rest

Day Five:
A 3 sets 8–10
C 3 sets 10–12
E 3 sets 12–15
G 3 sets 10–12
H 3 sets 12–15
I 3 sets 12–15
L 3 sets 10–12
N 3 sets 15–20

Day Six:
Cardio 30–45 minutes

Day Seven:
Rest

ADVANCED ROUTINE 1

Day One:
A 3 sets 8–10
C 3 sets 10–12
E 3 sets 12–15
G 3 sets 10–12
H 3 sets 12–15
I 3 sets 12–15
L 3 sets 10–12
N 3 sets 15–20
O 3 sets 12–15
S 3 sets 15

Day Two:
Cardio 30–45 minutes

Day Three:
A 3 sets 8–10
C 3 sets 10–12
E 3 sets 12–15
G 3 sets 10–12
H 3 sets 12–15
I 3 sets 12–15
L 3 sets 10–12
N 3 sets 15–20
O 3 sets 12–15
S 3 sets 15

Day Four:
Cardio 30–45 minutes

Day Five:
A 3 sets 8–10
C 3 sets 10–12
E 3 sets 12–15
G 3 sets 10–12
H 3 sets 12–15
I 3 sets 12–15
L 3 sets 10–12
N 3 sets 15–20
O 3 sets 12–15
S 3 sets 15

Day Six:
Cardio 30–45 minutes

Day Seven:
Rest

WORKOUT LEVEL 2

BEGINNER ROUTINE 2

Day One:
B 3 sets 12–15
D 3 sets 8–10
F 3 sets 8–10
J 3 sets 12–15
K 3 sets 12–15
M 3 sets 15–20

Day Two:
Rest

Day Three:
B 3 sets 12–15
D 3 sets 8–10
F 3 sets 8–10
J 3 sets 12–15
K 3 sets 12–15
M 3 sets 15–20

Day Four:
Rest

Day Five:
B 3 sets 12–15
D 3 sets 8–10
F 3 sets 8–10
J 3 sets 12–15
K 3 sets 12–15
M 3 sets 15–20

Day Six:
Cardio 30–45 minutes

Day Seven:
Rest

INTERMEDIATE ROUTINE 2

Day One:
B 3 sets 12–15
D 3 sets 8–10
F 3 sets 8–10
J 3 sets 12–15
K 3 sets 12–15
M 3 sets 15–20
P 3 sets 12–15
Q 3 sets 12–15

Day Two:
Cardio 30–45 minutes

Day Three:
B 3 sets 12–15
D 3 sets 8–10
F 3 sets 8–10
J 3 sets 12–15
K 3 sets 12–15
M 3 sets 15–20
P 3 sets 12–15
Q 3 sets 12–15

Day Four:
Rest

Day Five:
B 3 sets 12–15
D 3 sets 8–10
F 3 sets 8–10
J 3 sets 12–15
K 3 sets 12–15
M 3 sets 15–20
P 3 sets 12–15
Q 3 sets 12–15

Day Six:
Cardio 30–45 minutes

Day Seven:
Rest

ADVANCED ROUTINE 2

Day One:
B 3 sets 12–15
D 3 sets 8–10
F 3 sets 8–10
J 3 sets 12–15
K 3 sets 12–15
M 3 sets 15–20
P 3 sets 12–15
Q 3 sets 12–15
R 3 sets 25
T 3 sets 30–120 seconds

Day Two:
Cardio 30–45 minutes

Day Three:
B 3 sets 12–15
D 3 sets 8–10
F 3 sets 8–10
J 3 sets 12–15
K 3 sets 12–15
M 3 sets 15–20
P 3 sets 12–15
Q 3 sets 12–15
R 3 sets 25
T 3 sets 30–120 seconds

Day Four:
Cardio 30–45 minutes

Day Five:
B 3 sets 12–15
D 3 sets 8–10
F 3 sets 8–10
J 3 sets 12–15
K 3 sets 12–15
M 3 sets 15–20
P 3 sets 12–15
Q 3 sets 12–15
R 3 sets 25
T 3 sets 30–120 seconds

Day Six:
Cardio 30–45 minutes

Day Seven:
Rest

TABLE TENNIS WORKOUTS

A Lat Pulldown
page 42
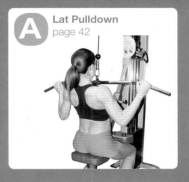

B Scapular Range of Motion
page 44
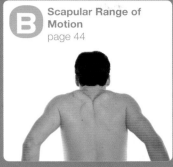

C Dumbbell Fly
page 64
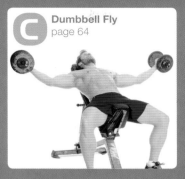

D Dumbbell Shoulder Press
page 74
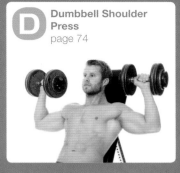

E External Rotation with Band
page 80
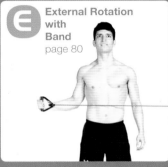

F Shoulder Raise and Pull
page 84
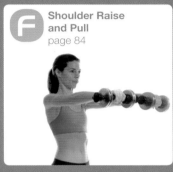

G Barbell Shoulder Shrug
page 94
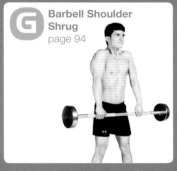

H Single-Arm Concentration Curl
page 102
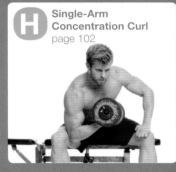

I Triceps Roll-Out
page 110
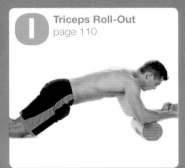

J Wrist Flexion
page 116
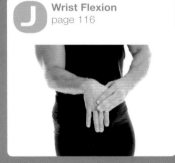

K Wrist Extension
page 117
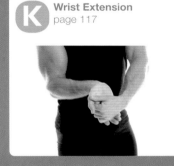

L Swiss Ball Wall Sit
page 134
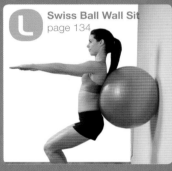

M Adductor Extension
page 162
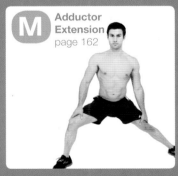

N Hamstring Abductor
page 163
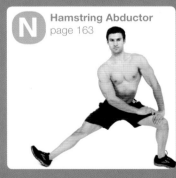

O Stiff-Legged Deadlift
page 174
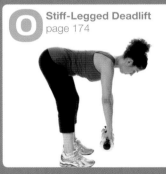

P Hamstring Pull-In
page 170
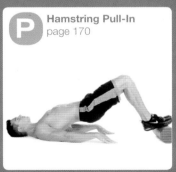

Q Dumbbell Shin Raise
page 180
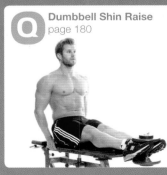

R Abdominal Kick
page 184
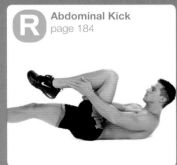

S Plank Press-Up
page 198
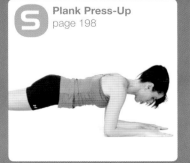

T Plank
page 120
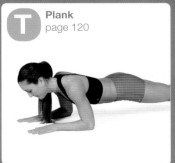

TENNIS

Tennis is a fast-paced, reactive sport that requires sharp reflexes and great stamina. Reactive power stems from the lower body. The calves, quadriceps, hamstrings and glutes transfer energy to the core and upward throughout the back and shoulders. Forehand strokes are reliant on pectorals, shoulders, biceps and forearms. The triceps, frontal deltoids and latissimus dorsi all contribute to the backhand swing. The serve is a throwing action that requires strong shoulder muscles.

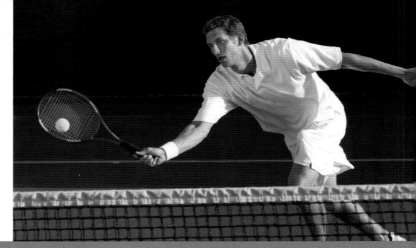

WORKOUT LEVEL 1

BEGINNER ROUTINE 1

Day One:
A 3 sets 8–10
B 3 sets 10–12
D 3 sets 15
F 3 sets 12–15
I 3 sets 12–15
K 3 sets 12–15

Day Two:
Rest

Day Three:
A 3 sets 8–10
B 3 sets 10–12
D 3 sets 15
F 3 sets 12–15
I 3 sets 12–15
K 3 sets 12–15

Day Four:
Rest

Day Five:
A 3 sets 8–10
B 3 sets 10–12
D 3 sets 15
F 3 sets 12–15
I 3 sets 12–15
K 3 sets 12–15

Day Six:
Cardio 30–45 minutes

Day Seven:
Rest

INTERMEDIATE ROUTINE 1

Day One:
A 3 sets 8–10
B 3 sets 10–12
D 3 sets 15
F 3 sets 12–15
G 3 sets 12–15
I 3 sets 12–15
J 3 sets 12–15
K 3 sets 12–15

Day Two:
Cardio 30–45 minutes

Day Three:
A 3 sets 8–10
B 3 sets 10–12
D 3 sets 15
F 3 sets 12–15
G 3 sets 12–15
I 3 sets 12–15
J 3 sets 12–15
K 3 sets 12–15

Day Four:
Rest

Day Five:
A 3 sets 8–10
B 3 sets 10–12
D 3 sets 15
F 3 sets 12–15
G 3 sets 12–15
I 3 sets 12–15
J 3 sets 12–15
K 3 sets 12–15

Day Six:
Cardio 30–45 minutes

Day Seven:
Rest

ADVANCED ROUTINE 1

Day One:
A 3 sets 8–10
B 3 sets 10–12
D 3 sets 15
F 3 sets 12–15
G 3 sets 12–15
I 3 sets 12–15
J 3 sets 12–15
K 3 sets 12–15
Q 20 per side
S 3 sets 15

Day Two:
Cardio 30–45 minutes

Day Three:
A 3 sets 8–10
B 3 sets 10–12
D 3 sets 15
F 3 sets 12–15
G 3 sets 12–15
I 3 sets 12–15
J 3 sets 12–15
K 3 sets 12–15
Q 20 per side
S 3 sets 15

Day Four:
Cardio 30–45 minutes

Day Five:
A 3 sets 8–10
B 3 sets 10–12
D 3 sets 15
F 3 sets 12–15
G 3 sets 12–15
I 3 sets 12–15
J 3 sets 12–15
K 3 sets 12–15
Q 20 per side
S 3 sets 15

Day Six:
Cardio 30–45 minutes

Day Seven:
Rest

WORKOUT LEVEL 2

BEGINNER ROUTINE 2

Day One:
C 3 sets 8–10
E 3 sets 10–12
H 3 sets 12–15
L 3 sets 12–15
M 3 sets 20
N 3 sets 30

Day Two:
Rest

Day Three:
C 3 sets 8–10
E 3 sets 10–12
H 3 sets 12–15
L 3 sets 12–15
M 3 sets 20
N 3 sets 30

Day Four:
Rest

Day Five:
C 3 sets 8–10
E 3 sets 10–12
H 3 sets 12–15
L 3 sets 12–15
M 3 sets 20
N 3 sets 30

Day Six:
Cardio 30–45 minutes

Day Seven:
Rest

INTERMEDIATE ROUTINE 2

Day One:
C 3 sets 8–10
E 3 sets 10–12
H 3 sets 12–15
L 3 sets 12–15
M 3 sets 20
N 3 sets 30
O 3 sets 15
P 3 sets 30–120 seconds

Day Two:
Cardio 30–45 minutes

Day Three:
C 3 sets 8–10
E 3 sets 10–12
H 3 sets 12–15
L 3 sets 12–15
M 3 sets 20
N 3 sets 30
O 3 sets 15
P 3 sets 30–120 seconds

Day Four:
Rest

Day Five:
C 3 sets 8–10
E 3 sets 10–12
H 3 sets 12–15
L 3 sets 12–15
M 3 sets 20
N 3 sets 30
O 3 sets 15
P 3 sets 30–120 seconds

Day Six:
Cardio 30–45 minutes

Day Seven:
Rest

ADVANCED ROUTINE 2

Day One:
C 3 sets 8–10
E 3 sets 10–12
H 3 sets 12–15
L 3 sets 12–15
M 3 sets 20
N 3 sets 30
O 3 sets 15
P 3 sets 30–120 seconds
R 3 sets 8–10
T 3 sets 25

Day Two:
Cardio 30–45 minutes

Day Three:
C 3 sets 8–10
E 3 sets 10–12
H 3 sets 12–15
L 3 sets 12–15
M 3 sets 20
N 3 sets 30
O 3 sets 15
P 3 sets 30–120 seconds
R 3 sets 8–10
T 3 sets 25

Day Four:
Cardio 30–45 minutes

Day Five:
C 3 sets 8–10
E 3 sets 10–12
H 3 sets 12–15
L 3 sets 12–15
M 3 sets 20
N 3 sets 30
O 3 sets 15
P 3 sets 30–120 seconds
R 3 sets 8–10
T 3 sets 25

Day Six:
Cardio 30–45 minutes

Day Seven:
Rest

TENNIS WORKOUTS

A Lat Pulldown
page 42
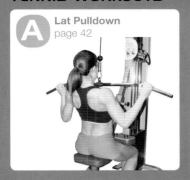

B Dumbbell Fly
page 64
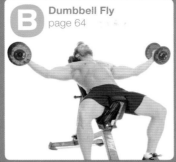

C Dumbbell Shoulder Press
page 74
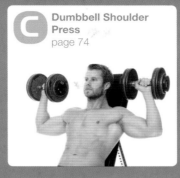

D Rotation Exercises
page 78
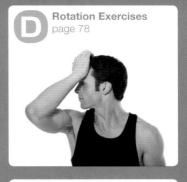

E Front-Plate Raise
page 92
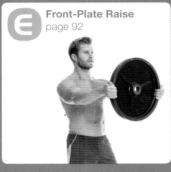

F Single-Arm Concentration Curl
page 102
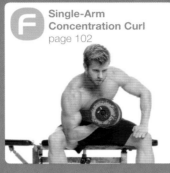

G Chair Dip
page 112
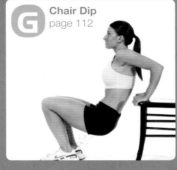

H Wrist Extension
page 117
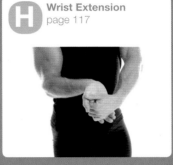

I Reverse Lunge
page 140
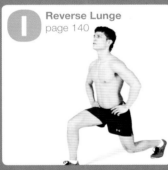

J Lateral Low Lunge
page 142
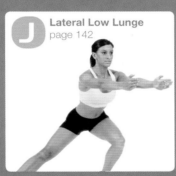

K Stiff-Legged Barbell Deadlift
page 168
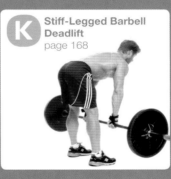

L Dumbbell Calf Raise
page 178
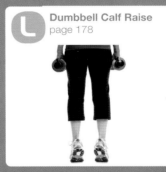

M Abdominal Hip Lift
page 186
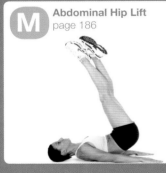

N Turkish Get-Up
page 188
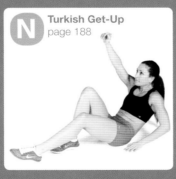

O Plank Press-Up
page 198
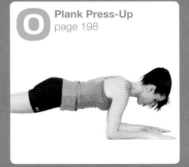

P Mountain Climber
page 158
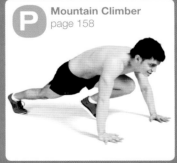

Q Medicine Ball Wood Chop
page 130
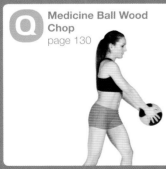

R Alternating Renegade Row
page 48
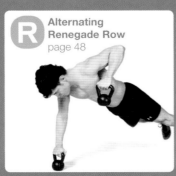

S Hip Abduction and Adduction
page 204
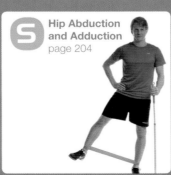

T Medicine Ball Slam
page 214
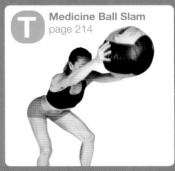

VOLLEYBALL

Volleyball uses most of the major muscle groups of the body. Serving, blocking, hitting and passing require a lot of upper-body strength. A strong core is paramount for delivering more power as well as explosive energy. The legs are used for positioning and jumping. To keep the muscles strong and pliable as well as preventing wrist sprains, knee problems and torn rotator cuffs, it is recommended to keep in good cardiovascular health as well as to strengthen the muscles regularly.

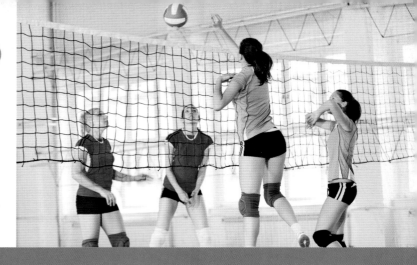

BEGINNER ROUTINE I

Day One:
A 3 sets 8–10
D 3 sets 20
F 3 sets 12–15
G 3 sets 8–10
O 3 sets 12–15
P 3 sets 12–15

Day Two:
Rest

Day Three:
A 3 sets 8–10
D 3 sets 20
F 3 sets 12–15
G 3 sets 8–10
O 3 sets 12–15
P 3 sets 12–15

Day Four:
Rest

Day Five:
A 3 sets 8–10
D 3 sets 20
F 3 sets 12–15
G 3 sets 8–10
O 3 sets 12–15
P 3 sets 12–15

Day Six:
Cardio 30–45 minutes

Day Seven:
Rest

INTERMEDIATE ROUTINE I

Day One:
A 3 sets 8–10
D 3 sets 20
F 3 sets 12–15
G 3 sets 8–10
I 3 sets 10–12
J 3 sets 10–12
O 3 sets 12–15
P 3 sets 12–15

Day Two:
Cardio 30–45 minutes

Day Three:
A 3 sets 8–10
D 3 sets 20
F 3 sets 12–15
G 3 sets 8–10
I 3 sets 10–12
J 3 sets 10–12
O 3 sets 12–15
P 3 sets 12–15

Day Four:
Rest

Day Five:
A 3 sets 8–10
D 3 sets 20
F 3 sets 12–15
G 3 sets 8–10
I 3 sets 10–12
J 3 sets 10–12
O 3 sets 12–15
P 3 sets 12–15

Day Six:
Cardio 30–45 minutes

Day Seven:
Rest

ADVANCED ROUTINE I

Day One:
A 3 sets 8–10
D 3 sets 20
F 3 sets 12–15
G 3 sets 8–10
I 3 sets 10–12
J 3 sets 10–12
O 3 sets 12–15
P 3 sets 12–15
Q 3 sets 15
T 3 sets 25

Day Two:
Cardio 30–45 minutes

Day Three:
A 3 sets 8–10
D 3 sets 20
F 3 sets 12–15
G 3 sets 8–10
I 3 sets 10–12
J 3 sets 10–12
O 3 sets 12–15
P 3 sets 12–15
Q 3 sets 15
T 3 sets 25

Day Four:
Cardio 30–45 minutes

Day Five:
A 3 sets 8–10
D 3 sets 20
F 3 sets 12–15
G 3 sets 8–10
I 3 sets 10–12
J 3 sets 10–12
O 3 sets 12–15
P 3 sets 12–15
Q 3 sets 15
T 3 sets 25

Day Six:
Cardio 30–45 minutes

Day Seven:
Rest

BEGINNER ROUTINE 2

Day One:
B 3 sets 8–10
C 3 sets 12–15
E 3 sets 8–10
H 3 sets 10–12
K 3 sets 12–15
L 3 sets 10–12

Day Two:
Rest

Day Three:
B 3 sets 8–10
C 3 sets 12–15
E 3 sets 8–10
H 3 sets 10–12
K 3 sets 12–15
L 3 sets 10–12

Day Four:
Rest

Day Five:
B 3 sets 8–10
C 3 sets 12–15
E 3 sets 8–10
H 3 sets 10–12
K 3 sets 12–15
L 3 sets 10–12

Day Six:
Cardio 30–45 minutes

Day Seven:
Rest

INTERMEDIATE ROUTINE 2

Day One:
B 3 sets 8–10
C 3 sets 12–15
E 3 sets 8–10
H 3 sets 10–12
K 3 sets 12–15
L 3 sets 10–12
M 3 sets 12–15
N 3 sets 12–15

Day Two:
Cardio 30–45 minutes

Day Three:
B 3 sets 8–10
C 3 sets 12–15
E 3 sets 8–10
H 3 sets 10–12
K 3 sets 12–15
L 3 sets 10–12
M 3 sets 12–15
N 3 sets 12–15

Day Four:
Rest

Day Five:
B 3 sets 8–10
C 3 sets 12–15
E 3 sets 8–10
H 3 sets 10–12
K 3 sets 12–15
L 3 sets 10–12
M 3 sets 12–15
N 3 sets 12–15

Day Six:
Cardio 30–45 minutes

Day Seven:
Rest

ADVANCED ROUTINE 2

Day One:
B 3 sets 8–10
C 3 sets 12–15
E 3 sets 8–10
H 3 sets 10–12
K 3 sets 12–15
L 3 sets 10–12
M 3 sets 12–15
N 3 sets 12–15
R 3 sets 20
S 3 sets 20

Day Two:
Cardio 30–45 minutes

Day Three:
B 3 sets 8–10
C 3 sets 12–15
E 3 sets 8–10
H 3 sets 10–12
K 3 sets 12–15
L 3 sets 10–12
M 3 sets 12–15
N 3 sets 12–15
R 3 sets 20
S 3 sets 20

Day Four:
Cardio 30–45 minutes

Day Five:
B 3 sets 8–10
C 3 sets 12–15
E 3 sets 8–10
H 3 sets 10–12
K 3 sets 12–15
L 3 sets 10–12
M 3 sets 12–15
N 3 sets 12–15
R 3 sets 20
S 3 sets 20

Day Six:
Cardio 30–45 minutes

Day Seven:
Rest

VOLLEYBALL WORKOUTS

A Lat Pulldown
page 42
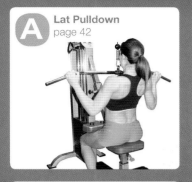

B Alternating Kettlebell Row
page 46
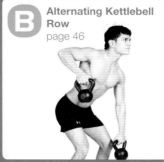

C Cable Fly
page 66
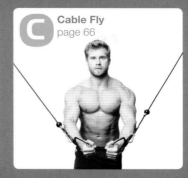

D Push-Up Hand Walk-Over
page 72
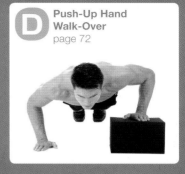

E Overhead Press
page 76
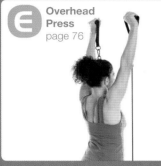

F External Rotation with Band
page 80
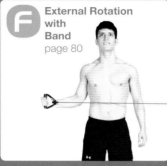

G Barbell Upright Row
page 86
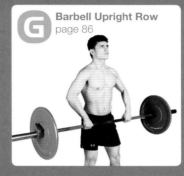

H Swiss Ball Reverse Fly
page 90
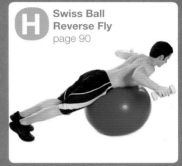

I Alternating Hammer Curl
page 98
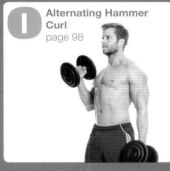

J Lying Triceps Extension
page 108
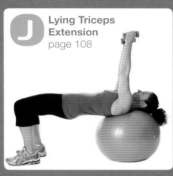

K Wrist Flexion
page 116
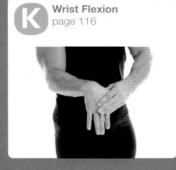

L Swiss Ball Wall Sit
page 134
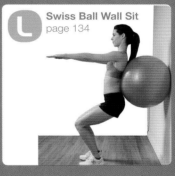

M Crossover Step
page 148
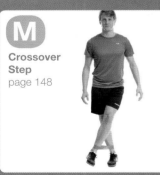

N Inverted Hamstring
page 166
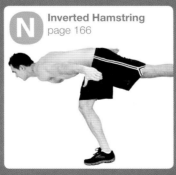

O Stiff-Legged Barbell Deadlift
page 168
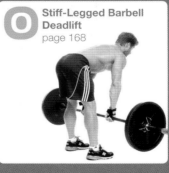

P Dumbbell Calf Raise
page 178
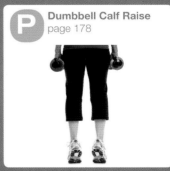

Q Star Jump
page 156
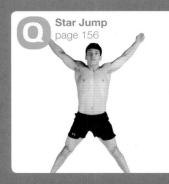

R Swiss Ball Roll-Out
page 206
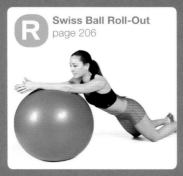

S Swiss Ball Hip Crossover
page 210
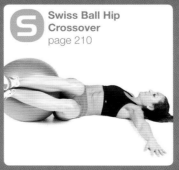

T Medicine Ball Slam
page 214
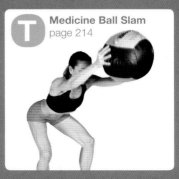

WATER POLO

Water polo is a game of multi-tasking in which you must fight to stay above water, head in the right direction and battle opponents to take — and keep — possession of the ball. As such, it requires strength, stamina and coordination. Shoulder strength is especially crucial, not just for throwing power but also because the shoulders are particularly susceptible to injury. Powerful legs and a strong core will help you navigate the waters more efficiently for improved performance.

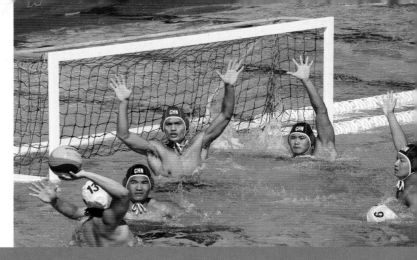

BEGINNER ROUTINE 1

Day One:
A 3 sets 8–10
B 3 sets 8–10
C 3 sets 8–10
F 3 sets 10–12
J 3 sets 12–15
Q 3 sets 8–10

Day Two:
Rest

Day Three:
A 3 sets 8–10
B 3 sets 8–10
C 3 sets 8–10
F 3 sets 10–12
J 3 sets 12–15
Q 3 sets 8–10

Day Four:
Rest

Day Five:
A 3 sets 8–10
B 3 sets 8–10
C 3 sets 8–10
F 3 sets 10–12
J 3 sets 12–15
Q 3 sets 8–10

Day Six:
Cardio 30–45 minutes

Day Seven:
Rest

INTERMEDIATE ROUTINE 1

Day One:
A 3 sets 8–10
B 3 sets 8–10
C 3 sets 8–10
D 3 sets 15
F 3 sets 10–12
I 3 sets 12–15
J 3 sets 12–15
Q 3 sets 8–10

Day Two:
Cardio 30–45 minutes

Day Three:
A 3 sets 8–10
B 3 sets 8–10
C 3 sets 8–10
D 3 sets 15
F 3 sets 10–12
I 3 sets 12–15
J 3 sets 12–15
Q 3 sets 8–10

Day Four:
Rest

Day Five:
A 3 sets 8–10
B 3 sets 8–10
C 3 sets 8–10
D 3 sets 15
F 3 sets 10–12
I 3 sets 12–15
J 3 sets 12–15
Q 3 sets 8–10

Day Six:
Cardio 30–45 minutes

Day Seven:
Rest

ADVANCED ROUTINE 1

Day One:
A 3 sets 8–10
B 3 sets 8–10
C 3 sets 8–10
D 3 sets 15
F 3 sets 10–12
I 3 sets 12–15
J 3 sets 12–15
P 30 per side
Q 3 sets 8–10
T 20 per side

Day Two:
Cardio 30–45 minutes

Day Three:
A 3 sets 8–10
B 3 sets 8–10
C 3 sets 8–10
D 3 sets 15
F 3 sets 10–12
I 3 sets 12–15
J 3 sets 12–15
P 30 per side
Q 3 sets 8–10
T 20 per side

Day Four:
Cardio 30–45 minutes

Day Five:
A 3 sets 8–10
B 3 sets 8–10
C 3 sets 8–10
D 3 sets 15
F 3 sets 10–12
I 3 sets 12–15
J 3 sets 12–15
P 30 per side
Q 3 sets 8–10
T 20 per side

Day Six:
Cardio 30–45 minutes

Day Seven:
Rest

BEGINNER ROUTINE 2

Day One:
E 3 sets 10–12
G 3 sets 12–15
H 3 sets 10–12
K 3 sets 12–15
L 3 sets 25
M 3 sets 20

Day Two:
Rest

Day Three:
E 3 sets 10–12
G 3 sets 12–15
H 3 sets 10–12
K 3 sets 12–15
L 3 sets 25
M 3 sets 20

Day Four:
Rest

Day Five:
E 3 sets 10–12
G 3 sets 12–15
H 3 sets 10–12
K 3 sets 12–15
L 3 sets 25
M 3 sets 20

Day Six:
Cardio 30–45 minutes

Day Seven:
Rest

INTERMEDIATE ROUTINE 2

Day One:
E 3 sets 10–12
G 3 sets 12–15
H 3 sets 10–12
K 3 sets 12–15
L 3 sets 25
M 3 sets 20
N 3 sets 30–60 seconds
O 3 sets 20

Day Two:
Cardio 30–45 minutes

Day Three:
E 3 sets 10–12
G 3 sets 12–15
H 3 sets 10–12
K 3 sets 12–15
L 3 sets 25
M 3 sets 20
N 3 sets 30–60 seconds
O 3 sets 20

Day Four:
Rest

Day Five:
E 3 sets 10–12
G 3 sets 12–15
H 3 sets 10–12
K 3 sets 12–15
L 3 sets 25
M 3 sets 20
N 3 sets 30–60 seconds
O 3 sets 20

Day Six:
Cardio 30–45 minutes

Day Seven:
Rest

ADVANCED ROUTINE 2

Day One:
E 3 sets 10–12
G 3 sets 12–15
H 3 sets 10–12
K 3 sets 12–15
L 3 sets 25
M 3 sets 20
N 3 sets 30–60 seconds
O 3 sets 20
R 3 sets 15
S 3 sets 20

Day Two:
Cardio 30–45 minutes

Day Three:
E 3 sets 10–12
G 3 sets 12–15
H 3 sets 10–12
K 3 sets 12–15
L 3 sets 25
M 3 sets 20
N 3 sets 30–60 seconds
O 3 sets 20
R 3 sets 15
S 3 sets 20

Day Four:
Cardio 30–45 minutes

Day Five:
E 3 sets 10–12
G 3 sets 12–15
H 3 sets 10–12
K 3 sets 12–15
L 3 sets 25
M 3 sets 20
N 3 sets 30–60 seconds
O 3 sets 20
R 3 sets 15
S 3 sets 20

Day Six:
Cardio 30–45 minutes

Day Seven:
Rest

WATER POLO WORKOUTS

A Rope Pulldown
page 52
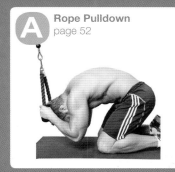

B Rope Overhead Extension
page 114
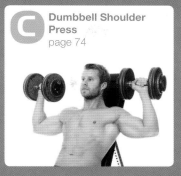

C Dumbbell Shoulder Press
page 74
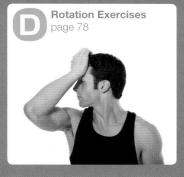

D Rotation Exercises
page 78
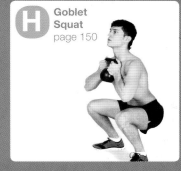

E Barbell Shoulder Shrug
page 94
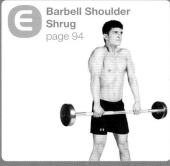

F Swiss Ball Wall Sit
page 134
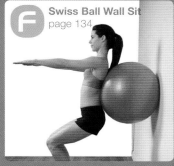

G High Lunge
page 146
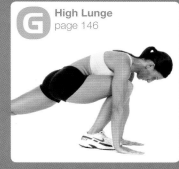

H Goblet Squat
page 150
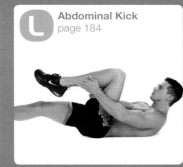

I One-Legged Step-Down
page 152
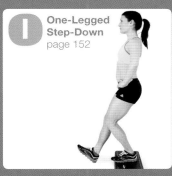

J Stiff-Legged Deadlift
page 174
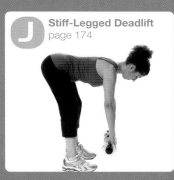

K Dumbbell Calf Raise
page 178
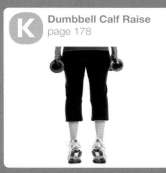

L Abdominal Kick
page 184
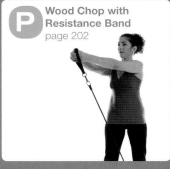

M Bicycle Crunch
page 190
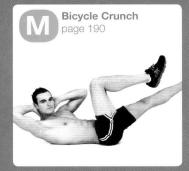

N Side Plank
page 122
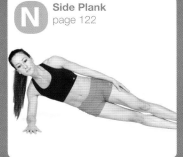

O Seated Russian Twist
page 200
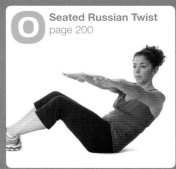

P Wood Chop with Resistance Band
page 202
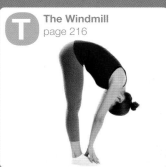

Q Alternating Renegade Row
page 48
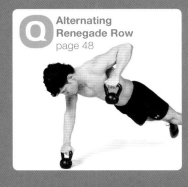

R Hip Abduction and Adduction
page 204
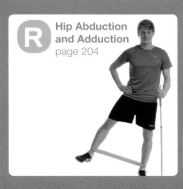

S Swiss Ball Hip Crossover
page 210
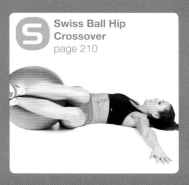

T The Windmill
page 216

WATER SKIING

Water skiing makes for a great workout. It requires endurance, balance, flexibility, coordination and good strength throughout the body. Your upper body especially must be strong enough to sustain long periods of contraction, while your hamstrings, quadriceps, hip flexors, glutes and calves are all vital for maintaining a strong frame and stabilizing your legs. Of course, the hands and forearms need to be strong to maintain a secure grip.

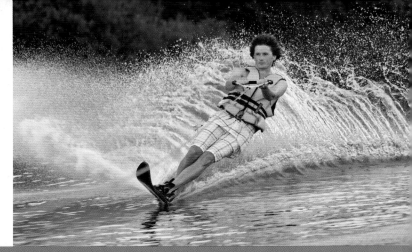

WORKOUT LEVEL 1

BEGINNER ROUTINE 1

Day One:
A 3 sets 8–10
D 3 sets 8–10
G 3 sets 10–12
I 3 sets 10–12
K 3 sets 10–12
O 3 sets 10–12

Day Two:
Rest

Day Three:
A 3 sets 8–10
D 3 sets 8–10
G 3 sets 10–12
I 3 sets 10–12
K 3 sets 10–12
O 3 sets 10–12

Day Four:
Rest

Day Five:
A 3 sets 8–10
D 3 sets 8–10
G 3 sets 10–12
I 3 sets 10–12
K 3 sets 10–12
O 3 sets 10–12

Day Six:
Cardio 30–45 minutes

Day Seven:
Rest

INTERMEDIATE ROUTINE 1

Day One:
A 3 sets 8–10
D 3 sets 8–10
E 3 sets 12–15
G 3 sets 10–12
I 3 sets 10–12
K 3 sets 10–12
O 3 sets 10–12
P 3 sets 12–15

Day Two:
Cardio 30–45 minutes

Day Three:
A 3 sets 8–10
D 3 sets 8–10
E 3 sets 12–15
G 3 sets 10–12
I 3 sets 10–12
K 3 sets 10–12
O 3 sets 10–12
P 3 sets 12–15

Day Four:
Rest

Day Five:
A 3 sets 8–10
D 3 sets 8–10
E 3 sets 12–15
G 3 sets 10–12
I 3 sets 10–12
K 3 sets 10–12
O 3 sets 10–12
P 3 sets 12–15

Day Six:
Cardio 30–45 minutes

Day Seven:
Rest

ADVANCED ROUTINE 1

Day One:
A 3 sets 8–10
D 3 sets 8–10
E 3 sets 12–15
G 3 sets 10–12
I 3 sets 10–12
K 3 sets 10–12
O 3 sets 10–12
P 3 sets 12–15
R 25 per side
T 3 sets 15

Day Two:
Cardio 30–45 minutes

Day Three:
A 3 sets 8–10
D 3 sets 8–10
E 3 sets 12–15
G 3 sets 10–12
I 3 sets 10–12
K 3 sets 10–12
O 3 sets 10–12
P 3 sets 12–15
R 25 per side
T 3 sets 15

Day Four:
Cardio 30–45 minutes

Day Five:
A 3 sets 8–10
D 3 sets 8–10
E 3 sets 12–15
G 3 sets 10–12
I 3 sets 10–12
K 3 sets 10–12
O 3 sets 10–12
P 3 sets 12–15
R 25 per side
T 3 sets 15

Day Six:
Cardio 30–45 minutes

Day Seven:
Rest

WORKOUT LEVEL 2

BEGINNER ROUTINE 2

Day One:
B 3 sets 12–15
C 3 sets 8–10
F 3 sets 10–12
H 3 sets 10–12
J 3 sets 10–12
L 3 sets 12–15

Day Two:
Rest

Day Three:
B 3 sets 12–15
C 3 sets 8–10
F 3 sets 10–12
H 3 sets 10–12
J 3 sets 10–12
L 3 sets 12–15

Day Four:
Rest

Day Five:
B 3 sets 12–15
C 3 sets 8–10
F 3 sets 10–12
H 3 sets 10–12
J 3 sets 10–12
L 3 sets 12–15

Day Six:
Cardio 30–45 minutes

Day Seven:
Rest

INTERMEDIATE ROUTINE 2

Day One:
B 3 sets 12–15
C 3 sets 8–10
F 3 sets 10–12
H 3 sets 10–12
J 3 sets 10–12
L 3 sets 12–15
M 3 sets 15–20
N 3 sets 15–20

Day Two:
Cardio 30–45 minutes

Day Three:
B 3 sets 12–15
C 3 sets 8–10
F 3 sets 10–12
H 3 sets 10–12
J 3 sets 10–12
L 3 sets 12–15
M 3 sets 15–20
N 3 sets 15–20

Day Four:
Rest

Day Five:
B 3 sets 12–15
C 3 sets 8–10
F 3 sets 10–12
H 3 sets 10–12
J 3 sets 10–12
L 3 sets 12–15
M 3 sets 15–20
N 3 sets 15–20

Day Six:
Cardio 30–45 minutes

Day Seven:
Rest

ADVANCED ROUTINE 2

Day One:
B 3 sets 12–15
C 3 sets 8–10
F 3 sets 10–12
H 3 sets 10–12
J 3 sets 10–12
L 3 sets 12–15
M 3 sets 15–20
N 3 sets 15–20
Q 3 sets 25
S sets 20

Day Two:
Cardio 30–45 minutes

Day Three:
B 3 sets 12–15
C 3 sets 8–10
F 3 sets 10–12
H 3 sets 10–12
J 3 sets 10–12
L 3 sets 12–15
M 3 sets 15–20
N 3 sets 15–20
Q 3 sets 25
S sets 20

Day Four:
Cardio 30–45 minutes

Day Five:
B 3 sets 12–15
C 3 sets 8–10
F 3 sets 10–12
H 3 sets 10–12
J 3 sets 10–12
L 3 sets 12–15
M 3 sets 15–20
N 3 sets 15–20
Q 3 sets 25
S sets 20

Day Six:
Cardio 30–45 minutes

Day Seven:
Rest

WATER SKIING WORKOUTS

A Lat Pulldown
page 42

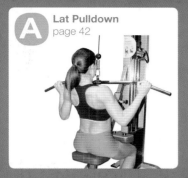

B Scapular Range of Motion
page 44

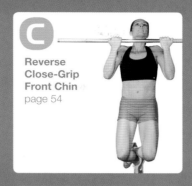

C Reverse Close-Grip Front Chin
page 54

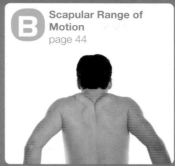

D Dumbbell Shoulder Press
page 74

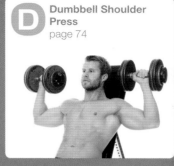

E External Rotation with Band
page 80

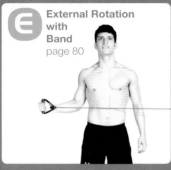

F Reverse Fly
page 88

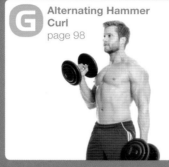

G Alternating Hammer Curl
page 98

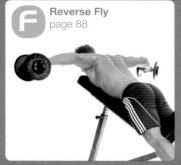

H Bicep Curl
page 96

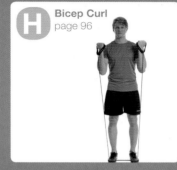

I Rope Pushdown
page 106

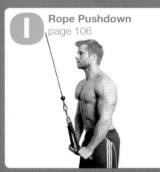

J Lying Triceps Extension
page 108

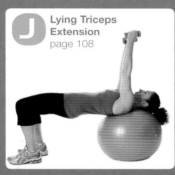

K Swiss Ball Wall-Sit
page 134

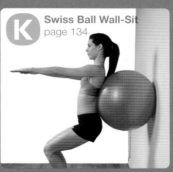

L One-Legged Step-Down
page 152

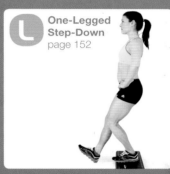

M Adductor Extension
page 162

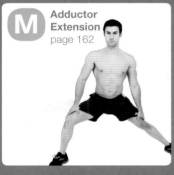

N Hamstring Abductor
page 163

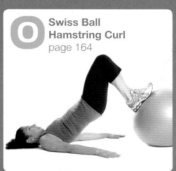

O Swiss Ball Hamstring Curl
page 164

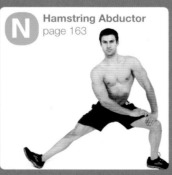

P Dumbbell Calf Raise
page 178

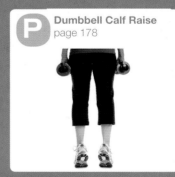

Q Crunch
page 118

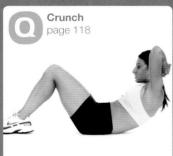

R Abdominal Kick
page 184

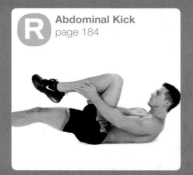

S Reverse Crunch
page 192

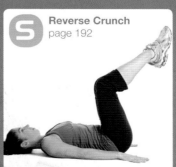

T Plank Press-Up
page 198

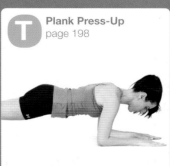

WRESTLING

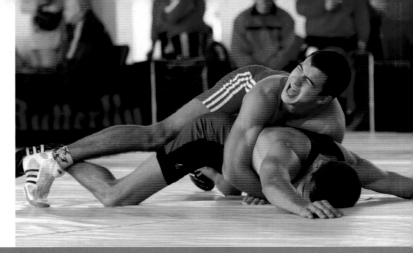

In wrestling, the biceps help to pull opponents to the mat as well as to pin them. The core muscles are engaged in every wresting maneuver; the abdominals especially need to be strong for the completion of a takedown, as well as for escaping being pinned. The neck and upper back work together for escaping pins as well as for getting out of holds such as the headlock. The thighs and glutes work together for pushing and lifting an opponent off the ground.

BEGINNER ROUTINE I

Day One:
C 3 sets 8–10
E 3 sets 10–12
F 3 sets 10–12
J 3 sets 12–15
K 3 sets 12–15
N 30–120 seconds

Day Two:
Rest

Day Three:
C 3 sets 8–10
E 3 sets 10–12
F 3 sets 10–12
J 3 sets 12–15
K 3 sets 12–15
N 30–120 seconds

Day Four:
Rest

Day Five:
C 3 sets 8–10
E 3 sets 10–12
F 3 sets 10–12
J 3 sets 12–15
K 3 sets 12–15
N 30–120 seconds

Day Six:
Cardio 30–45 minutes

Day Seven:
Rest

INTERMEDIATE ROUTINE I

Day One:
C 3 sets 8–10
E 3 sets 10–12
F 3 sets 10–12
J 3 sets 12–15
K 3 sets 12–15
N 30–120 seconds
O 30–60 seconds
P 30 per side

Day Two:
Cardio 30–45 minutes

Day Three:
C 3 sets 8–10
E 3 sets 10–12
F 3 sets 10–12
J 3 sets 12–15
K 3 sets 12–15
N 30–120 seconds
O 30–60 seconds
P 30 per side

Day Four:
Rest

Day Five:
C 3 sets 8–10
E 3 sets 10–12
F 3 sets 10–12
J 3 sets 12–15
K 3 sets 12–15
N 30–120 seconds
O 30–60 seconds
P 30 per side

Day Six:
Cardio 30–45 minutes

Day Seven:
Rest

ADVANCED ROUTINE I

Day One:
C 3 sets 8–10
E 3 sets 10–12
F 3 sets 10–12
J 3 sets 12–15
K 3 sets 12–15
N 30–120 seconds
O 30–60 seconds
P 30 per side
Q 3 sets 8–10
R 3 sets 15

Day Two:
Cardio 30–45 minutes

Day Three:
C 3 sets 8–10
E 3 sets 10–12
F 3 sets 10–12
J 3 sets 12–15
K 3 sets 12–15
N 30–120 seconds
O 30–60 seconds
P 30 per side
Q 3 sets 8–10
R 3 sets 15

Day Four:
Cardio 30–45 minutes

Day Five:
C 3 sets 8–10
E 3 sets 10–12
F 3 sets 10–12
J 3 sets 12–15
K 3 sets 12–15
N 30–120 seconds
O 30–60 seconds
P 30 per side
Q 3 sets 8–10
R 3 sets 15

Day Six:
Cardio 30–45 minutes

Day Seven:
Rest

BEGINNER ROUTINE 2

Day One:
A 3 sets 8–10
B 3 sets 12–15
D 3 sets 8–10
G 3 sets 10–12
H 3 sets 12–15
I 3 sets 10–12

Day Two:
Rest

Day Three:
A 3 sets 8–10
B 3 sets 12–15
D 3 sets 8–10
G 3 sets 10–12
H 3 sets 12–15
I 3 sets 10–12

Day Four:
Rest

Day Five:
A 3 sets 8–10
B 3 sets 12–15
D 3 sets 8–10
G 3 sets 10–12
H 3 sets 12–15
I 3 sets 10–12

Day Six:
Cardio 30–45 minutes

Day Seven:
Rest

INTERMEDIATE ROUTINE 2

Day One:
A 3 sets 8–10
B 3 sets 12–15
D 3 sets 8–10
G 3 sets 10–12
H 3 sets 12–15
I 3 sets 10–12
L 3 sets 25
M 3 sets 20

Day Two:
Cardio 30–45 minutes

Day Three:
A 3 sets 8–10
B 3 sets 12–15
D 3 sets 8–10
G 3 sets 10–12
H 3 sets 12–15
I 3 sets 10–12
L 3 sets 25
M 3 sets 20

Day Four:
Rest

Day Five:
A 3 sets 8–10
B 3 sets 12–15
D 3 sets 8–10
G 3 sets 10–12
H 3 sets 12–15
I 3 sets 10–12
L 3 sets 25
M 3 sets 20

Day Six:
Cardio 30–45 minutes

Day Seven:
Rest

ADVANCED ROUTINE 2

Day One:
A 3 sets 8–10
B 3 sets 12–15
D 3 sets 8–10
G 3 sets 10–12
H 3 sets 12–15
I 3 sets 10–12
L 3 sets 25
M 3 sets 20
S 3 sets 20
T 3 sets 20

Day Two:
Cardio 30–45 minutes

Day Three:
A 3 sets 8–10
B 3 sets 12–15
D 3 sets 8–10
G 3 sets 10–12
H 3 sets 12–15
I 3 sets 10–12
L 3 sets 25
M 3 sets 20
S 3 sets 20
T 3 sets 20e

Day Four:
Cardio 30–45 minutes

Day Five:
A 3 sets 8–10
B 3 sets 12–15
D 3 sets 8–10
G 3 sets 10–12
H 3 sets 12–15
I 3 sets 10–12
L 3 sets 25
M 3 sets 20
S 3 sets 20
T 3 sets 20

Day Six:
Cardio 30–45 minutes

Day Seven:
Rest

WRESTLING WORKOUTS

A Lat Pulldown
page 42
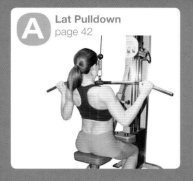

B Scapular Range of Motion
page 44
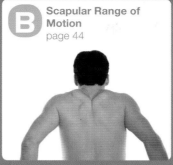

C Rope Pulldown
page 52
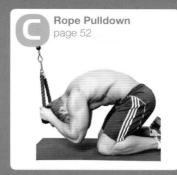

D Barbell Upright Row
page 86
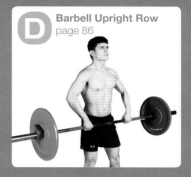

E Barbell Shoulder Shrug
page 94
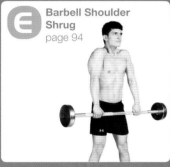

F Barbell Curl
page 100
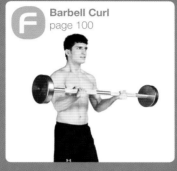

G Rope Hammer Curl
page 104
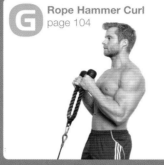

H Wrist Extension
page 117
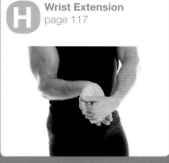

I Swiss Ball Wall Sit
page 134
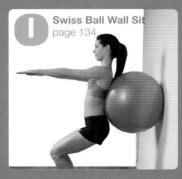

J Dumbbell Lunge
page 138
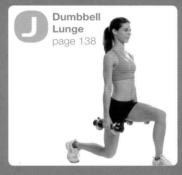

K Crossover Step
page 148
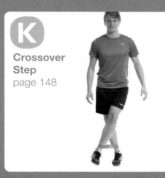

L Crunch
page 118
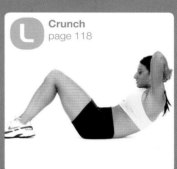

M Reverse Crunch
page 192
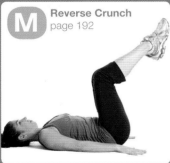

N Plank
page 120
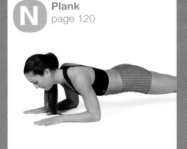

O Side Plank
page 122
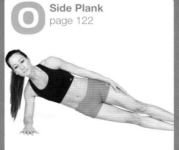

P Wood Chop with Resistance Band
page 202
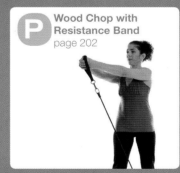

Q Alternating Renegade Row
page 48
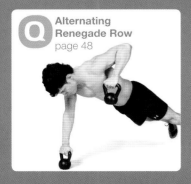

R Hip Abduction and Adduction
page 204
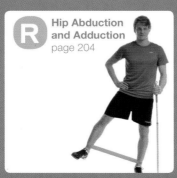

S Push-Up
page 70
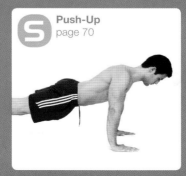

T V-Up
page 212
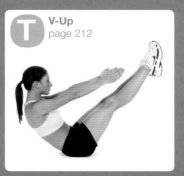

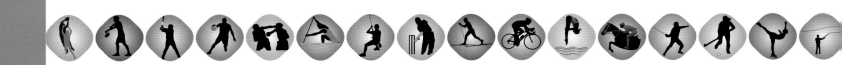

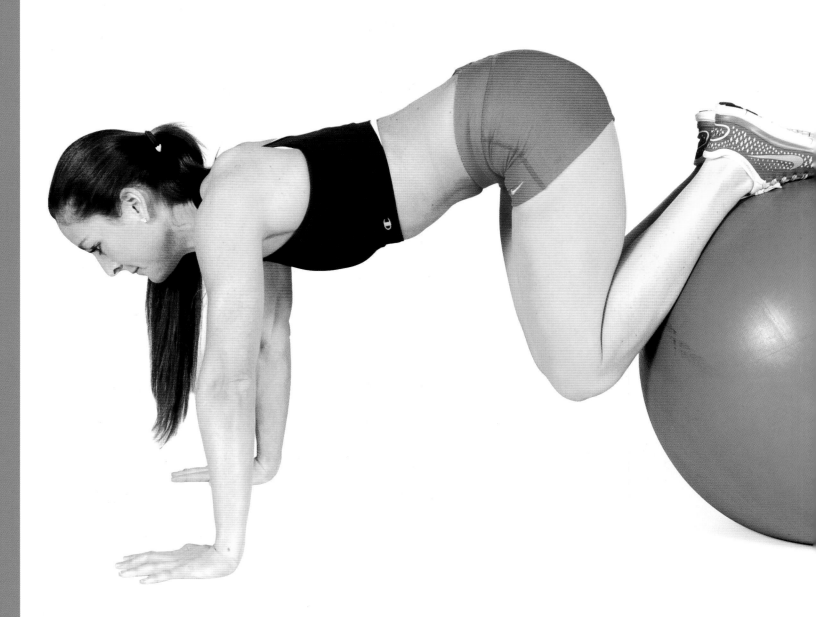

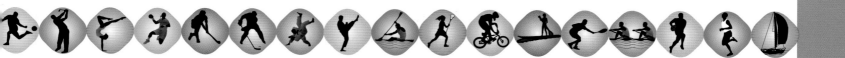

FUNCTIONAL WORKOUTS

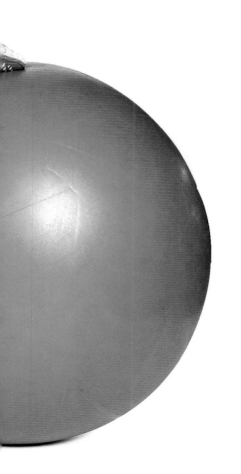

This is perhaps the most important section since it offers help in specific situations where stronger muscles can produce a better performance, help to avoid injuries or even help decrease recovery times where injuries already exist. Basic function and the reliability of the amazing machine that is the human body are more important than sporting achievement. The workouts provided here are suitable for people of all levels of fitness and with particular problems. Whether you have a bad back or weak knees there is an exercise routine to help. Attention to proper performance of each exercise at the correct speed, control and reach are important factors to consider and ultimately master if you are to get the most out of your body. These workouts will help to prepare it for all the challenges life throws at you.

HEALTHY BACK

A strong back helps stabilize the spine, making it easier to maintain correct posture and good mobility. And, as our mothers reminded us every day, posture is all important. From neck and back pain to blood flow and respiration, our posture has a major impact on how we live and how we feel. Good form is vital to perform proper lifting techniques and avoid putting unnecessary stress on the back. If you are receiving medical treatment for your back, check with your doctor before doing these exercises.

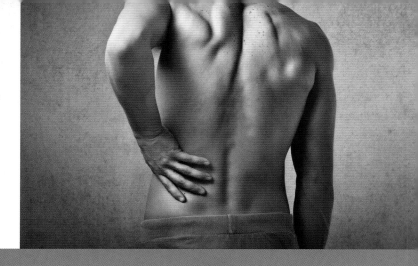

WORKOUT LEVEL 1

BEGINNER ROUTINE 1

Day One:
C 3 sets 8–10
D 3 sets 8–10
E 3 sets 8–10
H 3 sets 8–10
J 3 sets 8–10
M 3 sets 15

Day Two:
Rest

Day Three:
C 3 sets 8–10
D 3 sets 8–10
E 3 sets 8–10
H 3 sets 8–10
J 3 sets 8–10
M 3 sets 15

Day Four:
Rest

Day Five:
C 3 sets 8–10
D 3 sets 8–10
E 3 sets 8–10
H 3 sets 8–10
J 3 sets 8–10
M 3 sets 15

Day Six:
Cardio 30–45 minutes

Day Seven:
Rest

INTERMEDIATE ROUTINE 1

Day One:
C 3 sets 8–10
D 3 sets 8–10
E 3 sets 8–10
H 3 sets 8–10
J 3 sets 8–10
M 3 sets 15
N 3 sets 15
O 30–120 seconds

Day Two:
Cardio 30–45 minutes

Day Three:
C 3 sets 8–10
D 3 sets 8–10
E 3 sets 8–10
H 3 sets 8–10
J 3 sets 8–10
M 3 sets 15
N 3 sets 15
O 30–120 seconds

Day Four:
Rest

Day Five:
C 3 sets 8–10
D 3 sets 8–10
E 3 sets 8–10
H 3 sets 8–10
J 3 sets 8–10
M 3 sets 15
N 3 sets 15
O 30–120 seconds

Day Six:
Cardio 30–45 minutes

Day Seven:
Rest

ADVANCED ROUTINE 1

Day One:
C 3 sets 8–10
D 3 sets 8–10
E 3 sets 8–10
H 3 sets 8–10
J 3 sets 8–10
M 3 sets 15
N 3 sets 15
O 30–120 seconds
Q 30 per side
R 30–60 seconds per side

Day Two:
Cardio 30–45 minutes

Day Three:
C 3 sets 8–10
D 3 sets 8–10
E 3 sets 8–10
H 3 sets 8–10
J 3 sets 8–10
M 3 sets 15
N 3 sets 15
O 30–120 seconds
Q 30 per side
R 30–60 seconds per side

Day Four:
Cardio 30–45 minutes

Day Five:
C 3 sets 8–10
D 3 sets 8–10
E 3 sets 8–10
H 3 sets 8–10
J 3 sets 8–10
M 3 sets 15
N 3 sets 15
O 30–120 seconds
Q 30 per side
R 30–60 seconds per side

Day Six:
Cardio 30–45 minutes

Day Seven:
Rest

WORKOUT LEVEL 2

BEGINNER ROUTINE 2

Day One:
A 3 sets 6–8
B 3 sets 8–10
F 3 sets 12–15
G 3 sets 8–10
I 3 sets 8–10
K 3 sets 12–15

Day Two:
Rest

Day Three:
A 3 sets 6–8
B 3 sets 8–10
F 3 sets 12–15
G 3 sets 8–10
I 3 sets 8–10
K 3 sets 12–15

Day Four:
Rest

Day Five:
A 3 sets 6–8
B 3 sets 8–10
F 3 sets 12–15
G 3 sets 8–10
I 3 sets 8–10
K 3 sets 12–15

Day Six:
Cardio 30–45 minutes

Day Seven:
Rest

INTERMEDIATE ROUTINE 2

Day One:
A 3 sets 6–8
B 3 sets 8–10
F 3 sets 12–15
G 3 sets 8–10
I 3 sets 8–10
K 3 sets 12–15
L 3 sets 25
P 3 sets 30–60 seconds

Day Two:
Cardio 30–45 minutes

Day Three:
A 3 sets 6–8
B 3 sets 8–10
F 3 sets 12–15
G 3 sets 8–10
I 3 sets 8–10
K 3 sets 12–15
L 3 sets 25
P 3 sets 30–60 seconds

Day Four:
Rest

Day Five:
A 3 sets 6–8
B 3 sets 8–10
F 3 sets 12–15
G 3 sets 8–10
I 3 sets 8–10
K 3 sets 12–15
L 3 sets 25
P 3 sets 30–60 seconds

Day Six:
Cardio 30–45 minutes

Day Seven:
Rest

ADVANCED ROUTINE 2

Day One:
A 3 sets 6–8
B 3 sets 8–10
F 3 sets 12–15
G 3 sets 8–10
I 3 sets 8–10
K 3 sets 12–15
L 3 sets 25
P 3 sets 30–60 seconds
S 3 sets 25
T 3 sets 20

Day Two:
Cardio 30–45 minutes

Day Three:
A 3 sets 6–8
B 3 sets 8–10
F 3 sets 12–15
G 3 sets 8–10
I 3 sets 8–10
K 3 sets 12–15
L 3 sets 25
P 3 sets 30–60 seconds
S 3 sets 25
T 3 sets 20

Day Four:
Cardio 30–45 minutes

Day Five:
A 3 sets 6–8
B 3 sets 8–10
F 3 sets 12–15
G 3 sets 8–10
I 3 sets 8–10
K 3 sets 12–15
L 3 sets 25
P 3 sets 30–60 seconds
S 3 sets 25
T 3 sets 20

Day Six:
Cardio 30–45 minutes

Day Seven:
Rest

HEALTHY BACK WORKOUTS

A Barbell Deadlift
page 34
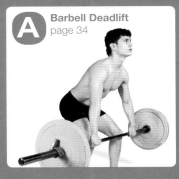

B Barbell Row
page 38
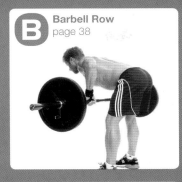

C Dumbbell Row
page 40
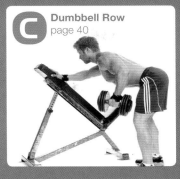

D Dumbbell Pullover
page 40
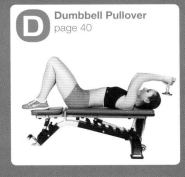

E Lat Pulldown
page 42
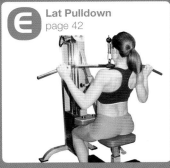

F Scapular Range of Motion
page 44
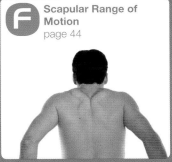

G Alternating Kettlebell Row
page 46
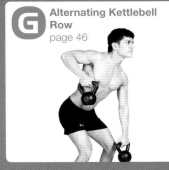

H Incline Bench Row
page 50
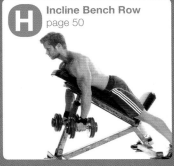

I Rope Pulldown
page 52
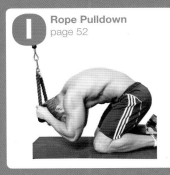

J Reverse Close-Grip Front Chin
page 54
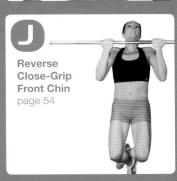

K Flat Bench Hyperextension
page 56
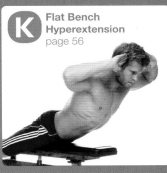

L Crunch
page 118
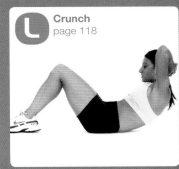

M Cobra Stretch
page 194
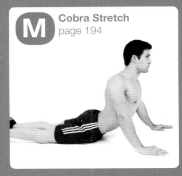

N Swiss Ball Pelvic Tilt
page 196
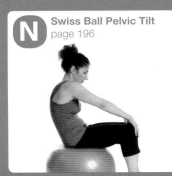

O Plank
page 120
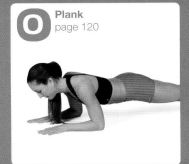

P Side Plank
page 122
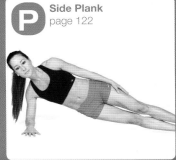

Q Wood Chop with Resistance Band
page 202
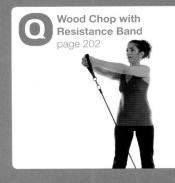

R T-Stabilization
page 124
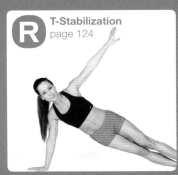

S Medicine Ball Slam
page 214
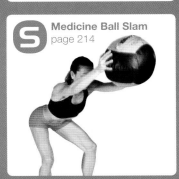

T The Windmill
page 216
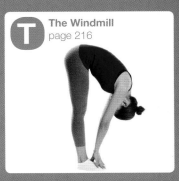

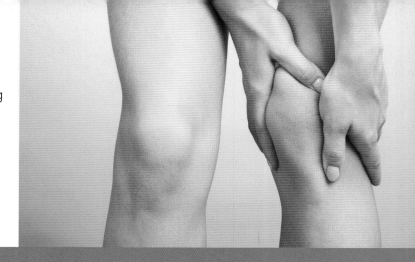

KNEE PROBLEMS

Knee rehabilitation can be helped through strengthening exercises. Rehab is important not only for lessening the burden on the knee joint, but also to prevent a weakening of the surrounding muscles. Stretching should be the first and last part of this workout. Low-impact cardiovascular exercise (eg, a session on a stationary bike) should be included after the strengthening portion of the program to increase endurance. Avoid strenuous or aggressive training.

WORKOUT LEVEL 1

BEGINNER ROUTINE 1

Day One:
A 20 seconds per leg
B 30 seconds per leg
C 3 sets 10–12
D 3 sets 12–15
G 3 sets 10–12
H 3 sets 12–15

Day Two:
Rest

Day Three:
A 20 seconds per leg
B 30 seconds per leg
C 3 sets 10–12
D 3 sets 12–15
G 3 sets 10–12
H 3 sets 12–15

Day Four:
Low Impact Cardio 30 minutes

Day Five:
A 20 seconds per leg
B 30 seconds per leg
C 3 sets 10–12
D 3 sets 12–15
G 3 sets 10–12
H 3 sets 12–15

Day Six:
Cardio 30–45 minutes

Day Seven:
Rest

INTERMEDIATE ROUTINE 1

Day One:
A 20 seconds per leg
B 30 seconds per leg
C 3 sets 10–12
D 3 sets 12–15
G 3 sets 10–12
H 3 sets 12–15
I 3 sets 12–15
J 3 sets 12–15

Day Two:
Low impact cardio 30 minutes

Day Three:
A 20 seconds per leg
B 30 seconds per leg
C 3 sets 10–12
D 3 sets 12–15
G 3 sets 10–12
H 3 sets 12–15
I 3 sets 12–15
J 3 sets 12–15

Day Four:
Low Impact Cardio 30 minutes

Day Five:
A 20 seconds per leg
B 30 seconds per leg
C 3 sets 10–12
D 3 sets 12–15
G 3 sets 10–12
H 3 sets 12–15
I 3 sets 12–15
J 3 sets 12–15

Day Six:
Rest

Day Seven:
Rest

ADVANCED ROUTINE 1

Day One:
A 20 seconds per leg
B 30 seconds per leg
C 3 sets 10–12
D 3 sets 12–15
G 3 sets 10–12
H 3 sets 12–15
I 3 sets 12–15
J 3 sets 12–15
K 30 seconds per leg
L 30 seconds per leg

Day Two:
Low Impact Cardio 30 minutes

Day Three:
A 20 seconds per leg
B 30 seconds per leg
C 3 sets 10–12
D 3 sets 12–15
G 3 sets 10–12
H 3 sets 12–15
I 3 sets 12–15
J 3 sets 12–15
K 30 seconds per leg
L 30 seconds per leg

Day Four:
Low Impact Cardio 30 minutes

Day Five:
A 20 seconds per leg
B 30 seconds per leg
C 3 sets 10–12
D 3 sets 12–15
G 3 sets 10–12
H 3 sets 12–15
I 3 sets 12–15
J 3 sets 12–15
K 30 seconds per leg
L 30 seconds per leg

Day Six:
Rest

Day Seven:
Rest

WORKOUT LEVEL 2

BEGINNER ROUTINE 2

Day One:
A 20 seconds per leg
B 30 seconds per leg
C 3 sets 10–12
D 3 sets 12–15
E 3 sets 15–20
F 3 sets 15–20

Day Two:
Rest

Day Three:
A 20 seconds per leg
B 30 seconds per leg
C 3 sets 10–12
D 3 sets 12–15
E 3 sets 15–20
F 3 sets 15–20

Day Four:
Low Impact Cardio 30 minutes

Day Five:
A 20 seconds per leg
B 30 seconds per leg
C 3 sets 10–12
D 3 sets 12–15
E 3 sets 15–20
F 3 sets 15–20

Day Six:
Rest

Day Seven:
Rest

INTERMEDIATE ROUTINE 2

Day One:
A 20 seconds per leg
B 30 seconds per leg
C 3 sets 10–12
D 3 sets 12–15
E 3 sets 15–20
F 3 sets 15–20
H 3 sets 12–15
J 3 sets 12–15

Day Two:
Low Impact Cardio 30 minutes

Day Three:
A 20 seconds per leg
B 30 seconds per leg
C 3 sets 10–12
D 3 sets 12–15
E 3 sets 15–20
F 3 sets 15–20
H 3 sets 12–15
J 3 sets 12–15

Day Four:
Low Impact Cardio 30 minutes

Day Five:
A 20 seconds per leg
B 30 seconds per leg
C 3 sets 10–12
D 3 sets 12–15
E 3 sets 15–20
F 3 sets 15–20
H 3 sets 12–15
J 3 sets 12–15

Day Six:
Rest

Day Seven:
Rest

ADVANCED ROUTINE 2

Day One:
A 20 seconds per leg
B 30 seconds per leg
C 3 sets 10–12
D 3 sets 12–15
E 3 sets 15–20
F 3 sets 15–20
H 3 sets 12–15
J 3 sets 12–15
K 30 seconds per leg
L 30 seconds per leg

Day Two:
Low Impact Cardio 30 minutes

Day Three:
A 20 seconds per leg
B 30 seconds per leg
C 3 sets 10–12
D 3 sets 12–15
E 3 sets 15–20
F 3 sets 15–20
H 3 sets 12–15
J 3 sets 12–15

Day Four:
Low Impact Cardio 30 minutes

Day Five:
A 20 seconds per leg
B 30 seconds per leg
C 3 sets 10–12
D 3 sets 12–15
E 3 sets 15–20
F 3 sets 15–20
H 3 sets 12–15
J 3 sets 12–15
K 30 seconds per leg
L 30 seconds per leg

Day Six:
Rest

Day Seven:
Rest

KNEE PROBLEMS WORKOUTS

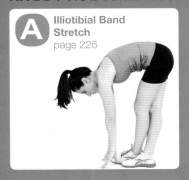

A Illiotibial Band Stretch
page 226

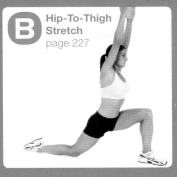

B Hip-To-Thigh Stretch
page 227

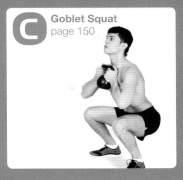

C Goblet Squat
page 150

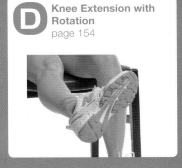

D Knee Extension with Rotation
page 154

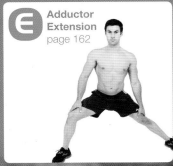

E Adductor Extension
page 162

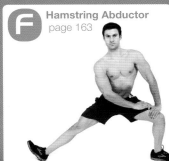

F Hamstring Abductor
page 163

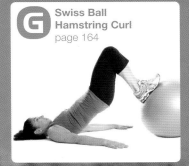

G Swiss Ball Hamstring Curl
page 164

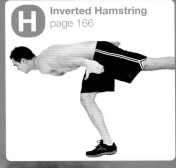

H Inverted Hamstring
page 166

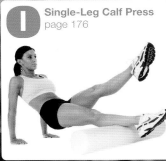

I Single-Leg Calf Press
page 176

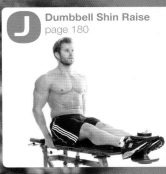

J Dumbbell Shin Raise
page 180

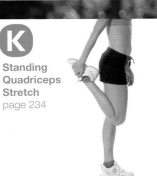

K Standing Quadriceps Stretch
page 234

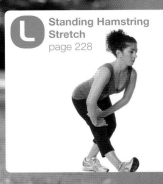

L Standing Hamstring Stretch
page 228

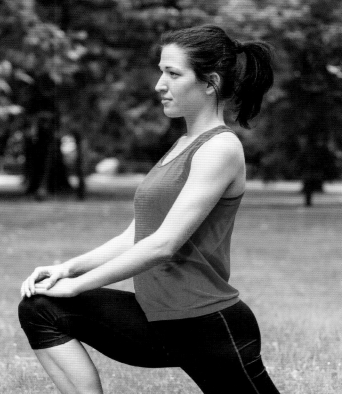

No equipment is needed for the stretches that can improve knee function — many of the exercises can be done anywhere, any time. Some exercises are commonly done for warm-ups before running or cool-downs afterward.

361

OFFICE FIT

Nowadays, millions of us spend the majority of our day sitting behind a desk for hours on end. Worse still, we often feel too mentally exhausted from work to make time to exercise later. The dangers are legion: weight gain, lethargy and bad posture to name but three (not to mention the host of health problems that can follow in their wake). This simple routine helps to counteract the negative effects of a sedentary lifestyle and is ideal for those of us who can't always make it to the gym.

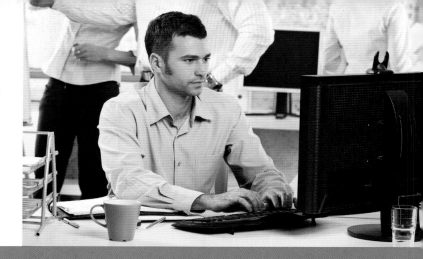

WORKOUT LEVEL 1

BEGINNER ROUTINE 1

Day One:
B 3 sets 20
C 3 sets 12–15
D 3 sets 10–12
F 3 sets 10–12
H 25 per side
I 3 sets 15

Day Two:
Rest

Day Three:
B 3 sets 20
C 3 sets 12–15
D 3 sets 10–12
F 3 sets 10–12
H 25 per side
I 3 sets 15

Day Four:
Rest

Day Five:
B 3 sets 20
C 3 sets 12–15
D 3 sets 10–12
F 3 sets 10–12
H 25 per side
I 3 sets 15

Day Six:
Cardio 30–45 minutes

Day Seven:
Rest

INTERMEDIATE ROUTINE 1

Day One:
B 3 sets 20
C 3 sets 12–15
D 3 sets 10–12
F 3 sets 10–12
H 25 per side
I 3 sets 15
J 3 sets 15
K 30–60 seconds

Day Two:
Cardio 30–45 minutes

Day Three:
B 3 sets 20
C 3 sets 12–15
D 3 sets 10–12
F 3 sets 10–12
H 25 per side
I 3 sets 15
J 3 sets 15
K 30–60 seconds

Day Four:
Rest

Day Five:
B 3 sets 20
C 3 sets 12–15
D 3 sets 10–12
F 3 sets 10–12
H 25 per side
I 3 sets 15
J 3 sets 15
K 30–60 seconds

Day Six:
Cardio 30–45 minutes

Day Seven:
Rest

ADVANCED ROUTINE 1

Day One:
B 3 sets 20
C 3 sets 12–15
D 3 sets 10–12
F 3 sets 10–12
H 25 per side
I 3 sets 15
J 3 sets 15
K 30–60 seconds
L 3 sets 20
N 3 sets 20

Day Two:
Cardio 30–45 minutes

Day Three:
B 3 sets 20
C 3 sets 12–15
D 3 sets 10–12
F 3 sets 10–12
H 25 per side
I 3 sets 15
J 3 sets 15
K 30–60 seconds

L 3 sets 20
N 3 sets 20

Day Four:
Cardio 30–45 minutes

Day Five:
B 3 sets 20
C 3 sets 12–15
D 3 sets 10–12
F 3 sets 10–12
H 25 per side
I 3 sets 15
J 3 sets 15
K 30–60 seconds
L 3 sets 20
N 3 sets 20

Day Six:
Cardio 30–45 minutes

Day Seven:
Rest

WORKOUT LEVEL 2

BEGINNER ROUTINE 2

Day One:
A 3 sets 12–15
C 3 sets 12–15
E 3 sets 12–15
F 3 sets 10–12
G 3 sets 25
H 25 per side

Day Two:
Rest

Day Three:
A 3 sets 12–15
C 3 sets 12–15
E 3 sets 12–15
F 3 sets 10–12
G 3 sets 25
H 25 per side

Day Four:
Rest

Day Five:
A 3 sets 12–15
C 3 sets 12–15
E 3 sets 12–15
F 3 sets 10–12
G 3 sets 25
H 25 per side

Day Six:
Cardio 30–45 minutes

Day Seven:
Rest

INTERMEDIATE ROUTINE 2

Day One:
A 3 sets 12–15
C 3 sets 12–15
E 3 sets 12–15
F 3 sets 10–12
G 3 sets 25
H 25 per side
I 3 sets 15
J 3 sets 15

Day Two:
Cardio 30–45 minutes

Day Three:
A 3 sets 12–15
C 3 sets 12–15
E 3 sets 12–15
F 3 sets 10–12
G 3 sets 25
H 25 per side
I 3 sets 15
J 3 sets 15

Day Four:
Rest

Day Five:
A 3 sets 12–15
C 3 sets 12–15
E 3 sets 12–15
F 3 sets 10–12
G 3 sets 25
H 25 per side
I 3 sets 15
J 3 sets 15

Day Six:
Cardio 30–45 minutes

Day Seven:
Rest

ADVANCED ROUTINE 2

Day One:
A 3 sets 12–15
C 3 sets 12–15
E 3 sets 12–15
F 3 sets 10–12
G 3 sets 25
H 25 per side
I 3 sets 15
J 3 sets 15
K 30–60 seconds
M 3 sets 15

Day Two:
Cardio 30–45 minutes

Day Three:
A 3 sets 12–15
C 3 sets 12–15
E 3 sets 12–15
F 3 sets 10–12
G 3 sets 25
H 25 per side
I 3 sets 15
J 3 sets 15

K 30–60 seconds
M 3 sets 15

Day Four:
Cardio 30–45 minutes

Day Five:
A 3 sets 12–15
C 3 sets 12–15
E 3 sets 12–15
F 3 sets 10–12
G 3 sets 25
H 25 per side
I 3 sets 15
J 3 sets 15
K 30–60 seconds
M 3 sets 15

Day Six:
Cardio 30–45 minutes

Day Seven:
Rest

OFFICE FIT WORKOUTS

A Push-Up
page 70
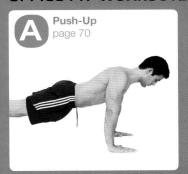

B Push-Up Hand Walk-Over
page 72
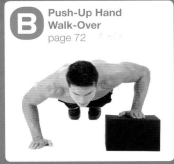

C Chair Dip
page 112
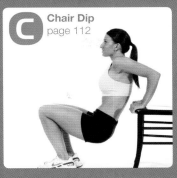

D Swiss Ball Wall Sit
page 134
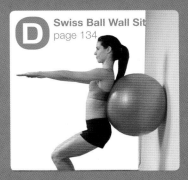

E Dumbbell Lunge
page 138
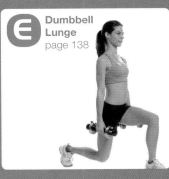

F Stiff-Legged Deadlift
page 174
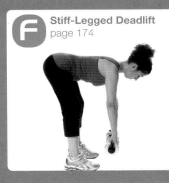

G Crunch
page 118
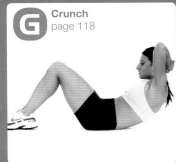

H Abdominal Kick
page 184
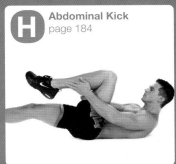

I Cobra Stretch
page 194
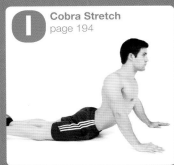

J Plank Press-Up
page 198
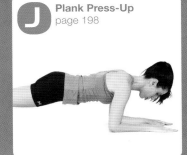

K Side Plank
page 122
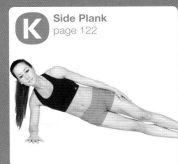

L Burpee
page 160
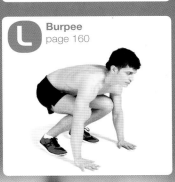

M Hip Abduction and Adduction
page 204
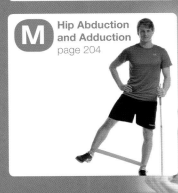

N V-Up
page 212
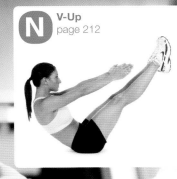

Many businesses offer organized exercise classes, including yoga and pilates, to their employees during lunch hours. Some companies give a financial incentive to join a health club.

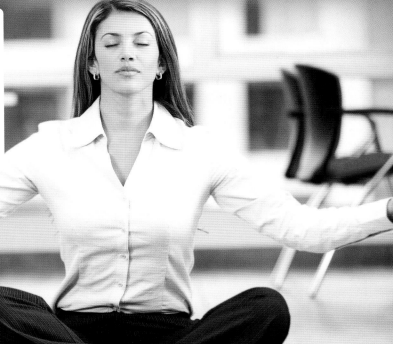

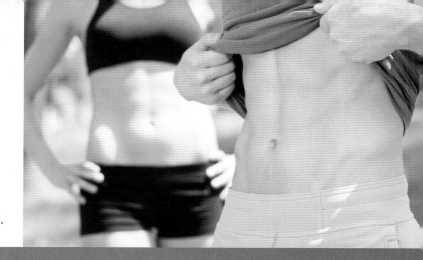

BELLY BUSTER

Of all of the showcase muscles in the human body, none receive more attention and admiration than the abdominals. It is the one muscle group that need not be increased in size, but rather should be toned and sculpted into that holy grail of health and athleticism — the six pack. Fab abs are only achieved through a combination of cardiovascular exercise, good nutrition and regular abdominal exercise. This belly-busting workout will set you on the right path in next to no time.

BEGINNER ROUTINE I

Day One:
A 3 sets 25
B 25 per side
C 3 sets 20
D 3 sets 15
E 3 sets 15
F 30 per side

Day Two:
Rest

Day Three:
A 3 sets 25
B 25 per side
C 3 sets 20
D 3 sets 15
E 3 sets 15
F 30 per side

Day Four:
Rest

Day Five:
A 3 sets 25
B 25 per side
C 3 sets 20
D 3 sets 15
E 3 sets 15
F 30 per side

Day Six:
Cardio 30–45 minutes

Day Seven:
Rest

INTERMEDIATE ROUTINE I

Day One:
A 3 sets 25
B 25 per side
C 3 sets 20
D 3 sets 15
E 3 sets 15
F 30 per side
G 30–60 seconds per side
H 3 sets 20

Day Two:
Cardio 30–45 minutes

Day Three:
A 3 sets 25
B 25 per side
C 3 sets 20
D 3 sets 15
E 3 sets 15
F 30 per side
G 30–60 seconds per side
H 3 sets 20

Day Four:
Rest

Day Five:
A 3 sets 25
B 25 per side
C 3 sets 20
D 3 sets 15
E 3 sets 15
F 30 per side
G 30–60 seconds per side
H 3 sets 20

Day Six:
Cardio 30–45 minutes

Day Seven:
Rest

ADVANCED ROUTINE I

Day One:
A 3 sets 25
B 25 per side
C 3 sets 20
D 3 sets 15
E 3 sets 15
F 30 per side
G 30–60 seconds per side
H 3 sets 20
I 3 sets 20
J 20 per side

Day Two:
Cardio 30–45 minutes

Day Three:
A 3 sets 25
B 25 per side
C 3 sets 20
D 3 sets 15
E 3 sets 15
F 30 per side
G 30–60 seconds per side
H 3 sets 20

I 3 sets 20
J 20 per side

Day Four:
Cardio 30–45 minutes

Day Five:
C 3 sets 8–10
D 3 sets 8–10
E 3 sets 8–10
H 3 sets 8–10
J 3 sets 8–10
M 3 sets 15
N 3 sets 15
O 30–120 seconds
Q 30 per side
R 30–60 seconds per side

Day Six:
Cardio 30–45 minutes

Day Seven:
Rest

The crunch strengthens all the muscles of the abdomen as well as improving core stability. Keep your elbows wide apart as you lift your upper body off the floor to avoid forcing the movement and ensure that the core muscles are fully engaged.

BELLY BUSTER WORKOUTS

A Crunch
page 118
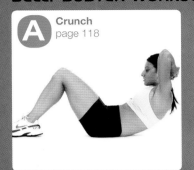

B Abdominal Kick
page 184
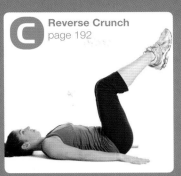

C Reverse Crunch
page 192
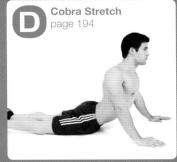

D Cobra Stretch
page 194
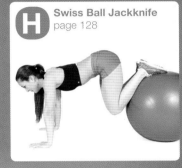

E Plank Press-Up
page 198
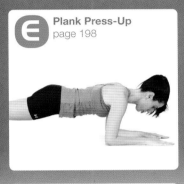

F Wood Chop with Resistance Band
page 202
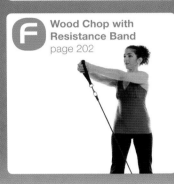

G T-Stabilization
page 124
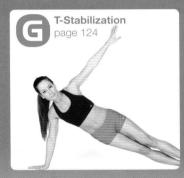

H Swiss Ball Jackknife
page 128
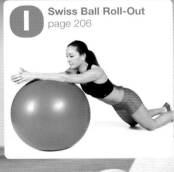

I Swiss Ball Roll-Out
page 206

J The Windmill
page 216
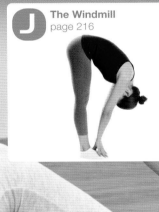

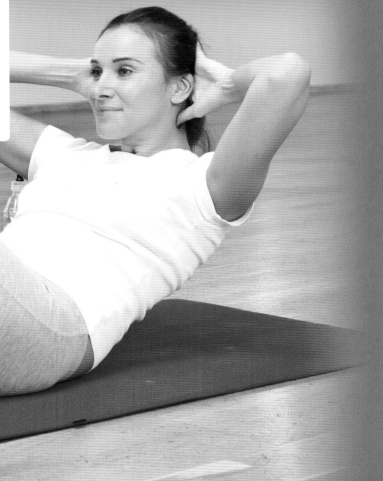

CARDIO PLAN

As well as providing an overall muscle-strengthening workout, the cardio plan also focuses on stamina by exercising the heart and lungs. It has a host of benefits: strengthening your heart (in the end it's a muscle and needs to be exercised like any other), increasing your metabolism to burn off calories (and excess fat) more quickly, releasing "feel good" hormones to relieve stress, and improving recovery time so you can get back in the gym more quickly and reboot the whole virtuous cycle.

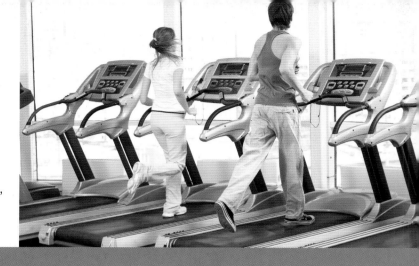

WORKOUT LEVEL 1

BEGINNER ROUTINE 1

Day One:
B 3 sets 10–12
D 3 sets 12–15
E 3 sets 10–12
G 3 sets 12–15
I 3 sets 15
P 3 sets 25

Day Two:
Rest

Day Three:
B 3 sets 10–12
D 3 sets 12–15
E 3 sets 10–12
G 3 sets 12–15
I 3 sets 15
P 3 sets 25

Day Four:
Cardio 45 minutes

Day Five:
B 3 sets 10–12
D 3 sets 12–15
E 3 sets 10–12
G 3 sets 12–15
I 3 sets 15
P 3 sets 25

Day Six:
Cardio 45 minutes

Day Seven:
Rest

INTERMEDIATE ROUTINE 1

Day One:
B 3 sets 10–12
D 3 sets 12–15
E 3 sets 10–12
G 3 sets 12–15
I 3 sets 15
J 3 sets 15
K 30–120 seconds
P 3 sets 25

Day Two:
Cardio 30–45 minutes

Day Three:
B 3 sets 10–12
D 3 sets 12–15
E 3 sets 10–12
G 3 sets 12–15
I 3 sets 15
J 3 sets 15
K 30–120 seconds
P 3 sets 25

Day Four:
Rest

Day Five:
B 3 sets 10–12
D 3 sets 12–15
E 3 sets 10–12
G 3 sets 12–15
I 3 sets 15
J 3 sets 15
K 30–120 seconds
P 3 sets 25

Day Six:
Cardio 45 minutes

Day Seven:
Rest

ADVANCED ROUTINE 1

Day One:
B 3 sets 10–12
D 3 sets 12–15
E 3 sets 10–12
G 3 sets 12–15
I 3 sets 15
J 3 sets 15
K 30–120 seconds
L 3 sets 20
O 3 sets 20
P 3 sets 25

Day Two:
Cardio 45 minutes

Day Three:
B 3 sets 10–12
D 3 sets 12–15
E 3 sets 10–12
G 3 sets 12–15
I 3 sets 15
J 3 sets 15
K 30–120 seconds
L 3 sets 20

O 3 sets 20
P 3 sets 25

Day Four:
Cardio 45 minutes

Day Five:
B 3 sets 10–12
D 3 sets 12–15
E 3 sets 10–12
G 3 sets 12–15
I 3 sets 15
J 3 sets 15
K 30–120 seconds
L 3 sets 20
O 3 sets 20
P 3 sets 25

Day Six:
Cardio 45 minutes

Day Seven:
Rest

WORKOUT LEVEL 2

BEGINNER ROUTINE 2

Day One:
A 3 sets 6–8
C 3 sets 12–15
E 3 sets 10–12
F 3 sets 12–15
H 3 sets 15
I 3 sets 15

Day Two:
Rest

Day Three:
A 3 sets 6–8
C 3 sets 12–15
E 3 sets 10–12
F 3 sets 12–15
H 3 sets 15
I 3 sets 15

Day Four:
Cardio 45 minutes

Day Five:
A 3 sets 6–8
C 3 sets 12–15
E 3 sets 10–12
F 3 sets 12–15
H 3 sets 15
I 3 sets 15

Day Six:
Cardio 45 minutes

Day Seven:
Rest

INTERMEDIATE ROUTINE 2

Day One:
A 3 sets 6–8
C 3 sets 12–15
E 3 sets 10–12
F 3 sets 12–15
H 3 sets 15
I 3 sets 15
K 30–120 seconds
L 3 sets 20

Day Two:
Cardio 30–45 minutes

Day Three:
A 3 sets 6–8
C 3 sets 12–15
E 3 sets 10–12
F 3 sets 12–15
H 3 sets 15
I 3 sets 15
K 30–120 seconds
L 3 sets 20

Day Four:
Cardio 45 minutes

Day Five:
A 3 sets 6–8
C 3 sets 12–15
E 3 sets 10–12
F 3 sets 12–15
H 3 sets 15
I 3 sets 15
K 30–120 seconds
L 3 sets 20

Day Six:
Cardio 45 minutes

Day Seven:
Rest

ADVANCED ROUTINE 2

Day One:
A 3 sets 6–8
C 3 sets 12–15
E 3 sets 10–12
F 3 sets 12–15
H 3 sets 15
I 3 sets 15
K 30–120 seconds
L 3 sets 20
M 3 sets 15
N 3 sets 20

Day Two:
Cardio 45 minutes

Day Three:
A 3 sets 6–8
C 3 sets 12–15
E 3 sets 10–12
F 3 sets 12–15
H 3 sets 15
I 3 sets 15
K 30–120 seconds
L 3 sets 20
M 3 sets 15
N 3 sets 20

Day Four:
Cardio 45 minutes

Day Five:
A 3 sets 6–8
C 3 sets 12–15
E 3 sets 10–12
F 3 sets 12–15
H 3 sets 15
I 3 sets 15
K 30–120 seconds
L 3 sets 20
M 3 sets 15
N 3 sets 20

Day Six:
Cardio 45 minutes

Day Seven:
Rest

CARDIO PLAN WORKOUTS

A Barbell Deadlift
page 34
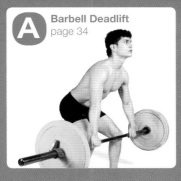

B Swiss Ball Wall Sit
page 134
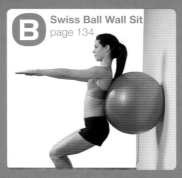

C Dumbbell Walking Lunge
page 144
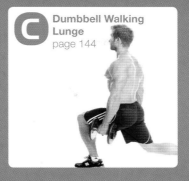

D One-Legged Step-Down
page 152
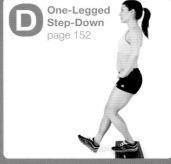

E Swiss Ball Hamstring Curl
page 164
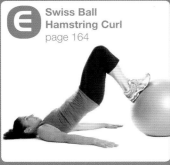

F Stiff-Legged Barbell Deadlift
page 168
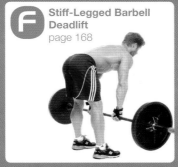

G Dumbbell Calf Raise
page 178
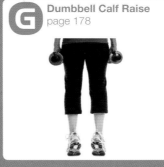

H Cobra Stretch
page 194
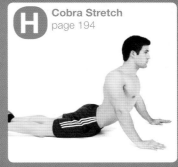

I Plank Press-Up
page 198
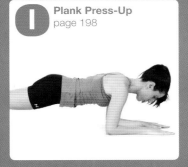

J Star Jump
page 156
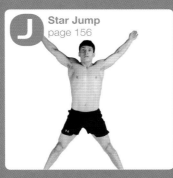

K Mountain Climber
page 158
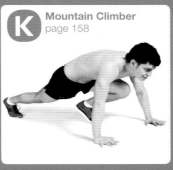

L Burpee
page 160
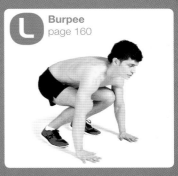

M Hip Abduction and Adduction
page 204
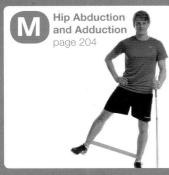

N Swiss Ball Hip Crossover
page 210
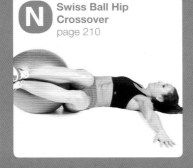

O V-Up
page 212
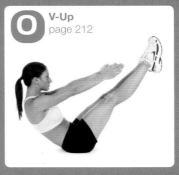

P Medicine Ball Slam
page 214
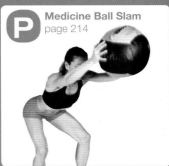

STRONGER LEGS

Toned legs look great, but we neglect our legs at our peril because weak legs (quite literally) undermine upper-body strength. Correct form for many lifts in training and daily life relies on the strength of the legs, and underdeveloped leg muscles can result in injuries — to the knees and lower back especially. Squats and deadlifts work your whole body, not just your legs, and should form a part of any good exercise regime.

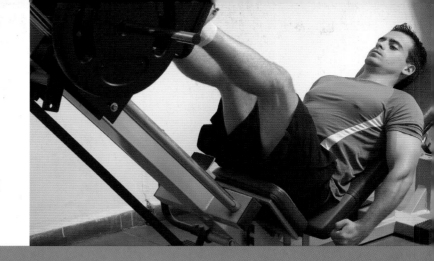

BEGINNER ROUTINE I

Day One:
A 3 sets 10–12
C 3 sets 10–12
E 3 sets 12–15
F 3 sets 10–12
H 3 sets 10–12
I 3 sets 12–15

Day Two:
Rest

Day Three:
A 3 sets 10–12
C 3 sets 10–12
E 3 sets 12–15
F 3 sets 10–12
H 3 sets 10–12
I 3 sets 12–15

Day Four:
Rest

Day Five:
A 3 sets 10–12
C 3 sets 10–12
E 3 sets 12–15
F 3 sets 10–12
H 3 sets 10–12
I 3 sets 12–15

Day Six:
Cardio 30–45 minutes

Day Seven:
Rest

INTERMEDIATE ROUTINE I

Day One:
A 3 sets 10–12
B 3 sets 12–15
C 3 sets 10–12
E 3 sets 12–15
F 3 sets 10–12
G 3 sets 12–15
H 3 sets 10–12
I 3 sets 12–15

Day Two:
Cardio 30–45 minutes

Day Three:
A 3 sets 10–12
B 3 sets 12–15
C 3 sets 10–12
E 3 sets 12–15
F 3 sets 10–12
G 3 sets 12–15
H 3 sets 10–12
I 3 sets 12–15

Day Four:
Rest

Day Five:
A 3 sets 10–12
B 3 sets 12–15
C 3 sets 10–12
E 3 sets 12–15
F 3 sets 10–12
G 3 sets 12–15
H 3 sets 10–12
I 3 sets 12–15

Day Six:
Cardio 30–45 minutes

Day Seven:
Rest

ADVANCED ROUTINE I

Day One:
A 3 sets 10–12
B 3 sets 12–15
C 3 sets 10–12
D 3 sets 12–15
E 3 sets 12–15
F 3 sets 10–12
G 3 sets 12–15
H 3 sets 10–12
I 3 sets 12–15
J 3 sets 12–15

Day Two:
Cardio 30–45 minutes

Day Three:
A 3 sets 10–12
B 3 sets 12–15
C 3 sets 10–12
D 3 sets 12–15
E 3 sets 12–15
F 3 sets 10–12
G 3 sets 12–15
H 3 sets 10–12
I 3 sets 12–15
J 3 sets 12–15

Day Four:
Cardio 30–45 minutes

Day Five:
A 3 sets 10–12
B 3 sets 12–15
C 3 sets 10–12
D 3 sets 12–15
E 3 sets 12–15
F 3 sets 10–12
G 3 sets 12–15
H 3 sets 10–12
I 3 sets 12–15
J 3 sets 12–15

Day Six:
Cardio 30–45 minutes

Day Seven:
Rest

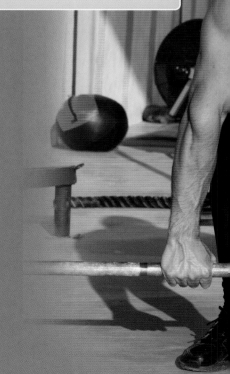

The deadlift activates muscles throughout the back, torso and legs as well as in the arms. Proper technique is critical to use the correct muscles and avoid injury to the back.

STRONGER LEGS WORKOUTS

A Swiss Ball Wall Sit
page 134
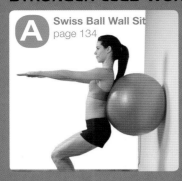

B Dumbbell Lunge
page 138
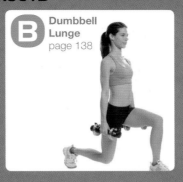

C Goblet Squat
page 150
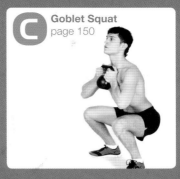

D One-Legged Step-Down
page 152
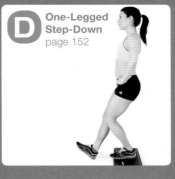

E Knee Extension with Rotation
page 154
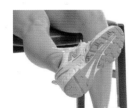

F Swiss Ball Hamstring Curl
page 164
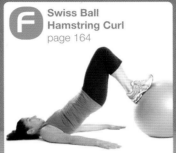

G Inverted Hamstring
page 166
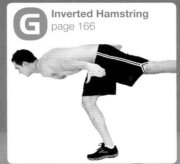

H Stiff-Legged Deadlift
page 174
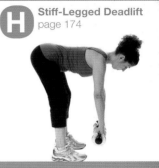

I Dumbbell Calf Raise
page 178
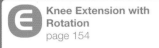

J Dumbbell Shin Raise
page 180

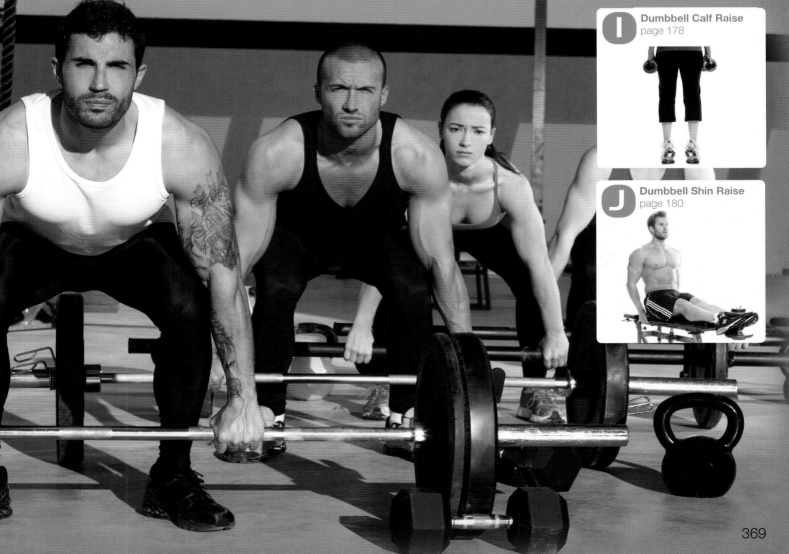

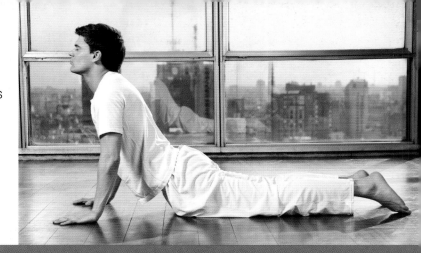

CORE STABILITY

Our sedentary lifestyles and the innumerable conveniences of modern living — even the artificial surfaces we walk on — come at a price. This routine focuses on building strength in the muscles that support the spine, shoulders and hips. It can be done in conjunction with the the belly buster workouts for all-round core fitness. Core work is vital because good alignment is essential to effective aerobic and weight training, as well as to every other aspect of your life.

BEGINNER ROUTINE I

Day One:
A 3 sets 12–15
C 3 sets 12–15
E 3 sets 15
H 30–60 seconds
I 30–60 seconds per side
J 3 sets 20

Day Two:
Rest

Day Three:
A 3 sets 12–15
C 3 sets 12–15
E 3 sets 15
H 30–60 seconds
I 30–60 seconds per side
J 3 sets 20

Day Four:
Rest

Day Five:
A 3 sets 12–15
C 3 sets 12–15
E 3 sets 15
H 30–60 seconds
I 30–60 seconds per side
J 3 sets 20

Day Six:
Cardio 30–45 minutes

Day Seven:
Rest

INTERMEDIATE ROUTINE I

Day One:
A 3 sets 12–15
B 3 sets 12–15
C 3 sets 12–15
E 3 sets 15
F 3 sets 15
H 30–60 seconds
I 30–60 seconds per side
J 3 sets 20

Day Two:
Cardio 30–45 minutes

Day Three:
A 3 sets 12–15
B 3 sets 12–15
C 3 sets 12–15
E 3 sets 15
F 3 sets 15
H 30–60 seconds
I 30–60 seconds per side
J 3 sets 20

Day Four:
Rest

Day Five:
A 3 sets 12–15
B 3 sets 12–15
C 3 sets 12–15
E 3 sets 15
F 3 sets 15
H 30–60 seconds
I 30–60 seconds per side
J 3 sets 20

Day Six:
Cardio 30–45 minutes

Day Seven:
Rest

ADVANCED ROUTINE I

Day One:
A 3 sets 12–15
B 3 sets 12–15
C 3 sets 12–15
D 3 sets 15
E 3 sets 15
F 3 sets 15
G 30–60 seconds
H 30–60 seconds
I 30–60 seconds per side
J 3 sets 20

Day Two:
Cardio 30–45 minutes

Day Three:
A 3 sets 12–15
B 3 sets 12–15
C 3 sets 12–15
D 3 sets 15
E 3 sets 15
F 3 sets 15
G 30–60 seconds
H 30–60 seconds
I 30–60 seconds per side
J 3 sets 20

Day Four:
Cardio 30–45 minutes

Day Five:
A 3 sets 12–15
B 3 sets 12–15
C 3 sets 12–15
D 3 sets 15
E 3 sets 15
F 3 sets 15
G 30–60 seconds
H 30–60 seconds
I 30–60 seconds per side
J 3 sets 20

Day Six:
Cardio 30–45 minutes

Day Seven:
Rest

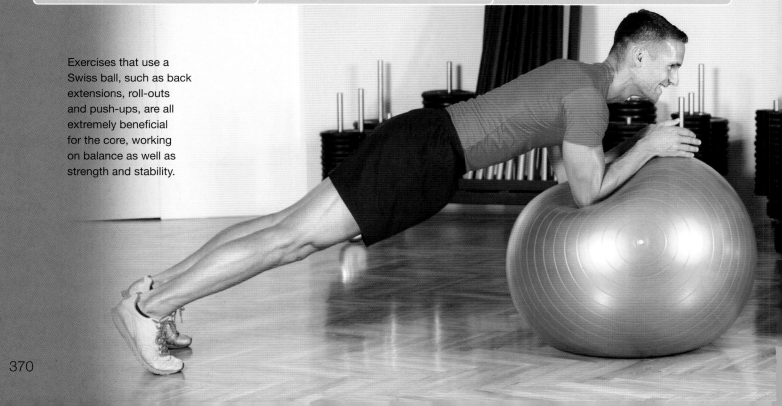

Exercises that use a Swiss ball, such as back extensions, roll-outs and push-ups, are all extremely beneficial for the core, working on balance as well as strength and stability.

CORE STABILITY WORKOUTS

A Flat Bench Hyperextension
page 56
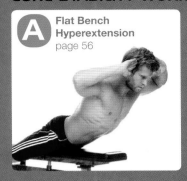

B Rotated Back Extension
page 58
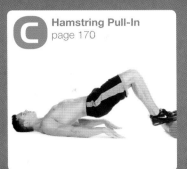

C Hamstring Pull-In
page 170
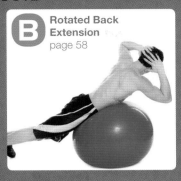

D Cobra Stretch
page 194
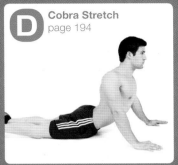

E Swiss Ball Pelvic Tilt
page 196
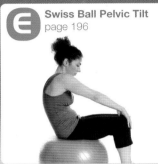

F Plank Press-Up
page 198
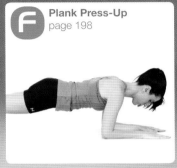

G Plank
page 120
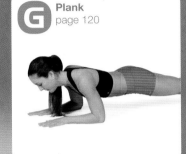

H Side Plank
page 122
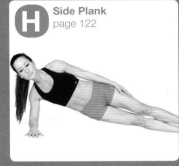

I T-Stabilization
page 124

J Swiss Ball Roll-Out
page 206
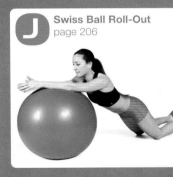

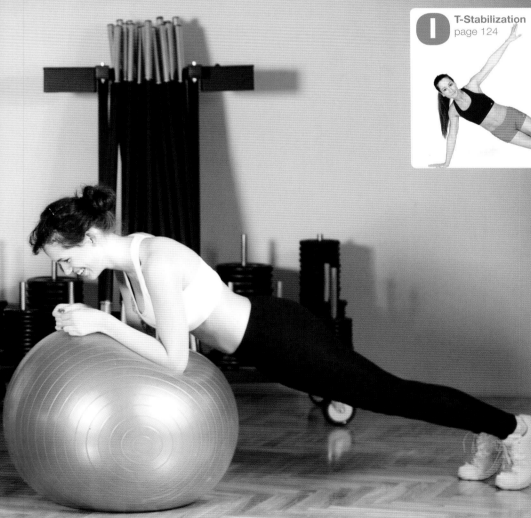

OVERALL STRENGTH

While a single-joint exercise such as a lateral raise will sculpt the side deltoid muscle, it will do little to increase your overall strength. Multi-joint, compound movements are instrumental to increasing strength. This power-packed workout is based around such exercises (deadlifts, presses and pulls). Where appropriate, work with the heaviest weight you can manage safely.

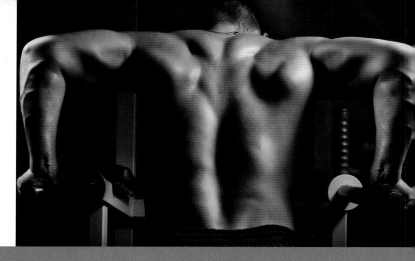

WORKOUT LEVEL 1

BEGINNER ROUTINE 1

Day One:
A 3 sets 6–8
B 3 sets 8–10
D 3 sets 8–10
F 3 sets 8–10
I 3 sets 10–12
J 3 sets 10–12

Day Two:
Rest

Day Three:
A 3 sets 6–8
B 3 sets 8–10
D 3 sets 8–10
F 3 sets 8–10
I 3 sets 10–12
J 3 sets 10–12

Day Four:
Rest

Day Five:
A 3 sets 6–8
B 3 sets 8–10
D 3 sets 8–10
F 3 sets 8–10
I 3 sets 10–12
J 3 sets 10–12

Day Six:
Cardio 30–45 minutes

Day Seven:
Rest

INTERMEDIATE ROUTINE 1

Day One:
A 3 sets 6–8
B 3 sets 8–10
D 3 sets 8–10
E 3 sets 8–10
F 3 sets 8–10
I 3 sets 10–12
J 3 sets 10–12

Day Two:
Cardio 30–45 minutes

Day Three:
A 3 sets 6–8
B 3 sets 8–10
D 3 sets 8–10
E 3 sets 8–10
F 3 sets 8–10
I 3 sets 10–12
J 3 sets 10–12
M 3 sets 20

Day Four:
Rest

Day Five:
A 3 sets 6–8
B 3 sets 8–10
D 3 sets 8–10
E 3 sets 8–10
F 3 sets 8–10
I 3 sets 10–12
J 3 sets 10–12
M 3 sets 20

Day Six:
Cardio 30–45 minutes

Day Seven:
Rest

ADVANCED ROUTINE 1

Day One:
A 3 sets 6–8
B 3 sets 8–10
D 3 sets 8–10
E 3 sets 8–10
F 3 sets 8–10
H 3 sets 10–12
I 3 sets 10–12
J 3 sets 10–12
L 30–60 seconds per side
M 3 sets 20

Day Two:
Cardio 30–45 minutes

Day Three:
A 3 sets 6–8
B 3 sets 8–10
D 3 sets 8–10
E 3 sets 8–10
F 3 sets 8–10
H 3 sets 10–12
I 3 sets 10–12
J 3 sets 10–12
L 30–60 seconds

per side
M 3 sets 20

Day Four:
Cardio 30–45 minutes

Day Five:
A 3 sets 6–8
B 3 sets 8–10
D 3 sets 8–10
E 3 sets 8–10
F 3 sets 8–10
H 3 sets 10–12
I 3 sets 10–12
J 3 sets 10–12
L 30–60 seconds per side
M 3 sets 20

Day Six:
Cardio 30–45 minutes

Day Seven:
Rest

WORKOUT LEVEL 2

BEGINNER ROUTINE 2

Day One:
A 3 sets 6–8
C 3 sets 8–10
D 3 sets 8–10
E 3 sets 8–10
G 3 sets 10–12
H 3 sets 10–12

Day Two:
Rest

Day Three:
A 3 sets 6–8
C 3 sets 8–10
D 3 sets 8–10
E 3 sets 8–10
G 3 sets 10–12
H 3 sets 10–12

Day Four:
Rest

Day Five:
A 3 sets 6–8
C 3 sets 8–10
D 3 sets 8–10
E 3 sets 8–10
G 3 sets 10–12
H 3 sets 10–12

Day Six:
Cardio 30–45 minutes

Day Seven:
Rest

INTERMEDIATE ROUTINE 2

Day One:
A 3 sets 6–8
C 3 sets 8–10
D 3 sets 8–10
E 3 sets 8–10
G 3 sets 10–12
H 3 sets 10–12
I 3 sets 10–12
J 3 sets 10–12

Day Two:
Cardio 30–45 minutes

Day Three:
A 3 sets 6–8
C 3 sets 8–10
D 3 sets 8–10
E 3 sets 8–10
G 3 sets 10–12
H 3 sets 10–12
I 3 sets 10–12
J 3 sets 10–12

Day Four:
Rest

Day Five:
A 3 sets 6–8
C 3 sets 8–10
D 3 sets 8–10
E 3 sets 8–10
G 3 sets 10–12
H 3 sets 10–12
I 3 sets 10–12
J 3 sets 10–12

Day Six:
Cardio 30–45 minutes

Day Seven:
Rest

ADVANCED ROUTINE 2

Day One:
A 3 sets 6–8
C 3 sets 8–10
D 3 sets 8–10
E 3 sets 8–10
G 3 sets 10–12
H 3 sets 10–12
I 3 sets 10–12
J 3 sets 10–12
K 3 sets 12–15
N 3 sets 20

Day Two:
Cardio 30–45 minutes

Day Three:
A 3 sets 6–8
C 3 sets 8–10
D 3 sets 8–10
E 3 sets 8–10
G 3 sets 10–12
H 3 sets 10–12
I 3 sets 10–12
J 3 sets 10–12
K 3 sets 12–15
N 3 sets 20

Day Four:
Cardio 30–45 minutes

Day Five:
A 3 sets 6–8
C 3 sets 8–10
D 3 sets 8–10
E 3 sets 8–10
G 3 sets 10–12
H 3 sets 10–12
I 3 sets 10–12
J 3 sets 10–12
K 3 sets 12–15
N 3 sets 20

Day Six:
Cardio 30–45 minutes

Day Seven:
Rest

OVERALL STRENGTH WORKOUTS

A Barbell Deadlift
page 34
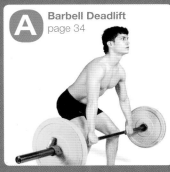

B Barbell Row
page 36
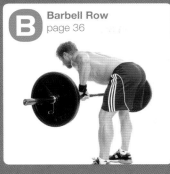

C Rope Pulldown
page 52
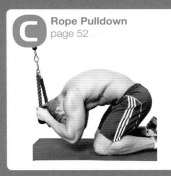

D Barbell Bench Press
page 60
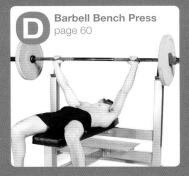

E Dips
page 68
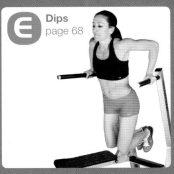

F Dumbbell Shoulder Press
page 74
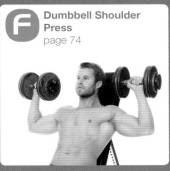

G Barbell Shoulder Shrug
page 94
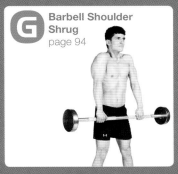

H Rope Hammer Curl
page 104
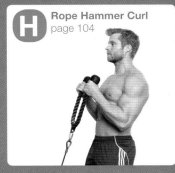

I Swiss Ball Wall Sit
page 134
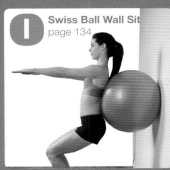

J Swiss Ball Hamstring Curl
page 164
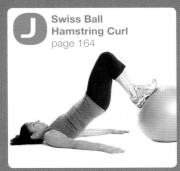

K Dumbbell Calf Raise
page 178
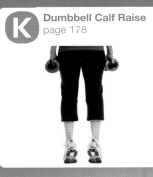

L T-Stabilization
page 124
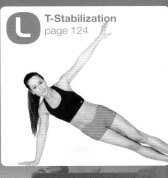

M Swiss Ball Jackknife
page 128
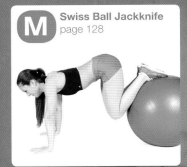

N V-Up
page 212
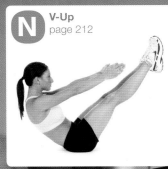

This variation on the traditional bench press provides resistance training that targets the muscles in the side of the abdomen as well as the arms.

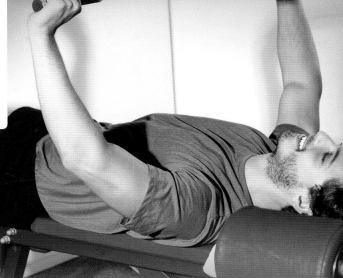

60+

You don't stop exercising because you get old, you get old because you stop exercising. Slacking off on healthy habits such as regular exercise and good nutrition is a major factor in age-related problems like excessive muscle loss, deteriorating bone density and declines in strength, aerobic fitness and flexibility. This workout will make your so-called "declining years" less about decline and more about helping to put the decades ahead among the best years of your life.

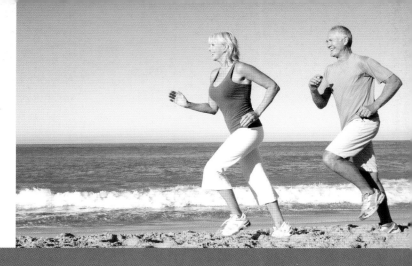

WORKOUT LEVEL 1

BEGINNER ROUTINE 1

Day One:
B 3 sets 8–10
D 3 sets 10–12
E 3 sets 15
F 3 sets 10–12
J 3 sets 12–15
K 3 sets 12–15

Day Two:
Rest

Day Three:
B 3 sets 8–10
D 3 sets 10–12
E 3 sets 15
F 3 sets 10–12
J 3 sets 12–15
K 3 sets 12–15

Day Four:
Rest

Day Five:
B 3 sets 8–10
D 3 sets 10–12
E 3 sets 15
F 3 sets 10–12
J 3 sets 12–15
K 3 sets 12–15

Day Six:
Cardio 30–45
minutes

Day Seven:
Rest

INTERMEDIATE ROUTINE 1

Day One:
A 3 sets 8–10
B 3 sets 8–10
D 3 sets 10–12
E 3 sets 15
F 3 sets 10–12
I 3 sets 10–12
J 3 sets 12–15
K 3 sets 12–15

Day Two:
Cardio 30–45
minutes

Day Three:
A 3 sets 8–10
B 3 sets 8–10
D 3 sets 10–12
E 3 sets 15
F 3 sets 10–12
I 3 sets 10–12
J 3 sets 12–15
K 3 sets 12–15

Day Four:
Rest

Day Five:
A 3 sets 8–10
B 3 sets 8–10
D 3 sets 10–12
E 3 sets 15
F 3 sets 10–12
I 3 sets 10–12
J 3 sets 12–15
K 3 sets 12–15

Day Six:
Cardio 30–45
minutes

Day Seven:
Rest

ADVANCED ROUTINE 1

Day One:
A 3 sets 8–10
B 3 sets 8–10
D 3 sets 10–12
E 3 sets 15
F 3 sets 10–12
I 3 sets 10–12
J 3 sets 12–15
K 3 sets 12–15
M 3 sets 15
O 3 sets 20

Day Two:
Cardio 30–45
minutes

Day Three:
A 3 sets 8–10
B 3 sets 8–10
D 3 sets 10–12
E 3 sets 15
F 3 sets 10–12
I 3 sets 10–12
J 3 sets 12–15
K 3 sets 12–15

M 3 sets 15
O 3 sets 20

Day Four:
Cardio 30–45
minutes

Day Five:
A 3 sets 8–10
B 3 sets 8–10
D 3 sets 10–12
E 3 sets 15
F 3 sets 10–12
I 3 sets 10–12
J 3 sets 12–15
K 3 sets 12–15
M 3 sets 15
O 3 sets 20

Day Six:
Cardio 30–45
minutes

Day Seven:
Rest

WORKOUT LEVEL 2

BEGINNER ROUTINE 2

Day One:
A 3 sets 8–10
C 30 per side
E 3 sets 15
F 3 sets 10–12
G 3 sets 10–12
H 3 sets 10–12

Day Two:
Rest

Day Three:
A 3 sets 8–10
C 30 per side
E 3 sets 15
F 3 sets 10–12
G 3 sets 10–12
H 3 sets 10–12

Day Four:
Rest

Day Five:
A 3 sets 8–10
C 30 per side
E 3 sets 15
F 3 sets 10–12
G 3 sets 10–12
H 3 sets 10–12

Day Six:
Cardio 30–45
minutes

Day Seven:
Rest

INTERMEDIATE ROUTINE 2

Day One:
A 3 sets 8–10
C 30 per side
E 3 sets 15
F 3 sets 10–12
G 3 sets 10–12
H 3 sets 10–12
I 3 sets 10–12
K 3 sets 12–15

Day Two:
Cardio 30–45
minutes

Day Three:
A 3 sets 8–10
C 30 per side
E 3 sets 15
F 3 sets 10–12
G 3 sets 10–12
H 3 sets 10–12
I 3 sets 10–12
K 3 sets 12–15

Day Four:
Rest

Day Five:
A 3 sets 8–10
C 30 per side
E 3 sets 15
F 3 sets 10–12
G 3 sets 10–12
H 3 sets 10–12
I 3 sets 10–12
K 3 sets 12–15

Day Six:
Cardio 30–45
minutes

Day Seven:
Rest

ADVANCED ROUTINE 2

Day One:
A 3 sets 8–10
C 30 per side
E 3 sets 15
F 3 sets 10–12
G 3 sets 10–12
H 3 sets 10–12
I 3 sets 10–12
K 3 sets 12–15
L 3 sets 12–15
N 3 sets 25

Day Two:
Cardio 30–45
minutes

Day Three:
A 3 sets 8–10
C 30 per side
E 3 sets 15
F 3 sets 10–12
G 3 sets 10–12
H 3 sets 10–12
I 3 sets 10–12
K 3 sets 12–15
L 3 sets 12–15
N 3 sets 25

Day Four:
Cardio 30–45
minutes

Day Five:
A 3 sets 8–10
C 30 per side
E 3 sets 15
F 3 sets 10–12
G 3 sets 10–12
H 3 sets 10–12
I 3 sets 10–12
K 3 sets 12–15
L 3 sets 12–15
N 3 sets 25

Day Six:
Cardio 30–45
minutes

Day Seven:
Rest

60+ WORKOUTS

A Dumbbell Row
page 38

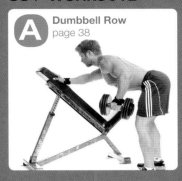

B Lat Pulldown
page 42

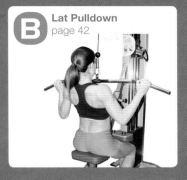

C Wood Chop with Resistance Band
page 202

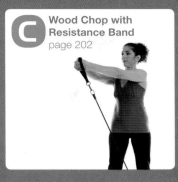

D Dumbbell Fly
page 64

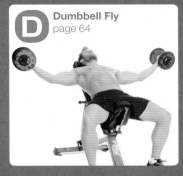

E Rotation Exercises
page 78

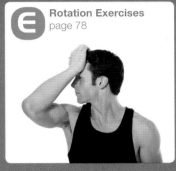

F Reverse Fly
page 88

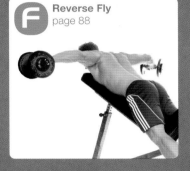

G Barbell Curl
page 100

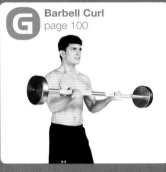

H Rope Pushdown
page 106

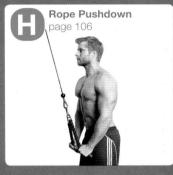

I Goblet Squat
page 150

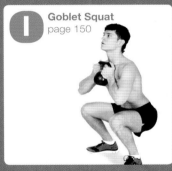

J Knee Extension with Rotation
page 154

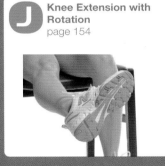

K Inverted Hamstring
page 166

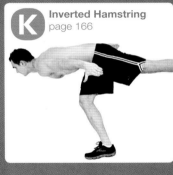

L Single-Leg Calf Press
page 176

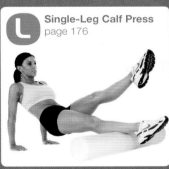

M Cobra Stretch
page 194

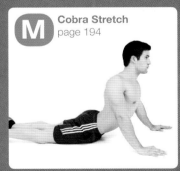

N Crunch
page 118

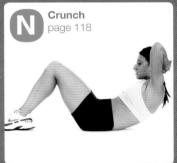

O Reverse Crunch
page 192

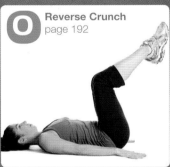

WEIGHT FREE

These exercises help you to achieve exceptional levels of strength and fitness, while avoiding the excessive muscle bulk that is often associated with weight training. Apart from the obvious financial advantage and convenience of training with minimal equipment, the exercises work the entire core and are generally more functional. If you can master push-ups, pull-ups, dips and squats (without weights), four demanding exercises, you can build real and lasting fitness.

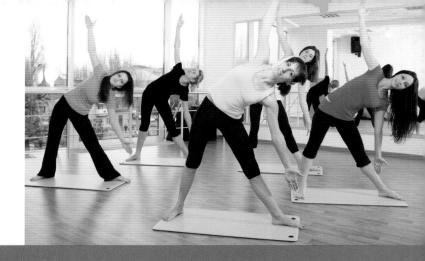

BEGINNER ROUTINE I

Day One:
A 3 sets 8–10
C 3 sets 8–10
D 3 sets 8–10
E 3 sets 12–15
G 3 sets 10–12
H 3 sets 10–12

Day Two:
Rest

Day Three:
A 3 sets 8–10
C 3 sets 8–10
D 3 sets 8–10
E 3 sets 12–15
G 3 sets 10–12
H 3 sets 10–12

Day Four:
Rest

Day Five:
A 3 sets 8–10
C 3 sets 8–10
D 3 sets 8–10
E 3 sets 12–15
G 3 sets 10–12
H 3 sets 10–12

Day Six:
Cardio 30–45 minutes

Day Seven:
Rest

INTERMEDIATE ROUTINE I

Day One:
A 3 sets 8–10
B 3 sets 8–10
C 3 sets 8–10
D 3 sets 8–10
E 3 sets 12–15
G 3 sets 10–12
H 3 sets 10–12
I 3 sets 15

Day Two:
Cardio 30–45 minutes

Day Three:
A 3 sets 8–10
B 3 sets 8–10
C 3 sets 8–10
D 3 sets 8–10
E 3 sets 12–15
G 3 sets 10–12
H 3 sets 10–12
I 3 sets 15

Day Four:
Rest

Day Five:
A 3 sets 8–10
B 3 sets 8–10
C 3 sets 8–10
D 3 sets 8–10
E 3 sets 12–15
G 3 sets 10–12
H 3 sets 10–12
I 3 sets 15

Day Six:
Cardio 30–45 minutes

Day Seven:
Rest

ADVANCED ROUTINE I

Day One:
A 3 sets 8–10
B 3 sets 8–10
C 3 sets 8–10
D 3 sets 8–10
E 3 sets 12–15
F 3 sets 20
G 3 sets 10–12
H 3 sets 10–12
I 3 sets 15
J 30–60 seconds per side

Day Two:
Cardio 30–45 minutes

Day Three:
A 3 sets 8–10
B 3 sets 8–10
C 3 sets 8–10
D 3 sets 8–10
E 3 sets 12–15
F 3 sets 20
G 3 sets 10–12
H 3 sets 10–12
I 3 sets 15

J 30–60 seconds per side

Day Four:
Cardio 30–45 minutes

Day Five:
A 3 sets 8–10
B 3 sets 8–10
C 3 sets 8–10
D 3 sets 8–10
E 3 sets 12–15
F 3 sets 20
G 3 sets 10–12
H 3 sets 10–12
I 3 sets 15
J 30–60 seconds per side

Day Six:
Cardio 30–45 minutes

Day Seven:
Rest

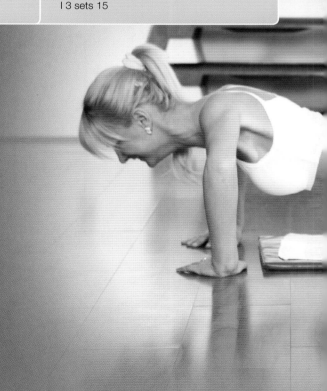

The push-up, and its various modifications, is one of the most familiar exercises to build chest strength. Doing push-ups works not only the muscles of the chest, but those of the arms, legs and core as well — and requires nothing more than an exercise mat.

WEIGHT FREE WORKOUTS

A Reverse Lunge
page 140

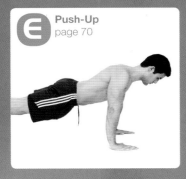

B Reverse Close-Grip Front Chin
page 54

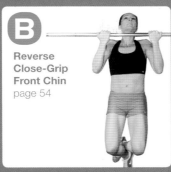

C Flat Bench Hyperextension
page 56

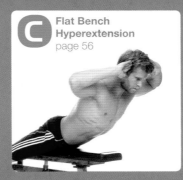

D Dips
page 68

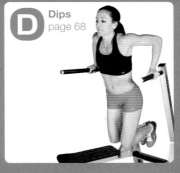

E Push-Up
page 70

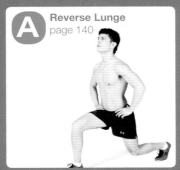

F Push-Up Hand Walk-Over
page 72

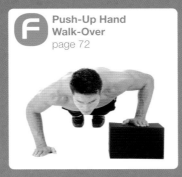

G Swiss Ball Wall Sit
page 134

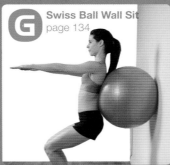

H Stiff-Legged Deadlift
page 174

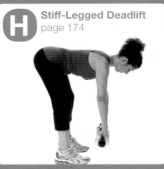

I Plank Press-Up
page 198

J T-Stabilization
page 124

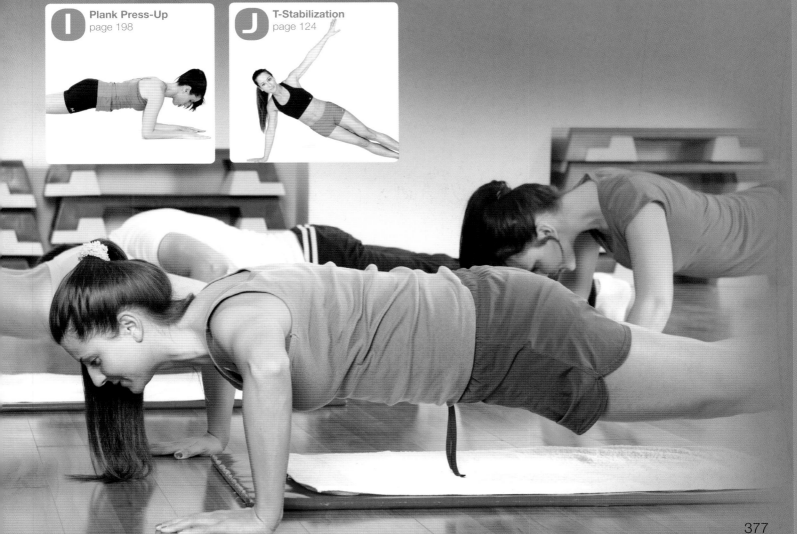

FULL-BODY RESISTANCE

The full-body resistance workout is beneficial for so many reasons: you're getting a cardiovascular, fat-burning, muscle-strengthening and toning workout in little time. By getting strong on several major lifts, you will be stimulating muscle growth without the need to use numerous exercises for each body part.

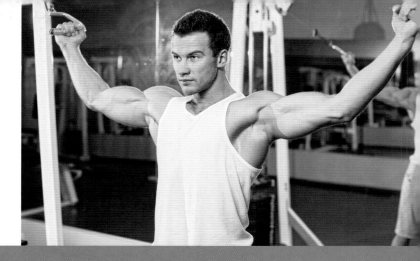

WORKOUT LEVEL 1

BEGINNER ROUTINE 1

Day One:
B 3 sets 8–10
C 3 sets 12–15
D 3 sets 8–10
F 3 sets 12–15
G 3 sets 12–15
K 3 sets 15

Day Two:
Rest

Day Three:
B 3 sets 8–10
C 3 sets 12–15
D 3 sets 8–10
F 3 sets 12–15
G 3 sets 12–15
K 3 sets 15

Day Four:
Rest

Day Five:
B 3 sets 8–10
C 3 sets 12–15
D 3 sets 8–10
F 3 sets 12–15
G 3 sets 12–15
K 3 sets 15

Day Six:
Cardio 30–45 minutes

Day Seven:
Rest

INTERMEDIATE ROUTINE 1

Day One:
A 3 sets 6–8
B 3 sets 8–10
C 3 sets 12–15
D 3 sets 8–10
F 3 sets 12–15
G 3 sets 12–15
I 3 sets 12–15
K 3 sets 15

Day Two:
Cardio 30–45 minutes

Day Three:
A 3 sets 6–8
B 3 sets 8–10
C 3 sets 12–15
D 3 sets 8–10
F 3 sets 12–15
G 3 sets 12–15
I 3 sets 12–15
K 3 sets 15

Day Four:
Rest

Day Five:
A 3 sets 6–8
B 3 sets 8–10
C 3 sets 12–15
D 3 sets 8–10
F 3 sets 12–15
G 3 sets 12–15
I 3 sets 12–15
K 3 sets 15

Day Six:
Cardio 30–45 minutes

Day Seven:
Rest

ADVANCED ROUTINE 1

Day One:
A 3 sets 6–8
B 3 sets 8–10
C 3 sets 12–15
D 3 sets 8–10
F 3 sets 12–15
G 3 sets 12–15
I 3 sets 12–15
J 3 sets 12–15
K 3 sets 15
L 3 sets 20

Day Two:
Cardio 30–45 minutes

Day Three:
A 3 sets 6–8
B 3 sets 8–10
C 3 sets 12–15
D 3 sets 8–10
F 3 sets 12–15
G 3 sets 12–15
I 3 sets 12–15
J 3 sets 12–15

K 3 sets 15
L 3 sets 20

Day Four:
Cardio 30–45 minutes

Day Five:
A 3 sets 6–8
B 3 sets 8–10
C 3 sets 12–15
D 3 sets 8–10
F 3 sets 12–15
G 3 sets 12–15
I 3 sets 12–15
J 3 sets 12–15
K 3 sets 15
L 3 sets 20

Day Six:
Cardio 30–45 minutes

Day Seven:
Rest

WORKOUT LEVEL 2

BEGINNER ROUTINE 2

Day One:
A 3 sets 6–8
B 3 sets 8–10
C 3 sets 12–15
D 3 sets 8–10
E 3 sets 10–12
F 3 sets 12–15

Day Two:
Rest

Day Three:
A 3 sets 6–8
B 3 sets 8–10
C 3 sets 12–15
D 3 sets 8–10
E 3 sets 10–12
F 3 sets 12–15

Day Four:
Rest

Day Five:
A 3 sets 6–8
B 3 sets 8–10
C 3 sets 12–15
D 3 sets 8–10
E 3 sets 10–12
F 3 sets 12–15

Day Six:
Cardio 30–45 minutes

Day Seven:
Rest

INTERMEDIATE ROUTINE 2

Day One:
A 3 sets 6–8
B 3 sets 8–10
C 3 sets 12–15
D 3 sets 8–10
E 3 sets 10–12
F 3 sets 12–15
H 3 sets 12–15
I 3 sets 12–15

Day Two:
Cardio 30–45 minutes

Day Three:
A 3 sets 6–8
B 3 sets 8–10
C 3 sets 12–15
D 3 sets 8–10
E 3 sets 10–12
F 3 sets 12–15
H 3 sets 12–15
I 3 sets 12–15

Day Four:
Rest

Day Five:
A 3 sets 6–8
B 3 sets 8–10
C 3 sets 12–15
D 3 sets 8–10
E 3 sets 10–12
F 3 sets 12–15
H 3 sets 12–15
I 3 sets 12–15

Day Six:
Cardio 30–45 minutes

Day Seven:
Rest

ADVANCED ROUTINE 2

Day One:
A 3 sets 6–8
B 3 sets 8–10
C 3 sets 12–15
D 3 sets 8–10
E 3 sets 10–12
F 3 sets 12–15
H 3 sets 12–15
I 3 sets 12–15
J 3 sets 12–15
K 3 sets 15

Day Two:
Cardio 30–45 minutes

Day Three:
A 3 sets 6–8
B 3 sets 8–10
C 3 sets 12–15
D 3 sets 8–10
E 3 sets 10–12
F 3 sets 12–15
H 3 sets 12–15
I 3 sets 12–15
J 3 sets 12–15
K 3 sets 15

Day Four:
Cardio 30–45 minutes

Day Five:
A 3 sets 6–8
B 3 sets 8–10
C 3 sets 12–15
D 3 sets 8–10
E 3 sets 10–12
F 3 sets 12–15
H 3 sets 12–15
I 3 sets 12–15
J 3 sets 12–15
K 3 sets 15

Day Six:
Cardio 30–45 minutes

Day Seven:
Rest

FULL-BODY RESISTANCE WORKOUTS

A Barbell Deadlift
page 34
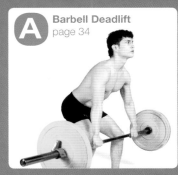

B Reverse Close-Grip Front Chin
page 54
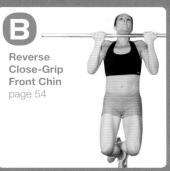

C Push-Up
page 70
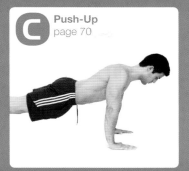

D Overhead Press
page 76
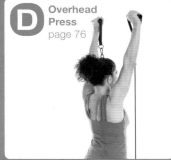

E Alternating Hammer Curl
page 98
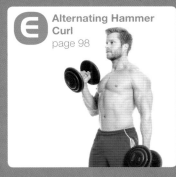

F Chair Dip
page 112
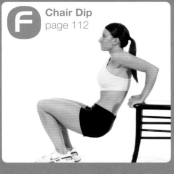

G Dumbbell Lunge
page 138
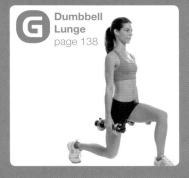

H One-Legged Step-Down
page 152
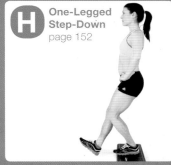

I Inverted Hamstring
page 166
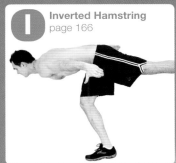

J Dumbbell Calf Raise
page 178
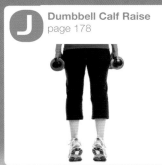

K Plank Press-Up
page 198
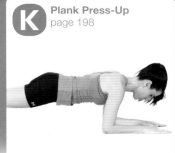

L V-Up
page 212
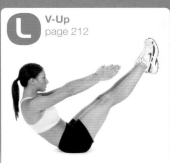

Resistance bands are a convenient training aid and an asset to any workout because they can be used anywhere and can be easily stored. Almost any weight-free exercise can be increased in difficulty by using a resistance band.

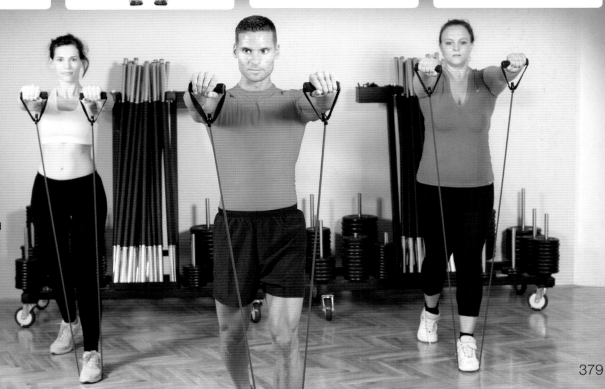

BIGGER ARMS

Second perhaps only to sculpted and prominent abdominals, the biceps — jokingly referred to as "guns" — are the main muscles that men want to develop. However, it's a common mistake to head straight for the dumbbell curls. To build bigger arms you must first increase your overall muscle mass by getting stronger and eating plenty of protein. So start this great arm-sculpting workout only after you have built up mass by following the Overall Strength program (see page 372).

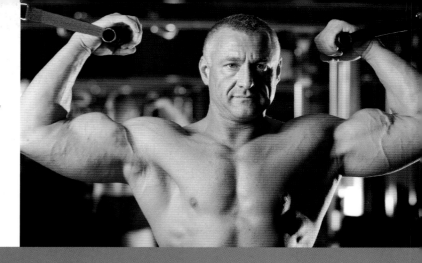

BEGINNER ROUTINE I

Day One:
A 2 sets 10–12
B 2 sets 10–12
E 2 sets 10–12
F 2 sets 10–12

Day Two:
Rest

Day Three:
A 2 sets 10–12
B 2 sets 10–12
E 2 sets 10–12
F 2 sets 10–12

Day Four:
Rest

Day Five:
A 2 sets 10–12
B 2 sets 10–12
E 2 sets 10–12
F 2 sets 10–12

Day Six:
Cardio 30–45 minutes

Day Seven:
Rest

INTERMEDIATE ROUTINE I

Day One:
A 2 sets 10–12
B 2 sets 10–12
D 2 sets 10–12
E 2 sets 10–12
F 2 sets 10–12
G 2 sets 12–15

Day Two:
Cardio 30–45 minutes

Day Three:
A 2 sets 10–12
B 2 sets 10–12
D 2 sets 10–12
E 2 sets 10–12
F 2 sets 10–12
G 2 sets 12–15

Day Four:
Rest

Day Five:
A 2 sets 10–12
B 2 sets 10–12
D 2 sets 10–12
E 2 sets 10–12
F 2 sets 10–12
G 2 sets 12–15

Day Six:
Cardio 30–45 minutes

Day Seven:
Rest

ADVANCED ROUTINE I

Day One:
A 2 sets 10–12
B 2 sets 10–12
C 2 sets 12–15
D 2 sets 10–12
E 2 sets 10–12
F 2 sets 10–12
G 2 sets 12–15
H 2 sets 10–12

Day Two:
Cardio 30–45 minutes

Day Three:
A 2 sets 10–12
B 2 sets 10–12
C 2 sets 12–15
D 2 sets 10–12
E 2 sets 10–12
F 2 sets 10–12
G 2 sets 12–15
H 2 sets 10–12

Day Four:
Cardio 30–45 minutes

Day Five:
A 2 sets 10–12
B 2 sets 10–12
C 2 sets 12–15
D 2 sets 10–12
E 2 sets 10–12
F 2 sets 10–12
G 2 sets 12–15
H 2 sets 10–12

Day Six:
Cardio 30–45 minutes

Day Seven:
Rest

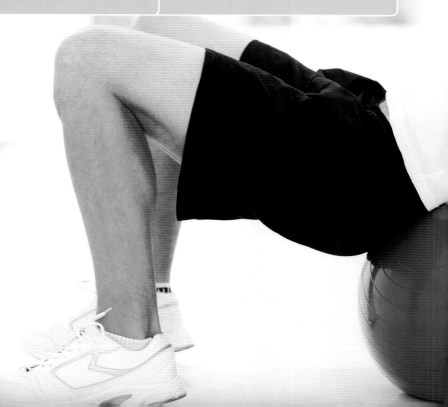

BIGGER ARMS WORKOUTS

A Barbell Curl
page 100
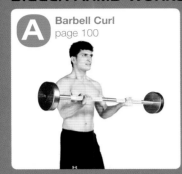

B Alternating Hammer Curl
page 98
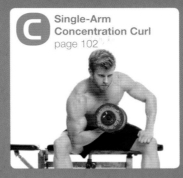

C Single-Arm Concentration Curl
page 102
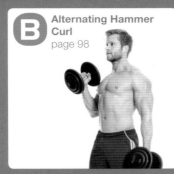

D Rope Hammer Curl
page 104
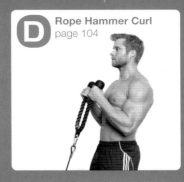

E Rope Pushdown
page 106
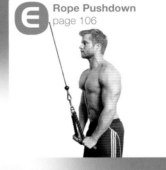

F Lying Triceps Extension
page 108
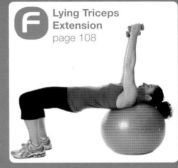

G Chair Dip
page 112
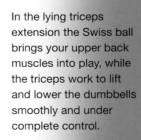

H Rope Overhead Extension
page 114
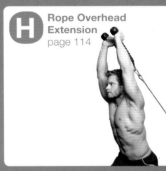

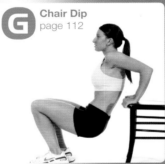

In the lying triceps extension the Swiss ball brings your upper back muscles into play, while the triceps work to lift and lower the dumbbells smoothly and under complete control.

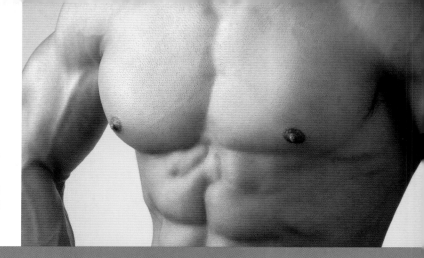

STRONGER CHEST

The key to building a powerful chest is to prioritize the upper portion, which will create a really solid, sculpted look. While many men are caught up in how much they can flat press, the incline press along with a fly motion, are just as critical. For women, too, this comprehensive chest workout — along with cardio work — can help to keep the chest firm and well-toned.

BEGINNER ROUTINE I

Day One:
B 3 sets 8–10
C 3 sets 8–10
E 2 sets 10–12
F 3 sets 10–12

Day Two:
Rest

Day Three:
B 3 sets 8–10
C 3 sets 8–10
E 2 sets 10–12
F 3 sets 10–12

Day Four:
Rest

Day Five:
B 3 sets 8–10
C 3 sets 8–10
E 2 sets 10–12
F 3 sets 10–12

Day Six:
Cardio 30–45 minutes

Day Seven:
Rest

INTERMEDIATE ROUTINE I

Day One:
A 3 sets 8–10
B 3 sets 8–10
C 3 sets 8–10
E 2 sets 10–12
F 3 sets 10–12
H 3 sets 8–10
J 2 sets 20

Day Two:
Cardio 30–45 minutes

Day Three:
A 3 sets 8–10
B 3 sets 8–10
C 3 sets 8–10
E 2 sets 10–12
F 3 sets 10–12
H 3 sets 8–10
J 2 sets 20

Day Four:
Rest

Day Five:
A 3 sets 8–10
B 3 sets 8–10
C 3 sets 8–10
E 2 sets 10–12
F 3 sets 10–12
H 3 sets 8–10
J 2 sets 20

Day Six:
Cardio 30–45 minutes

Day Seven:
Rest

ADVANCED ROUTINE I

Day One:
A 3 sets 8–10
B 3 sets 8–10
C 3 sets 8–10
D 3 sets 8–10
E 2 sets 10–12
F 3 sets 10–12
G 2 sets 12–15
H 3 sets 8–10
I 2 sets 12–15
J 2 sets 20

Day Two:
Cardio 30–45 minutes

Day Three:
A 3 sets 8–10
B 3 sets 8–10
C 3 sets 8–10
D 3 sets 8–10
E 2 sets 10–12
F 3 sets 10–12
G 2 sets 12–15
H 3 sets 8–10
I 2 sets 12–15
J 2 sets 20

Day Four:
Cardio 30–45 minutes

Day Five:
A 3 sets 8–10
B 3 sets 8–10
C 3 sets 8–10
D 3 sets 8–10
E 2 sets 10–12
F 3 sets 10–12
G 2 sets 12–15
H 3 sets 8–10
I 2 sets 12–15
J 2 sets 20

Day Six:
Cardio 30–45 minutes

Day Seven:
Rest

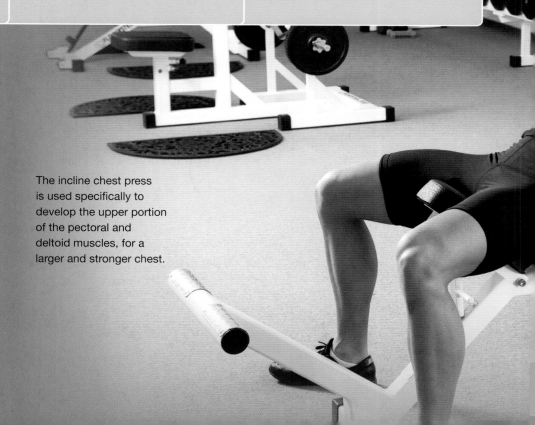

The incline chest press is used specifically to develop the upper portion of the pectoral and deltoid muscles, for a larger and stronger chest.

STRONGER CHEST WORKOUTS

A Barbell Bench Press
page 60
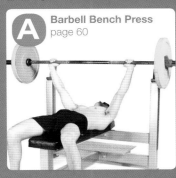

B Dumbbell Shoulder Press
page 74
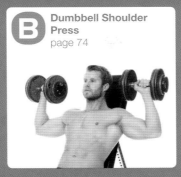

C Roller Push-Up
page 62
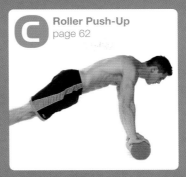

D Alternating Renegade Row
page 48
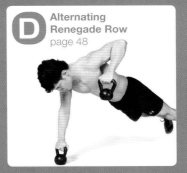

E Dumbbell Fly
page 64
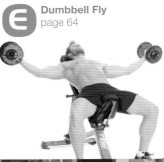

F Swiss Ball Reverse Fly
page 90
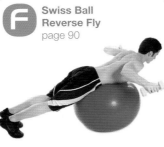

G Cable Fly
page 66
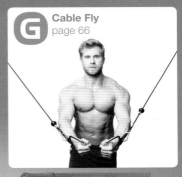

H Dips
page 68
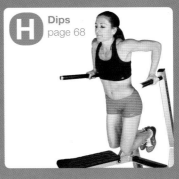

I Push-Up
page 70
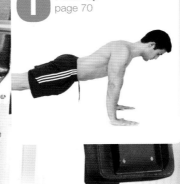

J Push-Up Hand Walk-Over
page 72
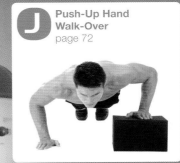

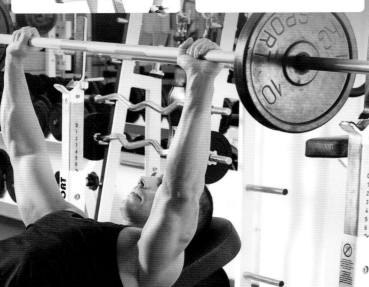

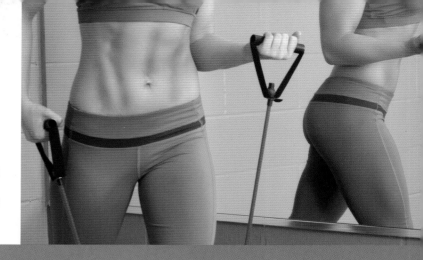

STRONG GLUTES

Although we are all born with a certain shape of glute muscles, we do have control over both the quality and ultimate size of those muscles. Glutes are the largest muscles in the human body and their function is hip extension, that is moving the thigh to the rear. However, your butt can also be a great asset aesthetically: for men the glutes play a supporting role, emphasizing a classic V-shaped back; for women having a strong toned butt is important as part of an overall fitness plan.

BEGINNER ROUTINE I

Day One:
A 3 sets 10–12
B 3 sets 12–15
C 2 sets 12–15
D 3 sets 10–12

Day Two:
Rest

Day Three:
A 3 sets 10–12
B 3 sets 12–15
C 2 sets 12–15
D 3 sets 10–12

Day Four:
Rest

Day Five:
A 3 sets 10–12
B 3 sets 12–15
C 2 sets 12–15
D 3 sets 10–12

Day Six:
Cardio 30–45 minutes

Day Seven:
Rest

INTERMEDIATE ROUTINE I

Day One:
A 3 sets 10–12
B 3 sets 12–15
C 2 sets 12–15
D 3 sets 10–12
E 3 sets 12–15
F 3 sets 12–15

Day Two:
Cardio 30–45 minutes

Day Three:
A 3 sets 10–12
B 3 sets 12–15
C 2 sets 12–15
D 3 sets 10–12
E 3 sets 12–15
F 3 sets 12–15

Day Four:
Rest

Day Five:
A 3 sets 10–12
B 3 sets 12–15
C 2 sets 12–15
D 3 sets 10–12
E 3 sets 12–15
F 3 sets 12–15

Day Six:
Cardio 30–45 minutes

Day Seven:
Rest

ADVANCED ROUTINE I

Day One:
A 3 sets 10–12
B 3 sets 12–15
C 2 sets 12–15
D 3 sets 10–12
E 3 sets 12–15
F 3 sets 12–15
G 3 sets 10–12
H 3 sets 15

Day Two:
Cardio 30–45 minutes

Day Three:
A 3 sets 10–12
B 3 sets 12–15
C 2 sets 12–15
D 3 sets 10–12
E 3 sets 12–15
F 3 sets 12–15
G 3 sets 10–12
H 3 sets 15

Day Four:
Cardio 30–45 minutes

Day Five:
A 3 sets 10–12
B 3 sets 12–15
C 2 sets 12–15
D 3 sets 10–12
E 3 sets 12–15
F 3 sets 12–15
G 3 sets 10–12
H 3 sets 15

Day Six:
Cardio 30–45 minutes

Day Seven:
Rest

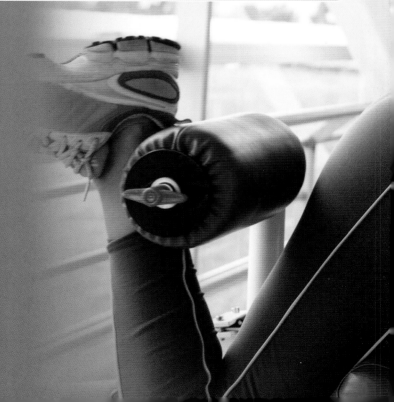

Hyperextension machines, used to strengthen the lower back, are also a fantastic way to tighten the glute muscles before the summer!

STRONG GLUTES WORKOUTS

A Swiss Ball Wall Sit
page 134

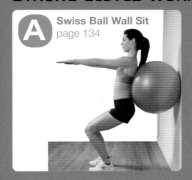

B Reverse Lunge
page 140

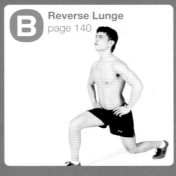

C One-Legged
Step-Down
page 152

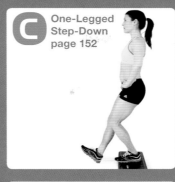

D Swiss Ball
Hamstring Curl
page 164

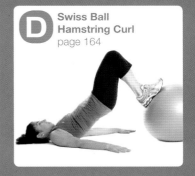

E Stiff-Legged Barbell
Deadlift
page 168

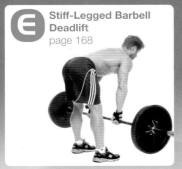

F Hamstring Pull-In
page 170

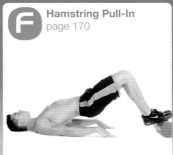

G Stiff-Legged Deadlift
page 174

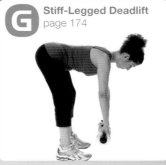

H Hip Abduction
and Adduction
page 204

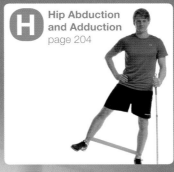

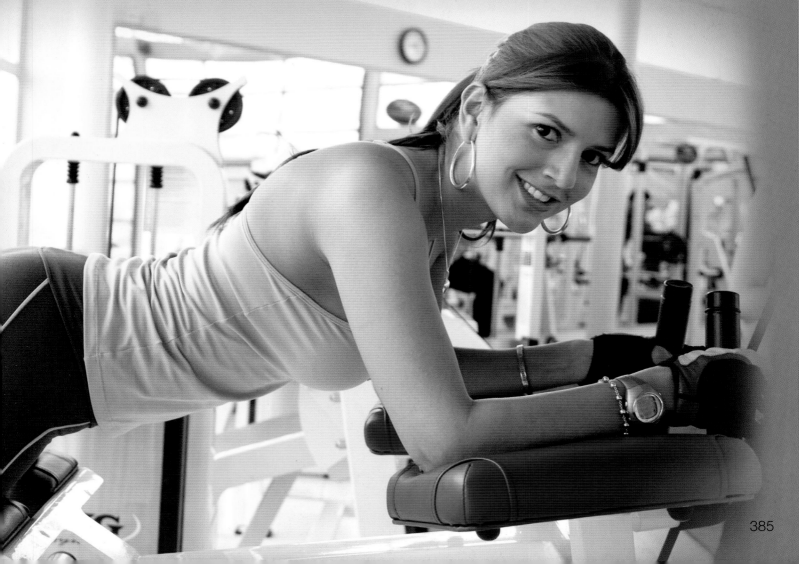

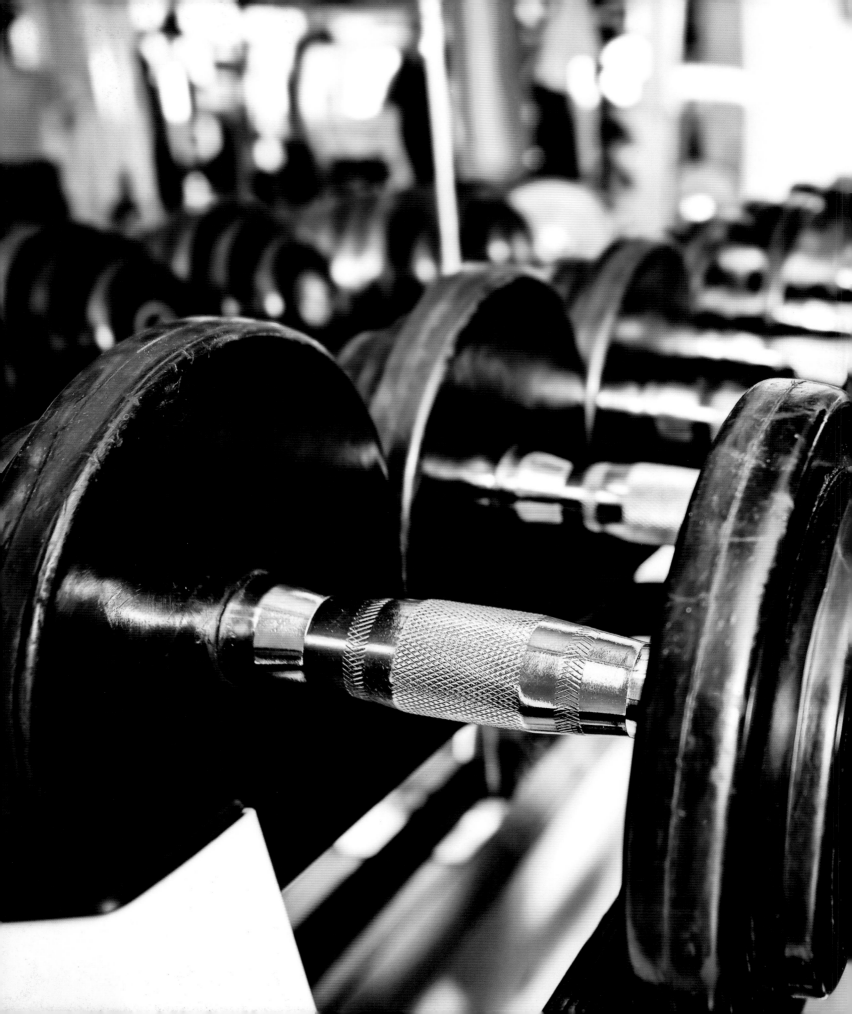

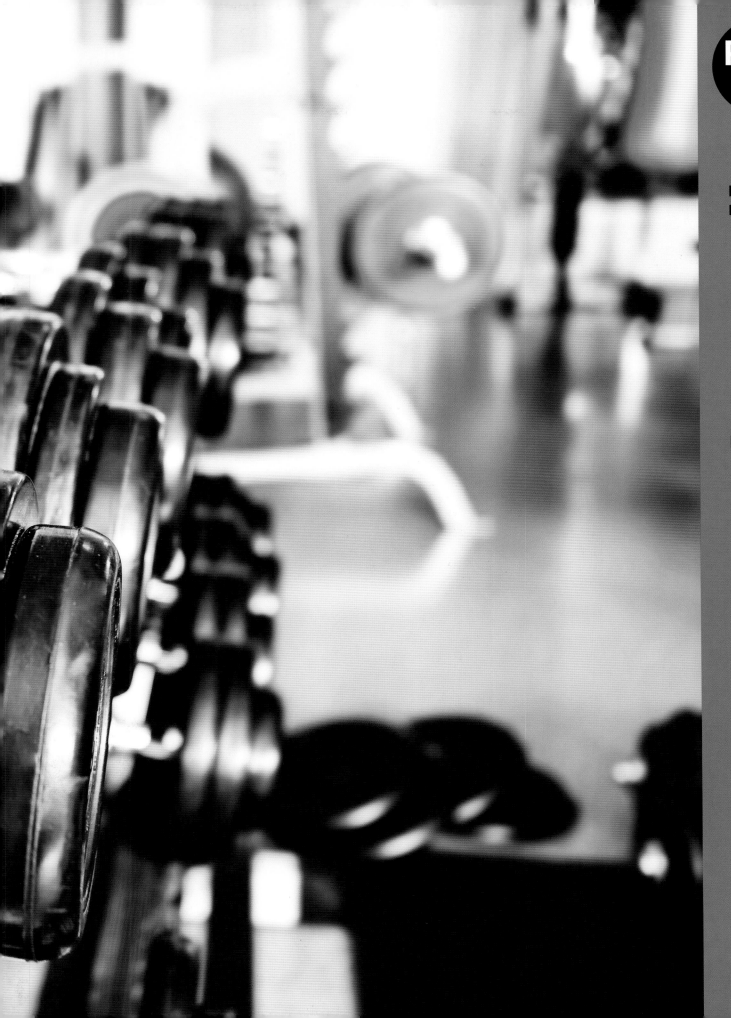

Part
4

Appendix

GLOSSARY: GENERAL TERMS

A

abdominals: The group of muscles that make up the abdomen. The rectus abdominis makes up the front of the abdomen and is known as the six-pack. The other muscles, from the outside of the body inward, are the obliquus externus (external oblique), obliquus internus (internal oblique) and transversus abdominis, the deepest muscle of the abdomen. See also *core*.

abduction: Movement away from the body.

adduction: Movement toward the body.

aerobic step: A portable step or platform with adjustable risers designed for cardiovascular exercising that also allows you to effectively work your calf muscles.

agonist muscle: See *antagonist muscle*.

anterior: Located in the front.

antagonist muscle: This is any muscle working in opposition to another, called the agonist. Most muscles work in antagonistic pairs, with one muscle contracting as the other expands; for example, when the biceps brachii contracts, the triceps brachii relaxes.

B

back: This provides the support system for most of the muscles of the body as well as having links to those of the legs, arms and neck. A healthy back is vital to fitness. During many exercises the back, or spine, must start by being straight but without tension. See also *neutral position*.

barbell: This is a training aid with weights placed at either end of a bar, which measures 4 to 7 feet (1.2–2.2 m) long or more. Various weights can be added to increase the power required to complete the exercise, and so increase the muscle workout.

C

cardiovascular exercise: Any exercise that increases the heart rate, making oxygen and nutrient-rich blood available to the working muscles.

core: This collective term refers to the deep muscle layers close to the spine that provide structural support for the entire body. Body stability comes from having a strong healthy core. The major core muscles reside on the trunk and include the belly area and the mid and lower back. This area encompasses the pelvic floor muscles (levator ani, pubococcygeus, iliococcygeus, puborectalis and coccygeus), the abdominals (rectus abdominis, transversus abdominis, obliquus externus and obliquus internus), the spinal extensors (multifidus spinae, erector spinae, splenius, longissimus thoracis and semispinalis), and the diaphragm. The minor core muscles include the latissimus dorsi, gluteus maximus and trapezius. Minor core muscles assist the major muscles when the body engages in activities or movements that require added stability.

crunch: A common abdominal exercise that calls for curling the shoulders toward the pelvis while lying supine with hands behind the head and knees bent.

curl: An exercise movement, usually targeting the biceps brachii, that calls for a weight to be moved through an arc, in a "curling" motion.

D

deadlift: An exercise movement that calls for lifting a weight, such as a dumbbell or barbell, off the floor from a stabilized bent-over position.

DOMS: This is short for delayed onset muscle soreness. DOMS is the muscle aching and weakness that may be experienced 24 to 72 hours after intense physical exercise such as a long-distance run or any exercise the body is not accustomed to. DOMS is a sign that the muscle cells have been damaged; as they repair they become stronger and bulkier. See also *lactic acid*.

dumbbell: A basic piece of equipment that consists of a short bar on which plates are secured. A person can use a dumbbell in one or both hands during an exercise. Most gyms offer dumbbells with the weight plates welded on and weight in pounds and kilos indicated on the plates, but many dumbbells intended for home use come with removable plates that allow you to adjust the weight.

E

exhale: Deep controlled breathing is important for many exercises, particularly where weights are involved. Breathe out as the weight is lifted. See also *inhale*.

extension: The act of straightening a joint, such as the knee results in the extension of the surrounding muscles.

extensor muscle: A muscle that extends a body part, such as an arm, away from the body.

F

flexion: The bending of a joint.

flexor muscle: A muscle that decreases the angle between two bones, such as when bending the arm at the elbow or raising the thigh toward the stomach.

foam roller: A tube that comes in a variety of sizes, materials and densities that can be used for stretching, strengthening, balance training, stability training and self-massage.

G

glutes: The group of powerful muscles that make up the buttocks and are responsible for keeping the body upright. There are

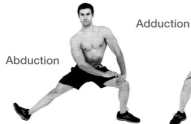
Abduction

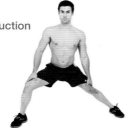
Adduction

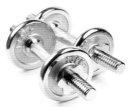
Dumbbells

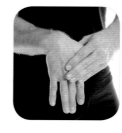
Flexion

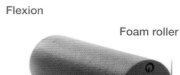
Foam roller

three key glutes: gluteus maximus, which is the one most commonly referred to and the one that gives the buttocks their curved shape, along with gluteus medius and gluteus minimus.

H

hammer-grip: Holding the weights, usually dumbells, with the palms facing inward and the thumbs upward. A hammer-grip is often used for lifts done using an incline bench with the body bending over so it is parallel with or at an angle to the floor. From this position, it helps to work the pecs, deltoids, trapezius and other muscles of the back. When done in an upright position it helps to work the biceps, brachialis and brachioradialis.

hamstrings: The three muscles of the posterior thigh (the semitendinosus, semimembranosus and biceps femoris) that work to flex the knee and extend the hip. Tight hamstrings are a common problem with many causes. Make sure you do plenty of leg stretches both before and after workouts and avoid excessive hard training. Tight hamstrings may also indicate back problems.

hand weight: Any of a range of free weights that are often used in weight training and toning. Small hand weights are usually cast iron formed in the shape of a dumbbell, sometimes coated with rubber or neoprene for comfort.

hyperextending: Extending the limbs or back beyond the point where the muscles can comfortably support them. This prevents the muscles from working correctly and may lead to injury.

I

iliotibial band (ITB): A thick band of fibrous tissue that runs down the outside of the leg, beginning at the hip and extending to the outer side of the tibia just below the knee joint. The band functions in concert with several of the thigh muscles to provide stability to the outside of the knee joint.

inferior: When referring to a muscle, one that is below or deeper. See also *superior*.

inhale: Slow deliberate inhaling is important for many of the exercises, especially where weights are included. It is usual to breathe in when lowering a weight and to exhale on lifting it.

isometric exercises: These are workouts that involve tensing the muscles then relaxing them without changing the position of any part of the body. They are good for working very specific areas of the body, and they can be done discretely even when you are sitting at a desk or driving, so are useful for exercising the muscles during the working day.

K

kettlebell: A weighted exercise aid with a rigid looped handle at the top. It looks a little like an old-fashioned kettle. The looped handle allows the weight to be swung, which creates a different range of strengthening exercises to a dumbbell, for example.

L

lactic acid: During intense exercise the body cannot supply enough oxygen to the blood stream for it to effectively work the muscles — this is anaerobic exercise — so it uses glucose to provide the energy. Breaking glucose down into a usable form also creates lactate (or lactic acid), which in turn produces "the burn." This is the body's self-defence system attempting to prevent overexertion. See also *DOMS*.

lateral: Located on, or extending toward, the outside.

lockout position: Straightening out the arm or leg to its furthest extent, without *hyperextending*.

lunge: Exercise movement that involves stepping forward and moving the body weight on to the forward leg. Lunges primarily target the quads and glutes as well as lower leg muscles.

M

medial: Located on, or extending toward, the middle.

medicine ball: A small weighted ball used in weight training and toning.

N

neutral position (spine): A spinal position resembling an S shape, consisting of a inward curve in the lower back, when viewed in profile.

O

obliques: Some of the muscles of the abdomen. See also *abdominals*.

overhand grip: Holding a barbell or other weight so that the backs of the hands are uppermost.

P

pelvis: Tucking the pelvis slightly under is important for body stability during many standing exercises. This helps to engage the abdominals and ensure the exercises are done correctly without straining the back. See also *starting position*.

plank position: Facing the floor with the back straight and the arms extended to support the head and upper body — as in a push-up. Alternatively, the body may be resting on the upper arms, with the forearms flat on the floor.

posterior: Located behind.

press: An exercise movement that calls for pushing a weight or other resistance away from the body.

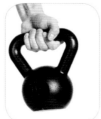

Hammer-grip

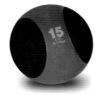

Kettlebell

Medicine ball

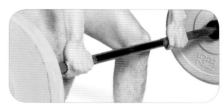

Overhand grip

primary muscle: One of the main muscles activated during a certain activity.

pronation: Turning inward. A pronated foot is one in which the heel bone angles inward and the arch tends to collapse. Opposite of *supination*.

Q

quadriceps (quads): A large muscle group (quadriceps femoris) that includes the four prevailing muscles on the front of the thigh: the rectus femoris, vastus intermedius, vastus lateralis and vastus medialis. It is the great extensor muscle of the knee, forming a fleshy mass that covers the front and sides of the femur muscle.

R

range of motion: The distance and direction a joint can move between the flexed position and the extended position. See also *lockout position*.

reactive power: This refers to the speed with which a body can react, particularly when playing a competitive sport, such as tennis, football and squash. The muscles of the lower body including the calves, quads, hamstrings and glutes are responsible for increasing speed of reaction.

repetitions: The number of times an exercise is done at any one time. Each repetition should be carried out carefully and under control to ensure it works on the groups of muscles in the way intended. Fast, careless repetitions are more likely to cause injury than increase fitness.

resistance: Resistance training works by making the muscles contract against a force, such as to lift a weight or move a resistance band. This develops their size and strength.

resistance band: Any rubber tubing or flat band device that provides a resistive force used for strength training. Also called a "fitness band," "Thera-Band," "Dyna-Band," "stretching band" and "exercise band."

roller: See *foam roller*.

rotator muscle: One of a group of muscles that assist the rotation of a joint, such as the hip or the shoulder.

S

scapula: The protrusion of bone on the mid to upper back, also known as the "shoulder blade."

secondary muscle: A muscle activated during a certain activity that usually works to support the primary muscles.

squat: An exercise movement that calls for moving the hips back and bending the knees and hips to lower the torso and an accompanying weight, and then returning to the upright position. A squat primarily targets the muscles of the thighs, hips, buttocks and hamstrings.

stability: This is the ability of the body to maintain its balance through a range of different positions. Core muscles, such as the abdominals, and the quads and hamstrings are used to increase body stability, which is needed in sports such as surfing, equestrianism and snowboarding.

stamina: With regular controlled exercise you increase your stamina, enabling you to make more repetitions, lift heavier weights or run further or faster. However, with increased stamina comes the need to do increase the level of exercise to continue to increase the benefit to your muscles and body.

starting position: Relaxed position from which to begin an exercise. When standing, this is usually with the feet parallel and shoulder-width apart, knees slightly flexed, pelvis tucked under and the spine in a *neutral position*. When lying down, the back should be flat without tension or any arching of the lower spine. The arms are usually relaxed by the side of the body and the head should be facing forward with no tension in the neck or jaw.

superior: When referring to a muscle, one that is above or on the surface. See also *inferior*.

supination: Turning outward. In running, supination is the insufficient inward roll of the foot after landing. This places extra stress on the foot and can result in iliotibial band syndrome, Achilles tendinitis or plantar fasciitis. Also know as "overpronation."

Swiss ball: A flexible, inflatable PVC ball measuring between 12 to 30 inches (30–76 cm) in circumference that is used for weight training, physical therapy, balance training and many other exercise regimens. It has other names, including "balance ball," "fitness ball," "stability ball," "exercise ball," "gym ball," "physioball," "body ball" and "therapy ball." Always use a ball that is the correct size for your height — when you sit on it, your thighs should be parallel to the ground — and properly inflated.

T

torso: This is the upper body from the hips to the shoulders. It is also referred to as the trunk.

W

waist: The most flexible, and usually the narrowest, part of the torso.

warm-up: Any form of light exercise of short duration that prepares the body for more intense exercises.

weight: Refers to the plates or weight stacks, or the actual weight in pounds or kilos listed on the bar or dumbbell.

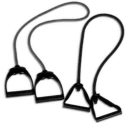
Resistance bands

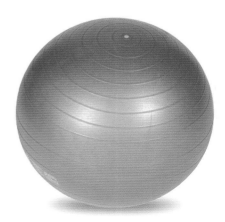
Swiss ball

GLOSSARY: LATIN TERMS

The following glossary explains the Latin scientific terminology used to describe the muscles of the human body. Certain words are derived from Greek, which is indicated in each instance.

CHEST
coracobrachialis: Greek *korakoeidés*, "ravenlike," and *brachium*, "arm"
pectoralis (major and minor): *pectus*, "breast"

ABDOMEN
obliquus externus: *obliquus*, "slanting," and *externus*, "outward"
obliquus internus: *obliquus*, "slanting," and *internus*, "within"
rectus abdominis: *rego*, "straight, upright," and *abdomen*, "belly"
serratus anterior: *serra*, "saw," and *ante*, "before"
transversus abdominis: *transversus*, "athwart," and *abdomen*, "belly"

NECK
scalenus: Greek *skalénós*, "unequal"
semispinalis: *semi*, "half," and *spinae*, "spine"
splenius: Greek *spléníon*, "plaster, patch"
sternocleidomastoideus: Greek *stérnon*, "chest," Greek *kleís*, "key," and Greek *mastoeidés*, "breastlike"

BACK
erector spinae: *erectus*, "straight," and *spina*, "thorn"
latissimus dorsi: *latus*, "wide," and *dorsum*, "back"
multifidus spinae: *multifid*, "to cut into divisions," and *spinae*, "spine"
quadratus lumborum: *quadratus*, "square, rectangular," and *lumbus*, "loin"
rhomboideus: Greek *rhembesthai*, "to spin"
trapezius: Greek *trapezion*, "small table"

SHOULDERS
deltoideus (anterior, medial, and posterior): Greek *deltoeidés*, "delta-shaped"
infraspinatus: *infra*, "under," and *spina*, "thorn"
levator scapulae: *levare*, "to raise," and *scapulae*, "shoulder [blades]"
subscapularis: *sub*, "below," and *scapulae*, "shoulder [blades]"

supraspinatus: *supra*, "above," and *spina*, "thorn"
teres (major and minor): *teres*, "rounded"

UPPER ARM
biceps brachii: *biceps*, "two-headed," and *brachium*, "arm"
brachialis: *brachium*, "arm"
triceps brachii: *triceps*, "three-headed," and *brachium*, "arm"

LOWER ARM
anconeus: Greek *anconad*, "elbow"
brachioradialis: *brachium*, "arm," and *radius*, "spoke"
extensor carpi radialis: *extendere*, "to extend," Greek *karpós*, "wrist," and *radius*, "spoke"
extensor digitorum: *extendere*, "to extend," and *digitus*, "finger, toe"
flexor carpi pollicis longus: *flectere*, "to bend," Greek *karpós*, "wrist," *pollicis*, "thumb," and *longus*, "long"
flexor carpi radialis: *flectere*, "to bend," Greek *karpós*, "wrist," and *radius*, "spoke"
flexor carpi ulnaris: *flectere*, "to bend," Greek *karpós*, "wrist," and *ulnaris*, "forearm"
flexor digitorum: *flectere*, "to bend," and *digitus*, "finger, toe"
palmaris longus: *palmaris*, "palm," and *longus*, "long"
pronator teres: *pronate*, "to rotate," and *teres*, "rounded"

HIP
gemellus (inferior and superior): *geminus*, "twin"
gluteus maximus: Greek *gloutós*, "rump," and *maximus*, "largest"
gluteus medius: Greek *gloutós*, "rump," and *medialis*, "middle"
gluteus minimus: Greek *gloutós*, "rump," and *minimus*, "smallest"
iliopsoas: *ilium*, "groin," and Greek *psoa*, "groin muscle"
iliacus: *ilium*, "groin"
obturator externus: *obturare*, "to block," and *externus*, "outward"
obturator internus: *obturare*, "to block," and *internus*, "within"
pectineus: *pectin*, "comb"
piriformis: *pirum*, "pear," and *forma*, "shape"
quadratus femoris: *quadratus*, "square, rectangular," and *femur*, "thigh"

UPPER LEG
adductor longus: *adducere*, "to contract," and *longus*, "long"
adductor magnus: *adducere*, "to contract," and *magnus*, "major"
biceps femoris: *biceps*, "two-headed," and *femur*, "thigh"
gracilis: *gracilis*, "slim, slender"
rectus femoris: *rego*, "straight, upright," and *femur*, "thigh"
sartorius: *sarcio*, "to patch" or "to repair"
semimembranosus: *semi*, "half," and *membrum*, "limb"
semitendinosus: *semi*, "half," and *tendo*, "tendon"
tensor fasciae latae: *tenere*, "to stretch," *fasciae*, "band," and *latae*, "laid down"
trachtus iliotibialis: *traho*, "to drag, extract," *ilium*, "groin," and *tibia*, "reedpipe"
vastus intermedius: *vastus*, "immense, huge," and *intermedius*, "between"
vastus lateralis: *vastus*, "immense, huge," and *lateralis*, "side"
vastus medialis: *vastus*, "immense, huge," and *medialis*, "middle"

LOWER LEG
adductor digiti minimi: *adducere*, "to contract," *digitus*, "finger, toe," and *minimum* "smallest"
adductor hallucis: *adducere*, "to contract," and *hallex*, "big toe"
extensor digitorum longus: *extendere*, "to extend," *digitus*, "finger, toe," and *longus*, "long"
extensor hallucis longus: *extendere*, "to extend," *hallex*, "big toe," and *longus*, "long"
flexor digitorum longus: *flectere*, "to bend," *digitus*, "finger, toe," and *longus*, "long"
flexor hallucis longus: *flectere*, "to bend," and *hallex*, "big toe," and *longus*, "long"
gastrocnemius: Greek *gastroknémía*, "calf [of the leg]"
peroneus: *peronei*, "of the fibula"
plantaris: *planta*, "the sole"
soleus: *solea*, "sandal"
tibialis anterior: *tibia*, "reed pipe," and *ante*, "before"
tibialis posterior: *tibia*, "reed pipe," and *posterus*, "coming after"
trochlea tali: trochlea, "pulley," and *tali*, "such, of a sort"

CREDITS & ACKNOWLEDGMENTS

key: l = left, r = right, c = center

5l YanLev/Shutterstock 5r wavebreakmedia/Shutterstock 6l holbox/Shutterstock 6r Kzenon/Shutterstock 7l stockyimages/Shutterstock 7r Martin Novak/Shutterstock 8l Gabriela Insuratelu/Shutterstock 8r Vanessa Nel/Shutterstock 9l Ipatov/Shutterstock 9r Natursports/Shutterstock 10–11 YanLev/Shutterstock 13 holbox/Shutterstock 17 Gemenacom/Shutterstock 22l ElenaGaak/Shutterstock 22c Africa Studio/Shutterstock 22r Mrs_ya/Shutterstock 23 Jiri Hera/Shutterstock 26–29 Linda Bucklin/Shutterstock 30–31 holbox/Shutterstock 246 holbox/Shutterstock 254–255 Kzenon/Shutterstock 258 Herbert Kratky/Shutterstock 260 Kravka/Shutterstock 262 Neale Cousland/Shutterstock 264 Jari Hindstroem/Shutterstock 266 Richard Paul Kane/Shutterstock 268 bikeriderlondon/Shutterstock 270 bikeriderlondon/Shutterstock 272 LesPalenik/Shutterstock 274 Vitalii Nesterchuk/Shutterstock 276 Ahmad Faizal Yahya/Shutterstock 278 Tatiana Dorokhova/Shutterstock 280 Ljupco Smokovski/Shutterstock 282 bikeriderlondon/Shutterstock 284 Marcel Jancovic/Shutterstock 286 Pavel L Photo and Video/Shutterstock 288 mooinblack/Shutterstock 290 testing/Shutterstock 292 Wolf Avni/Shutterstock 294 Ciaran McGuiggan 296 Vanessa Nel/Shutterstock 298 bikeriderlondon/Shutterstock 300 muzsy/Shutterstock 302 Sandra A Dunlap/Shutterstock 304 Laszlo Szirtesi/Shutterstock 306 Piotr Sikora/Shutterstock 308 testing/Shutterstock 310 Stas Volik/Shutterstock 312 James A Boardman/Shutterstock 314 Maxim Petrichuk/Shutterstock 316 Maridav/Shutterstock 318 Lisa F Young/Shutterstock 320 wheatley/Shutterstock 322 Eoghan McNally/Shutterstock 324 Maridav/Shutterstock 326 sainthorant daniel/Shutterstock 328 Jorge R Gonzalez/Shutterstock 330 pio3/Shutterstock 332 IM_photo/Shutterstock 334 Ipatov/Shutterstock 336 Natursports/Shutterstock 338 CHEN WS/Shutterstock 340 Natali Glado/Shutterstock 342 Aleksandr Markin/Shutterstock 344 muzsy/Shutterstock 346 bikeriderlondon/Shutterstock 348 dotshock/Shutterstock 350 luca85/Shutterstock 352 juliamcc/Shutterstock 354 muzsy/Shutterstock 358 ollyy/Shutterstock 360 Africa Studio/Shutterstock 361 Martin Novak/Shutterstock 362 StockLite/Shutterstock 363 Andresr/Shutterstock 364 Tyler Olson/Shutterstock 365 Cristi Lucaci/Shutterstock 366 Aleksandr Markin/Shutterstock 368 Orange Line Media/Shutterstock 369 holbox/Shutterstock 370 Tyler Olson/Shutterstock 370–371 Peter Bernik/Shutterstock 372 Wallenrock/Shutterstock 373 stockyimages/Shutterstock 374 Monkey Business Images/Shutterstock 376 George Dolgikh/Shutterstock 377 Lucky Business/Shutterstock 378 mashurov/Shutterstock 379 Peter Bernik/Shutterstock 380 Istvan Csak/Shutterstock 380–381 michaeljung/Shutterstock 382 Dave Kotinsky/Shutterstock 383 Mircea Netval/Shutterstock 384 Carl Stewart/Shutterstock 385 Andresr/Shutterstock 386–387 Kiselev Andrey Valerevich/Shutterstock 388c picamaniac/Shutterstock

All anatomical illustrations by Hector Aiza/3D Labz Animation India, except insets on pages 35, 39, 40, 43, 49, 51, 55, 57, 59, 61, 65, 67, 69, 71, 72, 75, 77, 78, 79, 81, 83, 85, 87, 89, 91, 93, 95, 97, 99, 101, 103, 107, 109, 110, 113, 115, 119, 121, 123, 125, 127, 129, 131, 135, 137, 139, 141, 143, 145, 147, 149, 151, 153, 155, 157, 159, 161, 162–163, 165, 167, 169, 171, 173, 175, 181, 187, 189, 193, 195, 197, 199, 201, 203, 205, 207, 209, 211, 213, 215, 217, 220–221, 222–223, 224–225, 226–227, 228–229, 231, 232, 238–239, 241, 244, 248–249, 250–251 and 252 by Linda Bucklin/Shutterstock

Additional photography by Jonathan Conklin/Jonathan Conklin Photography, Inc. and FineArtsPhotoGroup.com.

Thanks to models Nicolay Alexandrov, Elaine Altholz, David Anderson, Joseph Benedict, Sara Blowers, Miguel Carrera, Tara DiLuca, TJ Fink, Jenna Franciosa, Michael Galizia, Melissa Grant, Maria Grippi, Kelly Jacobs, Goldie Karpel, Jillian Langenau, Monica Ordonez, Michael Radon, Craig Ramsay and Peter Vaillancourt

Hollis Lance Liebman has been a fitness magazine editor, national bodybuilding champion, and author. He is a published physique photographer and has served as a bodybuilding and fitness competition judge. Currently a Los Angeles resident, Hollis has worked with some of Hollywood's elite, earning rave reviews. Visit his Web site, www.holliswashere.com, for fitness tips and complete training programs. This is his fifth book."

I dedicate this book to those who pursue their dreams with a relentless passion, honed vision and unwavering enthusiasm, for your unique voice must be heard.

Also available in this series

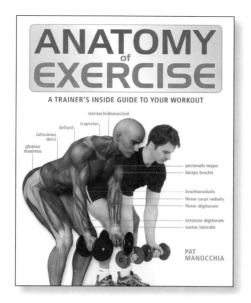

ANATOMY of EXERCISE
A TRAINER'S INSIDE GUIDE TO YOUR WORKOUT

PAT MANOCCHIA

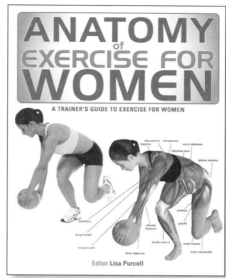

ANATOMY of EXERCISE FOR WOMEN
A TRAINER'S GUIDE TO EXERCISE FOR WOMEN

Editor Lisa Purcell

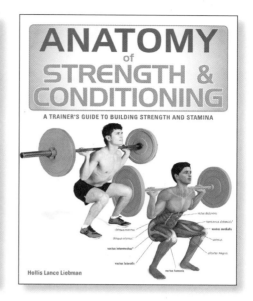

ANATOMY of STRENGTH & CONDITIONING
A TRAINER'S GUIDE TO BUILDING STRENGTH AND STAMINA

Hollis Lance Liebman

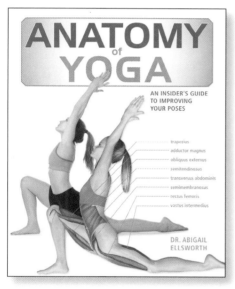

ANATOMY of YOGA
AN INSIDER'S GUIDE TO IMPROVING YOUR POSES

DR. ABIGAIL ELLSWORTH

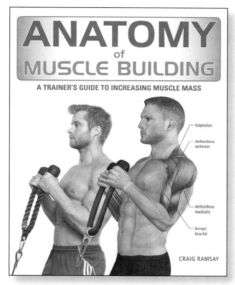

ANATOMY of MUSCLE BUILDING
A TRAINER'S GUIDE TO INCREASING MUSCLE MASS

CRAIG RAMSAY

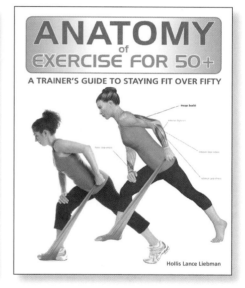

ANATOMY of EXERCISE FOR 50+
A TRAINER'S GUIDE TO STAYING FIT OVER FIFTY

Hollis Lance Liebman

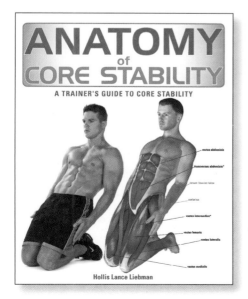

ANATOMY of CORE STABILITY
A TRAINER'S GUIDE TO CORE STABILITY

Hollis Lance Liebman

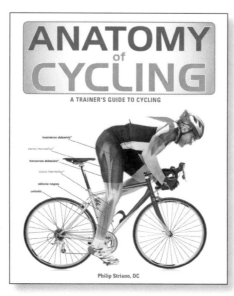

ANATOMY of CYCLING
A TRAINER'S GUIDE TO CYCLING

Philip Striano, DC

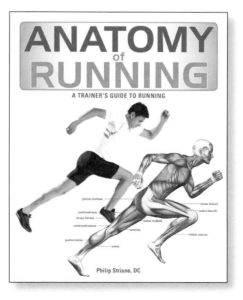

ANATOMY of RUNNING
A TRAINER'S GUIDE TO RUNNING

Philip Striano, DC